KT-486-855

Management of Advanced Disease

Fourth Edition

Edited by

Nigel Sykes MA BM BCh FRCGP ILTM
of Medicine and Consultant in Palliative Medicine, St Christopher's Hospice, Sydenham, London;
and Honorary Senior Lecturer in Palliative Medicine, King's College, London

Polly Edmonds MB BS FRCP
Consultant in Palliative Medicine, King's College Hospital NHS Trust, London;
and Honorary Clinical Senior Lecturer, King's College, London

and

John Wiles MB ChB MRCP D(Obst)RCOG DipTEd
Consultant in Palliative Medicine, Princess Royal University Hospital, Farnborough, Kent;
and Medical Director, Harris HospisCare, Orpington, Kent

ARNOLD
A member of the Hodder Headline Group
LONDON

616.029
SYK

First published in Great Britain in 2004 by
Arnold, a member of the Hodder Headline Group,
338 Euston Road, London NW1 3BH

http://www.arnoldpublishers.com

Distributed in the United States of America by
Oxford University Press Inc.,
198 Madison Avenue, New York, NY10016
Oxford is a registered trademark of Oxford University Press

© 2004 Arnold

All rights reserved. No part of this publication may be reproduced or transmitted in
any form or by any means, electronically or mechanically, including photocopying,
recording or any information storage or retrieval system, without either prior
permission in writing from the publisher or a licence permitting restricted copying.
In the United Kingdom such licences are issued by the Copyright Licensing Agency:
90 Tottenham Court Road, London W1T 4LP.

Whilst the advice and information in this book are believed to be true and accurate
at the date of going to press, neither the authors nor the publisher can accept any
legal responsibility or liability for any errors or omissions that may be made. In
particular (but without limiting the generality of the preceding disclaimer) every
effort has been made to check drug dosages; however, it is still possible that errors
have been missed. Furthermore, dosage schedules are constantly being revised and
new side-effects recognized. For these reasons the reader is strongly urged to
consult the drug companies' printed instructions before administering any of the drugs
recommended in this book.

British Library Cataloguing in Publication Data
A catalogue record for this book is available from the British Library

Library of Congress Cataloging-in-Publication Data
A catalog record for this book is available from the Library of Congress

ISBN 0 340 76313 2

1   2   3   4   5   6   7   8   9   10

Commissioning Editor: Joanna Koster
Development Editor: Sarah Burrows
Project Editor: Wendy Rooke
Production Controller: Lindsay Smith
Cover Design: Lee-May Lim

Typeset in 10/12 pt Sabon by Charon Tec Pvt. Ltd, Chennai, India
www.charontec.com
Printed and bound in Malta

What do you think about this book? Or any other Arnold title?
Please send your comments to **feedback.arnold@hodder.co.uk**

C O N T E N T S

SECTION 1   GENERAL

SECTION 2   A–Z OF SYMPTOMS

SECTION 3 CLINICAL CHALLENGES IN MALIGNANT DISEASE

SECTION 4 CLINICAL CHALLENGES IN NON-MALIGNANT DISEASE

SECTION 5 PSYCHOSOCIAL, SPIRITUAL AND ETHICAL ISSUES

SECTION 6 ORGANIZATIONAL ISSUES FOR PALLIATIVE CARE PROFESSIONALS

CONTRIBUTORS

Julia M. Addington-Hall PhD HonMFPHM
Senior Lecturer/Deputy Head of Department, Department of Palliative Care and Policy,
Guy's, King's and St Thomas' School of Medicine, King's College, London

Stephanie A. Amiel BSc MD FRCP
RD Lawrence Professor of Diabetic Medicine, Department of Diabetes, Endocrinology
and Internal Medicine, King's College, London

Fiona Aspinal RGN BA (Hons) MA
Research Associate, Department of Palliative Care and Policy, Guy's, King's and
St Thomas' School of Medicine, King's College, London

Emma Brown
Specialist Registrar, Western General Hospital, Edinburgh

Claire Butler
Guy's and St Thomas' Hospital, London

Colin W. Campbell DRCOG MRCGP
Consultant in Palliative Medicine, St Catherine's Hospice, Scarborough,
North Yorkshire

Irene Carey MSc MB BCh BAO MRCPI
Consultant in Palliative Medicine, Weston Park Hospital, Sheffield and
St Luke's Hospice, Sheffield

Sarah Cox BSc MRCP
Consultant in Palliative Medicine, Trinity Hospice, and Chelsea and Westminster
Hospital, London

Andrew N. Davies MB BS MSc MD FRCP
Consultant in Palliative Medicine, Royal Marsden Hospital, Sutton, Surrey

Polly Edmonds MB BS FRCP
Consultant in Palliative Medicine, King's College Hospital NHS Trust, London; and
Honorary Clinical Senior Lecturer, Department of Palliative Care and Policy,
King's College, London

Ann Elfred MCSP BSc (Hons)
Chartered Physiotherapist, Physiotherapy Manager, St Christopher's Hospice, Sydenham,
London

John Ellershaw MA FRCP
Medical Director/Consultant in Palliative Medicine, Marie Curie Centre Liverpool,
Woolton, Liverpool

Katie M. Emmitt BM BS MRCP
Specialist Registrar in Palliative Medicine, St Christopher's Hospice, Sydenham,
London

Louise Exton MB BS MRCP MSc
Consultant in Palliative Medicine, Haris Hospis Care, London

Brian Fisher MB BChir
General Practitioner, Wells Park Surgery, Sydenham, London; and Professional Executive
Committee and Board Member of Lewisham Primary Care Trust, London

J. Simon R. Gibbs MD FRCP
Senior Lecturer in Cardiology, Hammersmith Hospital, Imperial College, London

Louise M.E. Gibbs MA FRCP
Consultant in Palliative Medicine, St Christopher's Hospice, Sydenham, London

Patricia Grocott PhD BSc (Hons) DipN (Lon) RGN
Florence Nightingale School of Nursing and Midwifery, School of Health and Life
Sciences, King's College, London

Penny Hansford RN RM HV MSc
Director of Nursing, St Christopher's Hospice, Sydenham, London

Sarah Harris
Consultant Clinical Oncologist, Guy's and St Thomas' Cancer Centre, St Thomas'
Hospital, London

Max Henderson MB BS MRCP MRC Psych
Liaison Psychiatrist and Clinical Research Fellow, St Christopher's Hospice, Sydenham,
London

Irene J. Higginson BMedSci BM BS FFPHM PhD
Professor and Head, Department of Palliative Care and Policy, Guy's, King's and
St Thomas' School of Medicine, King's College, London

Matthew Hotopf PhD MRC Psych
Reader in Psychological Medicine, Institute of Psychiatry, King's College, London; and
Visiting Liaison Psychiatrist at St Christopher's Hospice, Sydenham, London

Allan Irvine MB MRCP FRCR
Consultant Radiologist, St Peter's Hospital, Chertsey, Surrey

Laura C. Kelly MB ChB MRCP
Specialist Registrar in Palliative Medicine, St Christopher's Hospice, Sydenham, London

Cynthia Kennett MCSP MSc BA
Formerly Day Centre Manager, St Christopher's Hospice, Sydenham, London

Jonathan Koffman BA (Hons) MSc
Lecturer in Palliative Care, Department of Palliative Care and Policy, Guy's, King's and St Thomas' School of Medicine, London

Luc Louette MD MCh Orth
Consultant Orthopaedic Surgeon, Kent and Canterbury Hospital, Canterbury, Kent

Barbara Monroe BA BPhil CQSW
Chief Executive, St Christopher's Hospice, Sydenham, London

John O'Dowd
Consultant Orthopaedic Surgeon, St Thomas' Hospital, London

David Oliver BSc FRCGP
Consultant Physician in Palliative Medicine, Wisdom Hospice, Rochester; and Honorary Senior Lecturer in Palliative Care, Kent Institute of Medicine and Health Sciences, University of Kent

David Oliviere MA BA CQSW
Director of Education and Training, St Christopher's Hospice, Sydenham, London

Brendan O'Neill
Macmillan Consultant in Palliative Medicine, Greenwich and Bexley Cottage Hospice, London

Victor Pace FRCS(Ed) LRCP LRCP&S
Consultant in Palliative Medicine, St Christopher's Hospice, Sydenham, London

Jeanette Parry-Crowther BTec Dipl (Pharm Sci)
Specialist Pharmacy Advisor for Palliative Care, Trinity Hospice, London

Jeremy Rees FRCP PhD
Senior Lecturer in Medical Neuro-oncology and Honorary Consultant Neurologist, Institute of Neurology, National Hospital for Neurology and Neurosurgery, London; and Royal Marsden Hospital, London

Dag Rutter MB BS MRCP
Clinical Research Fellow, Royal Marsden Hospital, London

Dame Cicely Saunders OM OBE FRCP
Founder/President, St Christopher's Hospice, Sydenham, London

Charles Shee MD FRCP
Consultant Physician, Queen Mary's Hospital, Sidcup, Kent

Frances Sheldon MA MPhil Dipl (Soc Admin) Dipl (App Soc Studies)
Formerly Macmillan Senior Lecturer in Psychosocial Palliative Care, Department of
Social Work Studies, University of Southampton, Highfield, Southampton. Francis
Sheldon died in February 2004

Anthony M. Smith MB BChir FRCSEd
Former Medical Director, Pilgrims Hospices of East Kent, Canterbury

Peter W. Speck MA BSc DPS
Former Chaplaincy Team Leader, Southampton University Hospitals NHS Trust,
Southampton, and Honorary Senior Research Fellow, Department of Palliative Care and
Policy, King's College London

Patrick Stone MA MD MRCP
MacMillan Senior Lecturer in Palliative Medicine, Department of Psychiatry, St George's
Hospital Medical School, London

Debra Swann MB BS MRCGP MA
Consultant in Palliative Medicine, Mayday Healthcare NHS Trust; and St Christopher's
Hospice, Sydenham, London

Nigel Sykes MA BM BCh FRCGP ILTM
Head of Medicine and Consultant in Palliative Medicine, St Christopher's Hospice,
Sydenham, London; and Honorary Senior Lecturer in Palliative Medicine, King's College,
London

Andrew Thorns MB BS MA MRCGP
Specialist Registrar, Guy's and St Thomas' NHS Trust, London; and Consultant and
Honorary Senior Lecturer in Palliative Medicine, Pilgrim Hospice, Margate and
the East Kent NHS Trust, University of Kent, Margate, Kent

Jennifer Todd BSc MBChB MRCP MA
Consultant in Palliative Medicine, Trinity Hospice, Clapham, London

Steven Wanklyn BSc (Hons) MSc MRPharms
Specialist Senior Pharmacist in Palliative Care and Oncology, Guy's and St Thomas' NHS
Trust and Trinity Hospice, London

John Wiles MB ChB MRCP D(Obst)RCOG DipTEd
Consultant in Palliative Medicine, Princess Royal University Hospital, Farnborough,
Kent; and Medical Director, Harris HospisCare, Orpington, Kent

Don Williams MD FRCPsych
Honorary Consultant Psychiatrist, Department of Old Age Psychiatry, Cefn Coed
Hospital, Cockett, Swansea

PREFACE

It is now more than 25 years since palliative care gained its first textbook. *The Management of Terminal Malignant Disease* was edited by Dame Cicely Saunders and had an authorship largely associated with St Christopher's Hospice, which she had founded. Since then, palliative care has developed hugely. It has spread far beyond hospices, into the community and into hospitals. It has spread far beyond Britain, with more than 90 countries around the world now having some form of palliative care service. More and more countries have incorporated palliative care provision into government health policy, with the UK making it the subject of guidance from the National Institute of Clinical Excellence (NICE). It has spread beyond the final stage of life, with the recognition that the need for palliative care may co-exist with potentially curative therapies. And it has spread far beyond cancer, with the discovery that the symptoms of advanced malignant disease that hospices were originally set up to tackle are in fact common to most progressive, life-shortening illnesses.

In these 25 years, textbooks of palliative care have moved on too, in both size and format. There is now a wide choice, from the voluminous to the pocket book and from the discursive to the bulleted list. The present book is the successor to that first landmark text of 1978. It aims to provide manageable and accessible coverage of all aspects of palliative care for a multi-professional readership. Much of it is still written out of the experience of clinicians who work at, or have associations with, St Christopher's Hospice in London. But it is not a book for or about hospices. Rather, it acknowledges that palliative care is practised in many settings, in different styles and for different conditions, facts recognized in its change of title from previous editions.

The symptom management section is arranged alphabetically, and details of drugs are collected in an appendix. Each chapter ends with a summary of key points. We hope these features will make the book a practical, day-to-day resource in the workplace. But palliative care is more than just symptom control, and this book provides useful guidance on meeting the psychological, social and spiritual needs of people with advanced disease and those close to them. It also recognizes that this work has an ethical context and affects staff in ways that must be dealt with if they are to be able to continue to work together to provide effective care. The cultural context has always helped determine how palliative care is practised in different countries; but even within one country, multiple cultures exist: unless services are sensitive to such differences, they will not be accessed by the whole range of people who could benefit from what they offer. The international spread of palliative care is de facto evidence of its success, but today there are legitimate calls for firmer research-based evidence for its practices, clearer outcome measures and a commitment to continued updating that can never be met by any book but only by harnessing electronic resources.

All these topics, and more, are covered in *The Management of Advanced Disease*. We hope that it will be useful, every day, to those who are providing palliation, no matter in what setting they do so. If that hope is fulfilled, this book will also have been useful to the people whose needs inspired palliative care in the first place – our patients, their families and their friends.

London
March 2004

Nigel Sykes
Polly Edmonds
John Wiles

SECTION 1

GENERAL

chapter 1

INTRODUCTION

Dame Cicely Saunders

The first edition of this book in 1978 was greeted warmly in a three-page review in *Pain*.[1] It was to be the first in a series on malignant disease planned by Professor Gordon Hamilton Fairley before his untimely death and was dedicated to his memory. The word 'malignant' was omitted from the title of the first edition, *The management of terminal disease*, which was published as part of the series, but was added to the second edition in 1984. The word was retained for the third edition in 1993, but a change has been made for this fourth volume that has important implications. The new emphasis, using the word 'advanced', implies a wider brief than malignant disease alone, although much of the research and practice upon which the book is based will have come from clinicians working among cancer patients in the multi-disciplinary specialty of palliative medicine. The focus in the earlier edition was on end-stage problems, but this new edition also looks at problems that may arise earlier in the disease process. The attitudes and skills involved are increasingly employed at earlier stages, often, indeed, from the moment of diagnosis of a life-threatening illness. This was recognized in the third edition and it stands alongside publications with emphasis both on palliative care for non-cancer patients[2] and its worldwide spread.[3]

Palliative care as both a specialty and a general challenge to all clinicians grew out of the research and much consultation that led up to the opening of St Christopher's Hospice (the first research and teaching hospice) in 1967. As Clark observed, '... it becomes apparent that to claim an arbitrary starting point for such a complex and far-reaching movement is unsatisfactory. Indeed it may be preferable to see the opening of St Christopher's in 1967 as a crucial *outcome* of ideas and strategies developed over the preceding decade, in which can be located the essential characteristics of the subsequent hospice movement'.[4] These beginnings and development are documented in extensive archives.[5]

The origins of modern palliative care include the first systematic study of the details of 1100 patients with advanced cancer who were being cared for in St Joseph's Hospice between 1958 and 1965. A qualitative, descriptive study, it was based on detailed clinical notes and tape recordings of patients. In these recordings, patients described their pain and its relief when they were transferred from drugs 'on demand' to a regular giving schedule. This work was to lead to the double-blind cross-over studies between morphine and diamorphine by Twycross in the 1970s, but it demonstrated, as Faull and Nicholson suggest,[6] a refutation of myths or sacred cows that were prevalent at that time regarding the use of opiates. A typical contemporary view comes in the Foreword to the 1956 American text *The management of pain in cancer*. Here, Cole writes: 'Unfortunately, practically all the drugs that are really effective in controlling pain are habit producing and must be used sparingly'.[7] Widely used medical textbooks tended to ignore the issue of pain in cancer and the use of opiates. Brief entries can be found, such as that in Davidson's *The principles and practice of medicine: a textbook for student doctors*: 'As in the management of other carcinomatous patients, analgesics should be given in sufficient amounts to control pain'.[8] The question of when and how to introduce these analgesics was not addressed.

The paper based on the first 900 patients of the St Joseph's series gave what was eventually to become accepted evidence that opiates were not addictive for patients with advanced cancer; that the regular giving of opiates did not cause a major problem of tolerance; that giving oral morphine worked and that it did so not by causing indifference to pain, but by relieving it. Set alongside the prevailing myths of tolerance and addiction, it is not surprising that a patient arriving at St Joseph's should say, 'The pain was so bad that if anyone came into the room, I would say: "Don't touch me, don't come near me" '. The regular giving of oral morphine balanced to that patient's need enabled her to say later, 'It felt as if something had come between me and the pain' (tape recording). She was alert and cheerful, as the recording suggests, and maintained her composure until her death some weeks later. At that stage and in the setting of St Joseph's Hospice, controlled clinical trials were not possible, but this was a ground-breaking first step in what has become a widely recognized field of peer-reviewed research and practice.[9] Twycross's later detailed studies provided the evidence base for the cardinal principles of the method of cancer pain relief endorsed by the World Health Organisation in its highly influential publication *Cancer pain relief* in 1986.[10]

This clinical exploration and the almost contemporary discovery of naturally occurring opiate-like substances and their receptors[11] had surprisingly little communication between them. The latter caused great scientific and lay interest but, whereas Iversen was to write, 'Perhaps the most important practical question is whether enkephalin offers the long sought approach to the development of a non addictive analgesic',[12] Faull and Nicholson, in their detailed study of the scientist/clinician divide,[6] quote Wall's perceptive comment that, 'It's astonishing to look at the basic pharmacologists still working on what *isn't* a problem'.

The second principle developed in the early work at St Joseph's was that 'We have to consider the whole person'. This emphasis led by 1964 to the concept of 'total pain', the complex of physical, psychological, social and spiritual elements that make up the patient's whole experience and that has proved important in the development of this specialty.[13]

THE IMMEDIATE PAST

The principles underlying the whole practice of palliative medicine were defined by a patient whose dying became its founding myth. In 1947, as a recently qualified medical social worker and former nurse, I met in my first ward a Jewish patient aged 40 called David Tasma, who had come originally from the Warsaw ghetto. He received a palliative colostomy for an inoperable and obstructed carcinoma of the rectum. After a few months' follow-up in out-patients, he was admitted to another hospital and I visited him frequently, in a well-run but extremely busy surgical ward, until he died 2 months later. Discussions of a setting that could have helped him find better symptom relief, and the time and space to make his own terms with an apparently unfulfilled and meaningless life, led not only to an initial inspiration but also to his own quiet peace.

Two key phrases from those long conversations were founding insights for the hospice movement. When David Tasma said of a small legacy, 'I'll be a window in your Home', he gave a commitment to openness. Seen first as openness to and from the world, it grew later to a commitment to all future challenges, to be open not only to patients and families but also among ourselves. In another, more personal exchange, he said: 'I only want what is in your mind and in your heart'. Again, later consideration led to a commitment to all that could be a combination of continually developing skills, understanding and research together with a readiness for personal concern. When he died, having made a quiet and personal peace with the God of his forefathers, he left me with the assurance that he had found his answers and that all our caring must give total freedom to others to make their own journey.

Hospice openness, scientific rigour together with personal concern, and freedom for the spirit were built on these foundations and led directly to the ever-widening impetus of the modern movement. Many of the teams have had Christian foundations, Catholic, Protestant and ecumenical. The early challenge to responsibility for openness and respect for differing perceptions of the right way to give the best and most appropriate care for dying patients and their families has led to various approaches coming from very different backgrounds. To suggest that such care could only be based in a separate building, still more only one with some form of religious foundation, would have been to close doors, when the commitment from the beginning was to open them and to spread such care as widely as possible and, in due course, earlier in the disease stage.

After St Christopher's Hospice opened for in-patient care in 1967 and for home care in 1969, pioneers visited from North America on sabbatical leave. Florence Wald, Dean of the Graduate School of Nursing at Yale, and the University Hospital Chaplain Ed Dobihal were among the founders of the first hospice home care team with no back-up beds of its own based in New Haven, Connecticut. Dr Sylvia Lack, from St Joseph's and St Christopher's, joined them as they began caring for patients at home in 1974. Chaplain Carleton Sweetser, from St Luke's Hospital, New York, became chairman of the committee that set up the first consulting team within a hospital later that same year, again with no designated beds of its own. Finally, Dr (now Professor) Balfour Mount, after a period of clinical experience at St Christopher's, founded the Palliative Care Service of the Royal Victoria Hospital, Montreal, early in 1975. Based in a small palliative care unit, it also included home care and a small hospital consulting team. That was the first use of the word 'palliative' as applied to this field, the older word 'hospice' having come to mean custodial, or less than optimal, care in French-speaking Canada.

Hence these three different patterns for planning palliative care, together with day centres (first established by St Luke's Hospice in Sheffield, England, in 1975), had been demonstrated by the mid-1970s. Together with the independent hospices – usually developing or working with a home care programme – these formed the impetus that has led to such a proliferation of services, now spread worldwide. Notable in the United Kingdom has been a series of far-reaching initiatives by the National Society for Cancer Relief, now the Macmillan Cancer Relief Fund, and the work of the Marie Curie Memorial Foundation. The spread has been remarkably fast.

EARLIER HISTORY

The word hospice dates from early in the Christian era when such institutions formed part of the spread of Christianity across Europe.[14] The first use of the ancient word specifically for dying people came long after many of these services in their often beautiful old buildings were closed following the Protestant Reformation. Others were changed and became almshouses for the elderly, while much of their earlier work was taken over by a number of new 'hospitals'. In 1842, Mme Jeanne Garnier, a young widow who had also lost her two children, opened the first of her refuges for the dying in Lyon. It was called both a Hospice and a Calvaire. Several more were opened later by her 'Dames de Calvaire' in other parts of France. Some remain and are becoming involved in today's growth of the palliative care movement in that country. The choice of a different name is due in part to the association with the changes in the mediaeval institutions noted above. If hospice denotes shelter for the elderly, or largely custodial care, it is not a word easily used for a modern home care or hospital team.

The Irish Sisters of Charity quite independently chose the same name when they founded Our Lady's Hospice for the Dying in Dublin in 1879. Mother Mary Aikenhead's Order, dating from much earlier in the century, had always been concerned with the poor, the sick and the dying, but this was their first institution founded specifically for such care. By the time the Order opened St Joseph's Hospice in London's East End in 1905, at least three Protestant homes had opened in the city under other titles: the Friedensheim Home of Rest (later St Columba's) in 1885, the Hostel of God in 1891 and St Luke's Home for the Dying Poor in 1893. The last, founded by Dr Howard Barrett and the Methodist West London Mission, published detailed and vivid annual reports that reveal how much of today's respect for personal worth to the end of life was present in this obviously lively institution. When I arrived there as a volunteer registered nurse in early 1948, the matron, Lilian Pipkin, was still giving copies of these reports to new members of staff as embodying the spirit of what was by then called St Luke's Hospital. From the beginning, Dr Barrett was telling compelling stories about individual people. He wrote little about symptom control, but gave vivid pictures of the courage and characteristics of his patients and showed a deep concern for the families left at home in dire poverty, unrelieved by any form of social security.

Few people had systematically observed this area of medicine before the first 900-patient analysis from St Joseph's Hospice was presented in 1962,[9] although several eminent late nineteenth and early twentieth-century physicians, such as Munk[15] and Snow,[16] had recounted anecdotal reports. Snow's work was based in the Cancer Hospital (later the Royal Marsden) and comprised the most detailed observations. In 1935, Alfred Worcester, a family doctor, published a small classic, *The care of the elderly, dying and the dead*,[17] based on three lectures he had been giving to Boston medical students. He was already 80 when it was printed, after a lifetime as a family doctor with a particular interest in nursing. He acknowledged that he owed much to observing the care given by the Protestant deaconesses of Kaiserswerth (founded in 1836) and the Augustine Sisters of Paris. He is rightly regarded as one of the pioneers in this field, and his book was one of the few writings on the subject when my first searches of the literature began in the 1950s.

A new turn to the history of end-of-life care came in the 1940s. Four social workers documented the many needs of the 200 patients with persistent disease: they tackled as what they referred to as an 'almost insurmountable problem'. Their detailed study, published in a prestigious medical journal, was the first objective study of the current unmet needs of dying patients and their families.[18]

Some years later, three reports added to this new dimension of systematic study. That published by the Marie Curie Foundation in 1952 documented much suffering among patients at home as seen by district nurses.[19] In 1960, Glyn Hughes' *Peace at the last* reviewed provision for end-of-life care nationwide,[20] and in 1963 Hinton reported on 'The physical and mental distress of the dying' in a London teaching hospital in a uniquely detailed study of 102 patients compared with a matched group who were seriously ill but not dying.[21]

The main gift of St Luke's to the hospice movement, and thence to the whole spectrum of palliative medicine, was the regime of the regular giving of oral morphine to control the constant pain of much far-advanced cancer. Lilian Pipkin dated this from before she had joined the staff in 1935, and believed it was a routine established by the matron of that time. This must have been soon after the Brompton Hospital had put together its Brompton Cocktail of opioids, cocaine and alcohol for patients with advanced tuberculosis. When I arrived in 1948, I had met such a cocktail before but not the regularity or the careful assessment in balancing the dose to the patient's need. Elsewhere one saw patients, as a medical student later expressed it, 'earning their morphine', with the doctors' and nurses' fear of drug dependence leading to the sadly common phrase, 'See if you can hang on a little longer'.

It was the first few years of experience at St Luke's and an awareness of much pain and isolation both in hospital and at home that led me to a medical training, with this area of need in mind. It was Mr Norman Barrett, a thoracic surgeon, who discussed the problem and suggested the following: 'Go and read medicine. It's the doctors who desert the dying. There is so much more to be learned about pain. You will only be frustrated if you don't do it properly, and they won't listen to you'. He was right – only a clinical and research base would persuade.

It is from the continuing multi-professional development of palliative care's clinical and research base that this fourth edition is presented.

REFERENCES

1. Madden EJ. Review: 'The management of terminal disease'. Saunders CM (ed.). London: Arnold, 1978. *Pain* 1979; 7(1), 95–9.
2. Addington Hall JM, Higginson IJ (eds). *Palliative care for non-cancer patients.* Oxford: Oxford University Press, 2001.
3. Saunders C, Kastenbaum R. *Hospice care on the international scene.* New York: Springer, 1997.
4. Clark D. Originating a movement: Cicely Saunders and the development of St Christopher's Hospice 1957–1967. *Mortality* 1998; 3(1), 43–63.
5. Clark D. *Cicely Saunders – founder of the hospice movement. Selected letters 1959–1999.* Oxford: Oxford University Press, 2002.
6. Faull C, Nicholson A. Taking the myths out of the magic: establishing the use of opioids in the management of cancer pain. In: Meldrum ML (ed.), *Opioids and pain relief: a historical perspective.* Seattle: IASP Press, 2003, 111–30.
7. Cole W. Foreword. In: Schiffin MJ (ed.), *The management of pain in cancer.* Chicago: Year Book, 1956, 7.
8. Davidson LSP (ed.). *The principles and practice of medicine: notes for Scottish medical students,* 6th edn. Edinburgh: Churchill Livingstone, 1962, 751.
9. Saunders C. The treatment of intractable pain in terminal cancer. *Proc R Soc Med* 1963a; 56, 195–7.
10. World Health Organisation. *Cancer pain relief.* Geneva: WHO, 1986.
11. Hughes J, Smith TW, Kosterlitz HW et al. Identification of two related pentapeptides from the brain with potent opiate agonist activity. *Nature* 1975; 258(5536), 577–80.
12. Iversen L. Chemical identification of a natural opiate receptor agonist in brain. News and views. *Nature* 1975; 258, 567–8.
13. Saunders C. The symptomatic treatment of incurable malignant disease. *Prescr J* 1964; 4, 68–73.
14. Phipps WE. The origin of hospices/hospitals. *Death Studies* 1988; 12, 91–9.
15. Munk W. *Euthanasia or medical treatment in aid of an easy death.* London: Longmans Green & Co., 1887.
16. Snow J. Opium and cocaine in the treatment of cancerous disease. *BMJ* 1896; II, 718–19.
17. Worcester A. *The care of the aged, the dying and the dead.* Springfield, Ill: Charles C Thomas, 1935; Oxford: Blackwells, 1961.
18. Abrams R, Jameson G, Poehlman M, Snyder S. Terminal care in cancer: A study of two hundred patients attending Boston clinics. *N Engl J Med* 1945; 232, 719–24.
19. Marie Curie Memorial Foundation. *Report on a national survey concerning patients nursed at home.* London: Marie Curie Memorial Foundation, 1952.
20. Hughes HLG. *Peace at the last. A survey of terminal care in the United Kingdom. A report to the Calouste Gulbenkian Foundation.* London: Calouste Gulbenkian Foundation, 1960.
21. Hinton JM. The physical and mental distress of the dying. *QJM* 1963; 32, 1–23.

chapter 2

COMMUNICATION

Frances Sheldon

INTRODUCTION

Every moment that professionals spend with a person who is dying or their carers is spent in communicating with them. Communication is about dialogue, to which each party brings assumptions, expectations and behaviour styles which influence both their contribution to and their interpretation of the dialogue and therefore its outcome. The first part of this chapter considers these issues, and the values and theoretical framework that underpin the skills that the professional brings. The second part discusses particular communication problems that often come up in this area of care. Communication with children when someone they love is dying is covered in Chapter 16.

WHAT DO PATIENTS AND CARERS BRING TO THE DIALOGUE?

Much of the research on communication skills and the most commonly used methods of counselling have been developed in Western cultures, and neither may apply to those who come from other cultures. Those working with dying people and their carers need to consider the following factors.

- *Expectations.* Western societies expect that the vast majority of children will live to adulthood and that death is reserved for those in late middle life and old age, and a few unlucky and poignant younger people. They expect doctors to have considerable power over life and death, and may therefore unrealistically credit doctors with knowledge about the course and length of an illness.

A funeral director discussed his dying wife's illness with her doctor and pressed him for the likely length of her life. This was all the more important to him because he was having an affair with another woman and wished to know how long it might be before he was free to marry her. The doctor carefully and honestly explained that it was not possible to say. Later, the funeral director commented to a social worker who had also been present at the interview, 'Of course he knows, all doctors do, he's just not saying'. Conditioned by his society's belief in the foreknowledge of the doctor and impelled by his own circumstances, this man could never be convinced that information was not being withheld.

- *Family history and life experience* shape people's beliefs about illness, death and bereavement. Personal experience of a death is relatively unfamiliar to those in Western societies, because it so frequently takes place in hospitals or other institutions. This inexperience can add to the common fear of the unknown which those facing death may feel, and can fuel anxieties about the inevitability of pain and suffering. These may have a basis in fact if a member of an earlier generation did indeed suffer greatly when dying because modern methods of symptom control were unavailable. It is always important for one member of the professional team to explore with the person who is dying or with the carers what past experience may be influencing the way this death is being approached.

- *Beliefs* about illness may affect the way the patient and carers feel and behave. A man said casually to his doctor, 'Of course, my wife and I have been sleeping in separate rooms since her cancer was diagnosed', and then revealed that they thought cancer was infectious and that he and the children might catch it. He opened up huge anxieties and guilt, which needed to be gently explored and challenged with both the husband and wife. Acquired immunodeficiency syndrome (AIDS) is another illness that brings real anxieties, but misconceptions too.

- The *meaning* atttributed to the disease will influence the way the situation is dealt with.

Mary was 54 when she developed bony metastases following a cancer of the breast. The palliative care team were puzzled by her great reluctance to take medication for her pain. Eventually she revealed that she saw her cancer as a punishment. As a child, she had worked in her father's small grocery shop on Saturdays without payment and used to steal money from the till. Forty years later she felt she was paying the price for this behaviour with her cancer, and that she should not try to avoid her punishment. The team were able to show her that there were other ways of understanding her pain, and she became more ready to be helped.

Barkwell[1] found that, of her sample of 100 patients in the community with cancer, 23 per cent saw their illness as a punishment and 36 per cent as a challenge. Those who saw it as a challenge had less pain and depression than those who saw it as a punishment. Professionals need to explore these beliefs and experiences with patients and their carers in order to enable them to use any help offered.

Research into communication has revealed the importance of recognizing that it is a dialogue and not a communication from an active professional to a passive, receptive patient. Patients make choices about what they communicate and with whom.[2,3] They may perceive a nurse as too busy to have a prolonged conversation from observing her rushing about the ward. So even if she sits down listening attentively, the patient will hold back from opening up sensitive issues. Patients may view different professionals as interested only in a narrow range of issues – nurses interested in physical symptoms, not emotional concerns, social workers in benefits, not spiritual conflicts – and not express their greatest concern. This makes it all the more important to use the resources of the whole team in communication and to ensure that each member tries to convey their readiness to hear the pressing issues even if they need to draw others into tackling them.

WHAT SHOULD PROFESSIONALS BRING TO THE DIALOGUE?

The success of communication depends crucially on the values that the professional brings to it.

- A *non-judgemental approach* that asserts the unique value of the individual and his or her experience is vital. Many people may behave in ways that the professional cannot endorse. Limits may need to be set by a team about, for example, the extent to which alcohol can be consumed by a patient in hospital. However, unacceptable behaviour should not alter the commitment to value the person. Stedeford comments: 'How a person lives depends on at least three factors: the way he has lived, the type of illness and the quality of care. Staff share grief about the first and second, but only the third is their responsibility'.[4]

- *Self-determination* for the patient within the limits set by the legitimate interests of others is an associated value. Balancing competing interests, for example between the patient who wishes to stay at home to die and the exhausted wife whose own health is suffering, or between the patient who feels safe in hospital and wishes to stay there and the patient in pain at home who needs admission, requires an open and honest approach with all those involved.

- The concept of *partnership* with patients and families builds on this value and has been influenced by improvements in education and access to a much wider range of information about illness and its treatments than in the past. So now there is often an expectation of joint decision-making about issues that might have been decided by the professional alone in the past. The extent to which each new patient wishes to exercise this right to self-determination requires careful negotiation.[5,6] Cultural factors will certainly influence this,[7] since in some cultures decision-making is seen as a family rather than an individual issue.

  Alongside these values, some particular qualities will assist the professional working in this field.

- The *ability to face reality but maintain hope* – not the hope of cure but a sense that life may still offer good things – can be sustaining to both patients and their carers. A positive belief in the potential of individuals for change, even when they face the crisis of death, is an asset.

- *Genuineness* is basic to this field of care. This was defined by Truax and Carkhuff as involving 'the very difficult task of being intimately acquainted with ourselves, and of being able to recognise and accept, as well as respect ourselves as a whole, containing both good and bad'.[8] Professionals need to understand which situations may be particularly challenging for them as individuals and with which they may need help, and conversely, those situations to which they may be able to make a unique contribution. Professionals, no less than those they wish to help, are formed by their society and their individual experience, and need to understand how this has happened to work sensitively with others. Such self-awareness will help in treading the narrow line between an over-involvement, which may destroy the professional and stifle the patient, and a cool detachment, which communicates 'I don't care' to patient and carers. This self-awareness needs to operate both at the general level and in particular situations. A critical self-monitoring at an interview – 'What exactly made me feel particularly sad at this moment?', 'Why am I finding eye contact difficult now?' – contributes to a full and sensitive evaluation of a situation.

- Alongside this, there must be an *ability to empathize*. Tuson suggests '... the experience of having someone empathise accurately and deeply implies the possibility of change. If someone understands my despair that well, but is not despairing themselves, and is regarding enough to spend time experiencing my despair, then change might be possible'.[9] Such deep empathy may bring pain. Those offering this must learn to take care of themselves and establish a network of support if they are not to suffer the battle fatigue described by Vachon.[10]

KUBLER-ROSS STAGE THEORY – AN EVALUATION

One of the most widely known models of the psychological response to the process of dying is that described by Elisabeth Kubler-Ross.[11] From interviews with 200 dying people in hospital, she identified five common experiences, which she called 'stages', in the process of dying:

- *denial* – a refusal to believe that death will be the outcome: 'No, not me!',

- *anger* – 'Why me?', 'It's not fair!', 'Someone is to blame',

- *bargaining* – an attempt to delay the disaster, maybe a secret pact with God,

- *depression* – the two manifestations of this were a reaction to the losses that the illness brought and preparatory withdrawal at a later stage,

- *acceptance* – peaceful resignation.

Kubler-Ross's findings were rapidly elevated into a prescription for the right way to die which still remains extraordinarily powerful, perhaps because it provided professionals with a way of distancing themselves from the suffering of the dying by checking off feelings against a list, rather than actually listening to the anguish.[12] So it is important to value Kubler-Ross's insights, but not to use them as a straitjacket, and to recognize that dying people may not experience all these emotions and may swing in and out of them.

DIFFERENT APPROACHES TO COMMUNICATION

There is value in a range of approaches to communication with people who are dying and their carers. Emphasizing communication *skills* alone is not enough. To be effective, and to sustain skills learnt, communication must take place within a structure that encourages openness and provides support for the communicator that recognizes their deep feelings and involvement. Moorey and Greer have described the use of cognitive therapy with cancer patients, which gives them the techniques to manage overwhelming feelings of anxiety and fear.[13] The use of the arts as a means of communication and exploration of feeling is increasing in many specialist palliative care services.

Parkes, Laungauni and Young suggest a framework for approaching dying or bereaved people from cultures different from our own.[14]

- Take time to get to know them before raising issues relating to death and bereavement, to find out whether such matters can be openly discussed in that culture.

- Ask them to explain their culture and where in a general pattern they would locate themselves. Are they members of a very traditional group? Have they adapted many customs through moving to a new country?

- Invite questions about the current situation.

- Recognize and set aside your own cultural prejudices and assumptions – this will in turn help others in the dialogue to do the same.

- Use non-verbal communication but be alert to reactions that indicate that what you have just done is inappropriate to that culture.

- Use interpreters if necessary, but make sure that the interpreter is acceptable to the family or individual. Make sure, too, that the interpreter can tolerate interpreting painful and difficult emotions and that he or she has support if needed. As a general rule, do not use children to interpret for adults.

WHAT SKILLS DO PROFESSIONALS NEED?

NON-VERBAL COMMUNICATION

In a typical interaction between two people, about one-third of what is exchanged is in words and two-thirds are non-verbal. There are some clear guidelines which are at their most essential when breaking bad news, but relevant in any communication.

- Make the environment as secure, comfortable and free from distraction as possible. Ask permission to turn off the television (having made sure this is not the start of a favourite programme). Shut the door, or draw the curtain at least part way round the bed.

- Concentrate on the other person, making eye contact comfortably.

- Use touch, but tentatively at first, until it is clear what this particular person feels comfortable with.

People in distress often initiate conversations in less than ideal circumstances. The relative who pounces on a nurse rushing with a bed pan to another patient with the anxious enquiry, 'My husband seems much worse today?', still needs the reassurance that the nurse will give her anxieties proper attention at another time. That reassurance is communicated as much by the non-verbal elements of the exchange – stopping for a moment, eye contact, smiling – as by any words used.

COUNSELLING SKILLS

A number of these skills must form part of the basic tool kit of any professional.

- Attentive listening hears not just the words themselves but also their tone, picks up additional clues to the meaning of what is being said from non-verbal behaviour, and conveys interest and concern by concentration which also encourages openness.

- Reflecting and summarizing build on this listening, checking that the interviewer's perceptions are accurate, focusing on key issues and thus moving discussion forward.

- Questioning can elicit information using closed questions – 'When did you have your operation?' – or attitudes, feelings and opinions by using open questions – 'What do you think the problem is now?'.

- Challenging unclear or distorted statements – 'You say your mother has always hated you; why does that make you a bad person?', 'How will you make sure that you have time for yourself at weekends as well as caring for your sick wife?' –- helps the interviewee to reassess situations and develop new strategies for managing them.

However, an important distinction needs to be made between the use of these skills as part of every interaction and the offer of counselling sessions to those who are dying or their carers. This distinction needs to be clear to both client and worker. Concern to offer a more personal and caring service to those facing their own death and their carers has sometimes led to the misconception that every patient or carer is looking for, or ought to be offered, formal counselling sessions.

Professionals have underrated the potential for the sensitive use of counselling *skills* while doing a wound dressing or arranging admission for a period of respite care. Formal counselling sessions should only be put in place after an assessment with the patient or carer has found that there are specific issues that need more intensive attention.

PRESENTING A CASE AND CO-OPERATING WITH OTHERS

Not all communication is with patients or their families. Working in the field of advanced disease means working with a wide variety of different professionals, perhaps with volunteers, or with public or charitable organizations whose services or interventions are needed. Negotiating skills and an ability to be appropriately assertive are a vital part of advocating on behalf of someone more vulnerable. Working in teams is discussed elsewhere in this book. Just as one-to-one communication needs to be underpinned by a value base, so teamwork needs to have a common ethical base and common aims for the overall work of the team, even if individuals within it have individual goals for their own. This is only likely to occur if the team takes time to have open discussion about the challenging ethical issues arising in this field separate from such issues arising in practice, and if team aims are regularly reviewed and not just assumed to be shared. Self-awareness and empathy are just as necessary in working with team members as in work with those who are dying and their carers. Wilkinson's research on nurse communication has shown how significant the attitudes of a team leader may be in enabling others to use their skills, or limiting their use.[15]

PARTICULAR COMMUNICATION PROBLEMS

BREAKING BAD NEWS

Breaking bad news poses both ethical and communication challenges. The key ethical decision, which must be clarified first, is: who has a right to the information about a particular person's diagnosis and prognosis? Attitudes in the UK and the USA have changed in recent years, influenced by an increased emphasis on patients' rights and by specialist palliative care practice, so it is now more common to share this information, particularly with the person suffering from cancer.[16] However, a review of research shows both that, in practice, professionals are still more likely to offer 'conditional openness', making judgements about the capacity of the patient, and that patients move in and out of open awareness, choosing sometimes to protect themselves from confronting a difficult reality.[17] It is important that professional judgements do not disenfranchise whole groups of patients, such as older people.[18] Here, the critical self-monitoring mentioned earlier is especially important. It should also be understood that people have a right *not* to know the truth, if this is their wish.

The doctor is the team member most likely to take the responsibility for breaking bad news about diagnosis or prognosis, but any member of the team may be drawn into discussion by patient or carer afterwards. Team members need to be clear about what the patient has been told, so that any member, be they physio-therapist, chaplain or nurse, may be able to respond appropriately if the patient wants to discuss it.

Breaking bad news too abruptly may disorganize the patient psychologically and provoke denial.[19] A step-wise approach is the best way to test the pace at which the individual wishes to understand what is happening.

- *Preparation.* The best moment to start to prepare to break bad news is at the start of the investigative process when the doctor has a suspicion that the outcome is unlikely to be good. This is the moment to discuss with the patient whether information about the disease should be shared with a spouse or partner or another family member, and in very general terms how much the patient wishes to know of the detail of any results of the investigations. This will begin to give the doctor a 'feel' for the style of communication the individual prefers.

- When there is some bad news to discuss, the doctor should secure as *safe and comfortable an environment* as possible, following the guidelines outlined above in the section on non-verbal communication. Acknowledging the well-established research finding that anxiety prevents patients retaining much of what they are told in a consultation, it is now common practice to ask the patient's permission (and the carer's, if present) for a nurse or social worker to be present at the interview. This second professional can then remain after the doctor has left and be available for both questions and support. Another well-received method is to tape the interview, with permission, and to offer the patient the tape to take away.[20]

- *Giving a warning shot* is one way to start the interview; 'We have now had the results of the tests, and I am afraid they are not as good as we hoped. Would you like me to tell you what we found?'. This gives the patient the option of asking for the detail or signalling that this is too threatening today by saying, for example, 'I'll leave the detail to you, doctor, just let me know what treatment you are going to give me'. If the patient asks for the information, a short, clear, jargon-free explanation is needed: 'I am sorry to tell you that we have found some cancer cells in your liver. I'm afraid this may be rather a shock'.

- *Allow time for expression of feelings* – bewilderment, terror, resignation. This may be the time to explore past experience of this disease, or particular fears about it. Once feelings and fears have been expressed, the doctor may introduce a discussion on the management of the situation: 'I'd like to discuss with you how we can tackle this problem'. Even if there are no options for curative treatment, the patient should be reassured that symptoms will be managed, though not given false reassurance that no pain or problems will be experienced, and that this team, or another more appropriate one, will continue to be concerned.

- *Continuing the process*. Ideally, after an opportunity has been given for asking any other questions, an appointment should be arranged with the same doctor in a day or two for further discussion. If this is not possible, it should be made clear that full information will be passed promptly to a doctor who will be able to give ongoing care, such as the general practitioner. This signals the doctor's commitment to the patient's future care and demonstrates that breaking and receiving bad news is a process for doctor and patient. A series of short interviews will take no longer and use time more effectively than a heroic session that attempts to tie everything up at once.

- *Deterioration* during the course of an illness can be handled slightly differently. Here, the patient has had some experience of the disease and is likely to be having some symptoms. It is then important to find out what the patient suspects or knows about what is happening to him or her. So starting with an open question – 'How do you think your illness is going?', 'How do you feel at the moment?' – or responding to the questions 'Am I getting worse?', 'Am I going to die?' by saying, 'Let's discuss that, but tell me what makes you think so?', will help professional and patient start from the same place. Again, a gentle, stepwise procedure can proceed at the patient's pace. Maguire and Faulkner suggest that 'this strategy of moving from acknowledging and exploring the nature and the basis of any strong feelings to identifying key concerns is essential if the breaking of bad news is to be managed effectively. It allows the patient to be "lifted" from being overwhelmed to feeling hopeful that something can be done'.[19]

THE PROTECTIVE CARER

The carer who buttonholes the professional at the front door or in the hospital corridor and firmly says 'He mustn't be told' is not uncommon. If the strategy of discussing with a patient at the start of an investigation how communication should be handled has been followed, the professional should have some idea of the patient's wishes, and can react accordingly. If not, then the ethical issue again comes to the fore: who has a right to this information? However, even if the professional wishes to assert the primacy of the patient's right to know, a stark statement of this principle is likely to be counter-productive.

The fears, anxieties and concern of the carer need to be explored first, and his or her more intimate knowledge of the person drawn out. Asking 'What would worry you particularly about him/her knowing?' gives the opportunity for this, and shows that the listener values the carer's opinions. The majority of carers with such anxieties will then accept a reassurance that the professional will undertake not to initiate any discussion on the outcome of the illness, but that if the dying person raises the issue, the professional will respond truthfully in order to maintain and deserve that person's trust.

ANGER

Buckman describes three main types of anger in this situation:[21]

- anger at the rest of the world who will survive when this person will not,

- anger at fate/God/destiny,

- anger at anyone who is trying to help, such as doctors or nurses.

Behind anger are feelings of powerlessness and a desperate search to regain some sort of meaning in a world out of control. Team members themselves may feel some of the second sort of anger from time to time and may be drawn into discussion on this topic with someone who is dying. The chapter on spiritual issues (Chapter 20) covers this area.

Professionals may be involved in situations in which people who are dying are making life difficult for their carers by their angry behaviour towards them. Here, the carer may need support and help in understanding why this previously loving person is so awkward now. Carers can be helped to set appropriate boundaries for the dying person. The odd episode of rudeness and rage can be understood and forgiven, but a constant battery will wear out love, and result in further loss for both parties. Professionals can strengthen carers to ask for proper consideration of their needs without feeling guilty.

Most professionals in this field have experienced being blamed by a dying person or a carer for failing to cure or to alleviate a problem. Defensiveness is never useful. Real shortcomings need to be honestly acknowledged, and it always helps to say 'I'm sorry that you feel things went so badly', even if everything possible has been done. Allowing angry people a chance to talk about their dissatisfaction will often help them to see things in proportion.

However, it has sometimes to be accepted that someone will need to hang on to anger as the only way of dealing with distress. Teams may then need to be supportive of a team member who is the focus of that anger.

DENIAL

Denial is a useful protective psychological mechanism in a dangerous situation, provided it does not prevent the person from taking action which could protect against further harm. So a woman who finds a lump in her breast but denies that it could damage her is denying inappropriately because it prevents her seeking treatment. A woman with well-established and untreatable cancer of the lung who asserts that she has another 20 years yet to make that round the world trip is distancing herself from an unbearable reality.

It is important to distinguish denial from conscious suppression, resorted to by many patients from time to time, and to recognize that there may be cultural or religious factors that promote denial in this individual.[22] Denial can be uncomfortable for professionals if they prefer to be open with those they work with. The secret is not to collude with the denial by pretending to share it, but to understand the individual's need for self-protection and to speak to the feelings underneath. To say 'When things are difficult it helps to think about something pleasant' recognizes the pain of the situation.

Less frequently, it is the carer who denies the illness is serious and continues to expect the sick person to carry on as usual. This desperate attempt to maintain normality needs a caring rather than a punitive response from professionals, whose first concern may be the effect on their patient.

There are some circumstances in which denial may need to be tackled – mainly where there are vulnerable family members *solely* dependent on the dying person and plans need to be made for their future care. Examples are:

- young children

- someone with a learning disability

- a frail elderly person.

A useful mechanism here is 'What if?'. Discussing with single parents what they would like to happen to their children if they were not around helps to maintain some of the protective distance.

However, if the dying person has a partner who is caring for the children or a frail parent, and will continue to be able to do so, then there is no need to breach the denial. Professionals may regret that those who are dying do not take opportunities to speak to those they love about their own death, but each person chooses a personal path to death. It will certainly be important for the parent who is going to survive to prepare the children for the death.

Another situation is which denial needs to be tackled is when someone is overtly denying what is happening but is displaying an unusual amount of distress or pain which is not responding to treatment. Again, this is best dealt with in a way that avoids direct confrontation. Kearney gives an interesting example of using image work successfully to relieve distress in a young man.[23] Image work can form part of a psychotherapeutic approach and uses imagery to help create a bridge between the conscious and unconscious self. The imaginary material is often visual, but may be auditory or tactile, or from the client's dreams. Kearney comments that 'because the imagery enabled emotional expression in symbolic form it did not challenge the protective shield of Sean's denial, which was allowed to remain intact'.

DEPRESSION AND DESPAIR

Standing alongside another human being in despair at their coming death is a real challenge. The usual methods for dealing with sadness and despair involve reassurance that in the long run things will improve. This is plainly untenable when someone is dying, and to a recently bereaved person seems so unlikely as to be insulting to the person who died.

Cyril was 56. He had taken early retirement, had a large lump sum in the bank and an ample pension. He had planned to travel and enjoy sun, good food and wine after a lifetime's hard work. Now he was lying in a palliative care bed with cancer of the stomach, unable to eat, his money useless to him. To jolly him along would have been insensitive. He needed an honest acknowledgement that life can be unfair, and empathy with his misery and sense of loss.

Given this understanding, the clear messages from the caring team that they value this despairing individual and have not given up their attempts to make the quality of life as good as possible, some patients may be enabled to recover their coping abilities or even find new ones. Some will never lift their spirits, and team members need to help each other not to be drawn down into the pit with the person in despair and thereby become ineffective. If such sadness does spill over into a clinical depression, antidepressant drugs may be considered as an adjunct to the strategies already described.

FEAR

The person who shows panic and fear in a final illness can create great unease in the caring team, in fellow patients in the ward, and in those who love them. Panic and fear provide a painful challenge to one of the basic assumptions of palliative care – that it is possible to enable people to have a good quality of life at the end of life. It reminds those who may soon follow of how much is unknown and how tenuous is the control they may have achieved. Like any other emotion, fear may be communicated in words or in behaviour. The patient who frequently calls for extra pain relief during the night when that level of medication is effective during the day may in reality be asking for help with fears in a way that is socially acceptable. The test will be if the patient can be helped to settle without medication if a nurse spends time in gentle exploration of anxieties and stays until the patient is calm.

Common fears are of the manner of death – sudden haemorrhage, being unable to breathe, choking to death, being buried alive – or of what may lie beyond the moment of death. The first essential is not to assume what the fear is, but to ask: 'You don't seem comfortable, and sometimes you look really scared. One of the team may be able to help. Is there anything that is frightening you particularly?'. A discussion of anxieties about the manner of death may bring reassurance about the way the distressing event can be handled. Patients may see that, for instance, the level of sedation as the end approaches is something that can be negotiated and be more under their control than they had expected. Some fears may be to do with after death:

Peter, aged 68 and knowing he was within a few weeks of death from cancer of the pancreas, seemed to be uneasy and unsettled. It became clear that he was ruminating for much of the time on what might happen after he died. His wife had died some years before and he now feared that he would not be allowed to join her in heaven because he had been a nominal rather than an active Christian. After discussion he agreed to a two-pronged approach. He would talk to the chaplain about these fears and, to help with his constant rumination, he would be supplied with some jigsaws. He had found these a good distraction in the past.

Much has been learnt in recent years about the ways those facing crises can be helped to gain greater control over their fears. Cognitive therapy has been mentioned already, and relaxation techniques, possibly incorporating music or guided imagery, can also help. Art therapy can offer a release. Massage and aromatherapy have become much more readily available in health care and can contribute to a sense of peace.

UNCERTAINTY

Common uncertainties faced by those who are dying and their carers are how much hope is there, how long before death comes, what will the intervening period be like and how will death come. For some, the uncertainty about the possibility of cure or remission may be with them until the day of death. For others, the knowledge that death is coming may be a sort of relief. In their efforts to deal with the tremendous anxiety that living with uncertainty creates, both those who are dying and their carers may press professionals to give them specific answers to these questions.

Studies have shown how unreliable forecasts of prognosis usually are, and that they are likely to be too optimistic. Maguire and Faulkner suggest 'it is better to acknowledge your uncertainty and the difficulties this will cause'.[24] They go on to describe a scheme of responses which checks if the enquirer would like to know what signs may herald further deterioration, encourages positive use of the present time, and shows a willingness to monitor the situation regularly and a readiness to respond to any emergency. This gives the security of feeling that someone with more experience recognizes the problem and can be called on if there are particular worries or difficulties.

For some, the strategy of 'hoping for the best and planning for the worst' is helpful. When carers come with such questions as 'Shall I take unpaid leave from my job now or later?', 'Shall I get my daughter over from Australia?', or when someone for whom there is no hope of cure asks 'Shall I take early retirement?', 'Shall I have more chemotherapy?', this strategy offers a framework for reviewing options. Thinking with the patient or carer about what the situation would be if the best happened and what they would need to consider if the worst happened enables them to take a variety of considerations into account without necessarily focusing too heavily on one scenario or the other.

THE UNCOMMUNICATIVE PATIENT

There is no such thing as an uncommunicative patient, though there may be patients who do not talk as professionals think they should, or do not choose to talk to a particular member of staff for the reasons discussed earlier. The issue here is not silence alone. A patient may not talk but a smile or squeeze of the hand may convey trust or grief. These are the patients who do not talk about their fears and sadness, patients who only converse in monosyllables, patients who shut their eyes when someone asks how they are, and who do this in a way that makes professionals feel uncomfortable and not in control. Some questions need to be asked here.

- How has this person dealt with life crises in the past?
- Can family or friends identify this as a common way of coping?

- Has every professional in the team in turn tried to start up a deep conversation about feelings and is the patient just plain irritated with intrusive questions? An unfortunate effect of the greater concern for the feelings of those who are dying and the increased openness in discussing them is that there may almost be an expectation that people *should* be ready to talk. They may be pressed to do so, as much to satisfy a professional's view of how people should die as to meet any real need or wish of the patient.

- Are the professionals picking up the patient's own feelings of angry hopelessness? Casement shows how valuable the therapist's own feelings are as a guide to the patient's experience.[25] If this seems the likely explanation, it should be tackled with the patient, who needs to be given some responsibility for his or her own feelings and the effect of them on others. One way might be: 'Mr Jones, recently I [the team] have felt very uncomfortable and helpless when with you, as if nothing I [we] do is any good. Is this how you are feeling?' This may produce an angry outburst that clears the air, or a continuing silence. In the latter case, a firm statement about appropriate boundaries may help: 'Mr Jones, I know this is a difficult time for you. I am sorry that we cannot cure you/relieve your pain as we would wish. We do want to go on trying to help but we need to work on it together. I won't press you to talk again unless you show me that you are ready to do so, but until then I won't be able to be as useful as I could be'.

Professionals need to be clear about what is properly their responsibility, which is not that of making everything right, but of working with the patient to the best of their ability.

ASKING FOR EUTHANASIA

Patients may ask for assistance in ending their lives directly or they may be more indirect: 'You wouldn't let a dog live like this'. The ethical aspects of this issue are dealt with in Chapter 9. The communication approach should be based on principles already outlined in this chapter:

- a readiness to explore with the patient or carer what particular aspects of the situation are most painful,

- acknowledgement of, and empathy with, the emotional pain.

Only after this should the professional gently outline the boundaries set by the law and conscience. This needs to be done in a way that does not make the person who has asked feel either ashamed or abandoned. It may well be appropriate to give an assurance that nothing will be done to prolong life. It can be painful to face the reproach or even anger that refusing such a request can bring. This is another situation in which the support of team members is vital.

AROUND THE DEATH

There is a particular need for good communication skills in the period around the actual death. People who are dying communicate increasingly through non-verbal means, but this should not stop professionals talking to them, describing what they are about to do, and treating them as individuals with feelings.

The carers are likely to be tense and distressed. Good preparation is the key here. If there has been open and honest discussion with the person who is dying and the carers at an earlier stage about possible wishes at the time of death, professionals will feel clearer about how to meet their needs. If someone in the later stages of a life-threatening disease is admitted, carers should be asked on admission about the degree of involvement they wish at the time of death and whether they wish to be called in the night. This should be done even when death is not immediately expected, since it is in practice so hard to predict.

If the death is planned to be at home, similar early exploration of all parties' views is needed. In addition, carers need to be aware of what actual sources and levels of help there may be. The vague promise 'You'll have all the help you need' may lead to unrealistic expectations of 24-hour care being provided when all that is available is a night sitter once a week.

Once the death is approaching, the carers' wishes should be reviewed with them regularly. What they expected they would wish may not turn out in practice to be so, or they may change their view if the death is particularly long and drawn out. Carers may suffer higher levels of distress than the patient at this time.[26] By now, the likely manner of death may be clearer, and the doctor or nurse should explore whether carers would like to be aware in more detail of what the event might be like. Special attention needs to be paid to those who may often be excluded at this time – children, those with learning disabilities and the mentally frail elderly. The professionals involved can give a lead in ensuring that they are properly informed and participating appropriately, for example by including them in family conferences or specifically asking their opinion of how things are going on home visits.

There is no 'right' amount of time for carers to spend with the body once the person has died, or any 'right' way to grieve. Here, different cultural practices need to be especially respected. At home, carers can be in control. It may be useful to point out to those unused to death at home that there is no need to rush the body out of the house immediately. Farewells can be taken slowly. Grandchildren can come to say goodbye to their grandmother after school in familiar surroundings. In hospital, there may be pressure on beds that means unlimited time is not available. If staff know they will soon need the space for another patient, they need to give some warning: 'In about a quarter of an hour we will need to move your husband elsewhere. You will be able to see him there if you wish or you can finish your goodbyes here in that time'. The procedures for obtaining the death certificate and recovering the patient's belongings from hospital may be a source of distress for the bereaved.[27] Making procedures clear and efficient, training staff to carry them out sensitively and providing something more presentable than a black plastic rubbish bag for the belongings communicate a great deal to carers about the degree of concern for them and the value of the person they cared for.

In hospital, there are other participants in the death besides the carers and the staff. Other patients will certainly be keen observers and may be more deeply involved if they have known the patient. On the positive side, they may learn from seeing how this death has been handled how caringly their own end may be dealt with. On the negative side, this death may be a terrifying reminder of their own mortality, especially if it has not been peaceful. So deaths on the ward should not be ignored. Staff can take the opportunity to say: 'Perhaps you saw that Mrs Brown died last night'. This gives permission to ask questions about the death and may lead to some discussion of that patient's own death. If the death was distressing, it gives an opportunity to reassure that not all deaths are like it.

CONCLUSION

This chapter attempts to establish some principles for good practice in communication with those who are dying and their carers, and discusses some particular issues. However, there can be no exact blueprint for this work. Egan observes: 'helpers tend to over-identify the helping process with the communication skills that serve it. Technique can replace substance. Communication skills are essential of course, but they still must serve the outcomes of the helping process'.[28] Communication is a creative process – herein is its excitement and its danger. It is not possible to be perfectly prepared for whatever comes. So courage is needed, with a solid value base and some understanding of basic skills. Most important though is a faith in the potential of the partner in the dialogue, whether that person is dying or bereaved, to change and grow in response to the crisis of loss and death.

KEY POINTS

- Explore expectations, family experience and beliefs about illness since these will influence patients' and carers' communication.
- Communication is a dialogue between two active partners, and there is now greater recognition of the choices patients may make about what and to whom they communicate.
- A non-judgemental approach, a belief in self-determination for people who are dying, and qualities of genuineness and empathy are essential for professionals working in this field.
- Breaking bad news should be a process that proceeds in a gentle stepwise manner at the patient's pace.
- The identification of denial is complex and requires a careful analysis and exclusion of cultural and religious factors. It is not always appropriate to try to breach denial.
- Around the time of death, maintaining a sensitive awareness towards the patient and regularly checking the changing needs of carers in the changing situation are key issues.

REFERENCES

1. Barkwell DP. Ascribed meaning: a critical factor in coping and pain attentuation in patients with cancer-related pain. *J Palliat Care* 1991; 7(3), 5–14.
2. Heaven C, Maguire P. Disclosure of concerns by hospice patients and their identification by nurses. *Palliat Med* 1997; **11**, 283–90.
3. Jarrett N, Payne S. A selective review of the literature on nurse–patient communication – has the patient's contribution been neglected? *J Adv Nurs* 1995; **22**, 72–8.
4. Stedeford A. *Facing death: patients, families and professionals.* Oxford: Heinemann Medical Books, 1984.
5. Payne S. Information needs for patients and families. *European Journal of Palliative Care* 2002; **9**, 112–14.
6. Grbich C, Parker D, Maddocks I. Communication and information needs of caregivers of adult family members at diagnosis and during treatment of terminal cancer. *Prog Palliat Care* 2000; 8(6), 345–50.
7. Akabayashi A, Kai I, Takemura H, Okazaki H. Truth telling in the case of a pessimistic diagnosis in Japan. *Lancet* 1999; **354**, 1263.
8. Truax CB, Carkhuff RR. *Towards effective counselling and psychotherapy.* Chicago: Aldine, 1967.
9. Tuson G. Schindler's Ark: a study in heroism, therapy and change. *J Fam Ther* 1985; 7, 161–73.
10. Vachon M. Battle fatigue in hospice/palliative care. In: Gilmore A, Gilmore S (eds), *A safer death.* New York: Plenum Press, 1988.
11. Kubler-Ross E. *On death and dying.* New York: Macmillan, 1969.
12. Kastenbaum R. Is death a life crisis? In: Datan N, Ginsberg LH (eds), *Lifespan developmental psychology: normative life crises.* New York: Academic Press, 1975.
13. Moorey S, Greer S. *Psychological therapy for cancer patients.* Oxford: Heinemann Medical Books, 1989.
14. Parkes CM, Laungauni P, Young B. *Death and bereavement across cultures.* London: Routledge, 1997.
15. Wilkinson S. Factors which influence how nurses communicate with patients. *J Adv Nurs* 1991; **16**, 677–88.
16. Seale CF, Addington-Hall JM, McCarthy M. Awareness of dying: prevalence, cause and consequences. *Soc Sci Med* 1997; **45**, 477–84.
17. Field D, Copp G. Communication and awareness about dying in the 1990s. *Palliat Med* 1999; **13**, 459–68.
18. Costello J. Truth telling and the dying patient: a conspiracy of silence? *Int J Palliat Nurs* 2000; 6(8), 398–405.
19. Maguire P, Faulkner A. How to do it. Communicate with cancer patients: 1. Handling bad news and difficult questions. *BMJ* 1988; **297**, 907–9.
20. Bruera E, Pituskin E, Calder K, Neuman CM, Hanson J. The addition of an audio cassette recording of a consultation to written recommendations for patients with advanced cancer: a randomised controlled trial. *Cancer* 1999; **86**(12), 2420–5.
21. Buckman R. *I don't know what to say.* London: Macmillan, 1988.
22. Ness D, Ende J. Denial in the medical interview. *JAMA* 1994; **272**(22), 1777–81.
23. Kearney M. Imagework in a case of intractable pain. *Palliat Med* 1992; 6, 152–7.

24. Maguire P, Faulkner A. How to do it. 2. Handling collusion, uncertainty and denial. *BMJ* 1988; **297**, 972–4.

25. Casement P. *On learning from the patient.* London; Tavistock, 1985.

26. Hinton J. Can home care maintain an acceptable quality of life for patients with terminal cancer and their relatives? *Palliat Med* 1994; **8**, 183–96.

27. Wright A, Cousins J, Upward J. *A study of bereavement support in NHS hospitals in England.* Kings Fund Project Paper No. 77. London: King Edward's Hospital Fund for London, 1988.

28. Egan G. *The skilled helper.* Belmont: Brooks Cole, 1990.

chapter 3

AUDIT, OUTCOMES AND QUALITY OF LIFE IN PALLIATIVE CARE

Fiona Aspinal and Irene J. Higginson

INTRODUCTION

This chapter defines audit and discusses some of the methods to measure the quality of palliative care services. It follows the development of quality assessment, from its roots in simple assessment of care towards a more scientific method of service quality assessment: audit. The interrelationship between audit, outcome measurements and quality of care and how these methods of quality assessment can affect the quality of a person's life are discussed. The chapter also considers why being able to monitor the quality and effectiveness of services is particularly important in today's health care climate, with particular emphasis placed on the UK perspective.

THE CONCEPT OF QUALITY IN HEALTH CARE

In recent years an extensive discourse has developed surrounding the concept of quality in health care. These discussions centre around two different, but closely related, ideas: quality of care and quality of life. The explicit emphasis on 'quality' in UK health service reforms is founded in the market-oriented approach to public services that came to the forefront of political and social policy debates in the 1980s.[1] Although the issue of quality of care may have surfaced as an explicit dimension of policy debates at this time, it was not a new notion in the clinical environment.

- In medicine, the Charter of the Royal College of Physicians (1518) recognized that one of the aims of medicine was to ensure that high standards were maintained for their own benefit, for the good of the profession and for the good of society.[2]

- In nursing, Florence Nightingale tried to identify interventions that could promote better quality of care by assessing the outcomes of nursing practice.[3]

This long-term commitment to ensuring quality of care and treatment is evident from the foundation of peer-led councils to monitor and regulate professionals' conduct and practice. In the UK these are:

- the General Medical Council (GMC), established in 1858 to monitor doctors' practice and conduct,

- the General Nursing Council (GNC), established in 1919 to monitor nurses' practice and conduct; these aims were continued by its superseding organization, the United Kingdom Central Council (UKCC) in 1979 and subsequently by the Nursing and Midwifery Council (NMC) in 2002.

It is clear, therefore, that health professionals have always placed a significant emphasis on quality in health care. This emphasis remains a high priority for most healthcare professionals today. However, during the 1970s and 1980s, quality moved from being an implicit concern of professionals to an explicit priority of funders, managers and policy makers. For example, in the UK, reviews of the National Health Service (NHS) during the 1980s showed that quality needed to be given higher priority in terms of healthcare management and policy. These reviews indicated that:

- inequality of access to high quality services existed,

- the type of services available varied from region to region and even within health care regions,

- between regions, similar interventions resulted in different outcomes.

Subsequently, a number of Government reports and legislative reforms in the UK aimed to deal with these issues. For example, the Griffiths Report (1983)[4] promoted the recruitment of senior officers to enhance quality assurance strategies within the health services; Working for Patients (1989)[5] was based on a NHS review that began in 1987 to address the public concern about cuts in services; The NHS and Community Care Act (1990)[6] introduced the idea of competition between services and established the internal market, NHS Trusts and fund-holding general practitioners; The Patient's Charter (1991)[7] gave patients formal choice and rights that could impact on the quality of services. These initiatives were often based on a growing parallel movement in the USA, promoting quality assurance and accountability for quality care. Other countries have also adopted these approaches.

These ideological movements towards an explicit concern with quality assessment and assurance in the political dimension of health care have influenced consecutive legislative reforms.

WHAT IS QUALITY?

What do we mean by quality? Quality, as defined in many dictionaries, pertains to 'degree of excellence' or 'general excellence'. However, numerous questions arise about the notion of quality in health care: namely, what constitutes excellence in the context of a service, who defines excellence and what components does it address? For example, should excellence be limited to clinical skills, or should it encompass broader aspects, such as whether the service reaches all those in need? We would argue that when measuring quality of a service all the features and characteristics that bear on its ability to satisfy the stated or implied needs of the users of that service should be assessed. As Donabedian asserts, quality in health care is a multi-dimensional concept and, as such, a multi-dimensional approach to measurement and assessment of that quality is required.[8]

Numerous authors have identified some of the dimensions that should be included when assessing the quality of a service. For example, Maxwell identifies the following as dimensions of care that need to be measured when monitoring quality:[9]

- effectiveness

- acceptability

- efficiency

- access

- equity

- relevance.

Black (1990) agrees that all these aspects of care require consideration when assessing quality, but adds a further dimension: humanity.[10]

So how do we determine whether we are offering a good-quality service if we have to consider all these dimensions? One method of assessing service quality is to conduct a clinical audit of the service that is provided.

WHAT IS CLINICAL AUDIT?

Clinical audit is the process of assessing, evaluating and improving service provision for its users. Professional organizations, suggests Shaw, agree that there are three main aims of audit:[11]

- education and training of staff,

- promotion of the effective use of resources,

- improvement of care to individual patients.

Clinical audit covers all aspects of clinical care and addresses the issue of quality of care for both direct and indirect users of a service. Thus, promoting audit benefits not only patients, families and services, but also staff. Audit is a cycle of monitoring care against goals, outcomes or standards, and feeding the results back into practice in order to change and improve care. This cycle is then repeated to assess the new system of practice. This is often different from evaluation, which

Table 3.1 Common differences between evaluation and audit

Evaluation	Audit
A linear process	A cyclical process
Aims to assess the service provided	Aims to provide evidence base for practice, standards and policy development
Is conducted as a single study	Is undertaken regularly
Cases are chosen for their specific case history or circumstances	Cases for review are selected at random or all patients are included
Assesses whether practitioners are doing the right thing at all and finds new information	Assesses whether practitioners are doing the right thing well

tends to occur once and where the emphasis tends to be on learning new facts and on providing generalizable information. However, components of audit can be similar to evaluation, and the results of evaluation can be used in a variety of ways, including informing care programmes for individuals and also improvements in local care. Common differences between audit and evaluation are shown in Table 3.1. In the USA, in end-of-life care, Lynn has developed continuous quality improvement, using a similar cycle of: plan, do, study, act.[12]

Audit provides a regular method of monitoring service provision and quality and enables checks into whether standards are being met. It provides a more systematic approach to practice review and aims to assess the overall quality of a service.

Audit entails:

- setting standards and targets for good practice and developing protocols within which to attain these standards; these standards, targets and protocols should be guided by best practice and peer review;

- gathering information in a systematic manner about the service;

- obtaining objective information about the service;

- comparing the findings of this data collection against the standards set;

- identifying areas where the service is weak or of poor quality and identifying methods of addressing these limitations of the services;

- monitoring the impact of these changes in care and service provision.

The process is then able to begin again, with review of standards and so on, thus completing the 'audit cycle'.

WHERE DID THE NOTION OF CLINICAL AUDIT COME FROM?

Clinical audit developed as a component of market strategies that were introduced into public services in the UK. This partnered a change in political ideology that had its foundation in the customer-oriented approach to public services proposed in the USA and Canada.

The idea of transposing management strategies directly from the private sector into public services was driven by contemporary common concerns in Western nations, those of constantly increasing demands on public expenditure and calls for extensions of financial support. Reducing public expenditure, or at least limiting it, was a high priority for the UK as well as for the USA. Given the political relationship between these two nations, it was inevitable that a system that was viewed as being effective in the USA would be adopted in the UK.

One problem that could potentially arise from reducing costs to a service is a reduction in the quality of that service. The introduction of the internal market and compulsory competitive tendering were other reasons for the increased emphasis on quality. If the NHS was having to pay for a service, it needed to know that it was paying for a high-quality service and that it could not get one of similar quality for less money.

These concerns were addressed with the introduction of 'total quality management' strategies alongside the market mechanisms. This not only balanced some of the worries about reduced quality of services, but also seemed to fit the UK government's drive towards a more accountable health care service. As lack of quality had been identified as a major cause of high costs, addressing this was seen as an alternative method of limiting demand on the public purse.

These new strategies in the UK also moved control and regulation of services towards the hands of NHS managers, giving them more control over agendas and budgets. However, with the perceived movement away from centrally directed health care provision, managers needed to find a method of determining where they would spend the money; thus a method of assessing outcomes and service quality was needed. This is where audit stepped into the political and clinical picture. Although this new political paradigm was, and remains today, controversial, it did reinforce the health service's pursuit of quality in more formal terms. The process of quality assurance can even be of assistance to health care practitioners, funding decision makers and policy makers, who are now able to base their practice and decisions on evidence. It is useful to note that several initiatives, such as quality assurance, audit, total quality management and, more recently, clinical governance, all focus on improving, in a systematic way, the quality of care.

WHY IS AUDIT IMPORTANT TODAY?

Quality remains a high priority in contemporary health care debates. Indeed, in the UK, the Labour administration has introduced a new vocabulary to describe the process of quality management and has established a number of organizations to reinforce the work of the national accreditation bodies in a more general service sense.

Clinical governance

The notion of clinical governance first entered the UK health care arena through the publication of the white paper *The new NHS – modern, dependable*.[13] Monitoring quality is a requirement of all service providers, but they are not always able to fulfil the requirements of clinical audits, complaint resolution and risk management.[14] Clinical governance has been introduced in an attempt to meet these requirements. In most cases, clinical governance begins with quality assessment of the services already in place. It proposes that quality can be attained by ensuring that:

- a patient-centred approach is adopted,
- there is a line of accountability for quality,
- high standards and safety are ensured,
- the organization and staff in the clinical environment aim to improve services and care for patients.

Clinical governance is closely related to *accountability*, a concept that has long been included within professional codes of conduct for all healthcare professionals. The main principles are:

- promotion of good practice,
- prevention of poor practice,
- intervening when unacceptable practice is evident.

Accountability has commonly focused on healthcare professionals' ability to demonstrate that they act in the best interests of the patient. However, clinical governance has extended this role from being simply an individual accountability to an organizational responsibility. Clinical governance can be defined as: '[a] framework through which NHS organisations are accountable for continually improving the quality of their services and safeguarding high standards of care by creating an environment in which excellence in clinical care will flourish'.[15] Clinical governance is closely related to clinical audit, as it emphasizes shared responsibility for quality assurance.

In England and Wales, several national organizations have been established to examine the quality of care: the Commission for Healthcare Audit and Inspection (CHAI, concerned with ensuring clinical governance) and the National Institute for Clinical Excellence (NICE, concerned with ensuring evidence-based practice).

WHY IS AUDIT IMPORTANT IN PALLIATIVE CARE TODAY?

These reasons for the importance of audit in general health care are also relevant to more specialist settings such as palliative care. The reasons for conducting audit in palliative care settings are wide and varied.

- Reassurance for healthcare professionals that they are providing patients with a high-quality service.
- The need to show that palliative care is effective in order to continue to receive funding.
- To provide evidence that there is a need for palliative care.

- To provide a method of ensuring that there is equitable access and quality of palliative care services across the UK.

- To monitor whether professionals and organizations are able to achieve the requirements imposed by government, and to investigate why not, if necessary.

- To provide the public with access to information regarding quality of palliative care.

- Purchasers of health care services, such as UK primary care trusts, need evidence upon which to base their decisions about where and how best to spend public money.

- The NHS Executive demand that organizations and their staff are involved in audit, producing guidelines and setting standards before they can be granted a 'specialist' title.[16]

WHAT DOES AUDIT LOOK LIKE?

Audit can focus on a single issue or multiple issues and can involve one group of professionals or the multi-disciplinary team.

- *Retrospective audit* utilizes clinical notes or discussion with family members to enable information to be collected about the past quality of care provided.

- *Prospective audit* is conducted whilst the patient is undergoing treatment or in receipt of care. It is a process where the standards of care to be met are agreed at the outset, as are the measures to be used.

- *Nursing audit* adopts a comparative approach. Nurses draw a parallel between their practice and pre-agreed guidelines of professional conduct. The aim of this form of audit is to identify areas where nursing care can be improved.

- *Medical audit* describes a more scientific approach to the assessment of services. It is a systematic critical review of the quality of medical care and aims to appraise the whole process of medical care. It therefore addresses procedures used for diagnosis and treatment, use of resources and the resulting outcomes and quality of life for patients.

- *Organizational audit* covers assessment of the more administrative aspects of service provision.

CLINICAL AUDIT AND PALLIATIVE CARE

There can sometimes be a reluctance to conduct audit in the palliative care setting. This is based on staff perceptions that 'palliative care cannot be measured' and 'there is no problem, since palliative care is of a high quality and is self auditing'.[17] However, palliative care lends itself very well to clinical audit. Some of the factors that make clinical audit the most appropriate method of quality assessment in palliative care are indicated below.

- The primary aim of palliative care is to improve quality of life. Clinical audit allows overall quality of care and life to be assessed.

- Palliative care practitioners do not only care for patients, but also for the patients' families and friends. Clinical audit enables direct and indirect users of palliative care services to be included in quality assessment.

- Palliative care is traditionally a multi-professional discipline. Clinical audit enables every professional's input to be assessed.

Although the aims of all members of the multi-professional team are similar, different palliative care environments, whilst using a holistic approach, may place greater emphasis on different aspects of quality of life or goals. In-patient units, for example, may place greater emphasis on the physical symptoms, whereas day-care units may place greater emphasis on emotional and social support. It may be necessary, therefore, to include some core and some complementary components in an audit, the latter being determined by local need. Although clinical audit may be the most obvious choice for service assessment in palliative care, the decision about which method to use depends on which component of the service, or which professional group, is being assessed. At times, it may be more appropriate to use one of the other types of audit discussed above.

WHAT POSITIVE OUTCOMES ARE THERE IN AUDITING PALLIATIVE CARE?

The benefits of audit, whilst being applicable to all areas of health care, are especially so in palliative care because they are so far-reaching. People who can benefit from clinical audit in palliative care include:

- patients
- families
- staff
- policy makers
- the general public
- palliative care organizations.

Some of the benefits that can arise from conducting clinical audit in palliative care include the following.

- All aspects of care can be assessed, thus preventing certain elements of care being overlooked and promoting a more holistic approach to care.

- Interventions that are most effective can be identified, ensuring better standards of care for patients and their families. This also provides evidence that can be used to attract financial resources to, and political support for, palliative care services.

- Individual critical appraisal of clinical practice can be promoted, enabling staff to identify areas where they may need further training.

- Due to the multi-disciplinary approach adopted when conducting clinical audit, better communication systems between professional groups and different clinical areas can result.

A project to study the extent of clinical audit in palliative care in the North Thames region of the UK confirmed that these benefits could result. Staff thought that the most significant advantage of conducting audit was the improvement or maintenance of quality of care, with other factors considered important including identifying areas where practice could be changed and promoting the function of palliative care.[17]

WHAT NEGATIVE OUTCOMES ARE THERE TO CONDUCTING CLINICAL AUDIT IN PALLIATIVE CARE?

This study also identified some of the disadvantages of being involved in audit, which included:

- clinical audit is time consuming,

- clinical audit increases workload,

- the implementation of the findings of the audit is lengthy,

- results may be used against the palliative care team.

Although there are some limitations and negative aspects of assessing the quality of palliative care services through clinical audit, correct implementation and adherence to guidance for audit can lead to the delivery of a more appropriate and higher quality palliative care service, with better-educated carers, in better-organized services. It can also ensure that the public has equity of access to palliative care services irrespective of location.

GUIDELINES FOR CONDUCTING AUDIT IN PALLIATIVE CARE

BEFORE YOU START

The management team needs to address the possible implications of the results of audit on staff. A review of audit activities in one region found that some staff were concerned that audit data may be used against them.[17] For this reason, it is important that clinical staff, with guidance and support from their managers, own and direct audit. This should ensure that staff are able to influence the audit process in the early stages and see the potential benefits, rather than focusing on the potential negative outcomes. In addition, staff can be made aware of negative findings and can develop strategies to manage these at an early stage. To ensure that the audit process is a positive experience for the staff involved, it is essential that staff provide positive feedback to questions such as the following.

- Am I willing to appraise my work and my contribution to the team critically?

- Am I willing to change my clinical practice if required?

- Do I want to enhance my professional knowledge and clinical skills?

- Is there anything that I would want to be changed?

- Do I want to improve the service that I provide?

- Am I interested in improving quality of life for patients and their families?

THE AUDIT PROCESS

When initiating and conducting audit, it is essential to bear in mind the aim and the cyclical process of audit. So, simply, when you are auditing your clinical practice, you need to follow the schedule outlined in Figure 3.1.

MAKING AUDIT EASIER

The audit process should be kept as simple as possible. Constraints on time and resources due to clinical demands can impact negatively on the introduction of clinical audit in palliative care. This can be addressed by adopting the following guidance (the mnemonics BRAVE and SPREE).[18]

- *Borrow*: borrow and adapt methods, measures and standards from similar organizations that are conducting clinical audit.

- *Reliability*: in most clinical audits, more than one member of staff will be collecting the information. It is necessary, therefore, to ensure that any measurement tool provides stable and consistent information when used by different people at different times.

- *Appropriate*: it is essential that whatever measurement tool is used and whatever standards are set, they are acceptable to staff and patients (if patients' perspectives will be collected). It is also important that the tool is able to represent and assess the work that is conducted in that setting.

- *Valid*: when it has been decided what aspect of care provision will be audited, it is important that the measures that are developed (or borrowed) are measuring what they set out to measure so that the goal of the audit can be achieved.

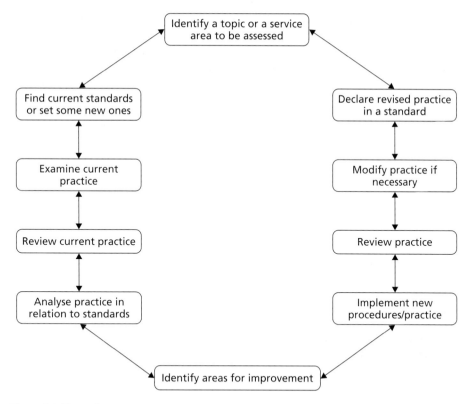

Figure 3.1 The audit process.

- *Easy*: this applies to all parts of the audit process. The methods used to collect information should be easy to understand and easy to do.

- *Small*: try not to audit the whole service from all perspectives and at all levels in the first instance, but focus on one aspect of a service or one intervention.

- *Plan*: plan to learn from experience, with lessons learnt about the audit process influencing consecutive audits.

- *Regular*: regular audit enables assessment of care over time, and adaptation of measurement tools for specific demands and services, and ensures that we are always providing the highest-quality care.

- *Exchange*: we can learn from the experience of other professionals conducting audits in a similar clinical environment. By sharing experiences, procedures and outputs, we should ensure that our audit is the most appropriate and of the highest standards that we are able to attain.

- *Enjoy*: most important of all, the experience of being able to discuss results and procedures with other professionals and the chance to evaluate our work can be rewarding and enjoyable.

OUTCOMES AND QUALITY OF LIFE IN PALLIATIVE CARE

Just as there are various ways to audit palliative care, there are also different levels of palliative care that can be assessed through audit.

- *Structure* is concerned with the stable resources within a service, such as bed numbers, numbers of staff and equipment available. Structural audit would be used to assess the skill mix of staff, for example.

- *Process* is concerned with the use of resources and the activities that take place between practitioners and patients. Audit of process would be conducted to assess aspects of care including prescribing, throughput, documentation and time taken for providing care.

- *Outcome* refers to the result of an intervention.[19] It is concerned with the patient's current and future health status and, in palliative care, also refers to the results for the family. This would include the assessment of clinical management of patients, covering, for example, symptom control, the extent to which needs have been met, levels, types and effectiveness of communication and patient and family satisfaction.

These aspects are interrelated. Structure influences, and makes possible, the process of care, which in turn affects outcomes. *Structural* audit is probably the easiest of these to conduct, as it is concerned with the more stable elements of care provision, whilst the *process* of providing care is less easy to measure, but is more closely related to direct patient care.[8] Neither of these levels of audit reflects the care actually given to a patient, or the way in which this has affected the patient or the family. Conducting audit of *outcomes* can enable assessments of patient-oriented or family-oriented aspects of care provision, but they are more difficult to measure.[8] As such, audit of the structural and process levels of health care is more common than audit of outcomes. However, for the complete assessment of the efficiency and effectiveness of a service or particular intervention, audit of outcomes is essential.[20]

OUTCOMES AND QUALITY OF LIFE IN PALLIATIVE CARE

Traditional indicators of outcomes of health care interventions, such as morbidity and mortality, are not useful in palliative care because they are not appropriate to our patient population. Different outcomes need to be used that reflect the specific goals of palliative care,[21] such as control of symptoms, support for the family, improving quality of life,[22] satisfaction,[8] achieving wishes for place of care, quality of death and identification and managements of abnormal bereavement. Quality of life is one of the most important and common measures of outcome in palliative care, although measures that include broader aspects are available.

Outcomes in palliative care are not easy to assess, as these aspects are less tangible than traditional measures of outcome. This makes it difficult both to measure these aspects of care and to find measures that will detect important changes in palliative care patients and their families. Nevertheless, significant effort has been employed in validating outcome measures that can be used to assess palliative care (examples are listed in Table 3.2).

Because some of the goals of palliative care can only be defined in terms of the individual patient, whenever we are measuring palliative care outcomes it is important to look at outcomes from the patient's perspective. Quality of life, for example, has a number of definitions. It is not an easy concept to measure, but can be defined as the level of attainment of personally set goals and standards for life. It is, therefore, a very personal concept and means different things for different people. Direct assessment of quality of life is, therefore, almost impossible, but it is possible to infer how good a patient's quality of life is from audit results.

Ideally, patients should always complete outcome measures because only they can truly know how interventions affect their quality of life.[24] However, it is often

Table 3.2 Examples of outcome and quality of life measures[22]

Outcome measures	Main domains
Palliative Care Core Standard	Symptom control Information giving Emotional support Bereavement support Collaboration with other organizations
The Palliative Care Assessment (PACA)	Symptom control Future care placements Insight
The McGill Quality of Life Questionnaire	Psychological symptoms Physical symptoms Outlook on life Global quality of life scale
The Edmonton Symptom Assessment Schedule (ESAS)	Physical and psychological symptoms including appetite, depression, dyspnoea, pain etc.
The European Organisation for Research on Cancer Treatment Quality of life Questionnaire (EORTC QLQ-C30)	Global quality of life scale Global physical condition Functioning ability Symptom scales including nausea, tiredness, worry, memory, pain etc.
The Support Team Assessment Schedule (STAS)	Symptoms Family needs Communication Psychosocial needs and support
The Palliative Care Outcome Scale (POS)[23]	Physical symptoms Patient psychological well-being Family psychological well-being Functioning ability

the case in palliative care that patients are too ill to complete questionnaires themselves and so it is also important to be able to collect views on the patient's behalf from a proxy.

Although collecting information on behalf of a patient from a proxy can sometimes be the only method of collecting information about dying people, the reliability of data collected in this way has not been fully determined.[25-27] Staff, family members or friends can act as proxies for the patient. However, staff ratings have been shown to be more similar to patients' than ratings provided by members of the patients' families.[28] The similarity between patient-generated and proxy-generated scores is strongest when measuring physical symptoms.[29] but validity studies of the Support Team Assessment Schedule (STAS) showed that staff may underestimate levels of pain.[28] Psychosocial aspects of quality of life seemed to be more difficult for proxies to assess and showed poor correlation with patients' own scores.[29] Nevertheless, research suggests that proxy assessments can provide valuable and valid data when evaluating services, when assessing observable symptoms, such as vomiting, and when measuring levels of satisfaction with services.[28]

One method of trying to obtain as much similarity between the results of these assessments as possible is to use the same assessment schedule for patients and for their proxies. One of the tools that has been used to measure palliative care outcomes from both the patients' and staff's perspectives is the Palliative care Outcome Scale (POS).[23] This 11-item questionnaire includes questions about physical, psychological, esoteric, social and emotional dimensions of care and has been used in a variety of specialist palliative care settings to evaluate the services provided. (See the POS below.)

So, outcome measures can be, and are, commonly used to assess and improve the quality of palliative care. Outcomes can also provide some insight into the quality of a patient's or family's life. Indeed, outcomes are probably the best method of gaining some insight into how patients' quality of life is influenced by the palliative care that they receive because they aim to assess the actual care that service users receive.

ENDNOTE

This version of the POS includes the most recent developments. However, other options are available, such as changing the time period being assessed or the order of the questions. The patient-centred open questions could be used at the beginning of the questionnaire, for example. Adding questions on specific symptoms or replacing existing questions with others that measure the same domain are further alternatives. Question 7, which asks about level of depression, could be replaced with the following example shown below. Further modifications are being tested.[30]

It is essential to remember, when comparing POS data between units or over time, that only similar questions asked in the same way can be compared.

Example – alternative question 7:

Over the past 3 days, have you felt that life was worthwhile?

- ❐   0 Yes, all the time
- ❐   1 Most of the time
- ❐   2 Sometimes
- ❐   3 Occasionally

CONCLUSION

The quality of a patient's life and other outcomes such as symptom control are clearly important to measure whenever assessing palliative care services because life-extending treatment is limited and life expectancy may be short. One of the best ways of ensuring that palliative care services are able to achieve this outcome is to conduct a clinical audit. Clinical audit allows service providers to ascertain where they are performing well and where changes are needed. It will determine areas of clinical care where staff may require further training and identify where management strategies need to change. Auditing palliative care service ensures that patients and families are able to receive high-quality care and that staff can be sure that their interventions are improving their patients' quality of life and other outcomes for the patient and family.

KEY POINTS

- Audit is an essential component of providing quality health care.
- Audit is the process of assessing, evaluating and improving service provision for its users.
- The structure – process – outcome framework is useful for understanding the audit process.
- Appropriate areas for audits of outcomes in palliative care may include symptom control, care of the family, improving quality of life, achieving wishes for place of care, quality of death and identification and management of abnormal bereavement.
- The use of validated outcomes measures, such as the POS, may identify whether patients' and families' needs are being met.

REFERENCES

1. Kendall I, Moon G. Health policy and the Conservatives. In: Savage P, Atkinson R, Robins L (eds), *Public policy in Britain*. Basingstoke: St Martin's Press, 1994, 162–81.
2. Shaw C. *Medical audit: a hospital handbook*. London: Kings Fund Centre, 1989.
3. Rosser RM. A history of the development of health indices. In: Smith GT (ed.), *Measuring the social benefits of medicine*. London: Office of Health Economics, 1995, 50–62.
4. Griffith's Report. *Department of Health and Social Security NHS Management Enquiry*. London: DHSS, 1983.
5. The Secretaries of State for Health. *Working for patients*. London: HMSO, 1989.
6. Department of Health. *The NHS and Community Care Act*. London: HMSO, 1990.
7. Department of Health. *The Patient's Charter*. London: HMSO. 1991.
8. Donabedian A. *Explorations in quality assessment and monitoring, Vol. 1: The definition of quality and approaches to its assessment*. Michigan: Health Administration Press, 1980.
9. Maxwell RJ. Dimensions of quality revisited: from thought to action. *Qual Health Care* 1992; **1**, 171–7.
10. Black N. Quality assurance of medical care. *J Public Health Med* 1990; **12**(2), 97–104.
11. Shaw CD. Introduction to audit in palliative care. In: Higginson I (ed.), *Clinical audit in palliative care*. Abingdon: Radcliffe Medical Press, 1993, 1–7.

12. Lynn J. Reforming care through continuous quality improvement. In: Addington-Hall JM, Higginson IJ (eds), *Palliative care for non-cancer patients*. Oxford: Oxford University Press, 2001, 210–6.

13. Department of Health. *The new NHS: modern, dependable*. London: HMSO, 1998.

14. Garland G. Governance: taking the first step. *Nursing Management* 1998; 5(6), 28–31.

15. United Kingdom Central Council for Nursing, Midwifery and Health Visiting. *Accountability in practice*. London: UKCC, 2001.

16. Menzies K, Murray J, Wilcock A. Audit of cancer pain management in a cancer centre. *Int J Palliat Nurs* 2000; 6(9), 443–7.

17. Higginson I, Webb D. What do palliative staff think about audit? *J Palliat Care* 1995; 11(3), 17–19.

18. Higginson I (ed.) *Clinical audit in palliative care*. Abingdon: Radcliffe Medical Press, 1993.

19. Wilkin D, Hallam L, Doggett M-A. *Measures for need and outcome for primary health care*. Oxford: Oxford University Press, 1992.

20. Bardsley MJ, Coles JM. Practical experiences in auditing patient outcomes. *Qual Health Care* 1992; 1, 124–30.

21. Persuelli C, Paci E, Franceschi P, Legori T, Mannucci F. Outcome evaluation in a home palliative care service. *J Pain Symptom Manage* 1997; 113(3), 158–65.

22. Hearn J, Higginson I. Outcome measures in palliative care for advanced cancer patients: a review. *J Public Health Med* 1997; 19(2), 193–9.

23. Hearn J, Higginson I. Development and validation of a core outcome measure for palliative care: the palliative care outcome scale. *Qual Health Care* 1999; 8, 219–27.

24. Higginson I, Romer AL. Measuring quality of care in palliative care services. *J Palliat Med* 2000; 3(2), 229–36.

25. Fakhoury WKH. Satisfaction with palliative care: what should we be aware of? *Int J Nurs Stud* 1998; 35, 171–6.

26. Higginson I, Priest P, McCarthy M. Are bereaved family members a valid proxy for a patient's assessment of dying? *Soc Sci Med* 1994; 38, 553–7.

27. Hinton J. How reliable are relatives' reports of terminal illness? Patients and relatives compared. *Soc Sci Med* 1996; 43, 1229–36.

28. Higginson IJ, McCarthey M. A comparison of two measures of quality of life; their sensitivity and validity for patients with advanced cancer. *Palliat Med* 1994; 8, 282–90.

29. Rothman ML, Hedrick SC, Bulcroft KA, Hickam DH, Rubenstein LZ. The validity of proxy-generated scores as a measure of patient health status. *Med Care* 1991; 29, 115–24.

30. Hughes R, Higginson IJ, Addington-Hall J, Aspinal F, Thompson M, Dunckley M. Project to imPROve Management Of Terminal illnEss (PROMOTE). *J Interprofessional Care* 2001; 15(4), 398–9.

FURTHER READING

Addington-Hall JM, Higginson IJ (eds). *Palliative care for non-cancer patients*. Oxford: Oxford University Press, 2001.

Higginson I (ed.). *Clinical audit in palliative care*. Abingdon: Radcliffe Medical Press, 1993.

APPENDIX: THE POS

PATIENT QUESTIONNAIRE

Care setting: .... Unique no: ....
Date: .... Date of birth: ....
Assessment no: ....

Please answer the following questions by ticking the box next to the answer that is most true for you. Your answers will help us to keep improving your care and the care of others. Thank you.

1. Over the past 3 days, have you been affected by pain?
   - ❐ 0 Not at all, no effect
   - ❐ 1 Slightly – but not bothered to be rid of it
   - ❐ 2 Moderately – pain limits some activity
   - ❐ 3 Severely – activities or concentration markedly affected
   - ❐ 4 Overwhelmingly – unable to think of anything else

2. Over the past 3 days, have other symptoms, e.g. feeling sick, having a cough or constipation, been affecting how you feel?
   - ❐ 0 No, not at all
   - ❐ 1 Slightly
   - ❐ 2 Moderately
   - ❐ 3 Severely
   - ❐ 4 Overwhelmingly

3. Over the past 3 days, have you been feeling anxious or worried about your illness or treatment?
   - ❐ 0 No, not at all
   - ❐ 1 Occasionally
   - ❐ 2 Sometimes – affects my concentration now and then
   - ❐ 3 Most of the time – often affects my concentration
   - ❐ 4 Can't think of anything else – completely preoccupied by worry and anxiety

4. Over the past 3 days, have any of your family or friends been anxious or worried about you?
   - ❐ 0 No, not at all
   - ❐ 1 Occasionally
   - ❐ 2 Sometimes – it seems to affect their concentration
   - ❐ 3 Most of the time
   - ❐ 4 Yes, always preoccupied with worry about me

5. Over the past 3 days, how much information have you and your family or friends been given?
   - ❐ 0 Full information – always feel free to ask what I want
   - ❐ 1 Information given but hard to understand
   - ❐ 2 Information given on request but would have liked more
   - ❐ 3 Very little given and some questions were avoided
   - ❐ 4 None at all

6. Over the past 3 days, have you been able to share how you are feeling with your family or friends?
   - ❐ 0 Yes, as much as I wanted to
   - ❐ 1 Most of the time
   - ❐ 2 Sometimes
   - ❐ 3 Occasionally
   - ❐ 4 No, not at all with anyone

7. Over the past 3 days, have you been feeling depressed?
   - ❐ 0 No, not at all
   - ❐ 1 Occasionally
   - ❐ 2 Some of the time
   - ❐ 3 Most of the time
   - ❐ 4 Yes definitely

If you have placed a tick in boxes 3 or 4 for this question, please speak with your nurse or doctor at your next appointment.

8. Over the past 3 days, have you felt good about yourself as a person?
   - ❐ 0 Yes, all the time
   - ❐ 1 Most of the time
   - ❐ 2 Sometimes
   - ❐ 3 Occasionally
   - ❐ 4 No, not at all

9. Over the past 3 days, how much time do *you* feel you have wasted on appointments relating to your health care, e.g. waiting around for transport or repeating tests?
   - ❐ 0 None at all
   - ❐ 1 Up to half a day wasted
   - ❐ 2 More than half a day wasted

10. Over the past 3 days, have any practical matters resulting from your illness, either financial or personal, been addressed?
    - ❐ 0 Practical problems have been addressed and my affairs are as up to date as I would wish
    - ❐ 1 Practical problems are in the process of being addressed
    - ❐ 2 Practical problems exist which were not addressed
    - ❐ 3 I have had no practical problems

11. If any, what have been your main problems in the last 3 days?

    1 ....

    2 ....

12. How did you complete this questionnaire?

    ❐　0　On my own

    ❐　1　With the help of a friend/relative

    ❐　2　With help from a member of staff

STAFF QUESTIONNAIRE

Care setting:　...................................　Unique no:　...

Date:　...　Assessment no:　.................................

Please answer the following questions by ticking the box next to the answer that you think most accurately describes how the patient has been feeling. Thank you.

1. Over the past 3 days, has the patient been affected by pain?

    ❐　0　Not at all, no effect

    ❐　1　Slightly – but not bothered to be rid of it

    ❐　2　Moderately – pain limits some activity

    ❐　3　Severely – activities or concentration markedly affected

    ❐　4　Overwhelmingly – unable to think of anything else

2. Over the past 3 days, have other symptoms, e.g. feeling sick, having a cough or constipation, been affecting how they feel?

    ❐　0　No, not at all

    ❐　1　Slightly

    ❐　2　Moderately

    ❐　3　Severely

    ❐　4　Overwhelmingly

3. Over the past 3 days, have they been feeling anxious or worried about their illness or treatment?

    ❐　0　No, not at all

    ❐　1　Occasionally

    ❐　2　Sometimes – affects their concentration now and then

    ❐　3　Most of the time – often affects their concentration

    ❐　4　Patient does not seem to think of anything else – completely preoccupied by worry and anxiety

4. Over the past 3 days, have any of their family or friends been anxious or worried about the patient?
   - ❒ 0 No, not at all
   - ❒ 1 Occasionally
   - ❒ 2 Sometimes – it seems to affect their concentration
   - ❒ 3 Most of the time
   - ❒ 4 Yes, they always seem preoccupied with worry

5. Over the past 3 days, how much information has been given to the patient and their family or friends?
   - ❒ 0 Full information – patient feels free to ask
   - ❒ 1 Information given but not always understood by patient
   - ❒ 2 Information given on request – patient would have liked more
   - ❒ 3 Very little given and some questions have been avoided
   - ❒ 4 None at all

6. Over the past 3 days, has the patient been able to share how they are feeling with family or friends?
   - ❒ 0 Yes, as much as they wanted to
   - ❒ 1 Most of the time
   - ❒ 2 Sometimes
   - ❒ 3 Occasionally
   - ❒ 4 No, not at all with anyone

7. Over the past 3 days, do you think the patient has been feeling depressed?
   - ❒ 0 No, not at all
   - ❒ 1 Occasionally
   - ❒ 2 Some of the time
   - ❒ 3 Most of the time
   - ❒ 4 Yes definitely

8. Over the past 3 days, do you think they have felt good about themselves?
   - ❒ 0 Yes, all the time
   - ❒ 1 Most of the time
   - ❒ 2 Sometimes
   - ❒ 3 Occasionally
   - ❒ 4 No, not at all

9. Over the past 3 days, how much time do you feel has been wasted on appointments relating to the health care of this patient, e.g. waiting around for transport or repeating tests?
   - ❒ 0 None at all
   - ❒ 1 Up to half a day wasted
   - ❒ 2 More than half a day wasted

10. Over the past 3 days, have any practical matters resulting from their illness, either financial or personal, been addressed?
    - ❒ 0 Practical problems have been addressed and their affairs are as up to date as they would wish
    - ❒ 1 Practical problems are in the process of being addressed
    - ❒ 2 Practical problems exist which were not addressed
    - ❒ 3 The patient has had no practical problems

11. If any, what have been the patient's main problems in the last 3 days?
    1 ....
    2 ....

12. What is the patient's ECOG scale performance status?
    - ❒ 0 fully active
    - ❒ 1 restricted
    - ❒ 2 ambulatory
    - ❒ 3 limited self-care
    - ❒ 4 completely disabled

SECTION 2

A–Z OF SYMPTOMS

SYMPTOM ASSESSMENT

Polly Edmonds

One of the main principles of managing patients with advanced disease is to improve the management of physical symptoms. Symptom control can be improved by accurate assessment of contributing factors in an individual patient at any given time. The general principles for the systematic assessment of symptoms can be summarized as follows.

- Detailed history and examination.

- Appropriate investigations to guide clinical decision-making.

- Treat potentially reversible causes.

- Explanation.

- Proactive treatment.

- Skilful prescribing.

- Regular monitoring.

HISTORY AND EXAMINATION

Symptoms in a patient with advanced disease may be caused by:

- the disease itself,

- the treatment,

- general debility,

- concurrent disorder.

It is important to take a detailed history and to examine patients in order to identify a pattern of symptoms that will inform subsequent investigations and management. This could include the identification of a specific pain syndrome in a cancer patient, or of the aetiology of nausea and vomiting, which will guide anti-emetic use.

APPROPRIATE INVESTIGATIONS

Investigations should be targeted at identifying the underlying cause of a symptom. Decisions to investigate or not should be individualized, and taken in the context of a patient's overall clinical condition. For example, a patient who has deteriorated suddenly, with nausea, vomiting and drowsiness, might be suspected to have developed hypercalcaemia. A serum calcium is a relatively non-invasive test that will be appropriate to perform in the majority of patients, unless it is seen as part of a terminal event. More invasive investigations, such as a computerized tomography (CT) scan of the head in a patient with headaches and vomiting, will only be appropriate if the patient is well enough for palliative treatment such as radiotherapy to be considered.

MANAGEMENT

GENERAL MEASURES

The majority of patients and their carers benefit from a full explanation of the reason(s) for a symptom occurring. Patients and carers may become more anxious when the aetiology of a symptom is unclear, and may also attach great importance to the development or progression of symptoms such as pain or breathlessness. Taking time to explain your thoughts to patients and their families and to outline a plan of action may alleviate anxiety.

It is considered good practice for healthcare professionals to discuss treatment options with patients and their carers. Patients may have clear opinions regarding their symptom management, which should be respected. Enlisting the co-operation of carers in treatment management strategies may improve compliance considerably.

SPECIFIC TREATMENTS

Where possible, treatment should be focused on identifying and treating any reversible underlying cause(s) of symptoms. Examples in a patient with breathlessness could include the drainage of a pleural effusion, a blood transfusion to correct symptomatic anaemia, or the use of antibiotics to treat a co-existent infection.

These treatment decisions need to be individualized. Some patients may be too unwell to tolerate or benefit from specific treatments, and in these situations treatment should be geared towards comfort measures.

SYMPTOMATIC TREATMENTS

Symptomatic treatments may be either non-pharmacological or pharmacological. Examples of non-pharmacological treatment approaches include:

- breathing control techniques for breathlessness,

- relaxation techniques for anxiety,

- dietary modifications for anorexia,

- provision of a pressure-relieving mattress for debilitated patients,

- acupuncture or trans-cutaneous electric nerve stimulation for the relief of pain,

- provision of a quiet and supportive environment for agitated or distressed patients.

PRINCIPLES OF PRESCRIBING IN ADVANCED DISEASE

There are several basic principles that should guide all prescribing for symptoms for patients with advanced disease.

- Prescribe drugs proactively for persistent symptoms.

- Each new drug should be perceived to have benefits that outweigh potential side effects (burdens) in the context of the patient's condition.

- Consider drug interactions.

- Consider the most appropriate route of administration.

- Avoid polypharmacy – stop medications that are no longer appropriate or have not worked.

- Undertake regular review.

Improving compliance in advanced disease

Both patients and carers need clear, concise guidelines to ensure maximum co-operation. Drug regimens should ideally be written out in full for patients and their carers to work from, and patients' self-medication charts are a useful adjunct to this (Fig. 4.1.1). Where patients and their families are easily confused by treatment regimens, this should be reviewed to reduce the number of drugs/tablets. Compliance may be further aided by the use of a dosette box, which can be filled by a relative, district nurse or pharmacist (Fig. 4.1.2).

Patients and their carers also benefit from a clear plan of action should a current management plan not be working and should know whom to contact and how to contact them.

Regular review is essential to effective symptom control.

A–Z OF SYMPTOMS

Date	Drug (approved name and strength)	Dose	Directions for taking your medicine				
			At break-fast	At mid-day meal	At evening meal	At bed-time	Additional information
31/5/02	MST	60 mg	8 am ✓		8 pm ✓		For pain
"	CODANTHRAMER	10 mls	✓		✓		For constipation
"	HALOPERIDOL	1.5 mg				✓	For nausea & vomiting
"	DICLOFENAC	75 mg	✓		✓		For pain
"	LANSOPRAZOLE	30 mg	✓				To protect stomach

Figure 4.1.1 Medication chart.

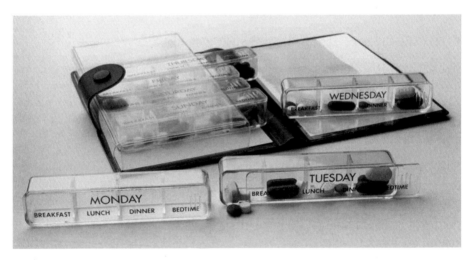

Figure 4.1.2 Dosette box.

KEY POINTS

- Ask why a symptom is occurring.
- Target investigations to identifying reversible underlying causes of symptoms.
- Treat the underlying cause wherever possible.
- Prescribe rationally.
- Review regularly.

ANOREXIA AND CACHEXIA

Brendan O'Neill

DEFINITION

Anorexia and cachexia can be defined as follows:

anorexia – loss of appetite (from the Greek *an* meaning not and *orexis* meaning appetite),
cachexia – wasting of physical appearance (from the Greek *Kakos* meaning bad and *hexis* meaning condition).

Anorexia and cachexia often coincide and the syndrome of cancer cachexia is well recognized, despite its precise cause being unclear.

Most research in this field revolves around cancer, with a small amount looking specifically at human immunodeficiency virus (HIV) infection and acquired immunodeficiency syndrome (AIDS). However, some of the points raised may be applied to patients suffering with advanced non-malignant conditions and these will be highlighted where possible.

PREVALENCE

Anorexia and cachexia are common in patients with advanced malignancy and may be a contributing factor to the cause of death in up to 50 per cent of such patients. The prevalence of anorexia in patients with advanced malignancies varies with disease type between 31 per cent and 87 per cent.[1]

Anorexia and cachexia are relatively uncommon in breast cancer but are seen more frequently in lymphoma (about a third of patients) and particularly in gastro-intestinal cancers (e.g. over 80 per cent of patients with advanced gastric carcinoma). In addition to the presence of the primary malignancy, cachexia may be the only other abnormality at post mortem in around 25 per cent of cases.[1] In general, prevalence is increased in advanced disease, with solid tumours, in the elderly and in the very young.

Both anorexia and cachexia are directly linked to marked morbidity and can have a devastating effect on patients. Patients who are markedly underweight tolerate oncological treatments less well, are more prone to side effects and suffer psychologically due to the dramatic change in the appearance of their body.

PATHOPHYSIOLOGY

The clinical hallmarks of cancer cachexia are profound weight loss accompanied by loss of appetite. Metabolic abnormalities are prominent and are reflected in anaemia, low levels of albumin/protein and impaired glucose tolerance. These metabolic changes may appear before weight loss is apparent and reflect a developing catabolic state, i.e. a state in which the patient's body is driven to increase consumption of nutrients. In some cases, development of the cancer cachexia syndrome may pre-date detection of the cancer. The precise mechanism for the cachexia syndrome has not been fully elucidated, but several metabolic abnormalities predominate.

MAIN METABOLIC ABNORMALITIES

Carbohydrate metabolism
- Increased glucose turnover/futile cycling.

- Insulin resistance.

Protein metabolism
- Catabolism of muscle.

- Hepatic synthesis of protein not able to match rate of loss.

- Negative nitrogen balance.

Lipid metabolism
- Decreased lipogenesis (due to down-regulation of lipoprotein lipase).

- Increased lipolysis causing a rise in serum lipids.

Energy expenditure
- Elevated at rest.

PROPOSED MECHANISMS FOR METABOLIC ABNORMALITIES

Food supplementation and artificial feeding do not reverse the weight loss of cancer cachexia, supporting the assertion that this is not a state induced by simple starvation. An early explanation suggested that consumption of nutrients by malignant cells led to weight loss, but this is unlikely, as malignant cells have a metabolic activity similar to that of normal tissues and may only account for 0.5–1 per cent of body weight. More recently, attention has focused on cytokines as mediators of cachexia and anorexia.

Cytokines are proteins that are released by cells when an antigen activates the cell. They are involved in cell-to-cell communications and act as enhancing mediators for immune responses via cell surface receptors.

Salient cytokines in anorexia and cachexia include tumour necrosis factor, interleukins 1 and 6, gamma interferon and leukaemia inhibitory factor. Anorexia and cachexia develop when cytokines are administered to animals; antibodies to some cytokines can reverse part of the weight loss.[2] Cytokines have been shown to alter metabolic processes in a fashion similar to that seen in the cancer cachexia syndrome. However, serum levels of cytokines in cancer patients do not correlate with degree of anorexia and weight loss.

One hypothesis suggests that cells of the patient's immune system interact, via cytokine production, with malignant cells, augmenting tumour production of cytokines that contribute to anorexia and cachexia. A final common pathway in the appetite regulatory centre in the hypothalamus via neuropeptide Y may be responsible for the loss of appetite, either by depressing the level of this peptide or by developing brain insensitivity to it.[3] Cytokines thus offer an attractive target for intervention in this condition.

CLINICAL FEATURES

The salient features of the cancer cachexia syndrome are:

- relative hypophagia

- profound weight loss

- increased resting metabolic rate

- metabolic abnormalities

- responds poorly if at all to nutritional supplementation.

Associated symptoms include chronic nausea, early satiety, immune dysfunction, decreased motor and mental skills, weakness and easy fatigue (asthenia).

INVESTIGATIONS AND EXAMINATION

The thorough assessment of anorexia and cachexia must include evaluation not only of these symptoms, but also of the wider context in which they present themselves. This will include acknowledging the psychological impact of the patient's illness: the distress of coming to terms with the diagnosis of an incurable illness and witnessing progressive weight loss may directly affect appetite or give rise to anorexia indirectly via the impact on the patient's mental health. Taking a full history, including co-existent medical problems, the chronology of the cancer and treatments tried with details of their success, will bring the problem into perspective.

A–Z OF SYMPTOMS

Concurrent symptoms should be noted which might directly impact on anorexia and cachexia (Table 4.2.1). The importance and impact of these symptoms must not be overlooked and examination and investigation should be tailored to search for reversible contributing factors.

The usual assessment of nutritional status, usually undertaken by dieticians, involves dietary intake questionnaires, height and weight measurements and estimations of percentage body fat by skin-fold measurements. Such assessments are not validated in the palliative care patient group and may not be appropriate to use. Simple serial body weighing is a crude way of assessing cachexia but will not reflect changes in lean body mass (a better measure of muscle bulk), as changes in fluid status, such as the development of peripheral oedema, lymphoedema and ascites, will mask the loss of lean body mass. Loss of lean body mass appears to be more important, as it will proceed hand in hand with muscle wasting and weakness, which will impact on the day-to-day quality of life experienced by our patients.

Table 4.2.1 Management of co-existing symptoms

Problem	Management
Dry mouth	Review prescribed drugs which may be responsible Correct dehydration Look for underlying diabetes or hypercalcaemia and treat Offer saliva replacements/stimulants
Oral candidiasis	Prescribe antifungal Correct xerostomia if co-existing
Mucositis	May resolve in time if treatment induced Analgesics Mouth care
Nausea	Find cause and correct if possible (e.g. gastric stasis) Offer appropriate food Trial of anti-emetics
Dysphagia	Correct if possible (stent, radiotherapy) Bypass (gastrostomy tube) Appropriate consistency of food Trial of steroids
Constipation	Look for underlying cause and correct if possible Appropriate choice of laxatives
Pain	Find cause and reverse if possible (e.g. radiotherapy and chemotherapy) Analgesic medications Anaesthetic interventions
Depression	Counselling/exploration of causes/drug treatment if appropriate
Dementia	Prompting and help with feeding

Assessment of appetite may be more troublesome. Assessment tools are not commonly used. Visual analogue scales have been employed, as have multi-item and single-item tools in order to assess appetite, but no one tool has come to the fore as most appropriate.

At the outset of managing anorexia and cachexia, one must be sure not to have missed a patient whose problem is starvation. Certain groups of patients are cachexic not through a loss of appetite but due to an inability to eat. In this group would fall patients with obstructing lesions preventing them from swallowing (e.g. head, neck and oesophageal tumours). Occasionally, patients restrict food intake for fear of diarrhoea (e.g. malabsorption states in pancreatic cancer and patents with short bowel after surgery).

Blood tests may confirm an anaemia (usually normochromic and normocytic), for which transfusing may be considered if symptomatic and the haemoglobin is less than 10 g/dL. Protein and albumin levels may be depressed.

MANAGEMENT

GENERAL

At the outset, the goals of managing anorexia and cachexia should be clear to the patient and the multi-professional team. The limitations of treatment should be emphasized. For example, appetite stimulants in advanced disease have not been proven to influence prognosis, and an improvement in appetite is not always associated with weight gain when induced by drugs. A full assessment will identify how advanced a patient's illness is and will aid in selecting the most appropriate management plan; only then can one decide the place of cancer treatments, nutritional measures and orexigenic agents. As anorexia and cachexia in themselves can be hard to treat successfully, attention should also be focused on co-existing symptoms that impact on both appetite and weight loss. Some of the important confounding factors are listed in Table 4.2.1.

SPECIFIC

Non-pharmacological measures

Aggressive management of anorexia with artificial nutritional supplementation is virtually always inappropriate for patients with advanced disease. Randomized trials have failed to demonstrate an increase in lean body mass, survival improvement or tolerance of chemotherapy when parenteral nutrition is given.[4] This reflects the complexity of the anorexia–cachexia syndrome that cannot be reversed purely by supplementing a low oral intake of nutrition. This is unlike the setting when radical treatment, aiming for cure, is deemed appropriate and low body weight precludes further treatment such as further chemotherapy. Enteral feeding (e.g. via nasogastric tube or percutaneous gastrostomy) is associated with complications such as aspiration pneumonia and diarrhoea and, with advanced disease, patients given parenteral nutrition (delivered intravenously) have higher rates of morbidity and mortality than those not receiving such treatment, due to infection and embolism.

Supplementation of existing oral intake should be the first line of management. This is ideal as it uses the gastrointestinal tract. Forcing an anorexic patient to eat will often cause nausea. Disappointingly, nutritional counselling via dieticians tends to improve intake by 450 cal/day for a few weeks only. A few simple measures, listed below, can maximize nutritional intake.

- Provide attractively presented food in smaller portions.

- Offer tempting foods or foods that a patient has a particular liking for.

- Only expect patients to eat when they are hungry, rather than sticking rigidly to set meal times.

- Use plastic utensils to avoid the unpleasant taste of metal cutlery.

- Eat and prepare food in separate areas to avoid food odours.

- Choose more palatable foods – non-spicy.

- Reduce the problem of early satiety by not drinking at meal times.

- Supplement foods with high-calorie substances, e.g. cream/sugar.

In certain settings it may be appropriate to offer supplemental foods, especially where the effort of preparing food at home is too daunting for an already lethargic patient. Similarly, patients may find it easier to take supplemental drinks than to tackle more solid food. Choosing the correct supplement is crucial and one should account for patients' taste preferences.

Throughout the assessment and management process, it is always pertinent to consider any underlying psychological stresses incumbent upon the patient and those close to them. The powerful psychosocial meaning of food must never be underestimated. Meal times are an important part of the day, when families and friends come together. Food is imbued with symbolism. It remains one area over which patients and those close to them have some control. Control becomes particularly important when medical treatments fail a patient and treatment options diminish. Eating and drinking are seen as salient to living: when patients are troubled by anorexia, those around them often feel they are giving up and are nearing death.

Pharmacological measures

Steroids   Steroids have been shown to improve well-being, appetite and quality of life in up to 80 per cent, but not to significantly improve nutritional status, performance status[5] or survival[6] when used to treat anorexia and cachexia. Steroids act quickly and a response should be expected in under a week if it is going to occur. The efficacy of steroids is short lived, however, and wears off over 4–8 weeks. This can be prolonged if the dose is escalated. Most commonly, dexamethasone is used in doses of 3–6 mg daily in the morning; prednisolone and methylprednisolone are alternatives. Due to the speed of onset of action, steroids are most often the appetite stimulant of choice, particularly when a patient's prognosis is limited.

The mode of action of steroids in cachexia and anorexia is unclear. Steroids are known to have analgesic, anti-emetic and mood-elevating properties. In addition, they inhibit the production of prostaglandins, a complex group of substances that interplay with cytokines.

As always, the risks of steroid use must be weighed against the benefits. The common side effects to consider with steroids include:

- gastrointestinal bleeding

- glucose intolerance

- psychosis/confusion

- proximal myopathy.

Megestrol acetate   During early oncological studies it was noted that megestrol acetate (MA) was associated with weight gain in both fat and lean body mass.[7] This effect was observed in both hormone-sensitive and non-sensitive tumours. Subsequent research has confirmed an improvement in appetite, food intake and occasionally nutritional status. However, this has not been shown to translate into an improvement in performance status. Weight gain with MA correlates with the dose used and the length of treatment. Benefits can be seen as early as 1 week, but maximal weight gain can take as long as 14 weeks. This contrasts with the faster action of steroids and renders MA less appropriate in patients with a short prognosis.

The mechanism of action may be by inhibition of cytokine release, perhaps via a direct action on neuropeptide Y, or MA may act in a steroid-like fashion. Megestrol acetate has been shown to have anti-emetic properties. Side effects include the development of peripheral oedema, hypercalcaemia and insulin resistance and, in small studies, decreased survival.

Megestrol acetate is more expensive to use compared to steroids. It has been used in doses ranging from 160 mg to more than 800 mg daily, and direct comparisons suggest higher doses to be more effective in improving appetite. Some authors advocate starting at low doses and increasing the dose whilst watching for the resolution of symptoms. It has been suggested that in non-responders, increasing above 480 mg per day is futile. Greatest benefit is often seen in patients treated earlier in the course of their disease (before overt cachexia develops).[7] Combining MA with non-steroidal anti-inflammatory drugs may be superior to the use of MA alone in treating cachexia.[8] In head-to-head comparisons of dexamethasone and MA, they were equally as effective in relieving anorexia and promoting weight gain, with MA being associated with fewer side effects.

Medroxyprogesterone acetate   As with MA, early oncological research found treatment with medroxyprogesterone acetate (MPA) was associated with weight gain. MPA promotes appetite and has anti-emetic properties and there is some evidence to confirm that treatment with MPA improves performance status and enables weight gain in doses of the order of 500 mg twice daily. It appears that the greatest benefit for cachexia is seen if MPA is used earlier on in the course of the illness.[9] Hypothesized mechanisms include inhibition of the release and production of cytokines, especially interleukin-6 and serotonin.

Cannabinoids The appetite-stimulating effect of cannabinoids may be attributable to the mood-altering effects of this group of compounds. There is also evidence for an anti-emetic effect of cannabinoids. Low doses of dronabinol have been found to stimulate appetite with tolerable mood alterations.[10]

Other agents Both hydrazine sulphate and cyproheptadine are no longer recommended for clinical use. Positive results for hydrazine sulphate from earlier studies have failed to be repeated and poorer survival and quality of life measures were also reported. Cyproheptadine has subsequently been shown to have no impact on progressive weight loss. Interest has been shown in pentoxifylline, a drug normally used in peripheral vascular disease, as it is shown to reduce one of the proteins (messenger ribonucleic acid) needed to produce tumour necrosis factor. However, trials failed to show a consistent improvement in weight or appetite when patients were treated with pentoxifylline.[11]

FUTURE DEVELOPMENTS

The mainstays of drug treatment are likely to remain steroids and progestogens for the foreseeable future However, in the future, safer and more efficacious drugs need to be found. The following compounds may be beneficial.

- *Melatonin.* The use of this well-tolerated drug at doses of 20 mg daily has been associated with a fall in levels of tumour necrosis factor and less weight loss.[12] Although expensive, it may well prove to be an alternative drug treatment for anorexia and cachexia when steroids and progestational agents are inappropriate.

- *Thalidomide.* This drug exerts a complex effect on the immune system via cytokine inhibition. In one study, administering 100 mg four times a day in patients with AIDS induced weight gain and improved performance status.

- *Eicosapentanoeic acid.* This polyunsaturated fatty acid has been shown to inhibit lipid-mobilizing factors and reduce the rate of protein degradation. It is found especially in fish-based products and could prove to be a dietary factor that could be manipulated in order to successfully treat anorexia and cachexia. A small study in pancreatic cancer patients demonstrated increased calorific intake and weight with improved performance status after 3 weeks on a diet enriched in fish oil. The proposed mechanism of action is one of altered cytokine production and reduced tissue responsiveness to circulating cytokines at a cell receptor level.

- *Cytokine antagonists*. There has been recent interest in the use of cytokine antagonists that are being developed for the treatment of inflammatory conditions, e.g. the tumour necrosis factor antagonists etanercept and infliximab for rheumatoid arthritis. Further research into the role of cytokines in the pathogenesis of cancer cachexia and the development of specific antagonist drugs offer exciting potential approaches towards treatment in the future.

ANOREXIA AND CACHEXIA IN ADVANCED NON-MALIGNANT CONDITIONS

Although the majority of research in the area of anorexia and cachexia has focused on patients with a diagnosis of cancer, these distressing symptoms are not solely the preserve of cancer patients. Lessons learnt from the cancer population can be applied to patients with AIDS and other non-malignancies.

The aetiology of anorexia and cachexia in AIDS and cancer may have a great deal in common, with cytokines again being of prime importance. Therapeutic studies have shown MA to promote non-fluid weight gain and improve appetite in AIDS patients with doses in the range of 320–800 mg daily.[13]

Weight gain and appetite improvement have been demonstrated in a small number of cystic fibrosis suffers with MA 400–800 mg per day.[14] Following a 12-week study of MA 800 mg daily, elderly nursing home residents with weight loss (not known to have cancer) reported improved appetite and well-being without significant changes in body composition.[15]

The management plan in these situations is much the same as in cancer patients. Where the aetiology of the anorexia and cachexia is cytokine dependent, strategies that target cytokine production and activity will be of value. General measures that address the importance of building on oral intake and dealing with the psychological distress are always appropriate.

KEY POINTS

- Anorexia and cachexia are common in advanced malignant disease.
- They are contributing factors in cancer mortality in up to two-thirds of patients.
- Communication between host and malignant cells via cytokines is thought to be salient to the aetiology of anorexia and cachexia, and there is some evidence that this is also the case in non-malignant conditions.
- Good management must involve open communication and realistic goal setting.
- Attempts should be made to build on oral intake.
- Drug therapies may improve appetite but tend rarely to influence loss of lean body mass and functional capacity. No effect on prognosis has been demonstrated with the use of pharmacological interventions.

A–Z OF SYMPTOMS

A–Z OF SYMPTOMS

REFERENCES

1. Wantanabe S, Bruera E. Anorexia and cachexia, asthenia, and lethargy. *Hematol Oncol Clin N Am* 1996; **10**, 189–206.
2. Noguchi Y, Yoshikawa T, Matsumoto A, Svaninger G, Gelin J. Are cytokines possible mediators of cancer cachexia? *Surg Today* 1996; **26**, 467–75.
3. Inui A. Neuropeptide Y: a key molecule in anorexia and cachexia in wasting disorders? *Mol Med Today* 1999; **5**, 79–85.
4. American College of Physicians. Parenteral nutrition in patients receiving cancer chemotherapy. *Ann Int Med* 1989; **110**(9), 734–6.
5. Bruera E. Pharmacological treatment of cachexia: any progress? *Support Care Cancer* 1998; **6**, 109–13.
6. Vansteenkiste JF, Simons JP, Wouters EF, Demedts MG. Hormonal treatment in advanced non-small cell lung cancer: fact or fiction. *Eur Respir J* 1996; **9**, 1707–12.
7. Beller E, Tattersall M, Lumley T *et al.* Improved quality of life with megestrol acetate in patients with endocrine-insensitive advanced cancer; a placebo-controlled trial. *Ann Oncol* 1997; **8**, 277–83.
8. Mcmillan D, O'Gorman P, Fearon KC, McArdle CS. A pilot study of megestrol acetate and ibuprofen in the treatment of cachexia in gastrointestinal cancer patients. *Br J Cancer* 1997; **76**, 788–90.
9. Simons JP, Aaronson NK, Vanstenkiste JF *et al.* Effects of medroxyprogesterone on appetite, weight and quality of life in advanced-stage non-hormone sensitive cancer. *J Clin Oncol* 1996; **14**, 1077–84.
10. Gorter R. Management of anorexia–cachexia associated with cancer and HIV infection. *Oncology* 1991; **5**(Suppl. 9), 15–17.
11. Puccio M, Nathanson L. The cancer cachexia syndrome. *Semin Oncol* 1997; **24**, 277–87.
12. Lissoni P, Paolorossi F, Tancini G *et al.* Is there a role for melatonin in the treatment of neoplastic cachexia? *Eur J Cancer* 1996; **32A**, 1340–3.
13. Von Roenn JH, Armstrong D, Kotler DP *et al.* Megestrol acetate in patients with AIDS-related cachexia. *Ann Int Med* 1994; **21**, 393–9.
14. Nasr SZ, Hurwitz ME, Brown RW, Elghoroury M, Rosen D. Treatment of anorexia and weight loss with megestrol acetate in patients with cystic fibrosis. *Pediatr Pulmonol* 1999; **28**, 380–2.
15. Yeh SS, Wu SY, Lee TP *et al.* Improvement in quality-of-life measures and stimulation of weight gain after treatment with megestrol acetate oral suspension in geriatric cachexia: results of a double-blind placebo controlled study. *J Am Geriatr Soc* 2000; **48**, 485–92.

A N X I E T Y

Max Henderson

Symptoms of anxiety, panic and fear are so common as to be universal human experiences – we have all been nervous at some point. Such symptoms are more common in those with physical illness generally, and more common still in the advanced and terminal stages of many diseases. However, and perhaps because of the universal nature of the experience, the point at which a symptom becomes an entity in itself, requiring an intervention, can be difficult to judge.

THE IMPACT OF ANXIETY

Anxiety symptoms are distressing and debilitating in their own right (Table 4.3.1). At the extreme end of the spectrum, panic attacks are – by definition – absolutely terrifying. However, such experiences can have a greater impact on the individual than just being unpleasant at the time. Quite understandably, most will want to avoid a repetition of their unpleasant episode or at least minimize its impact. Avoidance of situations that the person believes will trigger an attack is a common response, but this can itself cause great disability. What people avoid will depend both on the nature and occasion of the previous episode of anxiety, but also to some extent will reflect the greatest fear of that patient. Hence those with agoraphobia will want to avoid busy supermarkets and crowded buses, fearing perhaps that they will pass out or be incontinent. This may mean that their carer has to do the shopping, or accompany them out of the home.

Other anxious episodes may produce a need for someone to be close at all times and provide reassurance. In the longer term, this can be draining for family members and carers. Indeed, symptoms of anxiety in patients can be very distressing for carers, limiting opportunities for communication and producing feelings of helplessness or inadequacy. The physical nature of the symptoms of anxiety can also be confusing to both patient and carer alike, concerned that these represent sinister developments in the underlying disease.

The often overwhelming nature of anxiety symptoms means that tried and tested coping strategies cannot be implemented. Tolerance of physical symptoms can be reduced and there is often an increased vigilance for somatic symptoms. In such situations, the utilization of health care resources is greater. This includes the use of analgesic medication, but also calls to home care teams and even admissions increase.

Table 4.3.1 Symptoms of anxiety disorders

Group	Symptom	Comments
Physical	Dry mouth Frequent/loose motions Chest tightness Difficulty inhaling Over-breathing Palpitations Urinary frequency Reduced libido Erectile/orgasmic failure Tinnitus Blurred vision Dizziness Muscular tension Initial insomnia Waking unrefreshed Increased sensitivity to noise or light	These symptoms are largely a result of autonomic over-activity or muscular tension
Psychological	Dread Terror Irritability Poor concentration Anxious anticipation	There is a bi-directional relationship between psychological and physical symptoms
Behavioural	Avoidance Reassurance seeking Self-medication	Whilst initially reducing anxiety levels, these can often act to maintain the symptoms

Patients with terminal or chronic conditions are commonly more aware of changes in their body, and perhaps are more likely to draw catastrophic conclusions from perceived changes. For example, feeling an increase in heart rate might lead to the belief that a heart attack is imminent or shortness of breath that the patient is suffocating. The response of the autonomic nervous system to such a threat can increase both the underlying sensation and the patient's awareness of it (Fig. 4.3.1).

MAKING THE DIAGNOSIS

Accurate estimates of the prevalence of anxiety in advanced disease are hard to come by. Few studies have looked specifically at the question.[1,2] Those that have find markedly different results: prevalence ranges from 1.1 per cent[3] to more than 70 per cent.[4] There are many reasons for this. There is great methodological

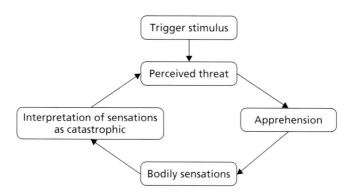

Figure 4.3.1 The cycle of anxiety.

heterogeneity within the studies – patient groups, diagnostic criteria and assessment tools all vary. Such confusion in the published literature to some degree reflects the confusion that can exist clinically: which patients? What diagnosis? Is it really pathological?

It has been suggested that 'loss' life events lead to depression, whereas 'threat'-type life events are more likely to lead to anxiety. Patients in a palliative care setting face the unusual situation of having to deal with both losses and threats.[5] The diagnosis itself, with the uncertain time course, the very thought of death and the process of dying can cause fear and concern. Anxiety can be worsened by intrusive physical symptoms, particularly pain, but also side effects from medications. Body changes from both the disease and its treatment can be an unwelcome reminder of the illness. Looking more widely, many patients are concerned at their changing roles, and what ultimately will happen to their families and loved ones. Fear of becoming dependent is common, but so is a fear of abandonment.

In order to diagnose an anxiety disorder, the presence of psychological distress must first be established. There is evidence that this does not happen as often as one might wish.[5] In some cases, patients are reluctant to disclose exactly how they feel. This may be due to embarrassment, or fear of what will happen, or a wish not to burden staff further. The very presence of anxiety can reduce patients' willingness to disclose any concerns.[6] Both doctors and nurses can be reluctant to ask about emotional issues. In one study it was shown that patients tend to be more willing to disclose physical concerns and nurses more willing to ask about areas in which they feel they can make a difference, such as pain, nausea or appetite loss.[7] Hospice staff can feel unskilled at asking about 'feelings' and concerned about where such a conversation will take them. Ideas that anxiety and depression are 'normal' in advanced disease, or at least understandable or appropriate, and that medications are unlikely to work still pervade.[8]

A further difficulty in the accurate diagnosis of anxiety is its differentiation from other conditions. The differential diagnosis of anxiety is given in Table 4.3.2. The most common is depression. Within the diagnostic hierarchy that exists in psychiatry, depression is given primacy and hence can be diagnosed in the presence of anxiety symptoms, whilst the converse is not the case. Many of the anxiety symptoms seen in advanced disease are part of a wider depressive condition. Where

Table 4.3.2 Differential diagnosis of anxiety

Major depressive disorder
Mixed anxiety and depression
Adjustment disorder
Alcohol/drug withdrawal
Delirium
Terminal agitation
Drug intoxication
Physical illness, e.g. thyrotoxicosis or phaeochromocytoma

anxiety and depression are of equal severity, a mixed depressive disorder can be diagnosed. This, too, may be more common than thought – indeed, there is a school of thought that no true point of rarification exists between depression and anxiety.

When symptoms are milder, an adjustment disorder may be present. Here, psychological distress and functional impairment are present following a recognizable stressor, though diagnostic criteria for neither depression nor anxiety are met. This is probably the most common psychiatric diagnosis in advanced disease. Less frequent, though no less important, are delirium, drug and alcohol withdrawal and terminal agitation occurring in the last days of life. Such situations require separate management strategies.

ANXIETY STATES

With so many competing and co-morbid diagnoses, pure anxiety states are relatively rare in palliative care (Table 4.3.3). They can be either episodic or continuous, episodic disorders being more discrete and easier to define. It has been suggested that generalized anxiety disorder is 'what is left over' in the pure anxiety category, bearing in mind that many anxiety symptoms are in fact part of a wider adjustment or depressive disorder. Post-traumatic stress disorder, obsessive–compulsive disorder and somatization disorder are often classified under the broad category of anxiety or neurotic disorders, but these fall outside the scope of this chapter.

PANIC DISORDER

Panic attacks include symptoms that are experienced with great intensity, to the point at which many patients feel they will pass out or even die. Asking about the worst fear during a panic attack is a key part of the assessment. Although these fears tend to appear out of the blue without any clear trigger, such is the extreme nature of the first attack that patients will often consciously avoid returning to the environment in which it occurred in case of repetition. *Panic attacks* can occur in a number of neurotic and affective disorders; when there is no mood or anxiety disorder between attacks, *panic disorder* is diagnosed.

Table 4.3.3 Subgroups of anxiety disorders

Disorder	Key diagnostic features
Panic disorder	Recurrent severe panic attacks Not restricted to specific situation
Phobias	Irrational fear out of proportion to actual threat Anxiety cannot be reasoned away
Agoraphobia	Leads to behavioural avoidance Fear of public places, enclosed spaces
Social phobia	Desire to escape is prominent Fear of being in front of other people, where they might form opinion of patient
Generalized anxiety disorder	Anxiety present most days for several weeks Criteria for phobias or panic not met

PHOBIC DISORDERS

In all phobic disorders there is a marked and persistent fear of an object or situation. Such fear is out of proportion to the objective threat of the situation and cannot be reasoned away. Avoidance of the object or situation occurs, which itself can lead to great disability and tends to increase the possibility of further anxiety on re-exposure. *Agoraphobia* is probably the most common in a palliative care setting. It incorporates a group of fears, best understood by having the fear of an *inability to escape* at its core. Hence the patient will be concerned about public, often crowded, places such as busy shops and buses, as well as tightly confined spaces such as lifts. Being alone or a long way from home typically exacerbates these feelings. In *social phobia*, the frightening situation is exposure to other people. This can be in the broad sense of meeting people or having to speak in public. Alternatively, there may be a more specific element such as a fear of eating in front of others. Often the patient will blush or tremble, the awareness of which makes their anxiety worse. *Simple phobias* include, for example, specific fears of spiders, cats or heights. They are most common in children, though needle phobia and phobia to computerized tomography (CT)/magnetic resonance imaging (MRI) scanners are seen in a number of adults and can interfere with symptom management, especially in a hospice setting.

GENERALIZED ANXIETY DISORDER

In contrast to the episodic disorders above, the diagnosis of generalized anxiety disorder requires anxiety symptoms to be present for most days for several weeks. The severity and intensity of symptoms will, of course, fluctuate, particularly with stress or physical symptoms, but the criteria for panic disorder or phobic disorders are not met.

MANAGEMENT

Anxiety deserves as detailed an assessment as, for example, pain or nausea. Obtaining a clear description of the patient's experience is vital – it can help to record this verbatim. Important triggers, both physical, such as pain or breathlessness, and emotional, should be sought. Any pattern linking physical symptoms, situations or treatments with the anxiety needs to be identified. The degree of functional day-to-day impairment produced by the symptoms must be examined; improvement in this disability should be a goal of treatment. Differential diagnoses should be explored. In particular, all patients who complain of anxiety symptoms should have their current mental state examined, looking specifically for evidence that their anxiety may be part of a depressive disorder.

Whilst anxiety *symptoms* are common, anxiety *disorders* are less so and hence treatment will often not be necessary. Fear and anxiety can arise from a misunderstanding regarding, for example, the illness or its treatment. Additional information and reassurance may suffice. A review of the management of symptoms exacerbating the anxiety, such as pain, may be enough to reduce the anxiety. Often just the opportunity to discuss feelings and concerns in a safe and supported environment will be beneficial. Nonetheless, there are times when symptoms are so severe and/or incapacitating that intervention is indicated.

DRUG MANAGEMENT[9]

Benzodiazepines

These remain a valuable treatment for short-term anxiety. They are particularly effective for an acute stress reaction and for panic. They also have a role in generalized anxiety disorders. Their great advantage is speed of action, with relief obtainable within minutes or hours. They are not without drawbacks though. The immediate relief can be seductive, and might mean that wider exploration of symptoms, particularly depressive symptoms, is missed. 'Indication drift' can occur whereby an initial prescription for acute stress can be used for much less severe symptoms as they occur. Patients then note the sedative effect and start to use the drugs as hypnotics. Sharp increases in intake can then occur.

Many patients are elderly and may have underlying cognitive impairment which can be worsened by sedating drugs. Benzodiazepines, especially short-acting drugs like lorazepam, easily induce dependence, and the increased tolerance to the anxiolytic effects produces a further increase in the dose taken. In those with a longer prognosis, it is advisable to prescribe small doses in small amounts and plan for early discontinuation.

Antidepressants

These drugs can treat depression with anxiety symptoms, mixed anxiety and depression, and can be useful for some pure anxiety states. They are most useful for panic disorder and for generalized anxiety disorder. As in the treatment of depression, the choice of antidepressant owes more to the particular side effects than to any difference in efficacy: serotonin-specific reuptake inhibitors such a sertraline or citalopram are as useful as tricyclic antidepressants such as dosulepin (dothiepin).[10]

There is less experience with newer drugs such a mirtazapine, but the early signs are promising.

The main advantages of antidepressant treatment are the effective treatment of co-morbid depressive symptoms and the lack of a dependence syndrome. The main disadvantage is the relatively slow onset of action, though this is less important in the management of, say, generalized anxiety disorder than in the management of an acute stress reaction.

Buspirone

This is a newer drug, indicated for use in generalized anxiety, which, in contrast to benzodiazepines that act at the gamma-amino butyric acid (GABA) receptor, acts as an agonist at the 5-hydroxytryptamine-1 (5HT-1) receptor. It is most effective in patients who have not been exposed to benzodiazepines. Its main advantages are the lack of sedation and dependence and its lack of interaction with alcohol. Unfortunately it has a slow onset (at least 2 weeks) and can induce nausea early in the course. This side effect profile will limit its use in a palliative care setting.

PSYCHOLOGICAL TREATMENTS

Behavioural therapy[11]

This is a well-established treatment for anxiety in which patients are exposed to the situations that have provoked their anxiety in a supported way, allowing the anxiety to subside. Triggers for anxiety are graded and approached in a hierarchical manner. This approach can be useful for agoraphobia, social phobia and other simple phobias.

Cognitive behavioural therapy[12]

This approach has been developed from the cognitive treatment of depression. At its core is the assertion that the patient's beliefs about symptoms and feelings are critical to their maintenance. By first getting the patient to understand the links, and then gradually testing out and challenging their 'negative automatic thoughts', the psychological symptoms can be improved. The main drawbacks of cognitive behavioural therapy are the difficulties in finding suitably qualified therapists, and that its impact might be slow. Nonetheless, familiarity with the principles and a willingness to explore underlying beliefs about symptoms can be helpful for all practitioners. Cognitive behavioural therapy has been used extensively and successfully with cancer patients and would seem an appropriate tool for use in many palliative care settings.

KEY POINTS

- Anxiety is common in advanced disease but is little researched.
- Pure anxiety states are less common than either mixed depression/anxiety or depression with anxiety features.
- Although dependence may not be a major concern, benzodiazepine should be used cautiously – antidepressants may be more effective.
- The role of non-pharmacological management requires further study.

REFERENCES

1. Chochinov H, Breitbart W (eds). *Handbook of psychiatry in palliative medicine.* New York: Oxford University Press, 2000.
2. Chochinov H. Psychiatry in terminal illness. *Can J Psychiatry* 2000; **45**, 143–50.
3. Minagawa H, Uchitomi Y, Yamawaki S, Ishitani K. Psychiatric morbidity in terminally ill cancer patients. A prospective study. *Cancer* 1996; **78**, 1131–7.
4. Breitbart W, Bruera E, Chochinov H, Lynch M. Neuropsychiatric syndromes and psychological symptoms in patients with advanced cancer. *J Pain Symptom Manage* 1995; **10**, 131–41.
5. Barraclough J. ABC of palliative care: depression, anxiety, and confusion. *BMJ* 1997; **315**, 1365–8.
6. Heaven C, Maguire P. The relationship between patients' concerns and psychological distress in a hospice setting. *Psycho-oncology* 1998; **7**, 502–7.
7. Heaven C, Maguire P. Disclosure of concerns by hospice patients and their identification by nurses. *Palliat Med* 1997; **11**, 283–90.
8. Massie J. Depression. In: Holland J, Rowland J (eds), *Handbook of psycho-oncology: psychological care of the patient with cancer.* New York: Oxford University Press, 1989.
9. Nutt D, Bell C, Potakar J. *Depression anxiety and the mixed conditions.* London: Martin Dunitz, 1997.
10. Kasper S, Resinger E. Panic disorder: the place of benzodiazepines and selective serotonin reuptake inhibitors. *Eur Neuropsychopharmacol* 2001; **11**, 307–21.
11. Marks I. Care and cure of neurosis. I: Cure. *Psychol Med* 1979; **9**, 629–60.
12. Moorey S, Greer S. *Cognitive behaviour therapy for people with cancer.* Oxford: Oxford University Press, 2002.

BREATHLESSNESS

Polly Edmonds

DEFINITION

Breathlessness (dyspnoea) has been defined as an 'uncomfortable awareness of breathing'.[1]

PREVALENCE

Breathlessness is a common symptom in patients with advanced cancer, with the prevalence reported to increase from referral to specialist palliative care services (15–55.5 per cent) to the last week of life (18–79 per cent).[2] In one study, a quarter of patients rated their breathlessness as 'horrible' or 'severe' in the last week of life.[3] Breathlessness is more common in patients with lung cancer and has been reported to be associated with shorter survival.[3] Patients with advanced non-malignant conditions such as respiratory and cardiac failure and motor neurone disease also experience disabling breathlessness.

PATHOPHYSIOLOGY

Breathlessness is a complex symptom involving physical, psychological, emotional and functional factors. Three main pathophysiological mechanisms can lead to breathlessness, all of which can co-exist:

1 an increase in respiratory effort to overcome a certain load (e.g. obstructive or restrictive lung disease, pleural effusion),
2 an increase in the proportion of respiratory muscle required to maintain normal workload (e.g. neuromuscular weakness, cancer cachexia),
3 an increase in ventilatory requirements (e.g. hypercapnia, anaemia).

In cancer patients, primary or secondary lung cancer and pleural disease are risk factors for breathlessness, but generalized muscle weakness may be the only apparent cause for up to a quarter of breathless cancer patients.[4]

Table 4.4.1 Causes of breathlessness

Cause	Examples
Pulmonary	Asthma
	Chronic obstructive pulmonary disease
	Infection
	Fibrotic lung diseases
	Pleural effusion
	Pneumothorax
	Bronchial obstruction
	Pulmonary embolism
Extra-pulmonary	Superior vena cava obstruction
	Tracheal obstruction
Chest wall	Involvement by malignancy
Cardiac	Heart failure
	Ischaemic heart disease
	Pericardial effusion/constriction
Neuromuscular	Motor neurone disease
	Cancer cachexia
Other	Anaemia
	Ascites
Psychological	Anxiety
	Hyperventilation

Table 4.4.1 outlines the common causes of breathlessness in patients with advanced disease.

INVESTIGATIONS AND EXAMINATION

The examination and investigations for patients with advanced disease will vary depending on the stage of the illness and the prognosis, but should be geared to identifying potentially reversible or treatable underlying causes.

HISTORY

- When does breathlessness occur – on moderate exertion, e.g. stairs; on minimal exertion, e.g. washing, dressing, eating or talking; at rest?

- Is there associated anxiety or panic attacks?

- Can the patient sleep? (Elicit fear of dying associated with insomnia.)

- Explore what the breathlessness means to the patient and carers.

- What are the practical implications for the patient, e.g. the effect of disability on activities of daily living; the use of or requirement for aids; the presence of carers or other support during day and night?

- Are there co-morbid conditions, e.g. chronic obstructive pulmonary disease (COPD), heart failure.

EXAMINATION

- Assess the degree of breathlessness. Is the patient breathless at rest or on talking? Is there cyanosis? Is the patient using the accessory muscles of respiration?

- Assess the degree of the patient's anxiety, distress and/or exhaustion.

- Identify clinical signs of potentially reversible causes: anaemia, pneumonia, pleural effusion, cardiac failure, COPD, superior vena cava obstruction, ascites, lobar collapse.

INVESTIGATIONS

These should be individualized, and will depend on the patient's performance status and ability to undergo treatment if reversible causes are identified. Investigations for patients in the last days of life are unlikely to be appropriate.

- Bloods, e.g. full blood count to exclude anaemia.

- Chest X-ray, e.g. to exclude collapse, effusion, consolidation, lymphangitis.

- Computerized tomography (CT) of the chest, e.g. to identify pulmonary metastatic disease, pleural disease, lymphangitis.

- Ventilation perfusion (VQ) scan or high-resolution chest CT to exclude pulmonary emboli.

- Lung function test, e.g. to identify obstructive or restrictive defects.

- Arterial blood gases, e.g. to identify clinically significant hypoxia or hypercapnia.

A–Z OF SYMPTOMS

MANAGEMENT

Management should focus on treating reversible underlying causes where these can be identified. The effectiveness of specific interventions should be evaluated on an individual basis and repeated as appropriate where symptom relief has been obtained. Where there are no obvious treatable factors, or for patients with poor performance status, the management should be symptomatic.

GENERAL MEASURES

Explanation and reassurance

Patients and carers need to be given as full an explanation as possible of the factors contributing to breathlessness and the possible management strategies. Breathlessness is a symptom frequently accompanied by fear and anxiety, which should be identified as part of developing an understanding of the patient's experience of breathlessness. Allowing patients to explore fears and difficulties associated with breathlessness, and identify losses with respect to activity levels and lifestyle, may assist in their relief.

Environment

Attention to a breathless patient's home or in-patient environment can improve quality of life. The following factors can be helpful.

- Easy access to fresh air or, if this is not possible, a fan.

- Some breathless patients need to be upright in order to be comfortable, and find it difficult to sleep in a bed. Aids such as a mattress variator or V-shaped pillow may improve comfort, but some patients will need to sleep in a chair. Adjustable chairs can be very useful in these circumstances.

- Breathless patients with significant anxiety also need to be supported in a calm environment, where possible, with carers available for reassurance and support.

SPECIFIC MEASURES

Disease-specific treatments

Cancer   A summary of the oncological treatments for breathlessness is shown in Table 4.4.2. The appropriateness of such treatments depends on the individual's disease status, performance status and wishes, and the aim should be to improve quality of life.

Patients with breathlessness secondary to an obstructing tumour can be palliated with minimal toxicity by radiotherapy, a standard regimen being a total dose of

Table 4.4.2 Summary of oncological treatments for breathlessness

Type of intervention	Site
Radiotherapy	External beam
	Endobronchial
Laser	Endobronchial
Chemotherapy	Systemic
Cryotherapy	Endobronchial
Stent	Endobronchial

Adapted from Ahmedzai (1998).[16]

17 Gy given in 2 weekly fractions. Patients with small cell lung cancer may experience marked improvements in symptoms such as breathlessness with chemotherapy, and recent evidence suggests that fit patients with non-small cell lung cancer may also achieve good symptom relief.[5]

Endobronchial therapies have developed in many centres, and may offer good palliation for selected patients. Endobronchial radiotherapy (or brachytherapy, where radioactive gold, caesium or iridium is implanted directly into the tumour via a bronchoscope), cryotherapy and expandable stents have all been used with success. A Medical Research Council trial[6] to compare the efficacy of endobronchial therapy with external beam radiotherapy failed to recruit an adequate number of patients, and the relative benefits of the conventional treatment versus the more innovative techniques remain unknown. The decision to employ endobronchial therapies in individual patients will depend on the clinical syndrome and local expertise.

Non-cancer therapies   Optimization of the medical management of medical conditions such as heart failure and COPD may improve breathlessness. Patients with type 2 respiratory failure from COPD or motor neurone disease, who are symptomatic from CO_2 retention, may benefit symptomatically from the use of non-invasive positive pressure ventilation (NIPPV). This is only available in selected centres at present, and not all patients tolerate the tight-fitting nasal mask. The use of NIPPV can complicate end-of-life decision-making in patients with far advanced disease.

Non-pharmacological strategies

Recent evidence suggests that breathless patients attending a nursing clinic (where the intervention included an exploration of the patient's experience of breathlessness, advice and support on managing breathlessness, and teaching breathing control and relaxation techniques) experience improvements in breathlessness, performance status, and physical and emotional states relative to controls.[7] This nursing intervention has close links with techniques that are successfully used by physiotherapists and in pulmonary and cardiac rehabilitation.

Acupuncture has been successfully used for breathless patients with cancer[8] and COPD,[9] with improvements demonstrated in both breathlessness and anxiety. Controlled trials in cancer patients have not been reported.

Pharmacological strategies

Clinical experience suggests that the risk/benefit ratio for many pharmacological strategies for breathlessness is quite narrow. It can be useful, therefore, to reserve symptomatic treatments for patients who are predominantly breathless on minimal exertion or at rest, or who are very distressed/disabled by their breathlessness.

Oxygen   The role of oxygen in reducing breathlessness is controversial. One randomized controlled trial (RCT) of 14 cancer patients with hypoxaemia showed symptomatic benefit from the administration of oxygen over air,[10] but a further single-blind controlled trial of 38 patients showed symptomatic benefits with both oxygen and air.[11] A recent RCT of supplemental oxygen versus air in non-hypoxaemic cancer patients failed to demonstrate any differences in breathlessness, fatigue or distance walked during a 6-minute walking test.[12] The majority of studies in COPD suggest that oxygen is of symptomatic benefit at rest and on exertion,[13] although care must be taken in patients with hypercapnia. Ahmedzai *et al.* recently reported a randomized study of heliox (a helium–oxygen mixture) in 12 lung cancer patients suggesting that this reduced exercise-induced breathlessness compared to air; larger studies including patients with non-cancer breathlessness are planned by the investigators.[14] Clinical experience at present supports the use of oxygen for symptom relief in breathless patients.

Opioids   Several studies have assessed the efficacy of opioids (by the oral, parenteral and nebulized routes) for breathlessness. Tables 4.4.3 and 4.4.4 outline some of these key studies in patients with non-malignant diseases and cancer. The limitations of interpreting these studies are the small patient numbers, lack of controlled studies in cancer patients, and differences in the reporting of outcome measures. However, a recently conducted systematic review has shown that oral and parenteral opioids are effective in palliating breathlessness for patients with advanced chronic disease.[15]

There is evidence for opioid receptors in the lungs, which stimulated interest in the use of nebulized opioids. Early studies in COPD suggested efficacy, but the systematic review identified no studies with improvements in breathlessness and only one in exercise tolerance.[15]

Current evidence would therefore support the use of oral or parenteral opioids for breathlessness. There is no clear consensus on which opioid to use or the optimal schedule or route of administration. My practice is to reserve opioids for patients who are disabled by breathlessness or are breathless at rest, and then to use low doses (e.g. 2.5 mg oral morphine 4 hourly) in opioid-naive patients, with gradual dose titration for maximum efficacy. Patients already requiring opioids for pain may benefit from breakthrough doses for breathlessness or an increase in the regular dose of up to a third.

Benzodiazepines   Benzodiazepines are respiratory sedatives. Current evidence is conflicting, but suggests that they do not improve breathlessness in patients with advanced disease[10–16] However, they have a key role to play in managing associated anxiety, especially where anxiety and panic precipitate increasing breathlessness. Short and quick-acting drugs, such as lorazepam given by the sublingual route (0.5–1 mg as required), can be very useful for managing episodes of panic, allowing patients to regain control in conjunction with breathing control and relaxation techniques. Longer-acting benzodiazepines, such as diazepam (2–5 mg), may be useful where there are high levels of anxiety, and especially at night where breathlessness and fear contribute to insomnia.

Other psychotropic agents   Nabilone is an anxiolytic with bronchodilator and respiratory stimulant activity.[17] There are few objective data to support its use in breathlessness, but clinical experience suggests that it can be useful to relieve anxiety and breathlessness for patients with type 2 respiratory failure, where symptomatic retention of CO_2 may limit the use of benzodiazepines. Local experience with nabilone suggests that is should be started at doses of 0.1 mg nocte, and the dose gradually titrated to minimize unpleasant psychomimetic effects, up to doses of 0.25 mg b.d. Similarly, buspirone is a drug that stimulates respiration; clinical experience at doses up to 20 mg q.d.s. again suggests efficacy in some patients.

A–Z OF SYMPTOMS

Table 4.4.3 Summary of clinical trials of opioids in non-malignant disease

Author and year	Drug	Number of patients	Placebo controlled	Disease group	Dose and schedule	Route	Outcome reduction in dyspnoea	Improved exercise tolerance
Woodcock 1981	DHC	12	Yes	COPD	1 mg/kg; single dose	p.o.	+	+
Johnson 1983	DHC	18	Yes	COPD	15 mg p.r.n. pre-exercise; 1 week	p.o.	+	−
					15 mg alternate days; 1 week	p.o.	−	−
Sackner 1984	Hydrocodone	17	No	COPD and restrictive lung disease	5 mg; single dose	p.o.	+	N/A
Robin 1986	Hydromorphone	1	n of 1	COPD	3 mg q.d.s.; 3 days	p.r.	+	N/A
Rice 1987	Codeine	11	No (promethazine)	COPD	30 mg q.d.s	p.o.	−	−
Browning 1988	Hydrocodone	7	Yes	Cystic fibrosis	20 mg/m² per day; 48 hours	p.o.	+	+
Light 1989	Morphine	13	Yes	COPD	0.8 mg/kg; single dose	p.o.	+	+
Eiser 1991	Diamorphine	10	Yes	COPD ('pink puffers')	2.5–5 mg q.d.s.; 2 weeks	p.o.	−	−
		8			7.5 mg; single dose	p.o.	−	−
Poole 1998	Morphine	16	Yes	COPD	10 mg o.d. titrating to mean dose 25 mg daily	p.o.	−	−
Abernethy 2003	Morphine	48	Yes	Predominantly COPD	20 mg sustained release o.d.	p.o.	+	N/A
Johnson 2002	Morphine	10	Yes	Heart failure	5 mg q.d.s.	p.o.	+	N/A

DHC, dihydrocodeine; COPD, chronic obstructive pulmonary disease; p.o., oral; p.r., rectal.

Table 4.4.4 Summary of clinical trials of opioids for breathlessness in malignant disease

Author and year	Number of patients	Drug	Route	Dose and schedule	Placebo controlled	Reduction in dyspnoea
Bruera 1990	20	Morphine	s.c.	4-hourly dose 5 mg or 2.5 × 4-hourly dose	No	Yes
Cohen 1991	8	Morphine	i.v.	Titrated versus response Continuous infusion Mean dose 5.6 mg/h	No	Yes
Bruera 1993	10	Morphine	s.c.	Single dose, 50% greater than 4-hourly dose Mean dose 34 ± 12 mg morphine	Yes	Yes
Boyd 1994	15	Morphine	p.o.	Regular oral preparation, MST 10 mg b.d. (13) or 30% increase in dose (2)	No	No
Allard 1998	15	Not specified	p.o./s.c.	15 successive pairs of patients, matched on route of administration, random allocation of two opioid doses (25% and 50% of 4-hourly dose)	Randomized, continuous sequential trial	Yes, both dose levels
Mazzocato 1999	9	Morphine	s.c.	5 mg in opioid-naive patients (7) 3.75 mg in addition to regular morphine dose of 7.5 mg 4-hourly (2)	Yes	Yes

s.c., subcutaneous; i.v., intravenous; p.o., oral; MST, morphine sulphate tablet (modified release); b.d., twice-daily.

Bronchodilators Many breathless patients may have underlying airflow obstruction, and a trial of bronchodilators may be beneficial. The combination of a beta-adrenergic stimulant (e.g. salbutamol) and anticholinergic agent (e.g. ipratropium bromide) appears to be most effective, given as required rather than regularly, as excessive use of beta-adrenergic agents can cause cardiac stimulation.[5] This combination is unlikely to be effective where there is fixed airway obstruction, e.g. by tumour.

Methylxanthines These bronchodilators (e.g. theophylline and aminophylline) have other effects, i.e. respiratory stimulation and augmentation of failing respiratory muscles. However, there is no evidence to suggest a role in breathlessness beyond that of bronchodilatation at present.

FUTURE DEVELOPMENTS

Breathlessness is a severe and complex symptom. It is likely that an increased understanding of the pathophysiology, combined with further research into the quantitative and qualitative aspects of breathlessness and its measurement, will aid the development of new non-pharmacological and pharmacological approaches.

KEY POINTS

- Breathlessness is a common and distressing symptom.
- Identify any potentially reversible underlying causes.
- Identify associated patient/carer anxiety and distress.
- Acknowledge its impact on function and social status.
- Explore non-pharmacological measures in all patients.
- Reserve symptomatic pharmacological management for patients who are breathless at rest or on minimal exertion.

REFERENCES

1. Gift A. Dyspnea. *Nurs Clin N Am* 1990; **25**(4), 955–65.
2. Edmonds PM, Higginson IJ, Altmann D, Sen-Gupta G, McDonnell M. Is the presence of dyspnea a risk factor for morbidity in cancer patients? *J Pain Symptom Manage* 2000; **19**, 15–22.
3. Reuben DB, Mor V, Hiris J. Clinical symptoms and length of survival in patients with terminal cancer. *Arch Int Med* 1988; **148**, 1586–91.
4. Dudgeon DJ, Lertzman M. Dyspnea in the advanced cancer patient. *J Pain Symptom Manage* 1998; **16**, 212–19.
5. Ellis PA, Smith IE, Hardy JR *et al*. Symptom relief with MVP chemotherapy in advanced non-small-cell lung cancer. *Br J Cancer* 1995; **71**(2), 366–70.

6. Moghissi K, Bond MG, Sambrook RJ, Stephens RJ, Hopwood P, Girling D. Treatment of endotracheal or endobronchial obstruction by non-small cell lung cancer: lack of patients in an MRC randomised trial leaves key questions unanswered. Medical Research Council Lung Cancer Working Party. *Clin Oncol* 1999; **1**(3), 179–83.

7. Bredin M, Corner J, Krishnasamy M, Plant H, Bailey C, A'Hern R. Multicentre randomised controlled trial of nursing intervention for breathlessness in patients with lung cancer. *BMJ* 1999; **318**, 901–4.

8. Filshie J, Penn K, Ashley S, Davis CL. Acupuncture for the relief of cancer-related breathlessness. *Palliat Med* 1996, **10**, 145–50.

9. Jobst K, Chen JH, McPherson K *et al*. Controlled trial of acupuncture for disabling breathlessness. *Lancet* 1986; **20**, 1416–18.

10. Bruera E, de Stoutz N, Velasco-Leiva A, Scholler T, Hanson J. The effects of oxygen on the intensity of dyspnoea in hypoxaemic terminal cancer patients. *Lancet* 1993; **342**, 13–14.

11. Booth S, Kelly MJ, Cox N, Adams L, Guz A. Does oxygen help dyspnea in patients with cancer? *Am J Respir Crit Care Rev* 1996; **153**, 1515–18.

12. Ripamonti C. Management of dyspnea in advanced cancer patients. *Support Care Cancer* 1999; **7**, 233–43.

13. Bruera E, Sweeney C, Willey J *et al*. A randomized controlled trial of supplemental oxygen versus air in cancer patients with dyspnea. *Palliat Med* 2003; **17**, 659–63.

14. Ahmedzai SH, Laude E, Hart A, Troy G. Randomised double blind study of oxygen/helium versus oxygen versus air for dyspnoea in lung cancer. Oral Abstract: Palliative Care Congress, 2002.

15. Jennings AL, Davies A, Higgins JPT, Broadley K. Systematic review of the effects of opioids on breathlessness in terminal illness. *Thorax* 2002; **57**(11), 939–44.

16. Ahmedzai S. Palliation of respiratory symptoms. In: Doyle D, Hanks G, MacDonald N (eds), *Oxford textbook of palliative medicine*, 2nd edn. Oxford: Oxford University Press, 1998, 582–616.

17. Ahmedzai S, Carter R, Mills RJ, Moran F. Effects of nabilone on pulmonary function. *Marihuana '84. Proceedings of the Oxford Symposium on Cannabis*. Oxford: IRL Press, 1984, 371–7.

SYSTEMATIC REVIEW

Jennings AL, Davies A, Higgins J, Broadley K. A systematic review of the use of opioids in the management of dyspnoea. *Thorax* 2002; **57**(11), 939–44.

chapter 4.5

CONFUSION AND PSYCHOSIS

Max Henderson and Matthew Hotopf

INTRODUCTION

There is a variety of reasons why patients with advanced disease may be disorientated or act strangely (Table 4.5.1). There is often considerable uncertainty surrounding the assessment and management of disturbed or disorientated patients. This chapter emphasizes the importance of making a clear assessment leading to a diagnosis. It first discusses the clinical syndromes of delirium and dementia, before describing three common presentations and going on to discuss the cognitive assessment and key aspects of management.

DELIRIUM

CLINICAL PICTURE

Delirium, also described as an acute confusional state, is characterized by the acute onset of symptoms. The core features of the syndrome consist of fluctuating

Table 4.5.1

New or acute confusion in patients with advanced disease
- Acute confusional state or delirium
- Dementia
- Functional psychiatric disorder (e.g. depression)

Chronic confusion in patients with advanced disease
- Dementia
- Subacute confusional state
- Functional psychiatric disorder

Existing psychotic illness in patients with advanced disease
- Schizophrenia
- Bipolar disorder
- Paranoid states

---

levels of both consciousness (though there are difficulties defining consciousness) and cognitive function, in particular attentional abnormalities. Patients with delirium appear perplexed, and when tested will usually be disorientated in time, place and person. They have a deficit in immediate or working memory, which translates into an inability to assimilate new information. This is demonstrated by eliciting a reduced digit span. Patients with delirium fluctuate between hypervigilance and drowsiness. There is often a profound disturbance of the sleep–wake cycle, sometimes with complete reversal. Patients show affective changes, appearing intensely anxious or, less commonly, fatuously elated. Alternatively, they may present with a hypoalert form with somnolence and reduced motor activity, which can be confused with sedation secondary to medications. They have alterations in the sensorium, often experiencing illusions and hallucinations, which occur in any modality, but are most characteristically visual. Insight is usually absent.

CAUSES

Delirium may be caused by almost any acute medical illness and affects up to 40 per cent of new admissions to hospices.[1] The majority of patients admitted to hospice with advanced cancer who die have 'terminal delirium'. However, about one half of all episodes of delirium in patients with advanced disease are reversible. The commonest causes are listed in Table 4.5.2. Particular attention should be paid to drug-induced delirium: anticholinergics, antidepressants, benzodiazepines and opioids are frequently implicated. There is evidence that delirium associated with medication use and dehydration is more likely to be reversible than other causes. Another important cause to identify is delirium tremens, associated with acute alcohol withdrawal, because the management of this is different from that of other types of delirium.

Rather than being regarded as a new or additional diagnosis, delirium is perhaps better thought of as a final common pathway following a number of insults. The insults are common and ubiquitous; the key variable is the individual's relative

Table 4.5.2 Possible causes of an acute confusional state

Infection – urinary tract/respiratory tract, but remember occult infections such as endocarditis or osteomyelitis
Drugs – anticholinergics/benzodiazepines/opiates
Alcohol
↑ intracranial pressure
Organ failure – liver/heart/kidney
Electrolyte imbalance – Ca^{2+}/Na^+
↑ or ↓ blood glucose
Dehydration
Hypoxia
New cerebrovascular event

resilience to delirium – his or her 'delirium threshold'. When the magnitude of the insult overwhelms the individual's ability to deal with it, delirium may result. The young and otherwise fit may become delirious, but the insult required to produce signs of acute confusion are more substantial than the straightforward urinary tract infection that can produce an identical constellation of symptoms and signs in an older person with pre-existing cerebral disease. It is important in the management of delirium to take into account the factors that might have impacted on the individual's threshold for delirium as well as the insult itself. An important randomized trial recently found that delirium could be prevented by ameliorating certain factors, such as sleep deprivation, immobility, visual and hearing impairments, and dehydration, and identifying patients with pre-existing cognitive impairments. By energetically intervening with groups thought to be at risk, the investigators reduced the incidence of delirium among elderly general hospital in-patients from 15 per cent to 9 per cent.[2]

MANAGEMENT

There are several strands to the management of delirium. First, a safe environment should be maintained. This may involve providing a nurse to sit with an agitated patient to prevent him or her coming to harm. Patients with delirium should be nursed in a side room, though with adequate lighting, and plenty of cues, such as a clock, to keep them orientated. Second, the underlying medical diagnosis should be identified. In patients with advanced disease, the management will vary according to how near to death the patient is judged to be. If death is thought to be imminent, it may be inappropriate to start an exhaustive search for causes of delirium. If death is not imminent, the search for causes should include a careful drug and alcohol history, and examination to determine hydration status and whether there is an obvious focus of infection. Investigations for infection, electrolyte imbalance, dehydration and hypoxia should be performed (Table 4.5.3). As delirium frequently

Table 4.5.3 Potential investigations in an acute confusional state

Full blood count

Urea and electrolytes

Calcium

Liver function tests

Blood glucose

Oxygen saturation ($\pm$ arterial blood gases)

Urinalysis ($\rightarrow$ MC + S)

Chest X-ray ($\pm$ sputum $\rightarrow$ MC + S)

$\pm$ Lumbar puncture

$\pm$ Further imaging, e.g. CT or MRI head/bone scan

$\pm$ EEG

MC + S, microscopy, culture and sensitivities; CT, computed tomography; MRI, magnetic resonance imaging; EEG, electroencephalogram.

A–Z OF SYMPTOMS

follows the natural history of the underlying cause, any abnormal findings should be corrected.

The third issue concerns whether patients with delirium should be medicated, and if so how? Given that the experiences in delirium are often extremely frightening, treatment may be a humane course of action. The only randomized controlled trial assessing the treatment of delirium compared benzodiazepines with low-dose neuroleptics in patients with human immunodeficiency virus (HIV), and found convincing evidence that neuroleptics were more effective in dealing with the troublesome affective and sensory symptoms.[3] Haloperidol may have theoretical advantages over chlorpromazine in terms of extra-pyramidal, sedative and hypotensive side effects. We recommend low doses of haloperidol (0.5–1 mg q.d.s.), which can then be built up steadily to achieve maximum effects. Patients with cerebral disease may be very sensitive to the extra-pyramidal side effects of neuroleptics. Alternatives to consider are benzodiazepines and atypical antipsychotics. There are a number of reports in the literature of the successful use of risperidone, olanzapine and quetiapine in delirium, though no controlled studies. Other drugs that offer potential benefit include the anticholinesterase drugs donepezil and rivastigmine and the 5-hydroxytryptamine-3 (5HT-3) antagonist ondansetron, more often used for the management of nausea.

Delirium tremens is an important diagnosis to make, and should be considered in all patients with delirium, even if their advanced disease status may suggest that they have been unable to drink alcohol recently. The syndrome is associated with acute withdrawal from alcohol, and usually manifests within 3–4 days of withdrawal, i.e. slightly after the 'typical' withdrawal signs of tremor and insomnia. It is characterized by the usual constellation of symptoms of delirium, but agitation is usually the predominant symptom, and there is often pronounced tremor. There is an increased risk of seizures. Patients frequently experience bizarre or frightening visual hallucinations. Classically, delirium tremens occurs in patients who have recently been admitted to a hospital or hospice when ill, and as a consequence have stopped consuming alcohol. Once the diagnosis is made, the emphasis should be on: (1) ensuring the fluid balance is maintained, (2) using chlordiazepoxide, initially at high doses (up to 40 mg q.d.s.) to sedate the patient, reducing over 5–10 days, and (3) giving parenteral vitamin B complex for at least 3 days or until a normal oral diet is resumed, followed by oral thiamine. If signs of Wernicke's encephalopathy remain, many would advise that parenteral B vitamins be continued.

DEMENTIA

Dementia is defined as an acquired, global impairment of memory, cognition and personality, which is usually, but not always, irreversible. The most common type of dementia is Alzheimer's disease, followed by vascular dementia.[4] The distinction between these two categories has blurred in recent years, as it has become clear that cardiovascular risk factors, such as smoking and hypertension, may be important risk factors for Alzheimer's disease.[5] Lewy body disease is an increasingly recognized form of dementia, characterized by fluctuating levels of consciousness and cognitive performance, such variations being apparent over the course of a day.

In addition, Parkinsonian features are prominent, including rigidity, bradykinesia and recurrent falls.[6] Other primary dementias include fronto-temporal dementia, Huntington's disease and Creutzfeld–Jakob disease, but these are relatively rare. Dementia is commonly seen in patients with cerebral disease, which may have been manifest with focal neurological signs for many years before the onset of cognitive impairment. Thus dementia complicates Parkinson's disease, multiple sclerosis, motor neurone disease and normal pressure hydrocephalus and may be a feature of cerebral space-occupying lesions. Less commonly, it may be a presenting feature of metabolic, endocrine and other medical conditions. Finally, there are so-called *pseudodementias* in which other psychiatric disorders masquerade as dementia. The most common psychiatric diagnosis to present in this way is depression (see Chapter 4.8).

CLINICAL FEATURES

The main features of dementia are of a gradual decline in cognitive functioning, which usually takes place insidiously over a matter of months. The patient (or a relative) notices loss of short-term memory as an early first sign. The clinical features depend on the predominant site of pathology: Alzheimer's disease is predominantly a disease of the cerebral cortex, and is characteristically associated with parietal lobe signs such as apraxias (difficulty carrying out motor tasks, such as dressing) and agnosias (difficulties in recognition, such as facial recognition or prosopagnosia). The subcortical dementias – for example that associated with Parkinson's disease – are characterized by a more general cognitive slowing and dulling with less specific cortical features. However, it should be noted that 'cortical' and 'subcortical' represent ends of a spectrum rather than distinct categories, and each may display the features of the other. As well as the cognitive symptoms and signs, dementia is associated with a coarsening of personality. Relatives may notice that subtle aspects of social interaction are less well managed, long before more obvious signs of frontal lobe damage, such as over-familiarity, disinhibition and a superficial or fatuous affect, become apparent.

ASSESSMENT

It is important to define the patient's cognitive impairments, rather than simply refer to him or her as 'demented'. The Abbreviated Mental Test Score[7] is a useful screening tool, and the Mini Mental State Examination[8] is widely used both in diagnosis and to assess progress. Although most cases of dementia are irreversible, the first aim of assessment should be to rule out the occasional reversible causes, such as hypothyroidism, or depressive pseudodementia. The second aim of assessment should be to gain a good understanding of the patient's functional limitations. What activities of daily living is he or she capable of? It is important to gain realistic assessments early on so that provision may be made for future care, including, perhaps, placement in a residential or nursing home. Whilst some dementias are best thought of as terminal diseases in their own right, most patients with dementia will be seen in palliative care settings for the management of symptoms related to other advanced physical disease. It is important to assess the extent to which patients with dementia can understand their diagnosis and the implications of treatment. Patients with mild depression sometimes present major problems when their poor memory makes it difficult for them to assimilate new information. They may understand and be distressed by the knowledge that they have advanced disease, but forget this information. The patient may keep asking the clinician for new information they have only recently been given, and be quite incapable of processing it. Where patients are incapable of understanding, there is a legal framework to assist (see below). It is also important to assess the patient's ability to communicate distress, including pain. Patients with dementia may show a sudden deterioration in their mental state, which turns out to be a manifestation of new pain. An added depressive illness can also complicate the clinical picture.

An essential angle to the management of dementia is the involvement of family members. Caring for a relative with dementia is associated with considerably increased rates of depression and anxiety. Carers whose relative has developed advanced physical disease may feel frustrated by their inability to communicate with them or 'say goodbye'.

The distinction between dementia and delirium is an important one (Table 4.5.4). This is mainly based on the onset and course of deterioration. Delirium usually has a rapid onset over a matter of hours or days, which is closely associated with a physical deterioration. Dementia is usually of more insidious onset over a matter of months. In vascular dementia, deteriorations may occur in a stepwise fashion. In delirium, there are marked psychomotor disturbances and prominent changes in conscious level, whereas these features only occur late in dementia. Patients with dementia frequently have a normal digit span, at least early in the disease. The two conditions also co-exist – indeed, dementia is a risk factor for delirium, and many patients with delirium will also have an underlying dementia.

Table 4.5.4 Distinguishing between delirium and dementia

	Delirium	Dementia
Onset	Acute, rapid	Insidious, occasionally step-wise
Course	Fluctuating	Progressive, but stable over course of the day
Natural history	Hours/weeks	Years
Alertness	Abnormally increased or decreased	Normal
Attention	Impaired	Normal
Working memory	Reduced digit span	Normal in early stages
Orientation	Impaired	Normal in early stages
Perception	Illusions and hallucinations common	Common only in later stages
Sleep	Disrupted	Normal
Reversibility	Often reversible	Rarely reversible

PSYCHOSIS

It is rare for patients to develop a new psychotic illness in the context of advanced disease. However, patients with chronic psychosis frequently require medical and nursing care for advanced disease. This means that patients with advanced disease who present with new psychotic symptoms (hallucinations and delusions) should be assumed to have an organic brain disorder (delirium or dementia) rather than a 'functional' psychosis such as schizophrenia or bipolar disorder, until proven otherwise.

Most patients with pre-existing psychotic illness can be successfully managed within normal hospital or hospice settings. Although this section emphasizes specific difficulties that may be encountered managing patients with psychotic illness, it is important to note that, in the majority of cases, patients with psychotic illness pose few additional problems. However, problems frequently arise when the 'psychiatric patient' is stigmatized in general medical settings, and assumptions are made that the patient is incapable of understanding his or her diagnosis or co-operating with treatment. This means psychotic patients are often not given sufficient information and can become isolated. This, in turn, may lead to avoidable behavioural difficulties.

Patients with psychotic illness may exhibit well-recognized 'positive' symptoms, such as hallucinations (predominantly auditory) and delusions. They may also have 'negative' symptoms that are more subtle and difficult to define. These include apathy, poverty of thought or speech, and loss of social skills. These symptoms may give the erroneous impression that the patient is depressed (although this is sometimes the case) and may also lead to frustration in carers, who may feel that the patient simply is not trying hard enough.

Psychotic phenomena may interfere with patients' understanding of their diagnosis. The diagnosis may become part of a delusional system, or – more commonly – be ignored or disbelieved. In these situations it may be difficult to obtain informed consent from the patient for treatments for his or her physical illness. However, the majority of patients with psychotic illness are capable of understanding information regarding their diagnosis.

COMMUNICATION WITH OTHER TEAMS

Most patients with an ongoing psychotic illness will be engaged on some level with mental health services. This often includes their general practitioner (GP). These teams will have substantial experience in managing this particular patient's problems and will be able to advise should management difficulties arise. It will be additionally important to liaise with these teams if the patient is discharged from the hospice, especially if alterations have been made to the medication regimen.

Alterations in psychotropic medication are rarely needed, and may produce a relapse in the psychotic illness. However, the side effects and interactions of antipsychotic medication need to be borne in mind at a time when patients have advanced disease and may be prescribed additional drugs. For example, the sedative effects of antipsychotics combined with those of opioid analgesics may be

A–Z OF SYMPTOMS

problematic, and the risk of Parkinsonism may be increased with domperidone and metoclopramide. If in doubt, specialist advice should be sought.

CAPACITY AND CONSENT WITH CONFUSED PATIENTS

In England and Wales, there are two important strands of law that affect acutely disturbed patients. First, statute law, which has been passed by Parliament, exists in the form of the Mental Health Act (MHA) 1983.[9] This act allows for the detention and treatment of patients with mental disorders against their will, provided the nature of their disorder is such that the health or safety of the patient, or the safety of others, is at risk. The MHA provides for treatment of mental disorder, but not physical illness. If a patient has a severe mental disorder such as schizophrenia and is not consenting to treatment of their advanced physical disease, the MHA cannot be used to compel them to have their advanced physical disease treated. However, there are situations in which a physical disease directly causes mental disorder (for example delirium) and it is acceptable to use the MHA under these circumstances. The MHA can usually only be applied to detain a patient in a hospital. Hospices and nursing homes do not have provision to administer the act – in the sense that they do not have a board of managers recognized under the act who would have the power to release patients.

Most commonly-used sections of the act require some combination of a psychiatrist, a second opinion doctor and a social worker. The agreement of the nearest relative is also sought, but in exceptional circumstances the MHA may be applied without their consent. Most sections of the act have built-in appeal procedures whereby patients may apply for their discharge. The exceptions are the very short sections used in emergencies.

The second main strand of law covering confused patients is the common law regarding mental capacity. This is based on case law from individual judgements, but has been subject to detailed review by the Law Commission[10] and the Lord Chancellor's Department.[11,12] It is presumed that all patients have capacity. There are some situations in which patients automatically do not have capacity, for example unconscious patients who cannot communicate. There are additional situations in which a patient with *mental disability* (as opposed to mental disorder) may be judged not to have capacity. The term mental disability is intentionally loose, as it allows not only for well-recognized mental disorders but also overwhelming but possibly temporary emotional states to be taken into account. Thus individuals with severe pain may be judged to have a mental disability that can cloud their judgement. If there is a mental disability, the next question is whether this interferes with the patient's decision-making abilities. It might do so in three ways: (1) by affecting the patient's retention of information regarding treatment, (2) by affecting the ability of the patient to believe the information being given, and (3) by affecting the patient's ability to weigh matters in the balance.

It is important to note that capacity is not an 'all-or-nothing' construct. Capacity relates to a specific question at a specific point in time. Thus a clinical team may judge that a patient with a chest infection and delirium lacks capacity to make a decision about being admitted to hospital, but the same patient may be able to make decisions regarding his or her finances or other treatment decisions. Obviously, if the same patient is treated, capacity may be regained.

Having made a decision regarding capacity, it is then necessary to determine whether the intervention planned is in the patient's best interests. Whilst members of the family are not able to consent on the patient's behalf, in weighing up the best interests it is good practice to take their views into account. It is also worth considering whether the patient expressed any views in the past. It is also important to involve the multi-disciplinary team and other health professionals (the GP is often a useful source of information) before making a decision. For decisions with very serious implications, it is good practice to request a second opinion.

The confused patient: history taking

1. *Description of disturbed behaviour*: whilst it is vital to obtain the patient's description of his or her behaviour as far as is possible, it is also crucial to get an account from either a relative or, if the patient is on the ward, a colleague such as a nurse. Are the patient's actions putting him or others at risk? Important considerations include the observation of interpersonal boundaries and the recognition of obvious dangers such as fires or stairs or roads. If the behaviour is goal directed, is the goal a safe and appropriate one? If the patient is wandering, can he return to his chair/bed independently?
2. *Onset of disturbance* (particularly from relatives): try to get to the key event that the relative recognized as abnormal. What was the run-up to this like? Looking back, were there subtle changes beforehand or did this come 'out of the blue'?
3. *Fluctuations in level of confusion*: do these occur hour by hour, day by day, or over a longer period? Is there a pattern within the day?
4. *Affect of patient whilst disturbed*: is the patient's mood reactive, fatuous or depressed?
5. *History of possible causes*: for example urinary tract infection, chest infection, alcohol consumption, current medication.
6. *Previous psychiatric history*.

The confused patient: cognitive assessment

GLOBAL FUNCTIONS

- *Orientation*
  1. Time: include year, season, month, day, date, how long in hospital.
  2. Place: include name *and type* of building (e.g. hospital/shop etc.).
  3. Person: it is rare for patients not to know their own name.

- *Attention/concentration*
  1. Digit span: ask the patient to repeat a list of numbers – start with, say, 4 and build up. Reverse digit span is an even better test: the patient is asked to repeat numbers in reverse order; normal scores = 6–8 forward and 4–6 backwards.

A–Z OF SYMPTOMS

2. Spell 'world' backwards.
3. Serial /s: ask the patient to subtract 7 from 100, then 7 from the result and so on to a maximum of 5 subtractions ($= 65!$).
4. Other backward lists: for example count down from 20 to 1/months of the year backwards.

- *Memory*
  1. Anterograde memory: name and address recall. This should ideally have five to seven parts. Ensure, by repetition if necessary, that registration has occurred.
  2. Retrograde memory: ask about autobiographical facts such as the street lived in as a child, name of school, first employer.
  3. Current affairs and important (appropriate) historical facts, e.g. date of the Second World War.

DISCRETE LOCALIZED FUNCTIONS

- *Frontal functions*
  1. Verbal fluency: maximum number of words beginning with the letter 'F' in 60 seconds; maximum number of words in a category, e.g. four-legged animals.
  2. Abstract thought: similarities between, for example, a table and a chair; differences between, for example, a child and a dwarf.

- *Language*
  1. Naming: ask the patient to identify everyday objects such as a pen or a tie.
  2. Comprehension: ask the patient to perform a simple but multi-stage task such as folding a piece of paper.

- *Calculation*
  Simple addition and subtraction.

- *Praxis*
  Ask the patient to mime simple tasks such as putting on a sock or brushing teeth.

- *Agnosias*
  1. Left–right agnosia: with the patient's eyes closed, ask him/her to indicate which palm you touch.
  2. Astereognosia: with the eyes closed, ask the patient to identify small objects such as a button or a pen-top in his/her palm.
  3. Agraphaesthesia: gently draw a number in the patient's palm with your finger and ask him/her to identify it.

- *Visuospatial abilities*
  1. Clock test: ask the patient to draw a clock face with all the numbers and the hands set to a certain time, say 'ten past eleven'.
  2. Ask the patient to copy a figure such as a three-dimensional cube.

KEY POINTS

- A clear assessment, leading to a diagnosis, is essential in the management of confusion.
- Delirium is characterized by an acute onset of fluctuating consciousness and cognitive function.
- Only about half of the cases of delirium in advanced disease are reversible: consider medication, hypercalcaemia, infection, dehydration and alcohol withdrawal among potential causes.
- Dementia is characterized by gradual onset of a global impairment of memory, cognition and personality. It is rarely reversible, but rule out hypothyroidism and depression.
- Onset of a new functional psychotic illness in the context of advanced physical disease is rare. Most patients with a pre-existing psychotic condition are capable of understanding information about their diagnosis and treatment.
- Decision-making capacity must be assessed in relation to a specific decision and not assumed to be generally impaired.
- Remember the information and support needs of relatives and carers of confused patients.

REFERENCES

1. Lawlor PG, Gagnon B, Mancini IL *et al.* Occurrence, causes, and outcome of delirium in patients with advanced cancer. *Arch Intern Med* 2000; **160**, 786–94.
2. Inouye SK, Bogardus ST Jr, Charpentier PA *et al.* A multi-component intervention to prevent delirium in hospitalized older patients. *N Engl J Med* 1999; **340**, 669–76.
3. Breitbart W, Marotta R, Platt MM *et al.* A double-blind trial of haloperidol, chlorpromazine, and lorazepam in the treatment of delirium in hospitalized AIDS patients. *Am J Psychiatry* 1996; **153**, 231–7.
4. Stewart R. Vascular dementia: a diagnosis running out of time. *Br J Psychiatry* 2002; **180**, 152–6.
5. Stewart R. Cardiovascular factors in Alzheimer's disease. *J Neurol Neurosurg Psychiatry* 1998; **65**, 143–7.
6. McKeith I. Dementia with Lewy bodies. *Br J Psychiatry* 2002; **180**, 144–7.
7. Hodkinson H. Evaluation of a mental test score for assessment of mental impairment in the elderly. *Age Ageing* 1972; **1**, 233–8.
8. Folstein M, Folstein S, McHugh P. 'Mini-mental state'. A practical method for grading the cognitive state of patients for the clinician. *J Psychiatr Res* 1975; **12**, 189–98.
9. *The Mental Health Act, 1995*. London: HMSO, 1995.
10. Law Commission. *Mental incapacity*. Report No. 231. London: HMSO, 1995.
11. Lord Chancellor's Department. *Who decides?* London: The Stationery Office, 1997.
12. Lord Chancellor. *Making decisions: the Government's proposals for making decisions on behalf of mentally incapacitated adults.* London: The Stationery Office, 1999.

A–Z OF SYMPTOMS

CONSTIPATION AND DIARRHOEA

Nigel Sykes

CONSTIPATION

BACKGROUND

Constipation affects around 60 per cent of palliative care patients who are not taking opioid analgesia and nearly 90 per cent of those who are.[1] The importance of the condition lies in the distress it causes as a symptom, which in some surveys has been more troublesome than pain.

Therefore it is appropriate that constipation is treated as a symptom, and patients define it themselves. External definitions, such as an average of less than three stools per week or the existence of straining during at least 25 per cent of defaecations, are of little clinical help. The range of normal bowel function is very wide and what matters is the deviation from what the individual considers normal rather than a deviation from a population average.

PATHOPHYSIOLOGY

A few palliative care patients will have a long history of idiopathic constipation, but for most the constipation is associated with their illness. The reasons why chronic illness produces constipation are multiple. Peristaltic activity in the colon is triggered by gastric emptying of meals and by general physical activity. As meals become smaller and less frequent, and mobility is reduced, both these triggers will become less effective. There is often reduced intake of fluid as well as of food, which results in more complete water absorption from the bowel and consequently a drier, harder stool. Whether constipation is exacerbated by physiological involvement of disease-induced cytokines in the control of gut motility and secretion remains to be determined.

Morphine and other opioids are probably the most important single constipating factor that can be isolated, but they operate against a background of widespread constipation arising from debility. Opioids reduce gut peristalsis and rectal sensitivity, increase sphincter tone throughout the bowel, and may increase net water absorption from the gut contents. Fentanyl is somewhat less constipating than morphine,[2] but so far there is no clear evidence for a difference between morphine and any other opioids in respect of constipating potency. Opioids are not the only constipating drugs, and anticholinergics and iron are also particularly prone to slow bowel function.

ASSESSMENT

Palliative medicine history-taking should include an enquiry about constipation and, if it is present, details about the patient's current bowel frequency and need to strain at stool and of how these differ from what has normally been experienced in the past. If there has been a change, a rectal examination is needed unless there is a clear report of a satisfactory evacuation within the past day or so. The purpose of the examination is to assess the consistency of the stool and, particularly, to uncover the existence of faecal impaction in the rectum which might need local intervention to remove it.

Occasionally there is doubt as to whether a patient has malignant intestinal obstruction or severe constipation. Erect and supine abdominal radiographs can help resolve this dilemma, but the distinction may not be clear, especially with very high or very low sites of obstruction.

PROPHYLAXIS

The pathophysiology of constipation suggests several prophylactic measures, but in practice strategies such as increasing dietary fibre, encouraging oral fluids and improving mobility are of limited value because the chance of making significant changes is small owing to the general effects of the disease. Conflicting reports have emerged of the effectiveness of abdominal massage, and there seems to be no evidence of the usefulness of other complementary approaches to constipation.

THERAPY

Most patients with advanced disease who are constipated will require laxative therapy. Most trials of laxative drugs have been carried out in idiopathic constipation or in geriatrics rather than in palliative medicine. The results do not allow a clear recommendation of one agent over another because of the small size of the studies, the number of different preparations, and the various endpoints and conditions involved. However, certain statements can be made.

- Systematic review evidence suggests that any kind of laxative can increase stool frequency by about 1.4 bowel actions per week compared with placebo.[3]

- There is limited experimental evidence that the optimal combination of effectiveness with few adverse effects and low dose is achieved by using a combination of stimulant and softening laxatives rather than either alone.[4]

- Laxative preparations vary significantly in price and physical characteristics. Ready-made combinations tend to be expensive. Given the lack of major differences in efficacy, cost and individual patient acceptability should both be strong influences in prescribing choice.[5]

- Bulk laxatives have been extensively tested in elderly patients and those with chronic constipation, but might not be so applicable to palliative care cancer patients. This is because in order to be used safely and effectively, these agents have to be taken with a volume of water that is often poorly tolerated by ill patients. Inadequate water can result in a gelatinous mass forming in the gut sufficient to precipitate intestinal obstruction. The risk is likely to be greater when the gut is affected by tumour, suggesting that bulk laxatives ought to be used with discretion in a palliative care setting.

The basic division of laxatives is between *stimulants* and *softeners*. This division seems useful in clinical practice, although in fact any drug that stimulates peristalsis will accelerate transit, allow less time for water absorption and so produce a softer stool. Similarly, softening the stool involves increasing its bulk, which will result in increased distension of the intestinal wall and a consequent stimulation of reflex enteric muscle contraction.

Oral laxatives
Stimulant laxatives   Examples: senna, bisacodyl, sodium picosulphate, dantron (only available in combination preparations).

- Act directly on the myenteric nerves to evoke gut muscle contraction.

- Reduce gut water absorption.

- Evidence for intestinal damage from these agents is poor.

- Can produce marked colic, particularly if not combined with a softening agent.

- Onset of action 6–12 hours.

- Dantron causes red urinary discolouration and perianal rashes.

Softening laxatives   *Osmotic laxatives*   Examples: magnesium sulphate, magnesium hydroxide; lactulose; polyethylene glycol (PEG).

- Magnesium sulphate and hydroxide have stimulant as well as osmotic actions at higher doses. The sulphate is the more potent. They are cheap.

- Magnesium sulphate used alone can be useful for resistant constipation. There is a risk of hypermagnesaemia with chronic use.

- Lactulose:
  is expensive,
  is needed in large volumes if used alone in marked constipation,
  causes flatulence in around 20 per cent of users.

- PEG has been reported to be effective as an oral treatment for faecal impaction.[6] However, it has to be taken in substantial volumes (500–1000 mL per day), which can prove unacceptable to frailer patients.

Surfactant laxatives   Examples: docusate sodium, poloxamer (available only in combination with dantron [danthron]).

- These drugs increase water penetration of the stool.

- Evidence for laxative efficacy is limited.

Lubricant laxative: liquid paraffin
- Chronic paraffin use can cause fat-soluble vitamin deficiencies and has been associated with anal faecal leakage. Neither adverse effect has been linked with the emulsion of liquid paraffin with magnesium hydroxide, which is currently the most common form in which it is used in Britain.

- It is cheap.

Rectal laxatives

Most patients prefer oral rather than rectal laxatives, and use of the latter should therefore be minimized by optimizing laxative treatment by mouth. There is a particular role for enemas and suppositories in the relief of faecal impaction and in bowel management in paraplegic patients. Evidence to guide their use is scantier even than that for oral laxatives. Anything introduced into the rectum can stimulate defaecation via the anocolonic reflex, but among rectal laxatives only bisacodyl suppositories have a pharmacological stimulant action. Glycerine suppositories, and arachis or olive oil enemas, soften and lubricate the stool, as do proprietary mini enemas which contain mixtures of surfactants.

An approach to the use of laxatives

- Exclude intestinal obstruction if possible.
- If obstruction remains a possibility, use a softening laxative alone. Avoid bulk laxatives.
- Rectal examination is needed unless there has been a recent complete bowel action.
- If the rectum is impacted with hard faeces, it might be necessary to soften the mass with an oil-retention enema before evacuation is possible.
- If manual rectal evacuation proves necessary, ensure adequate sedation with diazepam or midazolam.

A–Z OF SYMPTOMS

- If the rectum is loaded with soft faeces, an oral stimulant laxative alone may be adequate. The addition of a softener is likely to be needed in due course.
- If the rectum is largely empty, a combination of softening and stimulant laxatives should be given and the doses titrated according to response. Particularly when opioids are also being given, a b.d. or t.d.s. laxative dose schedule is likely to be needed. Remember patient acceptability and cost.
- There is no clear hierarchy of laxatives but, clinically, sodium picosulphate or magnesium hydroxide appear helpful for more resistant constipation.
- Paraplegic patients, who lack anal sensation and sphincter tone, are best managed by use of a softening laxative orally and the induction of defaecation every second or third day by means of suppositories or a mini enema.

DIARRHOEA

Diarrhoea, defined as the passage of loose stool frequently or with urgency, is much less common in palliative care than constipation, affecting about 10 per cent of patients. The most common cause has been reported to be laxatives. Early intestinal obstruction can produce alternating diarrhoea and constipation, but also relatively frequent in palliative care is malabsorptive diarrhoea secondary to pancreatic insufficiency, partial gastrectomy or ileal resection. Colonic resection rarely gives prolonged diarrhoea. Iatrogenic diarrhoea may be caused by pelvic irradiation or a variety of drugs other than laxatives, including antibiotics, nonsteroidal anti-inflammatory drugs, cytotoxics, diuretics, antacids and disaccharide-containing elixirs.

As in the population as a whole, diarrhoea may arise from intestinal infections. These may be viral, but in ill patients are probably more likely to be bacterial. *Clostridium difficile*, pathogenic *Escherichia coli* and *Salmonella* occur, but so do anaerobes, which are more difficult to isolate. The last are more common in bowel damaged by surgery or tumour.

ASSESSMENT

The fundamental distinction is between diarrhoea and the leakage of liquid stool past a faecal impaction. Most impactions are rectal and will be revealed by rectal examination. A history of 'diarrhoea' occurring after a period of constipation and characterized more by incontinence than urgency is suggestive.

Pale, offensive-smelling, buoyant stools reflect pancreatic insufficiency. Any diarrhoea lasting more than about 72 hours merits a stool specimen for culture and antimicrobial sensitivities.

MANAGEMENT

Although intravenous rehydration and electrolyte replacement might be needed, encouragement of oral fluid intake (especially fruit juices and salty soups) can

Table 4.6.1 Specific treatments for diarrhoea

Fat malabsorption	Pancreatin (give with H2 antagonist)
Radiation-induced diarrhoea	Aspirin
Pseudomembranous colitis	Vancomycin *or* metronidazole

usually satisfactorily accomplish the same result. A carbohydrate source, such as biscuits, bread or pasta, should also be provided.

Some specific anti-diarrhoeal therapies are listed in Table 4.6.1. A trial of metronidazole could also be considered for persistent diarrhoea for which no cause has been identified.

The most effective general treatments are based on opioids.

Approximate equivalent anti-diarrhoeal doses are 200 mg/day of codeine, 10 mg/day of diphenoxylate and 4 mg/day of loperamide.[7] Trials show loperamide to be more effective and have fewer adverse effects than either diphenoxylate or codeine.[8] However, codeine is cheaper and, idiosyncratically, may sometimes work better and be well tolerated.

KEY POINTS FOR MANAGING DIARRHOEA

- Distinguish between diarrhoea and overflow.
- Remember the possible role of drugs, especially laxatives.
- Identify malabsorption and treat.
- Consider the possibility of bacterial infection.
- Supportive therapy is important:
  fruit juices and salty, savoury drinks provide fluid and electrolytes,
  bread, savoury biscuits and pasta are sources of carbohydrate,
  intravenous fluid and electrolyte replacement is only occasionally necessary.
- Codeine is the cheapest effective general treatment, but loperamide has fewer systemic effects.

REFERENCES

1. Sykes NP. The relationship between opioid use and laxative use in terminally ill cancer patients. *Palliat Med* 1998; **12**, 375–82.
2. Radbruch L, Sabatowski R, Loick G *et al*. Constipation and the use of laxatives: a comparison between transdermal fentanyl and oral morphine. *Palliat Med* 2000; **14**, 111–19.
3. Petticrew M, Watt I, Sheldon T. Systematic review of the effectiveness of laxatives in the elderly. *Health Technol Assess* 1997; **1**, 1–52.
4. Sykes NP. A volunteer model for the comparison of laxatives in opioid-induced constipation. *J Pain Symptom Manage* 1997; **11**, 363–9.

5. NHS Centre for Reviews and Dissemination. Effectiveness of laxatives in adults. *Effective Health Care* 2001; 7(1), 1–12.
6. Culbert P, Gillett H, Ferguson A. Highly effective new oral therapy for faecal impaction. *Br J Gen Pract* 1998; **48**, 1599–600.
7. Twycross RG, Lack SA. Diarrhoea. In: *Control of alimentary symptoms in far advanced cancer.* London: Churchill Livingstone, 1986, 208–29.
8. Palmer KR, Corbett CL, Holdsworth CD. Double-blind cross-over study comparing loperamide, codeine and diphenoxylate in the treatment of chronic diarrhoea. *Gastroenterology* 1980; **79**, 1272–5.

FURTHER READING

Mancini I, Bruera E. Constipation. In: Ripamonti C, Bruera E (eds), *Gastrointestinal symptoms in advanced cancer patients.* Oxford: Oxford University Press, 2002, 193–206.
Mercadante S. Diarrhea, malabsorption. In: Ripamonti C, Bruera E (eds), *Gastrointestinal symptoms in advanced cancer patients.* Oxford: Oxford University Press, 2002, 207–22.
Sykes NP. Constipation and diarrhoea. In: Doyle D, Hanks G, Cherny N, Calman K (eds), *Oxford textbook of palliative medicine*, 3rd edn. Oxford: Oxford University Press, 2004, 483–96.

COUGH

Polly Edmonds

DEFINITION

Cough has been defined as 'to expel air from the lungs with a sudden sharp sound to remove an obstruction or congestion'.[1]

PREVALENCE

Cough is a common symptom, accounting for up to 50 per cent of consultations with general practitioners, and reported in between 29 and 83 per cent of palliative care patients.[2] It is frequently associated with breathlessness, syncope and vomiting.

PATHOPHYSIOLOGY

Cough is a normal mechanism for maintaining airway patency and cleanliness. It enables the ciliated airways to bring mucus, fluid and inhaled foreign bodies up to the larynx, where they can be expelled into the pharynx and either swallowed or spat out.

Sensory nerves in the pharynx, larynx and upper airways join the vagus nerve; mediation of the cough reflex is thought to occur in the 'cough centre' in the medulla. Important receptors in the mediation of cough are 5-hydroxytryptamine-1A (5HT-1A) and the opioid receptors mu-2 and kappa.[3]

INVESTIGATIONS AND EXAMINATION

HISTORY

Several factors in the history may be useful in the assessment of chronic cough:

- association with sputum production,
- sputum quality
  mucoid in chronic bronchitis

purulent in infection
thick/viscid and difficult to expectorate,

- occurrence, e.g. posture-related, paroxysmal, nocturnal,

- associated neuromuscular problems, e.g. bulbar palsy in motor neurone disease,

- effects of medication,

- drugs, e.g. angiotensin-converting enzyme (ACE) inhibitors,

- heartburn or regurgitation suggestive of oesophageal reflux,

- history of asthma or chronic obstructive pulmonary disease (COPD).

EXAMINATION

Features contributing to cough may be evident on examination, e.g. lobar collapse suggestive of a central tumour.

INVESTIGATION OF CHRONIC COUGH

Investigations that may alter management include:

- sputum microscopy and culture to exclude infection,

- chest X-ray (CXR) – infection, heart failure, primary or secondary lung malignancy, mediastinal nodes, effusion,

- computerized tomography (CT) of the thorax – as above,

- video fluoroscopy – to exclude bulbar palsy and aspiration,

- respiratory function tests – to assess airway obstruction.

MANAGEMENT

GENERAL MEASURES

Wherever possible, the management of cough should involve treating reversible underlying causes. Cough can be a very distressing symptom, and patients may be helped by:

- explanation of the cause(s),

- reassurance where appropriate,

- sedative medication at night if troubled by nocturnal cough,

- positioning, e.g. upright if aggravated by diaphragmatic irritation or oesophageal reflux.

SPECIFIC MEASURES

Table 4.7.1 outlines specific treatment strategies for cough.

Cough suppressants
- Simple linctus – useful for soothing the throat for a dry, irritating cough.

- Opioids:
   codeine, pholcodine and dihydrocodeine are all appropriate first-line opioids
   for managing cough, and all are available as an elixir;
   oral morphine preparations are useful where weak opioids are not effective
   or the patient has other indications for morphine, e.g. pain;
   methadone linctus (2 mg in 5 mL) is a strong opioid that is long acting and
   can therefore be used once or twice a day.

- Oral local anaesthetic lozenges – may be effective if cough is caused by an
   irritated pharynx.

Nebulized local anaesthetics
There are reports of the efficacy of nebulized lidocaine (lignocaine) (5 mL of 2 per
cent solution) and bupivacaine (5 mL of 0.25 per cent solution) in relieving cough,

Table 4.7.1 Management of cough by aetiology

Cause	Management strategy
Respiratory infection	Antibiotic
	Cough suppressant
	Expectorant, e.g. steam inhalation, nebulized saline
	Physiotherapy
Asthma/chronic obstructive pulmonary disease	Bronchodilators
	Corticosteroids
	Physiotherapy
Malignant airways obstruction	Cough suppressant
	Physiotherapy
	Nebulized local anaesthetics
Drug induced	Stop or change drug
	Cough suppressant
Oesophageal reflux	Upright position
	Antireflux agent
Aspiration of saliva	Anticholinergic (to reduce saliva volume)
	Mucolytic agent (to thin viscous sputum)
	Nebulized local anaesthetic

Adapted from Ahmedzai (1998).[2]

although the effect may be short lived.[4] Local anaesthetics will reduce the sensitivity of the gag reflex, so patients should be advised not to eat or drink for up to half an hour after the nebulizer to avoid the risk of inhalation. These agents can cause bronchospasm, so medical attention and bronchodilators should be available for the first dose.

Anticholinergic agents

Anticholinergic agents will thicken mucus, and may therefore be helpful where patient have a large volume of thin mucus. However, they will also reduce ciliary motion, thereby potentially making mucus more difficult to cough up.

Mucolytic agents

Anecdotal reports suggest that mucolytic agents, such as carbocisteine (Mucodyne) 750 mg t.d.s., can be helpful where patients are experiencing difficulties expectorating thick, viscous sputum. This author has found these agents to be particularly useful for patients with end-stage fibrotic lung disease and COPD.

Nebulized hypertonic saline may also be used to thin viscous sputum. Phosphorylated glycosylated recombinant human deoxyribonuclease 1 (rhDNase, Dornase Alfa) is used via a jet nebulizer (2500 units = 2.5 mg o.d.) in patients with cystic fibrosis as a mucolytic agent to improve pulmonary function.

The potential problem with the use of mucolytic agents is the production of copious liquid sputum that a weak patient is still not able to expectorate.

HAEMOPTYSIS

Haemoptysis is the coughing up of blood. It is important to differentiate haemoptysis from haematemesis (vomiting blood), and to exclude bleeding from the nose or oropharynx. Common causes of haemoptysis include: lung cancer, pulmonary embolism, pneumonia and bronchiectasis.

If haemoptysis persists despite appropriate treatment of the underlying cause, symptomatic treatment is warranted.

- Haemostatic agents, e.g. ethamsylate and tranexamic acid. There are no controlled trials of efficacy, but clinical use suggests benefit in mild to moderate haemoptysis.

- Radiotherapy – indicated for haemoptysis related to lung cancer, with response rates of up to 90 per cent reported for external beam therapy.[5]

- Endobronchial laser has been reported to be effective in controlling bleeding, and can be repeated.

KEY POINTS

- Cough is a common symptom.
- Opioids are effective cough suppressants.
- Nebulized local anaesthetics can be useful for persistent cough.

REFERENCES

1. *Oxford English dictionary.* Oxford: Oxford University Press, 1996.
2. Ahmedzai S. Palliation of respiratory symptoms – cough. In: Doyle D, Hanks G, MacDonald N (eds), *Oxford textbook of palliative medicine*, 2nd edn. Oxford: Oxford University Press, 1998, 602–4.
3. Kamei J. Mechanisms of central antitussives. *Nippon Yakurigaku Zasshi* 1998; **111**(6), 345–55.
4. Hansson L, Midgren B, Karlsson J-A. Effects of inhaled lignocaine and adrenaline on capsaicin-induced cough in humans. *Thorax* 1994; **49**, 1166–8.
5. Lung Cancer Working Party. Inoperable non-small cell lung cancer (NSCLC): a Medical Research Council randomised trial of palliative radiotherapy with two fractions or ten fractions. *Br J Cancer* 1991; **63**, 265–70.

chapter 4.8

DEPRESSION, SADNESS, HOPELESSNESS AND SUICIDE

Matthew Hotopf

DEFINITIONS – DEPRESSED OR SAD?

Clinicians in palliative care are frequently presented with patients who are low in mood, unmotivated and appear to have 'given up'. When confronted by such patients, it may be tempting to 'explain away' their symptoms as a natural reaction to advanced disease. Clearly, most people experiencing advanced disease will have spells of feeling sad about the many losses they face, and most especially their imminent loss of life. At what point does such sadness become the syndrome psychiatrists recognize as depression?

Psychiatric classifications[1,2] define depression as a syndrome of low mood, loss of enjoyment (anhedonia) and fatigue, with a number of characteristic additional features to do with biological functions (sleep, appetite and weight), and alterations in the content of thought (depressive thinking with thoughts of guilt, self-harm and hopelessness) and the form of thought (subjective memory disturbance, cognitive slowing, poor concentration and mental fatigability). The symptoms have to be present for at least 2 weeks, and not be in the context of a recent bereavement (Table 4.8.1).

There are obvious problems when applying such a definition in patients with advanced disease. First, some mood change is understandable. Second, some of the biological and cognitive symptoms of depression may be a direct consequence of physical disease. Various alternatives have been raised to deal with this problem. It has been argued that certain 'substitution' criteria can be used. Endicott proposed using a series of criteria whereby biological symptoms of depression are replaced with more mood-based symptoms (Table 4.8.2).[3] Other alternatives are to raise the diagnostic threshold for depression.[4] Finally, it has been argued that

Table 4.8.1 Diagnostic criteria for depression

DSM-IV Five or more symptoms in past 2 weeks	ICD-10 moderate depressive episode Two of first three symptoms, plus three of remainder for past 2 weeks
Persistent depressed mood	Low mood
Persistent decreased interest or pleasure	Loss of interest
Fatigue	Fatigue
Weight loss or gain	Disturbed appetite
Insomnia or hypersomnia	Disturbed sleep
Psychomotor agitation or depression	
Feelings of worthlessness or excessive guilt	Ideas of guilt or unworthiness
Diminished concentration or indecisiveness	Reduced concentration and attention
Recurrent thoughts of death, suicidal ideation or attempt	Ideas or acts of self-harm or suicide
	Bleak pessimistic view of future
	Reduced self-esteem and self-confidence

Table 4.8.2 Endicott substitution criteria for DSM-IV criteria for major depression

Conventional criteria		Substitution criteria
1. Change in appetite/weight	$\rightarrow$	Tearfulness, depressed appearance
2. Sleep disturbance	$\rightarrow$	Social withdrawal, decreased talkativeness
3. Fatigue/loss of energy	$\rightarrow$	Brooding self-pity, pessimism
4. Diminished concentration	$\rightarrow$	Lack of reactivity

depression is simply a syndrome – in other words, a collection of certain symptoms – and if patients have these symptoms, they have depression.[5]

In practice, depressive symptoms form a continuum – with at one end of the spectrum the most severe cases in whom depression may represent a life-threatening illness, and at the other end individuals with minor symptoms that blend into normality. The main reason for making the diagnosis of depression is to ensure that the patient receives adequate treatment and makes a recovery. Whilst the physical treatments described at the end of this chapter are undoubtedly effective in moderate or severe depression, it is much less clear whether they are useful for milder symptoms. The threshold at which treatments are associated with clear benefits is not known, even in patients whose depression is not associated with severe physical disease. Hence, when patients fall into the grey area where they may be troubled by a variety of depressive symptoms, which are not especially severe, the diagnosis of depression is not straightforward. It is often best under these circumstances to agree with the patient to treat his or her symptoms empirically, and keep an open mind.

CLINICAL ASSESSMENT AND DIAGNOSIS

HISTORY

The clinical assessment of a patient with depression requires time and patience. The interview is best conducted away from a busy ward. The content of the interview will depend to some extent on who is performing it. However, even if the patient is well known to the interviewer, it is worth considering how much is known about the patient's own *narrative* of his illness (see box below). It is extremely common to find that a withdrawn, depressed patient nurses a grievance about a perceived or real delay in diagnosis or believes that the intractable pain is an inevitable consequence of their diagnosis. Eliciting this history may in its own right be therapeutic. Many patients will have personal experience of witnessing a relative or friend die, and may have many preconceptions about the meaning of their illness. Such fears may be dispelled by a frank discussion with the clinical team.

A detailed family and personal history is helpful to understand the patient's previous life, sources of support and reactions to past crises. The technique of developing a life chart dealing with important biographical details may be helpful to both the patient and clinician. The patient's description of past crises (such as bereavements and other serious life events) is often very helpful in gaining an understanding of the techniques he or she has used in the past to cope. An account of interpersonal relationships is vital in assessing the depressed patient – in particular the quality of any marital relationship, and the reaction of close members of the family to the diagnosis. It is always important to determine in whom the patient has been able to confide fears about the illness.

Key questions in a patient's narrative of illness

- How did you first know you were ill?
- What did you think was the problem?
- How long was it before you were given the diagnosis?
- How did you react to the diagnosis?
- (If appropriate) Did you feel that your symptoms were not taken seriously early on?
- When did you realize that your illness was not going to get better?
- How did you discover this?
- How did you react when you realized this?

Having developed an understanding of the patient's reaction to his or her physical illness, it is much easier to ask about psychological symptoms. It is useful to acknowledge how difficult things must have been, and to ask directly about low mood. Special emphasis should be placed on the *reactivity* of mood and *anhedonia*. Does the patient cheer up during the interview? Do activities he/she used to enjoy still bring pleasure? The biological symptoms of depression should not be dismissed. Whilst in many cases pain, fatigue and loss of appetite can be directly attributed to the advanced disease, this does not always follow – it is not uncommon to find patients whose pain or fatigue seems out of proportion with their disease status, or in whom conventional remedies do not work. In some cases these symptoms may be an indication of depression or anxiety.

EXAMINATION

The mental state examination starts with a description of appearance and behaviour, paying particular attention to evidence of self-neglect, psychomotor slowing, tearfulness and reactivity of mood. Some of the best evidence of depression may come from those who are caring for the patient on a day-to-day basis. Patients often complain of low mood, but are observed to brighten when they get visitors. Conversely, patients may deny depression but remain withdrawn at all times. The talk in depression is often slow and laborious, and there may be poverty of speech or even mutism. Patients with depression should always be asked about suicidal ideas or plans (see below). They should also be asked about psychotic symptoms, such as auditory hallucinations or delusional beliefs. Psychotic symptoms in depression are typically *mood congruent*, i.e. they make sense in terms of the mood of the patient (derogatory auditory hallucinations; delusions of poverty or guilt). The cognitive assessment is also important, as many elderly patients with depression present with *depressive pseudodementia* characterized by cognitive impairments related to mental slowing. Dementia may also present with depressive symptoms.

RECOGNITION OF DEPRESSION AND SCREENING FOR CASES

There is a wealth of literature from general practice suggesting that depression often goes unrecognized. The same applies to patients with depression in general hospitals and palliative care settings. Patients with depression often do not complain openly about their low mood, and it is important always to be sensitive to the possibility that a patient may have depression. Case-finding questionnaires have been used in palliative care settings,[6,7] but many patients who are very frail will not be able to complete such questionnaires, and there is some evidence that simply asking patients 'Have you been depressed most of the time in the last 2 weeks?' is a sensitive and specific means of identifying cases.[8]

Apart from overt low mood, there are a number of typical presentations of depression in palliative care:

- 'giving up' – the patient becomes withdrawn, apathetic and unco-operative with treatment plans,

- cognitive impairment – depressive pseudodementia,

- anger and irritability,

- complaints of intractable pain, fatigue or other symptoms, which seem out of proportion to what would be expected.

Table 4.8.3 'Silent' presentations of depression

Endocrine: hypercalcaemia, hypothyroidism, Cushing's syndrome, hypoglycaemia
Infective: AIDS, syphilis, encephalitis
Neurological: cerebral space-occupying lesion, Parkinson's disease, chronic subdural haematoma,
  cerebral ischaemia
Drugs: steroids, beta-blockers, L-dopa, digoxin, diuretics
Alcohol
Dementias

DIFFERENTIAL DIAGNOSIS OF DEPRESSION

There are several medical conditions that are easy to overlook and can present with classical symptoms of depression (Table 4.8.3). Such conditions are common in patients with advanced disease, and endocrine disorders and drugs should always be considered, as they may be very easily remedied. Other psychiatric diagnoses should be distinguished from depression. In withdrawn elderly patients with poor self-care, the most relevant differential diagnosis is dementia, which, like depression, often goes unrecognized. Medical teams will usually be aware of pre-existing psychotic illness. Anxiety states overlap considerably with depression, but distinguishing one from the other is often of limited clinical importance as their management may be very similar.

PREVALENCE OF DEPRESSION IN ADVANCED DISEASE

How common is depression in advanced disease? A recent systematic review suggested the simple answer to this question is 'very'.[9] Studies that simply ask about depression as a symptom find as many as 40 per cent of patients endorsing the symptom, with 93 per cent judged to have some degree of psychological distress.[10] Other studies that have used questionnaires such as the Hospital Anxiety and Depression Scale[6] find rates of patients scoring above threshold of between 16 and 50 per cent.[11,12]

Studies that use more robust psychiatric interviews to make operationally defined diagnoses of depression have found up to one-third of patients with advanced disease suffer from depression. One of the best studies applied several definitions of depression to 130 hospice patients, and found the prevalence of major depression to be 8 per cent, with a further 5 per cent suffering from minor depression.[4] When the threshold was lowered, this increased to 26 per cent for all depressions. Similar results have also been shown elsewhere in palliative care patients.[13]

IMPACT AND PROGNOSIS OF DEPRESSION

We have seen that depression is common, and readily missed. Why recognize it? There are very few studies of prognosis of depression in patients with advanced

A–Z OF SYMPTOMS

disease, but in one study it was the most persistent of a number of different physical and psychological symptoms.[10] Depression may have a range of consequences in the context of advanced disease.

PHYSICAL CONSEQUENCES

Patients with depression in the absence of physical illness are more sensitive to bodily sensations and invariably report more pain, fatigue and other common symptoms.[14] In advanced disease, patients with depression often appear to have intractable pain, which may not respond adequately to conventional strategies. Depression may also affect compliance with medical treatment, and there is a growing body of research indicating that patients with depression in the context of serious disease may have a shorter life expectancy.[15,16]

PSYCHOSOCIAL CONSEQUENCES

Apart from the obviously unpleasant nature of depressive symptoms, they may also cause profound difficulties with other aspects of the patient's psychological and social worlds. People with depression are less able to communicate with close family members and this may impede not only their adaptation to their illness, but also that of their family – in turn possibly leading to more complicated bereavement. Depression may reduce the ability of the patient and his or her family to cope with the final illness, and it is likely – though it has not been demonstrated – that patients with depression are more likely to die in a hospice or hospital than at home.

ECONOMIC CONSEQUENCES

For all these reasons, depression may significantly increase the costs of caring for patients with advanced disease. Patients with depression consume many more resources, both for the treatment of the depression itself and for the treatment of their physical ailments. Given that depression increases symptoms and may worsen physical outcome, this is not necessarily surprising. There is some evidence that treating depression in patients with physical illness reduces the costs associated with their physical care.[17]

MANAGEMENT OF DEPRESSION

A number of obstacles confront the successful management of depression in patients with advanced disease: time is often short; the physical condition of patients may alter rapidly, making it difficult to assess change; and there is very little adequate research evidence for interventions. This means that clinical practice often has to be informed by knowledge from other patients without physical disease. Hence the number of randomized trials of treatments for depression in this group is small.[18]

A–Z OF SYMPTOMS

PHARMACOLOGICAL APPROACHES

Antidepressants

Antidepressants are the mainstay of the pharmacological management of depression. Tricyclics and selective serotonin reuptake inhibitors (SSRIs) are the two main groups in common use and are described in more detail below. The antidepressants all act to increase the availability of central monoamines in the synapse, mainly by blocking reuptake into the presynaptic neurone. The antidepressants all take 2 weeks to start having an effect on mood, but their side effects are usually experienced much sooner. It is therefore important to explain this to patients. Some side effects, such as sedation, may be useful in agitated depression, and in these cases sleep and anxiety may improve earlier. Overall, antidepressants are effective in approximately 60–70 per cent of patients, as opposed to remission rates on placebo of 30–40 per cent. Systematic review evidence indicates that this sort of effect size also applies to patients with physical disease.[19]

Tricyclic antidepressants

These drugs have a wide range of pharmacological actions and block both noradrenaline and serotonin reuptake. They have anticholinergic actions, causing dry mouth, blurred vision, constipation and delirium. The anticholinergic side effects rule out their use in patients with narrow angle glaucoma and prostatic symptoms. They have alpha$_1$-adrenoreceptor blocking effects leading to postural hypotension. Some tricyclics are sedating (dosulepin [dothiepin], amitriptyline) due to antihistaminergic effects. They also have a quinidine-like action on the heart, and should be avoided in patients with conduction defects such as heart block. With the exception of lofepramine, they are cardiotoxic in overdose.

These features have made tricyclics an increasingly unpopular choice, especially in frail patients with severe physical disease. Nonetheless, they still have an important role in the treatment of patients with advanced disease. Despite all their side effects, they are surprisingly well tolerated in the majority of patients. A systematic review of discontinuation rates from randomized trials indicated patients given tricyclics as opposed to SSRIs were only about 10 per cent more likely to drop out from treatment.[20] The SSRIs (see below) cause nausea, a side effect that is less common in tricyclics. As many patients with advanced disease have experienced chemotherapy, they are often highly sensitive to this side effect. Also, tricyclics are effective adjuvant analgesics and are more effective than SSRIs for the treatment of neuropathic pain.[21] Finally, the sedating side effects of some tricyclics may be welcomed in patients with agitated depression.

Patients should be prescribed tricyclics in low doses to start (25 mg), especially if they are frail. Doses can be built up over the first 2 weeks, titrating against any side effects. In frail or cachectic patients or those with impaired liver function, the usual advice to aim for a dose of 150 mg is unreasonable. It is better to gain a level the patient can readily tolerate. The plasma levels of some antidepressants can be monitored to check that the therapeutic range has been achieved.

Selective serotonin reuptake inhibitors

The SSRIs include fluoxetine, sertraline, fluvoxamine, citalopram and paroxetine. As the name implies, they are selective blockers of the reuptake of serotonin and

A–Z OF SYMPTOMS

are considerably 'cleaner' drugs than the tricyclics. They are probably as effective and slightly better tolerated. They have the major advantage of being safe in overdose. The main side effects are nausea, diarrhoea, agitation and insomnia. Sexual dysfunction may occur, and a small proportion of patients develop an idiosyncratic adverse drug reaction. Fluoxetine has a prolonged half-life, which makes it a less attractive option in patients with advanced disease. The SSRIs may theoretically interact with other drugs using the P450 cytochrome system, although reports of confirmed interactions are scarce. Sertraline and citalopram are probably the safest in this regard.

Psychostimulants

The psychostimulants (methylphenidate, dexamphetamine and pemoline) have been used in the management of depression in advanced disease, especially in North America. Their advantages are said to be their rapid action and effectiveness against severe psychomotor slowing and fatigue. Good-quality randomized controlled trials into their efficacy are lacking, but they have their enthusiasts. The treatment should be given in the morning to avoid causing sleep disturbance at night. Other side effects include nervousness, raised blood pressure, motor tics, dyskinesias and psychotic symptoms.

Lithium

Lithium carbonate is widely used in psychiatric practice as a mood stabilizer for bipolar affective disorder. Its other main use is to augment antidepressants in the management of treatment-resistant depression. It is one of very few treatments that have been demonstrated to help when patients have resistant depression. Lithium has a narrow therapeutic index, making it a drug for the specialist.

Electroconvulsive therapy

Electroconvulsive therapy (ECT) is sometimes appropriate in advanced disease. Before the SSRIs were available, it was often described as a safe alternative to pharmacotherapy, and is generally safe and well tolerated. It is indicated in patients with severe depression that is life threatening (for example due to extreme suicidal risk, or when the patient is not consuming sufficient fluids).

PSYCHOLOGICAL APPROACHES

A comprehensive summary of the main psychological treatments for depression is outside the scope of this chapter. A range of psychotherapeutic treatments may be helpful in patients with advanced disease, but very few have been evaluated specifically in this group. Therapies range from non-directive approaches that attempt to explore and clarify feelings, through to structured therapies such as cognitive behavioural therapy (CBT). There is some work that suggests that approaches informed by CBT are helpful in patients with depression and early cancer.[22] A few trials have shown that group therapies may be helpful in patients with physical disease,[23,24] but it is unclear from these whether it is the social support offered by the group or specific active ingredients of the intervention that are important.

The following section describes some useful psychotherapeutic techniques that all clinicians may use when managing patients with depression.

A–Z OF SYMPTOMS

Listening, understanding and clarifying

These skills are key to all psychotherapies as well as most routine clinical practice. The first role of the clinician is to engage the patient and, to do this, it is necessary to make sure he or she feels understood. Patients are often profoundly relieved to disclose painful emotions of which they may feel ashamed, and it is helpful to reassure patients about the nature of their symptoms.

Education

Many patients with depression or anxiety may think they are 'going mad' or 'losing my mind', and it is helpful to break their distress into its component symptoms, and to label these. Reassurance in these circumstances is often helpful. Although clinicians frequently think that patients are fully aware of their physical disease diagnosis and its implications, the patient may not have understood everything he or she has been told, or may have denied its full implications. Being aware of these gaps in understanding is an important aspect of clinical care.

Problem solving

'Problem solving' has been successfully used as a treatment for depression.[25] The technique involves identifying the full range of problems, choosing those that may be soluble, brainstorming solutions, and setting goals based on these solutions. For example, patients with advanced disease may have a range of 'unfinished business' such as making their will, discussing their diagnosis with close friends and so on, which they may feel unable to confront. In problem solving, the therapist works with the patient to identify a specific problem that could be tackled. The therapist then encourages the patient to generate as many possible solutions to the problem as possible, and to choose one solution that seems achievable. The patient is then left to complete the task, which is later reviewed. The active ingredient of this approach is probably not tackling the problem per se, but making the patient feel more in control.

Facilitating communication in couples and families

Communication difficulties are key to many of the psychological problems that present in palliative care settings.[26] Patients may try to protect their families from their own emotions. In turn, their partners may fear to discuss painful emotions lest they upset them. In practice, airing such feelings is usually very helpful, and seeing patients with their families is often a powerful tool in managing depression in palliative care settings.

Managing anger appropriately

Many patients with advanced disease have a powerful and often undisclosed sense of grievance. This may be a general grievance about the injustice of their predicament ('why me?') or a more specific grievance about aspects of their care. Psychodynamic understandings of depression often emphasize the importance of anger, and view depression as anger turned inwards. When such anger is not explicit, it may lead to problems in communication between patients and their carers. It is important under these circumstances to tackle anger openly, both with the patient and with other staff who may have become exasperated and feel their efforts to help the patient have been rejected or denigrated.

SOCIAL CARE

Social care is difficult to define, but covers a range of interventions whereby the patient's social circumstances may be improved. These include basic social work, such as helping to improve housing circumstances. Other facilities that provide supportive networks for patients, such as day hospitals, may be very helpful.

SPIRITUAL CARE

For patients with religious convictions, it may be helpful to explore their need for spiritual support, and to suggest contact with chaplains or other spiritual leaders.

ASSESSMENT OF DELIBERATE SELF-HARM AND THREATS OF SUICIDE

Many patients with advanced disease will have had thoughts that their lives are not worth living, and some make more direct statements about suicidal intent. These are best thought of as a spectrum, from thinking life is not worth living, to a sense that one would be better off dead, to actively planning suicide. Such thoughts usually have to be elicited with direct questions. A high proportion of patients with depression will have suicidal ideas, and may be greatly relieved by discussing them. As with any sensitive subject, it is important to approach the discussion of suicide from an unthreatening general perspective, and to ask gradually more specific questions.

A–Z OF SYMPTOMS

Suitable questions to ask about suicidal intent

- It sounds as though you've been feeling pretty low lately. Do you feel hopeless?
- Is life worth living?
- Do you go to sleep at night wishing you weren't going to wake up?
- Have you had any thoughts of harming yourself?
- What sort of things have you thought about doing to harm yourself?
- How often do you have these sorts of thoughts?
- How close have you come to acting on them?
- What has stopped you from acting on these thoughts?

What should be done when suicidal ideas have been uncovered? A high proportion of patients with depression will report fleeting feelings that they might be better off dead. If the patient has recently made a suicide attempt, or has persistent powerful thoughts that are accompanied by a plan, it is reasonable to consider hospital admission in order to provide a safe environment. The clinician is then left with the dilemma as to whether to admit to a psychiatric unit, hospice or even general hospital.

Many patients with advanced disease have considered euthanasia or physician-assisted suicide,[27,28] and a few request it. To many patients who have a life-shortening diagnosis, but who may be many months or even years from dying, euthanasia is a comforting possibility that allows them to maintain a sense of control over a destiny that is seen as terrifying. Requests for euthanasia or physician-assisted suicide should be explored in a similar way to threats of suicide. It is particularly important to assess what patients have considered doing and whether this is driven by their appreciation of their current predicament or is more a reflection of their fears of what might become of them. Patients who desire death are considerably more likely to have a depressive illness, and this should be actively treated when found.

CONCLUSION

Depression is a common clinical problem in patients with advanced disease. It is frequently missed, and this may have wide-ranging physical and psychological consequences. Early recognition and treatment should be the aim.

KEY POINTS

- Depression in palliative care settings is common, with a prevalence of at least 15 per cent.
- Depression is frequently not detected, or detected too late in the course of illness.
- Depression is associated with a number of adverse outcomes, including suicide, reduced will to live, disability, and poor symptom control.
- A range of approaches, including pharmacological, psychotherapeutic, social and spiritual, may be helpful for depressed patients in palliative care settings, although research evidence of effectiveness is very limited.

REFERENCES

1. World Health Organisation. *The tenth revision of the International Classification of Diseases and Related Health Problems (ICD-10)*. Geneva: World Health Organisation, 1992.
2. American Psychiatric Association. *Diagnostic and statistical manual of mental disorders: DSM IV*, IVth edn. Washington DC: APA, 1994.
3. Endicott J. Measurement of depression in patients with cancer. *Cancer* 1984; 53(Suppl.), 2243–8.
4. Chochinov HM, Wilson KG, Enns M, Lander S. Prevalence of depression in the terminally ill: effects of diagnostic criteria and symptom threshold judgements. *Am J Psychiatry* 1994; **151**, 537–40.
5. House A. Mood disorders in the physically ill – problems of definition and measurement. *J Psychosom Res* 1988; **32**, 345–53.

6. Zigmond AS, Snaith RP. The Hospital Anxiety and Depression Scale. *Acta Psychiatr Scand* 1983; **67**, 361–70.

7. Beck AT, Ward CH, Mendelson M. An inventory for measuring depression. *Arch Gen Psychiatry* 1961; **4**, 561–71.

8. Chochinov HM, Wilson KG. 'Are you depressed?' Screening for depression in the terminally ill: reply. *Am J Psychiatry* 1998; **155**, 994–5.

9. Hotopf M, Ly KL, Chidgey J, Addington Hall J. Depression in advanced disease – a systematic review: 1 Prevalence and case finding. *Palliat Med* 2002; **16**, 81–97.

10. Edmonds PM, Stuttaford JM, Peny J, Lynch AM, Chamberlain J. Do hospital palliative care teams improve symptom control? Use of a modified STAS as an evaluation tool. *Palliat Med* 1998; **12**, 345–51.

11. Faull CM, Johnson IS, Butler TJ. The Hospital Anxiety and Depression (HAD) Scale: its validity in patients with terminal malignant disease. *Palliat Med* 1994; **8**, 69.

12. Fulton CL. The physical and psychological symptoms experienced by patients with metastatic breast cancer before death. *Eur J Cancer Care (English Language Edition)* 1997; **6**, 262–6.

13. Power D, Kelly S, Gilsenan J et al. Suitable screening tests for cognitive impairment and depression in the terminally ill – a prospective prevalence study. *Palliat Med* 1993; **7**, 213–18.

14. Hotopf M, Mayou R, Wadsworth MEJ, Wessely S. Temporal relationships between physical symptoms and psychiatric disorder. Results from a national birth cohort. *Br J Psychiatry* 1998; **173**, 255–61.

15. Frasure-Smith N, Lesperance F, Talajic M. Depression following myocardial infarction: impact on 6-month survival. *JAMA* 1993; **270**, 1819–25.

16. Watson M, Haviland JS, Greer S, Davidson J, Bliss JM. Influence of psychological response on survival in breast cancer: a population-based case control study. *Lancet* 1999; **354**, 1331–6.

17. Thompson D, Hylan TR, McMullen W, Romeis ME, Buesching D, Oster G. Predictors of a medical-offset effect among patients receiving antidepressant therapy. *Am J Psychiatry* 1998; **155**, 824–7.

18. Ly KL, Chidgey J, Addington Hall J, Hotopf M. Depression in palliative care – a systematic review: 2 Treatment. *Palliat Med* 2002; **16**, 279–84.

19. Gill D, Hatcher S. A systematic review of the treatment of depression with antidepressant drugs in patients who also have a physical illness. *J Psychosom Res* 2000; **47**, 131–43.

20. Hotopf M, Hardy R, Lewis G. Discontinuation rates of SSRIs and tricyclic antidepressants: a meta-analysis and investigation of heterogeneity. *Br J Psychiatry* 1997; **170**, 120–7.

21. McQuay HJ, Tramer M, Nye BA, Carroll D, Wiffen PJ, Moore RA. A systematic review of antidepressants in neuropathic pain. *Pain* 1996; **68**, 217–27.

22. Greer S, Moorey S, Baruch J. Evaluation of adjuvant psychological therapy for clinically referred cancer patients. *Br J Cancer* 1991; **63**, 257–60.

23. Evans RL, Connis RT. Comparison of brief group therapies for depressed cancer patients receiving radiation treatment. *Public Health Rep* 1995; **110**, 306–11.

24. Larcombe NA, Wilson PH. An evaluation of cognitive–behaviour therapy for depression in patients with multiple sclerosis. *Br J Psychiatry* 1984; **145**, 366–71.

A–Z OF SYMPTOMS

25. Mynors-Wallis LM, Gath GH, Lloyd-Thomas AR, and Tomlinson D. Randomised controlled trial comparing problem-solving treatment with amitriptyline and placebo for major depression in primary care. *BMJ* 1995; **310**, 441 5.

26. Stedeford A. Psychotherapy of the dying patient. *Br J Psychiatry* 1979; **135**, 7–14.

27. Breitbart W, Rosenfeld BD, Passik SD. Interest in physician-assisted suicide among ambulatory HIV-infected patients. *Am J Psychiatry* 1996; **153**, 238–42.

28. Chochinov HM, Wilson KG, Enns M *et al*. Desire for death in the terminally ill. *Am J Psychiatry* 1995; **152**, 1185–91.

DROWSINESS AND FATIGUE

Patrick Stone

DEFINITIONS

Drowsiness may be defined as a feeling of sleepiness or diminished wakefulness. It is a sensation that most people experience on a regular basis and when it occurs in context (e.g. at the end of a long day) it is not usually regarded as a problem. When it becomes excessive or when it impacts on individuals' quality of life, it should be regarded as a 'symptom'.

The term 'fatigue' can be used to refer to both a subjective sensation and an objective decrease in physical performance. These two meanings need to be clearly distinguished. Subjective fatigue is a sensation of feeling easily tired, lacking energy or being exhausted. Objective fatigue is a decrease in performance with repeated or prolonged activity, for instance a loss of muscle strength with repeated muscular contractions or a diminution in attention with prolonged concentration.

Cella and co-workers have lamented the fact that most researchers have not distinguished between the symptom of fatigue (which is common to a host of medical and physical illnesses) and the syndrome of 'cancer-related fatigue'. They have produced draft diagnostic criteria for the diagnosis of cancer-related fatigue and have piloted the use of a fatigue diagnostic interview.[1,2] The concept of producing diagnostic criteria for cancer-related fatigue is an attractive one, as it would allow investigators to agree on what constitutes a 'case' of fatigue. However, in the absence of any widely accepted definition of what constitutes a *case*, this chapter focuses on the prevalence, pathophysiology and management of the *symptoms* of drowsiness and fatigue respectively.

PREVALENCE

Uncontrolled studies among patients with advanced cancer have reported a prevalence of fatigue of 33–89 per cent.[3–9] Fatigue is also a common complaint among the general population. Thus it is difficult to interpret fatigue prevalence figures for advanced cancer patients without reference to the background level of fatigue pre-existing in the community. One study has reported that the prevalence of 'severe fatigue' among patients with advanced cancer was 78 per cent, whereas the corresponding figure for elderly adults without cancer was 5 per cent.[10] Similar controlled studies to determine accurately the prevalence of drowsiness among patients with advanced cancer have not yet been undertaken.

PATHOPHYSIOLOGY

Drowsiness and fatigue are usually multifactorial problems. It is rare to identify a single cause for either symptom. One way in which to categorize the causes of these symptoms is to divide them into disease-related factors, patient-related factors and treatment-related factors.

DISEASE-RELATED FACTORS

- *Tumour type.* Certain types of cancer are more likely to be associated with fatigue or drowsiness. For example, higher levels of fatigue have been reported among patients with non-small cell lung cancer than among patients with gynaecological malignancies.[11] Primary or secondary brain tumours are often associated with increased drowsiness due to their anatomical position.

- *Stage of disease.* Patients with advanced cancers generally complain of greater fatigue than patients with localized disease.[11,12] The pre-terminal phase is often associated with a period of increased drowsiness leading to stupor or coma.[7,13]

- *Inter-current medical problems.* Patients with advanced cancer are at risk of developing inter-current medical problems as a result of their disease. Many of these problems can cause drowsiness or fatigue in their own right (e.g. pneumonia, urinary tract infection, steroid-induced diabetes, renal failure, liver failure, heart failure). Patients may also have medical problems unrelated to their primary cancer (e.g. multiple sclerosis, rheumatoid arthritis or chronic fatigue syndrome) and these in turn may lead to fatigue.

- *Anaemia.* Some degree of anaemia is a frequent finding among patients with advanced cancer. However, the correlation between fatigue severity and haemoglobin concentration among such patients is relatively weak.[12] It may be that fatigue severity is more related to the rate and size of the change in haematocrit than to the haemoglobin level per se. In support of this, a large study (n = 2289) of the use of erythropoietin for treating anaemia in cancer patients receiving chemotherapy reported that quality of life improvement (including fatigue) was significantly related to the size of the increase in haemoglobin concentration.[14]

- *Biochemical abnormalities.* A number of biochemical abnormalities can be associated with symptoms of drowsiness or fatigue (e.g. hypercalcaemia, hypomagnesaemia). Impaired renal or liver function can also aggravate drowsiness by reducing the metabolism of sedative drugs.

- *Hormonal abnormalities.* Cancer treatments can result in ovarian dysfunction and premature menopause, which can in turn lead to fatigue. A similar pattern has been reported in patients with prostate cancer receiving hormone therapy.[15] Adrenal metastases or abrupt steroid withdrawal can lead to hypoadrenalism and consequent fatigue.

PATIENT-RELATED FACTORS

- *Depression.* Fatigue and disordered sleep are cardinal features of a major depressive illness. All three are common in patients with advanced cancer.[10,16,17] However, this does not necessarily imply that cancer-related fatigue is 'caused' by depression. Not all patients with fatigue are depressed, and vice versa. Furthermore, depression and fatigue do not always vary together. One study has reported that whereas fatigue tended to increase after radiotherapy treatment, depression tended to decrease.[18] The precise nature of the association between these two constructs still needs to be defined.

- *Sleep disorders.* Patients with cancer suffer from disruption to both the quantity and the quality of their sleep, but may not always report the full extent of their difficulties.[16] Disturbed sleep may be an important cause of drowsiness and fatigue in patients undergoing chemotherapy.[19]

- *The severity of other symptoms.* Pain, dyspnoea and nausea/vomiting are all associated with higher levels of fatigue.[12,20] It is possible that patients with uncontrolled symptoms suffer from disturbed sleep and that this in turn leads to drowsiness and fatigue. Another possibility is that fatigue and drowsiness are caused by the use of sedative drugs to treat the co-existing pain, nausea or dyspnoea.

- *Cachexia.* Patients with cancer cachexia lose muscle protein and body fat. Loss of muscle bulk eventually leads to decreased strength and easy fatigue. Thus, one would expect that cachectic patients would experience more fatigue.[21] However, the correlation between fatigue severity and cachexia among a heterogeneous group (mixed diagnoses) of cancer patients was not found to be very strong.[12]

- *Immobility.* Even in otherwise healthy individuals, bed-rest can rapidly lead to loss of muscle bulk and physical de-conditioning. It has been postulated that physical de-conditioning, secondary to reduced mobility, may be a unifying explanation for the development of cancer-related fatigue in a number of different clinical situations.[22]

A–Z OF SYMPTOMS

TREATMENT-RELATED FACTORS

- *Anti-cancer therapies.* Fatigue is a frequent complication of radiotherapy,[23–25] chemotherapy[26,27] and hormone therapy.[15] Not all anti-cancer therapies cause fatigue. A study of palliative chemotherapy for non-small cell lung cancer, for instance, demonstrated a significant reduction in fatigue with cytotoxic treatment.[28] The mechanism by which particular treatments result in fatigue has not yet been identified, and is likely to be treatment specific. Drowsiness is less often reported as a side effect of cancer treatment. This is partly a consequence of the fact that the quality-of-life questionnaires that are commonly used in cancer clinical trials do not routinely contain questions about drowsiness.

- *Medication.* This is probably a common contributory factor to drowsiness and fatigue among patients with advanced cancer. Opioids, benzodiazepines, tricyclic antidepressants and phenothiazines are all commonly-used drugs with potentially sedating side effects.

INVESTIGATIONS AND EXAMINATION

Investigation of the problem should start with the taking of a thorough history. As with any symptom, attention should be paid to its onset, timing, duration, character, exacerbating or relieving factors and its impact on the individual. It is important to ascertain exactly what the patient means by fatigue or drowsiness. Fatigue that is associated with a low mood, feelings of worthlessness and guilt, or a history of previous psychiatric problems should alert one to the possibility of clinical depression. Where symptoms of drowsiness predominate, the interview should be directed more towards eliciting the therapeutic drug history or sleep pattern. Clinical examination should focus on excluding potentially reversible causes of fatigue or drowsiness.

For many patients, the taking of a thorough history, scrutiny of the drug chart and a physical examination are all that is required in order to reach an educated guess about the cause of the drowsiness or fatigue. For some patients, it will also be advisable to undertake a few simple screening tests. A full blood count and routine biochemistry will identify patients with anaemia, hypercalcaemia, renal or liver failure. In patients in whom drowsiness is predominant (particularly if associated with confusion), checking a midstream specimen of urine is advisable. Unless there are other reasons to suspect a specific remediable cause for the drowsiness or fatigue (e.g. cerebral metastases), there is probably little justification for routinely undertaking more complex investigations in patients with advanced disease.

MANAGEMENT

GENERAL MANAGEMENT

Before a patient is labelled as having cancer-related fatigue or drowsiness, it is important to be satisfied that easily treatable conditions have been excluded. An important place to start in this regard is with the patient's prescription chart. Each drug should be scrutinized and a decision made as to whether it could be omitted altogether or replaced by a less sedating alternative.

Since depression and fatigue are so closely linked, it is important that a diagnosis of depression is always entertained in a patient presenting with fatigue. If necessary, a therapeutic trial with an antidepressant should be considered.

Anaemia is a common finding among patients with advanced cancer and is commonly assumed to be a frequent cause of fatigue in this population. Blood transfusion has been reported to improve the symptom of 'weakness' in anaemic cancer patients,[29] but the effect is transient. As with all treatments, it is important to document the patient's symptomatic response and avoid transfusing again if there has been no improvement. For patients with earlier stage disease, or patients undergoing chemotherapy, erythropoietin may be an alternative to transfusion.[14,30-32]

Even after the appropriate management of reversible causes of fatigue or drowsiness, most patients will probably still not be symptom free. What options are available to treat this residual degree of cancer-related fatigue or drowsiness?

SPECIFIC MANAGEMENT

Non-pharmacological

It is important to be honest with patients about the lack of reliable evidence for the effectiveness of most interventions. Reassurance that no correctable cause for the condition has been identified and some general advice about a 'healthy' lifestyle can go a long way towards helping patients to cope with their fatigue.

Exercise   Exercise is probably one of the best-studied non-pharmacological interventions for cancer-related fatigue. Undertaking a brisk 30-minute walk three times per week has been shown to reduce fatigue significantly in patients with early-stage breast cancer undergoing postoperative radiotherapy.[33] Exercise has also been shown to prevent the development of fatigue among patients undergoing high-dose chemotherapy.[34] The largest study in this area has been conducted by Segal and co-workers,[35] who studied 123 patients with early-stage breast cancer who were undergoing adjuvant chemotherapy. They found that patients who participated in an exercise programme had better physical functioning at the end of the intervention than those patients who received usual care. However, the intervention did not result in improved quality of life or 'vitality'. The role of exercise in managing fatigued patients with advanced cancer is less clear. Porock has undertaken a small pilot study of an exercise intervention among palliative care patients.[36] Although the results of this study were encouraging, randomized controlled trials are needed to clarify the role of regular exercise in this population.

Diet   Many patients believe that their fatigue is a result of a poor diet and to a certain extent this may be true. If appropriate, simple advice about the constituents of a balanced diet or referral to a dietician may be necessary. However, for patients with advanced disease and progressive cachexia, it is not always helpful to dwell on the importance of nutritional intake, as this may simply lead to increased anxiety and distress.

A-Z OF SYMPTOMS

Improving sleep quality   Disturbed sleep is probably an important cause of day-time drowsiness among cancer patients. When specific causes for disrupted sleep are identified (e.g. pain, anxiety or depression), these should be treated appropriately. When no such causes are identified, improving sleep quality may be a matter of attending to sleep hygiene (e.g. maintaining a regular sleeping routine, limiting the amount of time spent in bed, creating a peaceful night-time environment, maintaining a suitable room temperature, avoiding unnecessary daytime naps and avoiding stimulants or excessive alcohol before bedtime).

Fatigue diary   It has been suggested that keeping a 'fatigue diary' (in which patients record the pattern and severity of their fatigue, along with the presence of aggravating and relieving factors) can be a therapeutic experience in itself.[26] The fatigue diary can help healthcare professionals identify lifestyle changes that may improve fatigue and can also be used to monitor the responsiveness of the patient's symptoms to any therapeutic interventions.

Pharmacological

Corticosteroids   Corticosteroids are almost certainly the most widely prescribed drugs for cancer-related fatigue. Their side effects are well documented. Evidence for their effectiveness in the management of cancer-related fatigue is lacking. There have been no randomized controlled studies in which fatigue has been a primary endpoint. One study has reported a transient (2-week) improvement in 'weakness' among female cancer patients given intravenous methylprednisolone,[37] whereas other studies have reported no such improvements. Indeed, an earlier study actually reported a higher mortality rate among female patients receiving corticosteroids than among patients receiving placebo.[38] In the light of this, it seems prudent to prescribe corticosteroids only as a therapeutic trial, and for a specified period of time. It is the author's current practice to prescribe dexamethasone 4 mg once/day for 5 days and then to review. Treatment should be stopped immediately if the patient shows no improvement. For responders, treatment should be continued at a lower dose and reviewed at regular intervals.

Psychostimulants   Psychostimulants (such as methylphenidate and dexamfetamine [dexamphetamine]) are central nervous system stimulants. As such, they have been investigated as potential treatments for drowsiness and fatigue in a variety of illnesses. Weinshenker and colleagues reported that pemoline provided good or excellent relief of fatigue in 46 per cent of patients with multiple sclerosis compared to 20 per cent of patients receiving placebo, although this difference failed to reach statistical significance ($p = 0.06$).[39] A later study similarly failed to find any benefit for pemoline over placebo in this patient population.[40] In contrast, Breitbart and colleagues reported that both pemoline and methylphenidate were superior to placebo for the treatment of fatigue associated with human immunodeficiency virus (HIV) disease.[41] There have been a few studies of the use of psychostimulants in cancer patients. Bruera and co-workers reported that methylphenidate (compared to placebo) increased 'activity levels' and decreased 'drowsiness' in patients ($n = 28$) with chronic cancer pain who were taking opioids.[42] Meyers and colleagues conducted an open-label study in 30 patients with primary brain tumours and reported that methylphenidate improved cognitive function, mood (including energy levels) and physical functioning.[43] Most recently, Sarhill and colleagues reported promising results (in terms of improved fatigue and drowsiness) with the use of methylphenidate in 11 patients with advanced cancer in an open-labelled, uncontrolled pilot study.[44] However, randomized controlled trials are needed to determine the proper place for these drugs in the management of fatigue and drowsiness in advanced cancer.

Progestational steroids Progestational steroids (such as medroxyprogesterone acetate and megestrol acetate) have demonstrated benefits in the management of cancer cachexia.[45,46] In short-term (7–10 days) placebo-controlled, cross-over studies, Bruera's group has also reported that megestrol acetate can improve 'energy' and 'activity levels'.[47,48] However, these improvements have not been confirmed in larger-scale, longer-term (4–12 weeks) studies.[45,46]

Antidepressants Given the close association that has been reported between the symptoms of depression and fatigue, one might expect that antidepressants would have a role to play in the alleviation of fatigue. Morrow and colleagues investigated this hypothesis in 549 fatigued cancer patients who were receiving chemotherapy.[49] They reported that although paroxetine was more effective than placebo at reducing depression, it was no more effective than placebo at reducing fatigue. Whether different antidepressants or different patient populations would result in a better outcome still needs to be evaluated.

FUTURE DEVELOPMENTS

Relatively little research has been undertaken to assess the effectiveness of clinical interventions for drowsiness or fatigue. Aerobic exercise has been shown to have a limited role in the management of fatigue in patients with early-stage cancers undergoing radiotherapy or chemotherapy. Questions remain about the precise form that this exercise should take, which patients stand to benefit most, and how long the effectiveness of the intervention lasts. Corticosteroids, the most widely prescribed drugs for cancer-related fatigue, have not yet been adequately evaluated. It will be important for future research to determine whether any benefits that these drugs might have are outweighed by the potentially serious side effects. Studies are also required to determine the underlying pathophysiology of cancer-related fatigue and drowsiness, since this will inform the development of new and more 'targeted' treatment strategies.

A–Z OF SYMPTOMS

KEY POINTS

- Fatigue and drowsiness are common problems in patients with advanced cancer.
- Management should focus on identifying treatable causes for these symptoms.
- Aerobic exercise can help in the management of fatigue in patients with early-stage disease.
- The role of other interventions still needs to defined.

REFERENCES

1. Cella D, Peterman A, Passik S, Jacobsen P, Breitbart W. Progress toward guidelines for the management of fatigue. *Oncology (Huntington)* 1998; **12**(11A), 369–77.
2. Cella D, Davis K, Breitbart W, Curt G, The Fatigue Coalition. Cancer-related fatigue: prevalence of proposed diagnostic criteria in a United States sample of cancer survivors. *J Clin Oncol* 2001; **19**(14), 3385–91.
3. Hardy J, Turner R, Saunders M, A'Hern R. Prediction of survival in a hospital-based continuing care unit. *Eur J Cancer* 1994; **30a**(3), 284–8.
4. Dunphy K, Amesbury B. A comparison of hospice and homecare patients: patterns of referral, patient characteristics and predictors of place of death. *Palliat Med* 1990; **4**, 105–11.
5. Walsh D, Donnelly S, Rybicki L. The symptoms of advanced cancer: relationship to age, gender, and performance status in 1,000 patients. *Support Care Cancer* 2000; **8**(3), 175–9.
6. Vainio A, Auvinen A. Prevalence of symptoms among patients with advanced cancer: an international collaborative study. Symptom Prevalence Group. *J Pain Symptom Manage* 1996; **12**(1), 3–10.
7. Coyle N, Adelhardt J, Foley KM, Portenoy RK. Character of terminal illness in the advanced cancer patient: pain and other symptoms during the last four weeks of life. *J Pain Symptom Manage* 1990; **5**(2), 83–93.
8. Dunlop G. A study of the relative frequency and importance of gastrointestinal symptoms, and weakness in patients with far advanced cancer: a student paper. *Palliat Med* 1989; **4**, 37–43.
9. McCarthy M. Hospice patients: a pilot study in 12 services. *Palliat Med* 1990; **4**, 93–104.
10. Stone P, Hardy J, Broadley K, Tookman AJ, Kurowska A, A'Hern R. Fatigue in advanced cancer: a prospective controlled cross-sectional study. *Br J Cancer* 1999; **79**(9–10), 1479–86.
11. Glaus A. The relationship between fatigue and type and stage of cancer. In: Glaus A (ed.), *Recent results in cancer research: fatigue in patients with cancer; analysis and assessment.* New York: Springer, 1998, 105–50.
12. Stone P, Richards M, A'Hern R, Hardy J. A study to investigate the prevalence, severity and correlates of fatigue among patients with cancer in comparison with a control group of volunteers without cancer. *Ann Oncol* 2000; **11**(5), 561–7.
13. Lichter I, Hunt E. The last 48 hours of life. *J Palliat Care* 1990; **6**(4), 7–15.
14. Demetri G, Kris M, Wade J, Degos L, Cella D. Quality-of-life benefit in chemotherapy patients treated with epoetin alfa is independent of disease response or tumour type: results from a prospective community oncology study. *J Clin Oncol* 1998; **16**(10), 3412–25.
15. Stone P, Hardy J, Huddart R, A'Hern R, Richards M. Fatigue in patients with prostate cancer receiving hormone therapy. *Eur J Cancer* 2000; **36**(9), 1134–41.
16. Savard J, Morin C. Insomnia in the context of cancer: a review of a neglected problem. *J Clin Oncol* 2001; **19**(3), 895–908.
17. Hotopf M, Chidgey J, Addington-Hall J, Ly KY. Depression in advanced disease: a systematic review. *Palliat Med* 2002; **16**(2), 81–97.
18. Visser MRM, Smets EMA. Fatigue, depression and quality of life in cancer patients: how are they related? *Support Care Cancer* 1998; **6**(2), 101–8.

19. Berger AM, Farr L. The influence of daytime inactivity and night-time restlessness on cancer-related fatigue. *Oncol Nurs Forum* 1999; **26**(10), 1663–71.

20. Smets E, Visser M, Willems-Groot A *et al.* Fatigue and radiotherapy: (A) experience in patients undergoing treatment. *Br J Cancer* 1998; **78**(7), 899–906.

21. Watanabe S, Bruera E. Anorexia and cachexia, asthenia, and lethargy. *Hematol Oncol Clin North Am* 1996; **10**(1), 189–206.

22. Winningham ML, Nail LM, Burke MB *et al.* Fatigue and the cancer experience: the state of the knowledge. *Oncol Nurs Forum* 1994; **21**(1), 23–36.

23. Stone P, Richards M, A'Hern R, Hardy J. Fatigue in patients with cancers of the breast or prostate undergoing radical radiotherapy. *J Pain Symptom Manage* 2001; **22**(6), 1007–15.

24. Hickok JT, Morrow GR, McDonald S, Bellg AJ. Frequency and correlates of fatigue in lung cancer patients receiving radiation therapy: implications for management. *J Pain Symptom Manage* 1996; **11**(6), 370–7.

25. Munro AJ, Potter S. A quantitative approach to the distress caused by symptoms in patients treated with radical radiotherapy. *Br J Cancer* 1996; **74**(4), 640–7.

26. Richardson A, Ream E, Wilson Barnett J. Fatigue in patients receiving chemotherapy: patterns of change. *Cancer Nurs* 1998; **21**(1), 17–30.

27. Jacobsen PB, Hann DM, Azzarello LM, Horton J, Balducci L, Lyman GH. Fatigue in women receiving adjuvant chemotherapy for breast cancer: characteristics, course, and correlates. *J Pain Symptom Manage* 1999; **18**(4), 233–42.

28. Smith IE, O'Brien ME, Talbot DC *et al.* Duration of chemotherapy in advanced non-small cell lung cancer: a randomized trial of three versus six courses of mitomycin, vinblastine, and cisplatin. *J Clin Oncol* 2001; **19**(5), 1336–43.

29. Gleeson C, Spencer D. Blood transfusion and its benefits in palliative care. *Palliat Med* 1995; **9**(4), 307–13.

30. Case D, Bukowski R, Carey R *et al.* Recombinant human erythropoietin therapy for anaemic cancer patients on combination chemotherapy. *J Natl Cancer Inst* 1993; **85**(10), 801–6.

31. Henry D, Abels R. Recombinant human erythropoietin in the treatment of cancer and chemotherapy-induced anaemia: results of double-blind and open-label follow-up studies. *Semin Oncol* 1994; **21**(2 (Suppl. 3)), 21–8.

32. Glaspy J, Bukowski R, Steinberg D, Taylor C, Tchekmedyian S, Vadhan-Raj S. Impact of therapy with epoetin alfa on clinical outcomes in patients with nonmyeloid malignancies during cancer chemotherapy in community oncology practice. *J Clin Oncol* 1997; **15**(3), 1218–34.

33. Mock V, Dow KH, Meares CJ *et al.* Effects of exercise on fatigue, physical functioning, and emotional distress during radiation therapy for breast cancer. *Oncol Nurs Forum* 1997; **24**(6), 991–1000.

34. Dimeo F, Stieglitz R, Novelli-Fischer U, Keul J. Effects of physical activity on the fatigue and psychologic status of cancer patients during chemotherapy. *Cancer* 1999; **85**(10), 2273–7.

35. Segal R, Evans W, Johnson D *et al.* Structured exercise improves physical functioning in women with stages I and II breast cancer: results of a randomized controlled trial. *J Clin Oncol* 2001; **19**(3), 657–65.

36. Porock D, Kristjanson LJ, Tinnelly K, Duke T, Blight J. An exercise intervention for advanced cancer patients experiencing fatigue: a pilot study. *J Palliat Care* 2000; **16**(3), 30–6.

A–Z OF SYMPTOMS

37. Popiela T, Lucchi R, Giongo F. Methylprednisolone as palliative therapy for female terminal cancer patients. The Methylprednisolone Female Preterminal Cancer Study Group. *Eur J Cancer Clin Oncol* 1989; 25(12), 1823–9.

38. Robustelli Della Cuna G, Pellegrini A, Piazzi M *et al*. Effect of methylprednisolone sodium succinate on quality of life in preterminal cancer patients: a placebo-controlled, multicenter study. *Eur J Cancer Clin Oncol* 1989; 25(12), 1817–21.

39. Weinshenker BG, Penman M, Bass B, Ebers GC, Rice GPA. A double-blind randomised crossover trial of pemoline in fatigue associated with multiple sclerosis. *Neurology* 1992; 42, 1468–71.

40. Krupp LB, Coyle PK, Doscher C *et al*. Fatigue therapy in multiple sclerosis: results of a double-blind, randomized, parallel trial of amantadine, pemoline, and placebo. *Neurology* 1995; 45(11), 1956–61.

41. Breitbart W, Rosenfeld B, Kaim M, Funesti-Esch J. A randomized, double-blind, placebo-controlled trial of psychostimulants for the treatment of fatigue in ambulatory patients with human immunodeficiency virus disease. *Arch Intern Med* 2001; 161(3), 411–20.

42. Bruera E, Chadwick S, Brenneis C, Hanson J, MacDonald RN. Methylphenidate associated with narcotics for the treatment of cancer pain. *Cancer Treat Rep* 1987; 71(1), 67–70.

43. Meyers CA, Weitzner MA, Valentine AD, Levin VA. Methylphenidate therapy improves cognition, mood, and function of brain tumor patients. *J Clin Oncol* 1998; 16(7), 2522–7.

44. Sarhill N, Walsh D, Nelson KA, Homsi J, LeGrand S, Davis MP. Methylphenidate for fatigue in advanced cancer: a prospective open-label pilot study. *Am J Hospice Palliat Care* 2001; 18(3), 187–92.

45. Simons JP, Aaronson NK, Vansteenkiste JF *et al*. Effects of medroxyprogesterone acetate on appetite, weight, and quality of life in advanced-stage non-hormone-sensitive cancer: a placebo-controlled multicenter study. *J Clin Oncol* 1996; 14(4),: 1077–84.

46. Westman G, Bergman B, Albertsson M *et al*. Megestrol acetate in advanced, progressive, hormone-insensitive cancer. Effects on the quality of life: a placebo-controlled, randomised, multicentre trial. *Eur J Cancer* 1999; 35(4), 586–95.

47. Bruera E, Macmillan K, Kuehn N, Hanson J, MacDonald RN. A controlled trial of megestrol acetate on appetite, caloric intake, nutritional status, and other symptoms in patients with advanced cancer. *Cancer* 1990; 66(6), 1279–82.

48. Bruera E, Ernst S, Hagen N *et al*. Effectiveness of megestrol acetate in patients with advanced cancer: a randomized, double-blind, crossover study. *Cancer Prev Control* 1998; 2(2), 74–8.

49. Morrow GR, Hickok JT, Roscoe JA *et al*. Differential effects of paroxetine on fatigue and depression: a randomized, double-blind trial from the University of Rochester Cancer Center Community Clinical Oncology Program. *J Clin Oncol* 2003; 21(24), 4635–41.

FURTHER READING

Armes J, Krishnasamy M, Higginson I (eds). *Fatigue in cancer*. Oxford: Oxford University Press, 2004.

Winningham ML, Barton-Burke M (eds). *Fatigue in cancer – a multidimensional approach*. Sudbury, MA: Jones and Bartlett Publishers, 2000.

A–Z OF SYMPTOMS

DYING

Nigel Sykes

At the very end of life, the needs of patients tend to converge. Conscious level diminishes, preventing explicit communication; swallowing deteriorates, necessitating a change away from oral medication for most people; and symptom control becomes concerned with a small number of key issues:

- pain
- retained bronchial secretions
- agitation,

and sometimes:

- nausea and vomiting
- breathlessness.

Acute, distressing symptoms do not occur often near death, but may be very frightening for patients and for those close to them when they do. The principal symptoms to try to anticipate are:

- severe haemorrhage
- respiratory obstruction.

Because of this limited range of concerns, it is natural that this was the first area of palliative care practice for which a care pathway was designed.[1]

HOW IS DYING IDENTIFIED?

A person who shows at least two of the following signs has a mean of 2 days to live:[2]

- bedridden
- semi-comatose

A–Z OF SYMPTOMS

- able to take only sips of fluids

- no longer able to take tablets.

SYMPTOM CONTROL

There is some evidence that pain might become more severe towards the end of life, but not that it becomes any more difficult to control. The crucial issue in symptom control at the end of life is preparedness. It is a wholly inadequate response to the onset of a distressing symptom if control has to wait for a doctor's order or the pharmacist's acquisition of the medication required. If drugs are to be used at home, locally agreed paperwork must be filled out to enable community nurses to give the drugs when needed.

The following categories of drug need to be available for symptom control in a dying person:

- analgesics

- sedatives

- anti-emetics

- anticholinergic agents.

FAMILY AND CARER SUPPORT

A vital element of preparedness in caring for a dying person is adequate and timely communication with family and others who are close, whether or not the patient is at home. Family members may not realize that death is close or, noticing the signs, may attribute them to medication effects (which might be correct, and should be considered when deterioration is noted). Even if they do recognize that the patient is dying, this is likely to be a situation they have not met before, and they will not know what to expect. Some patients and families fear that death will be heralded by an inevitable crescendo of pain, and need reassurance that there is no reason for such a thing to occur.

It can be helpful to be forewarned of the likely course of dying, in particular:

- a reduction in conscious level, irrespective of the use of sedative drugs,

- the cessation of eating and drinking, and the futility of assisted hydration and nutrition,

- increasing irregularity of breathing pattern,

- the possibility of noisy breathing as a result of retained secretions,

- the possibility of some restlessness, and the assurance that this is usually controllable with adjustments to medication,

- the fact that death occurs through the cessation of breathing, but that this does not imply the presence of feelings of suffocation or drowning.

It can also be valuable for family members to know what they can do to help, if they are not greatly involved in nursing the patient. The regular moistening of the lips and mouth with sponge sticks is an example. Whilst dying patients may not be able to respond, it is still plausible that they can experience touch and can hear. Relatives and carers should therefore feel free to keep gentle physical contact with the patient if they wish, and to speak to them (but not to talk in front of them about matters that they previously would not have discussed in their presence).

CHANGES IN MEDICATION

The main changes involving medication take the form of stopping treatments that have become irrelevant (see the box below) and adjusting others to a parenteral form because the person's deteriorating condition means that he or she can no longer swallow effectively. Two-thirds of cancer patients are able to take oral analgesia until within the last 24 hours of life, but during that last day, 84 per cent will need some medication to be given parenterally.[3]

Inappropriate interventions

- Any drug that is not controlling or preventing symptoms.
  Drugs that can be stopped:
  diuretics
  cardiovascular agents
  antibiotics
  hypoglycaemics
  hormones
  iron and vitamins
  steroids.
  Other interventions that can be stopped:
  blood tests
  artificial hydration or nutrition.

NB. Careful explanation is needed for relatives.

PAIN

Pain is not generally a problem at the end of life if it has been adequately controlled previously. In patients who can no longer indicate their feelings, carers interpret non-verbal signs of distress, for example groaning, grimacing or restlessness. Before increasing medication, it should be checked whether there are remediable causes of discomfort, particularly a full bladder or rectum.

Morphine or diamorphine is the mainstay of analgesia at the end of life. Liquid morphine can be given from a sponge stick or a syringe to a very ill patient who is still able to swallow sufficiently, and in this way oral analgesia might be maintained until death. Other liquid preparations, for instance haloperidol, chlorpromazine or diazepam, can be given in the same way. However, it is usually easier to use a parenteral route: subcutaneous, rectal or transdermal. There is no clinical advantage to intravenous administration.

Morphine can be given subcutaneously or rectally, and diamorphine subcutaneously. Fentanyl is available as a patch for transdermal delivery. Conversion ratios for the change from oral to parenteral routes are given in the appendix on page 205. It is generally appropriate to provide an equivalent dose to that previously given by mouth (although conversion ratios are only approximations, and in the individual the theoretical dose may need adjustment either up or down according to response). However, if other analgesics that can only be given orally – for example most neuropathic pain agents – have to be stopped, an increase in the opioid dose might be needed in order to compensate. Any resulting drowsiness is, in the circumstances, likely to be helpful rather than problematic.

A proportion of dying patients will develop myoclonus, even at usual morphine doses,[4] presumably as a result of deteriorating renal function causing accumulation of metabolites. Resolution may occur with a reduction in morphine dose but may require the addition of a benzodiazepine, for instance either midazolam or clonazepam. Phenothiazines can also precipitate or exacerbate myoclonus, and if this occurs it is worthwhile replacing them entirely by a benzodiazepine or reducing the dose to an anti-emetic level.

If there has been particular analgesic benefit from a non-steroidal anti-inflammatory drug (NSAID), this can be continued by suppository (e.g. in the form of diclofenac or naproxen) or syringe driver. Ketorolac will mix in a syringe with diamorphine and haloperidol, but diclofenac is not miscible with other drugs for syringe-driver use.

RESTLESSNESS AND AGITATION

A generalized restlessness, as distinct from co-ordinated myoclonic jerks, is seen quite often as death approaches. This, and a more pronounced disturbance that amounts to agitation, is the most usual reason for the introduction of sedation towards the end of life, and such therapy is used in about half of palliative care patients prior to their death. Because of the increased potential of phenothiazines to cause myoclonus in the dying, diazepam rectally or midazolam subcutaneously is a more appropriate sedative choice. There is no evidence that these agents precipitate death when given in doses just sufficient to control evidence of restlessness.[5] However, before introducing a sedative, it is important to check for a remediable cause of disturbance such as a full bladder or rectum. It is also worth remembering that a heavy smoker may undergo nicotine withdrawal when no longer able to smoke, and restlessness is sometimes eased by application of a transdermal nicotine patch.

Agitation at the end of life may be severe, amounting to a terminal delirium. There is a clinical impression that this is more likely to arise in those who have resisted facing the reality of their illness, or have previously shown marked anxiety. In this situation, midazolam, or even a combination of midazolam and levomepromazine (methotrimeprazine), can be insufficient. An alternative is phenobarbital [phenobarbitone], 100–300 mg subcutaneously/intravenously *stat* and 600–3000 mg/24 hours by subcutaneous infusion (not combined in the same syringe with other drugs). Potentially, a more accurate matching of dose and response can be obtained by a variable-rate intravenous infusion of propofol, because of its very rapid onset (30 seconds) and short duration (5 minutes) of action.

NAUSEA AND VOMITING

Where an anti-emetic has been an important part of symptom control before the dying phase, this should be continued when drugs are changed to a parenteral form. Appropriate formulations are given in Appendix 1. Should sedation be needed, this is likely to obscure any sense of nausea, and a benzodiazepine alone may then be sufficient.

RETAINED SECRETIONS

Any severely ill patient with reduced ability to cough can accumulate secretions in the upper airways, resulting in noisy breathing, which, if not always a distress to the patients themselves, may well be to attending relatives. This problem is best treated promptly, as it is not easy to get rid of secretions that have already gathered. Approximately half of dying patients have been reported to develop rattly breathing, and resolution is possible in about two-thirds of these.[6] It is not possible to stop noisy breathing altogether because in some cases it is due to infective exudate that cannot be prevented.

The first step in management is to explain to the patient's family the mechanism of the noisy breathing, what is being done and what its limitations are, and also to reassure them that by this stage of their illness the dying person is unlikely to be nearly as aware of the sounds as they are themselves.

An anticholinergic drug (e.g. hyoscine butylbromide or glycopyrronium bromide) or the generally more sedating (and, in Britain, significantly more expensive) hyoscine hydrobromide, can be given subcutaneously by syringe driver in combination with diamorphine and midazolam or levomepromazine (methotrimeprazine).[7] It is not clear that intravenous diuretics or antibiotics have a role to play at this stage.

HYDRATION AND NUTRITION

It is a common experience that patients can die with dignity and peacefully without artificial hydration. No relationship has been demonstrated between hydration

A-Z OF SYMPTOMS

and the symptoms of thirst and dry mouth in a palliative care population. These are likely to be related to non-specific disease-related effects, the anticholinergic actions of opioids and many anti-emetics, and to the mouth breathing that is common in the very ill. A more effective way of management is frequent, direct moistening using sponge sticks soaked in water or a drink the person has liked. Also, most dying patients not receiving hydration have relatively normal biochemical profiles, suggesting that the physiological mechanisms of the body are compensating for the decreased fluid intake. Hence the ongoing provision of assisted hydration to dying patients is likely to be futile, whilst continuing to have the potential to cause morbidity.

Advanced illness radically alters cellular metabolism, and in this situation there are no evident benefits of either enteral or parenteral nutrition when patients can no longer eat.[8]

The cessation of eating and drinking is hard for many families to accept, and this is an area of management that requires particularly careful explanation. (For a further consideration of feeding and hydration, see Chapter 21, 'Ethical issues'.)

FITS

Patients who have required anticonvulsant treatment for fits (as opposed to pain) should have continued anti-epileptic medication after they have become unable to take oral drugs, as any perception that they have died in convulsions is very distressing for relatives. Midazolam is an appropriate choice and, as at earlier stages of the illness, the use of phenothiazines should be minimized because of their risk of lowering the fit threshold.

CRISES

Acute haemorrhage or respiratory obstruction is frightening for patients and for those around them. Prodromal bleeds or progressive stridor may allow these events to be foreseen. In this case, provision should be made for adequate sedation to be available and, in the case of haemorrhage, red or green towels to soak up the blood and mask its amount. Rapid sedation can be achieved using midazolam 5–20 mg slowly intravenously if possible, subcutaneously if not (the buccal route is effective, but difficult in these circumstances). At home, a family may be able to administer diazepam 10 mg as an enema, but in order to be able to face the situation will need careful preparation and an assurance of prompt back-up from the professional team.

CONCLUSION

Management of the dying patient is a crucial part of palliative care because it provides some of the most powerful memories for those left behind. The future attitudes of the patient's family and friends towards severe illness in themselves or others, and towards death itself, will be moulded by this experience. Good symptom control and good communication with the patient as long as this is possible, and with the family, are crucial, not only for their direct benefit to the person who is dying, but also as a public health measure for all those who are bereaved.

KEY POINTS

- Anticipate the onset of the dying phase.
- Have parenteral medication, and the means of giving it, available in advance.
- Prepare the patient's family for what is happening.
- Stop inappropriate medications and interventions (including assisted hydration).
- Sedation may be needed for restlessness, but check for remediable causes first.
- Try to anticipate the possibility of fits, massive haemorrhage and respiratory obstruction, and make provision to deal with them.
- Remember that good care for the dying is a public health measure for the survivors.

REFERENCES

1. Ellershaw J, Foster A, Murphy D, Shea T, Overill S. Developing an integrated care pathway for the dying patient. *Eur J Palliat Care* 1997; **4**, 203–7.
2. Ellershaw JE, Sutcliffe JM, Saunders CM. Dehydration and the dying patient. *J Pain Symptom Manage* 1995; **10**, 192–7.
3. Lombard DJ, Oliver DJ. The use of opioid analgesics in the last 24 hours of life of patients with advanced cancer. *Palliat Med* 1989; **3**, 27–9.
4. Olarte JM. Opioid-induced myoclonus. *Eur J Palliat Care* 1995; **2**, 146–50.
5. Sykes NP, Thorns A. The use of opioids and sedatives at the end of life in palliative care. *Lancet Oncol*, 2003; **4**, 312–18.
6. Morita T, Tsunoda J, Inoue S, Chihara S. Risk factors for death rattle in terminally ill cancer patients; a prospective exploratory study. *Palliat Med* 2000, **14**, 19–23.
7. Bennett M, Lucas V, Brennan M, Hughes A, O'Donnell V, Wee B. Using anti-muscarinic drugs in the management of death rattle: evidence-based guidelines for palliative care. *Palliat Med* 2002; **16**, 369–74.
8. Vigano A, Watanabe S, Bruera E. Anorexia and cachexia in advanced cancer patients. *Cancer Surv* 1994; **21**, 99–115.

DYSPHAGIA

Debra Swann and Polly Edmonds

DEFINITION

Dysphagia means difficulty swallowing, which results in swallowed material being held up in its passage from the mouth to the stomach.

PREVALENCE

The prevalence of dysphagia in palliative care ranges from 9 to 55 per cent.[1,2] In one study of 797 consecutive admissions to a large hospice, 12 per cent of patients were found to have dysphagia as a presenting complaint.[3] Patients with head and neck malignancies have a much higher prevalence: in a retrospective study of 38 patients with head and neck cancer admitted to a hospice over a 3-year period, dysphagia was noted in 28 (74 per cent).[4] The prevalence of dysphagia in patients with motor neurone disease is around 60 per cent.

PATHOPHYSIOLOGY

The mechanism of swallowing is complex, involving the brainstem, five cranial nerves (V, VII, IX, X, XII) and skeletal muscles. The result is the smooth and easy passage of a bolus from the mouth to the stomach in three phases.

- *Oral phase*: after chewing and mixing with saliva, the bolus of food or fluid is passed to the back of the throat by the voluntary action of the tongue and oropharynx.

- *Pharyngeal phase*: this commences once the bolus being swallowed reaches the back of the tongue. There follows a pause in the respiratory cycle as the epiglottis closes over the larynx to prevent aspiration via the trachea, and the peristaltic wave moves the bolus on into the oesophagus.

- *Oesophageal phase*: peristalsis propels the bolus from the oesophagus to the stomach.

AETIOLOGY OF DYSPHAGIA

In palliative care patients there are multiple possible causes of dysphagia (Table 4.11.1), which can occur alone or in combination with each other. These can be grouped together as follows:

- oral problems,
- pharyngeal or oesophageal pathology,
- neurological problems,
- other.

INVESTIGATIONS AND EXAMINATION

HISTORY

Some patients may be able to localize the level of dysphagia.[5] Direct questions concerning the consistency of food that is easiest to swallow, sticking of food, episodes of choking or regurgitating (especially nasal regurgitation), and the presence of any pain on swallowing may be helpful. Some patients have certain positions in which they find it easier to eat and have modified their diet to avoid certain food types that are more difficult to swallow. The consistency of substances that are difficult to swallow may suggest the aetiology: neuromuscular disorders tend to cause difficulties with both liquids and solids at the outset, whereas obstructing lesions usually cause dysphagia for solids initially and liquids later.

A history of painful swallowing (odynophagia), classically after hot drinks, is associated with oesophageal candidiasis, reflux oesophagitis and acute mucositis. Acute mucositis is a recognized side effect following chemotherapy or radiotherapy to the mediastinum and chest.

The degree of weight loss associated with the dysphagia and associated weakness is also relevant, as dietetic advice on easy-to-swallow, high-calorie-containing foods may be relevant.

EXAMINATION

Initial examination should start with the mouth, looking for signs of dryness, ulceration, mucositis, candidiasis, hypersalivation and drooling. The state of dentition, or dentures if worn, is important: dentures that no longer fit because of significant weight loss can rub, causing sore gums, or be non-functioning, resulting in an inability to chew food.

Neurological evaluation of the relevant cranial nerves, looking for evidence of muscle weakness, examination of the anterior and posterior tongue movements and checking for stridor may be beneficial, but a more formal swallowing assessment should be done by a speech and language therapist.

A-Z OF SYMPTOMS

Table 4.11.1 Causes of dysphagia in palliative care

Oral problems	Neurological problems
Xerostomia (dry mouth) Reduced saliva secretion Drugs, e.g. morphine, anticholinergics Post-irradiation (head and neck region) Poor oral intake Anxiety	**Upper motor neurone damage** Cerebral tumour Infarction Surgery
Mucosal infection Candidiasis Cytomegalovirus Herpes simplex virus Zoster infection in the mouth Aphthous ulceration	**Lower motor neurone damage** Motor neurone disease Multiple sclerosis Surgery Radiation-induced neuronal fibrosis
Mucositis Chemotherapy Radiotherapy Immunodeficiency Non-steroidal anti-inflammatory drugs	**Direct nerve damage** Malignant linear infiltration of pharyngo-oesophageal wall resulting in nerve plexus damage
Surgery Hemiglossectomy Submandibular glands	**Damage to motor or sensory components of lower cranial nerves** Base of skull metastases Leptomeningeal infiltration Brainstem lesions Motor neurone disease Multiple sclerosis
Dentition Ill-fitting dentures Dental caries	**Cerebellar damage** Infarction Surgery Tumour
Post-radiation fibrosis Difficulty opening the mouth or moving the tongue	**Paraneoplastic** Neuropathies Cerebellar damage Myasthenia (Eaton–Lambert syndrome)
Dystonic reactions Drugs, e.g. metoclopramide, haloperidol	**Neuromuscular** Parkinson's disease Polymyositis
Pharyngeal/oesophageal pathology	**Other causes**
Intraluminal obstruction Local tumour in pharynx or oesophagus Over-growth of tumour above the stent Displacement of oesophageal stent	**Concurrent diseases** Benign oesophageal strictures Reflux oesophagitis
External compression Mediastinal nodes Aortic aneurysm	**Drowsiness** Level of alertness may affect swallowing

(continued)

Table 4.11.1 (continued)

Oral problems	Neurological problems
Treatment related Stricture post-surgery/radiotherapy Mucositis secondary to chemotherapy	**Pain** **Extreme weakness** Common in the dying phase
Infection Pharyngo-oesophageal candidiasis[a,b,c] Pharyngitis	**Depression** **Hypercalcaemia** Rare, causes severe functional dysphagia
Drugs altering upper oesophageal tone Dantrolene	
Drugs increasing lower oesophageal sphincter tone Metoclopramide Domperidone	
Anxiety Oesophageal spasm	

[a] In 50% of cases of oesophageal candidal infection there is no evidence of oral infection.
[b] Associated with a classical history of pain when taking hot drinks.
[c] Classical barium swallow images.

INVESTIGATIONS

An observation of the degree of dehydration may warrant emergency intervention before further investigations are appropriate. Serum biochemistry for urea and electrolytes will help assess the degree of dehydration. Other investigations may be required, as determined by the nature of the dysphagia, especially if pharyngeal or oesophageal pathologies are suspected.

Chest X-ray

• Demonstrates evidence of stricture in oesophagus.

• Visualizes the hilar structures if external compression is thought to be the underlying cause.

• Detects radiological evidence of aspiration, if oral or pharyngeal swallowing phases are felt to be impaired and aspiration pneumonia has developed.

Barium swallow

• First investigation for dysphagia thought to be due to oesophageal pathology.

• Safe and easy to perform.

- Demonstrates the level and position of an intraluminal lesion, external compression or an irregular stricture.

- 'Moth-eaten' appearance associated with oesophageal candidiasis and oesophageal ulceration due to herpes simplex virus or cytomegalovirus infection.

Upper gastrointestinal endoscopy

- Usually performed if oesophago-gastric pathology suspected and biopsy of the lesion is necessary. More appropriately performed as first line investigation if dilatation or stenting is being considered or a food bolus needs to be removed.

- May help to differentiate between intraluminal and extraluminal pathology.

- More invasive than the barium swallow.

Computed tomography (CT) scan

- To establish the stage and position of the primary disease and regional lymph node involvement.

- Used for assessment of operability rather than investigation of dysphagia.

Endoscopic ultrasound

- More recent technique that determines the thickness of oesophageal tumours and depth of invasion and detects any regional lymph node involvement.

Test swallow

- Crude bedside test of a patient's actual functional swallow.

- Initial test (dry swallow): the examiner's fingers are gently placed over the thyroid cartilage and behind the chin and the patient is asked to swallow.

- Allows oropharyngeal transit time (i.e. how long it takes between the first movement of the tongue and the last movement of the larynx) to be observed. This is usually less than 1 second.

- Repeat test above with 5 mL of water (wet swallow).

- A prolonged transit time warrants speech and language therapy referral and consideration of the non-oral route for feeding, usually if >10 seconds.

Speech and language therapy (SALT) assessment

A SALT professional with a special interest in swallowing disorders should do a formal swallowing assessment, especially in cases of neurological causes of dysphagia and cancers of the head and neck. Most neurological centres have a speech and language therapist working as part of the multi-professional team. Their assessment of a patient's swallowing may include video-assisted fluoroscopy, which is a modified barium swallow designed to observe the oral and pharyngeal phases of swallowing.

The following are indicators that aspiration is occurring:

- lip, tongue or voice impairment, especially a 'gurgly' or 'wet' voice,

- coughing on own secretions,

- recurrent chest infections,

- dehydration or poor oral intake,

- patient complains of effort or fear with swallowing,

- choking/coughing before, during or after swallow,

- eyes watering post-swallow,

- significant increase in respiratory rate post-swallow.

MANAGEMENT

GENERAL MEASURES

- Education and explanation to carers.

- Mouth care.

- Dentures and dentition assessment.

- Frequent small meals, which are presentable and of a suitable consistency.

- Soft diets, e.g.:
  use of liquidizer/blender to prepare food of correct consistency,
  ice-cream, custards and jellies are easy to swallow.

- Add calories to food, e.g. fresh cream, full-fat milk.

- Add high-calorie supplements to food, e.g. Maxijul.

- Thickened liquids may be swallowed more easily.

- Review unnecessary medications that may exacerbate swallowing difficulties (anticholinergics: tricyclic antidepressants, hyoscine, morphine).

- Psychological support for issues arising as a result of inability to eat.

- Where appropriate, a SALT professional can advise patients and carers about modifying the swallowing technique to minimize the risk of aspiration (see box overleaf).

> **Speech and language therapy guidelines for swallowing given to patients (courtesy of SALT Department, King's College Hospital)**
>
> 1. Make sure your back is straight and chin tucked down.
> 2. Don't turn round or talk while eating and drinking as it could send food down the wrong way.
> 3. Take plenty of time over eating and drinking and remember to take small mouthfuls of food and small sips of drink.
> 4. Chew the food well, then do a strong purposeful swallow. Try to do 2 swallows per mouthful to make it less likely for food to remain in your throat.
> 5. Make sure your mouth is clear of food before taking the next mouthful. Check along your gums and your cheeks to make sure there are no collections of debris.
> 6. If swallowing then triggers coughing, stop and rest. Check in the mouth for evidence of debris.
> 7. Eye watering, change in voice quality or fatigue during the swallowing process may imply aspiration is taking place.
>
> NB. **The gag reflex is not relevant.** Patients with a gag may aspirate and many patients without a gag do not aspirate.

SPECIFIC MEASURES

Endoscopic dilatation of oesophageal obstruction

- Relieves dysphagia in more than 50 per cent of patients.

- Generally lasts less than 2 weeks in malignant obstruction.

- Useful as a short-term measure before other treatment modalities begin.

Oesophageal intubation

- Older rigid stent (Cilastin) but high risk of perforation – useful for oesophago-bronchial fistulae.

- Self-expanding metal stents (SEMS – Wall Stents, Nitinol stents, Gianturco stents) – preferred over rigid stents, especially if there is a high risk of perforation.[6]
  Problems of migration of SEMS, especially at the gastric cardia-oesophageal junction in 50 per cent of cases.
  Gastro-oesophageal reflux associated with SEMS crossing the cardia in 22 per cent of cases.
  May become dislodged or block with solids.

Endoscopic NdYAG laser therapy

- Lower complication rate than other endoscopic treatment modalities.[7]

- First treatment choice for dysphagia in patients with a short life expectancy.

- Better relief of dysphagia than intubation.

- Improvement may last several months; can be repeated.

- Plays a complementary role to other palliative treatment modalities for dysphagia.[8]

- Useful for small polypoid intraluminal tumours.

Alcohol injection into malignant lesion
- Similar results to laser therapy.

- Increased analgesic requirements during treatment.[9]

External beam radiotherapy
- Takes several weeks to achieve maximum effect.

- Radiation oesophagitis may worsen symptoms in the short term.

- Suitable for patients with a prognosis of more than a few months.

Brachytherapy
- Endoscopically directed radiotherapy.

- Given as a single dose.

- More rapid onset of tumour control compared with external beam radiotherapy.

- Can be used even if external beam radiation has been given previously.

- Prolongs the first therapeutic interval.

- Effects last up to median 4 months.

Chemotherapy
- Limited role in palliation of squamous cell carcinoma of oesophagus.

- Relief of dysphagia (61 per cent) and increased survival following ECF (epirubicin, cisplatin and 5-fluorouracil) chemotherapy compared with laser therapy alone for adenocarcinoma of oesophagus.[6]

Percutaneous endoscopic gastrostomy (PEG) feeding
Fine-bore nasogastric feeding tubes are a short-term solution to the problem of alternative nutrition but are poorly tolerated and can displace, leading to aspiration of the feed and a chest infection. PEG feeding is a safer alternative with a low complication rate, and should be considered:

- when the oral route is inappropriate or nutritional intake inadequate but continued feeding is indicated;

- when the oropharyngeal transit time is >10 seconds;

Table 4.11.2 Pharmacological treatments for dysphagia

Oesophageal candidiasis	Fluconazole 150 mg p.o. (single dose) or 50 mg p.o. (o.d. for 5 days)
Viral oesophageal ulceration	Acyclovir at treatment doses
Oesophageal mucositis	Patient-controlled analgesia (PCA)
	Sucralfate 10 mL p.o. (2–4 hourly)
	Maalox 5–10 mL p.o. (q.d.s.)
	Cocaine mouthwash
Peritumour oedema	Dexamethasone 16 mg s.c./i.v. (o.d.)
Bleeding from primary tumour	Tranexamic acid 1 g q.d.s.
Sialorrhoea and drooling secondary to total obstruction or neurological disorders of swallowing	Low-dose tricyclic antidepressants (e.g. amitriptyline 10 mg nocte)
	Transdermal hyoscine hydrobromide
	Glycopyrollate/hyoscine butylbromide
	Via continuous s.c. infusion
	Radiation of salivary glands in neurological cases

p.o., orally; o.d., on demand; q.d.s., four times a day; s.c., subcutaneously; i.v., intravenously.

- when aspiration of >10 per cent of swallowed material (as assessed by a SALT) is occurring;

- for patients with a neurological cause of their dysphagia with a longer prognosis: motor neurone disease, multiple sclerosis;

- for nutritional support before radical surgery of head and neck tumours or chemotherapy;

- for nutritional support prior to prolonged radiotherapy treatment to the head and neck area to cover the period of associated mucositis.

Pharmacological strategies
See Table 4.11.2.

FUTURE DEVELOPMENTS

The increasing utilization of radiologically inserted gastrostomy (RIG) tubes (the use of a radiological technique for the insertion of gastrostomy feeding tubes) is likely to be beneficial for patients with neurological problems where sedation needs to be avoided. For patients with oesophageal or head and neck cancers, further developments with respect to combined chemo-irradiation techniques may lead to improvements in survival and better local palliation.

KEY POINTS

- Obtaining a careful history may help identify the level of obstruction.
- The advice of a speech and language therapist is invaluable in cases where the oral and pharyngeal phases of swallowing are impaired.
- Dietary advice is important.
- Newer palliative techniques, including laser therapy and brachytherapy, may improve symptoms of local obstruction.

REFERENCES

1. Curtis ER, Krech R, Walsh TD. Common symptoms in patients with advanced cancer. *J Palliat Care* 1991; **7**, 25–9.
2. Donnelly S, Washing D. The symptoms of advanced cancer: identification of clinical research priorities by assessment of prevalence and severity. *J Palliat Care* 1995; **11**(1), 27–32.
3. Sykes NP, Baines M, Carter RL. Clinical and pathological study of dysphagia conservatively managed in patients with advanced malignant disease. *Lancet* 1988; **2**, 726–8.
4. Forbes K. Palliative care in patients with cancer of the head and neck. *Clin Otolaryngol* 1997; **22**, 117–23.
5. Regnard CFB, Tempest S. *A guide to symptom relief in advanced disease*, 4th edn. Cheshire: Hochland and Hochland, 1998, 37.
6. Mason R. Palliation of malignant dysphagia: an alternative to surgery. *Ann R Coll Surg Engl* 1996; **78**, 457–62.
7. Gevers AM, Macken E, Hiele M, Rutgeerts P. A comparison of laser therapy, plastic stents and expandable metal stents for palliation of malignant dysphagia in patients without fistula. *Gastrointest Endosc* 1998; **48**(4), 383–8.
8. Abdel-Wahab M, Gad-Elhak N, Denewer A *et al.* Endoscopic laser treatment of progressive dysphagia in patients with advanced oesophageal carcinoma. *Hepato-Gastroenterology* 1998; **45**(23), 1509–15.
9. Carazzone A, Bonavina L, Segalin A, Ceriani C, Peracchia A. Endoscopic palliation of oesophageal cancer: results of a prospective comparison of Nd: YAG laser and ethanol injection. *Eur J Surg* 1999; **165**(4), 361–6.

A–Z OF SYMPTOMS

HICCUP

Victor Pace

Hiccups are usually annoying trivial events of unknown physiological significance, but they can also signal significant underlying illness. Occasionally they cause serious complications (operative wound breakdown, dehydration, fatigue, depression, sleep deprivation, stroke, heart block), and even death.[1] Hiccups lasting more than 24 hours or recurring frequently may indicate serious pathology.[2] The incidence of hiccups in palliative care is unknown.

PATHOPHYSIOLOGY

During a hiccup, a forceful inspiration, caused by sudden contraction of the diaphragm, external intercostals and scaleni, is suddenly interrupted by closure of the glottis, which produces the hiccup and characteristic sound. The reflex arc is thought to involve phrenic and vagus nerves and thoracic sympathetic fibres stimulating a hiccup centre. This entails complex connections between brainstem (respiratory centre, phrenic nerve nuclei, reticular formation) and midbrain (hypothalamus), linked in turn with cerebral hemispheres and cerebellum. Cranial nerves V–XII (excluding VIII), and nerve roots C3–C5 and T6–T12 are involved in the efferent arm of the reflex.[3] Hiccups are said to occur in runs of less than 7 or more than 63,[4] and often stop during sleep but resume on waking. They are more common in men than in women.

The process is most commonly caused by:

- gastric distension (overeating, fizzy drinks),

- alcohol or tobacco excess,

- emotion (shock, laughter),

- sudden change in temperature (cold drink, cold shower),

- psychogenic problems (but beware of bias: one early paper ascribed hiccup to psychogenic causes in 36 out of 39 women, as compared to 12 out of 181 men!).

PATHOLOGICAL CAUSES RELEVANT TO PALLIATIVE CARE

(See Launois *et al.*[1] for a full list.)

GASTROINTESTINAL

Oesophageal tumours, oesophagitis, gastric distension and bowel obstruction have all been associated with hiccups, as have pancreatic cancer, pancreatitis and biliary disease.

METABOLIC

Hiccups are a recognized symptom of renal failure. They also occur with diabetes, a low serum sodium, hypocalcaemia and Addison's disease. Hyperventilation produces hiccups through carbon dioxide washout.

NEUROGENIC

Lesions in the brain – tumours, strokes, infection, demyelinating disorders – cause hiccups, particularly when around the vagal nuclei or the nucleus tractus solitarius in the medulla (close to the area responsible for control of breathing); here they may presage respiratory arrest.[2] Problems with the afferent and efferent nerves to the respiratory muscles, such as pressure from mediastinal tumours, or diaphragmatic irritation (hepatic distension, pleural effusion, diaphragmatic hernia) are another possible cause. Foreign bodies or tumours in the ear give hiccups through irritation of the auricular branch of the vagus. Hiccups are also common under light general anaesthesia.

DRUGS

Drugs rarely cause this symptom, but the most commonly reported ones have uses in palliative care. Most commonly held responsible[5–7] are corticosteroids (dexamethasone, methylprednisolone) and benzodiazepines (midazolam, chlordiazepoxide). Megestrol, methandrostenolone (an anabolic steroid), opioids, phenobarbitone and co-trimoxazole have also been suggested as causes. Steroids are particularly interesting as causes; they are thought to facilitate hiccups by lowering the synaptic transmission threshold in the brainstem. Yet lack of steroids in Addison's disease also produces hiccups,[2] and in palliative care steroids have been known to relieve the symptom (was this in cases of undiagnosed steroid deficiency, one wonders?).

A–Z OF SYMPTOMS

TREATMENT

NON-PHARMACOLOGICAL TREATMENT

Non-pharmacological remedies are numerous (Launois *et al.*[1] list 69); Lewis even quotes one unfortunate who, having hiccupped for more than 8 years and having received more than 60 000 letters suggesting possible cures, ultimately responded only to prayers to St Jude, patron saint of lost causes![5] For those still intent on trying other methods, Lewis classifies non-pharmacological treatments as:

- irritation of uvula or nasopharynx (swallowing granulated sugar, catheter stimulation),

- interruption of respiratory rhythm (Valsalva manoeuvre, breath holding, sudden fright)

- counter-irritation of the diaphragm (pulling knees up to chest),

- relief of gastric distension (emesis, nasogastric aspiration),

- respiratory centre stimulation (breath holding, hyperventilation),

- disruption of phrenic nerve (electrical stimulation, transection),

- counter irritation of vagus (carotid sinus massage),

- psychiatric (behavioural treatments, hypnosis),

- miscellaneous (acupuncture).

PHARMACOLOGICAL TREATMENT

Numerous drugs have been proposed to treat hiccups, but for most of these the literature consists of case reports covering fewer than five patients. Chlorpromazine was tried out in the 1950s on large numbers of patients; it is best given as intravenous boluses of 25–50 mg and works putatively through dopamine blockade in the hypothalamus. Unfortunately, it causes sedation, postural hypotension and other disabling symptoms in the elderly. Metoclopramide is another dopamine antagonist with gastrointestinal and central actions, which, in a group of 14 patients with diverse serious illnesses, controlled hiccups in all.

Baclofen is the only drug tested in a double-blind, randomized, controlled crossover trial. It did not achieve resolution but did extend the hiccup-free period and the effect was dose dependent; the trial involved only four patients, but the results were statistically significant. In an open study of 37 patients, baclofen controlled hiccups in 18. A combination of baclofen, cisapride (now withdrawn) and omeprazole stopped hiccups in 11/29 patients with idiopathic chronic hiccup and improved the hiccups in a further seven. The addition of gabapentin if this regime fails has also been suggested.[3] Interestingly, midazolam, amongst the commonest drugs listed in the literature to cause hiccups, also figures in the palliative care literature as a possible treatment for this condition.

Table 4.12.1 lists some of the drugs used for treatment.

Table 4.12.1 Some drugs used for hiccups

More than five case reports
Chlorpromazine 25–50 mg i.v.
Metoclopramide 5–10 mg i.m./i.v., 10 mg q.d.s. p.o.
Baclofen 5–60 mg q.d.s. p.o.
Nifedipine 30–60 mg
Cisapride[a] 30 mg/day + omeprazole 20 mg/day + baclofen 45 mg/day

Fewer than five case reports

Central nervous system depressants
Morphine
Diamorphine
Ketamine
Magnesium sulphate

Drugs with dopamine-related effects
Haloperidol
Amphetamines
Amitriptyline

Anticonvulsants
Valproate
Carbamazepine
Phenytoin
Clonazepam
Barbiturates

Calcium-channel blockers
Lidocaine (lignocaine)
Quinidine
Amitriptyline
Cisapride[a]
Midazolam
Nimodipine

Skeletal muscle relaxants
Orphenadrine
Anticholinergics
Atropine
Hyoscine

Anti-inflammatories
Dexamethasone
Naproxen

Drugs acting on the gastrointestinal tract
Cisapride[a]
Simethicone
Amyl nitrate
Glyceryl trinitrate

Drug combinations
Cisapride[a] + omeprazole + gabapentin
Cisapride[a] + omeprazole + baclofen + gabapentin

For a fuller list see Friedman (1996).[5]
[a] Now withdrawn. i.v., intravenous; i.m., intramuscular; p.o., oral; q.d.s., four times a day.

A–Z OF SYMPTOMS

KEY POINTS

- Distressing hiccups can arise in end-stage disease from a multitude of causes.
- Many non-pharmacological treatments have been proposed, which can work well for the individual run of hiccups; however, frequently recurring hiccups will usually need drugs to prevent them or reduce their frequency.
- The evidence base for any pharmacological treatment of hiccup is particularly scanty. Chlorpromazine, metoclopramide, baclofen, nifedipine and a combination of baclofen, cisapride (now withdrawn) and omeprazole have the best evidence for success. Numerous other drugs have been reported as successful in a handful of cases. Some drugs appear to both cause hiccups in some contexts and relieve them in others.

REFERENCES

1. Launois S, Bizec JL, Whitelaw WA, Cabane J, Derenne JP. Hiccup in adults: an overview. *Eur Respir J* 1993; **6**(4), 563–75.
2. Dickerman RD, Sivakumar, J. The hiccup reflex arc and persistent hiccups with high dose anabolic steroids: is the brainstem the steroid-responsive locus? *Clin Neuropharmacol* 2001; **24**(1), 62–4.
3. Petroianou G, Hein G, Stegmeier-Petroianu A, Bergler W, Rufer R. Gabapentin 'add-on therapy' for idiopathic chronic hiccup (ICH). *J Clin Gastroenterol* 2000; **30**(3), 321–4.
4. Howard RS. Persistent hiccups: if excluding or treating any underlying pathology fails, try chlorpromazine. *BMJ* 1992; **305**, 1237–8.
5. Friedman NL. Hiccups: a treatment review. *Pharmacotherapy* 1996; **16**(6), 986–95.
6. Lewis JH. Hiccups: causes and cures. *J Clin Gastroenterol* 1985; **7**(6), 539–52.
7. Thompson DF, Landry JF. Drug-induced hiccups. *Ann Pharmacother* 1997; **31**, 367–9.

chapter 4.13

INSOMNIA

Laura C. Kelly

DEFINITION

In the tenth edition of the *International classification of diseases (ICD-10)* diagnosis of insomnia requires the presence of the following key features:

- difficulty in falling asleep or maintaining sleep, or poor quality of sleep;
- the sleep disturbance has occurred at least three times per week for at least a month;
- preoccupation with the sleeplessness and excessive concern over the consequences of insomnia;
- unsatisfactory quantity and/or quality of sleep either causes marked distress or interferes with ordinary activities.[1]

Insomnia is not defined by a particular *quantity* of sleep: many people function well with much less than the proverbial 8 hours a night. Advancing age tends to lead towards a pattern of multiple sleep episodes spread over 24 hours, rather than a single stretch of nocturnal sleep. Provided the quality of wakefulness is good, complaints of this change should evoke reassurance rather than a hypnotic prescription.

PREVALENCE

Insomnia is a common symptom, with a reported prevalence of 40 per cent in cancer patients and 15 per cent in healthy controls.[2] It is more common in women, the older population, and those with a previous history of insomnia or a co-existing psychiatric diagnosis.

AETIOLOGY

Multiple factors are liable to contribute to insomnia, such as:

- uncontrolled symptoms, for example pain and delirium;

- undergoing cancer treatments, which can cause insomnia through both their emotional and physical burdens;

- co-morbidities, including hyperthyroidism, congestive cardiac failure and obstructive sleep apnoea;

- caffeine and alcohol intake – although alcohol may reduce sleep latency, it also fragments sleep and, overall, is not a good hypnotic;

- stress.

Once insomnia is present, abnormal beliefs and maladaptive sleep patterns can prevent it being treated successfully. The consequences of insomnia have not been studied in an ill population, but in healthy subjects it leads to fatigue, impaired quality of diurnal wakefulness, cognitive impairment, mood disturbance and physical symptoms such as headache, diarrhoea and pain. There is some thought that insomnia can lead to an impaired immunity,[3] and a link has even been proposed between insomnia and early mortality.[4]

NON-PHARMACOLOGICAL TREATMENTS

TREATMENT OF UNDERLYING CAUSE

Insomnia should be treated as a symptom rather than a diagnosis, so underlying causes must be explored and treated where possible. Any underlying psychiatric or medical diagnosis needs to be excluded, and history-taking should include the caffeine and alcohol intake of the patient.

SLEEP HYGIENE EDUCATION

These relatively simple measures have been validated only in a healthy population, and may be less applicable in people who are ill. They include recommendations such as:

- regular daytime exercise; avoidance of large meals at night;

- avoidance of caffeine and alcohol;

- maintaining a constant wake-up time and avoidance of bright lights, noise and temperature extremes.[5]

COMPLEMENTARY THERAPIES

A variety of complementary therapies has been reported to be beneficial in the management of insomnia, including acupuncture, hypnotherapy, aromatherapy and reflexology. However, there are no systematic reviews looking at their efficacy for insomnia in a population with advanced disease.

COGNITIVE BEHAVIOURAL THERAPY

There is meta-analysis evidence that cognitive behavioural therapy (CBT) will benefit 70–80 per cent of people with insomnia in the general population, with sleep improvement continuing for up to 2 years, but this is derived from studies that excluded medically unwell patients.[3] However, a randomized trial of CBT for insomnia in a cancer population found that sleep latency was significantly improved in the experimental group compared with the control group.[6]

Given the potential adverse effects of pharmacological treatments for insomnia, a recent Cochrane Review recommended that CBT be considered in the management of sleep disturbance in the elderly.[7] There are, however, no reliable predictors of the success of this treatment, and palliative care patients, who are often not only elderly but also very ill, would need to be fit enough to undergo it.

PHARMACOLOGICAL TREATMENTS

BENZODIAZEPINES

Benzodiazepines are the most popular class of medication for insomnia. In a study of 1579 cancer patients, just over half were prescribed a benzodiazepine, and in 86 per cent of these cases the indication was insomnia.[8] In the general population, benzodiazepines are effective for the acute and short-term treatment of insomnia, a meta-analysis of studies finding that sleep was increased by 61.8 minutes.[9]

There are no studies of long-term follow-up and no placebo-controlled trials of the efficacy of benzodiazepines for insomnia in cancer patients. A Cochrane Review failed to identify any randomized controlled trials in palliative care and was therefore unable to draw any conclusions.[10] Despite this, these drugs are widely used in the treatment of insomnia in terminally ill patients, temazepam 10–30 mg at night being a common choice in the UK.

The risks include hangover effects the following day, an increase in falls and hip fractures in the elderly, and dependency, although this is less likely to be a problem in the palliative care population. It is important to select a drug with a short half-life. However, benzodiazepine half-lives are extended in older people and in renal failure, so that an initially helpful hypnotic dose may be the cause of confusion and an apparent clinical deterioration 2 or 3 weeks later.

ZOPICLONE

Zopiclone differs structurally from the benzodiazepines but acts on the same receptors. It has a half-life of 5–6 hours, compared with around 11 hours for temazepam, and can be taken in doses of 3.75 mg or 7.5 mg. Zopiclone is contraindicated in liver failure and may cause gastrointestinal disturbance, low mood and drowsiness.

BARBITURATES

Once frequently used as hypnotics, barbiturates have a high abuse potential and are dangerous in overdose. Consequently their use for this indication is no longer recommended.

CHLORAL HYDRATE

Chloral hydrate and its derivative triclofos exert barbiturate-like depressant effects on the central nervous system. As a liquid, chloral hydrate has an unpleasant taste and in any formulation it can cause nausea and vomiting. Although supposedly useful for insomnia in the elderly, this group is particularly prone to the nightmares it can cause. Hangover is possibly less of a problem than with some benzodiazepines, but the use of these drugs has declined.

CLOMETHIAZOLE

Clomethiazole has muscle relaxant and anticonvulsant properties as well as being a hypnotic. It has a higher therapeutic index than barbiturate-like drugs and is relatively free from hangover effects. As a result, it may be considered in those who do not tolerate benzodiazepines, particularly older patients.

MELATONIN

Melatonin is a synthetic derivative of a natural hormone produced by the pineal gland that has a role in the regulation of the circadian rhythm. It is an 'over-the-counter' medication, available in the USA but not in the UK. Melatonin has a direct soporific effect and lowers not only alertness but also body temperature.

There are no large trials of the efficacy of melatonin, but it has been shown to be effective in the treatment of jet lag. Side effects include abdominal cramps, dizziness, headaches and loss of appetite. The safety of this medication is uncertain and there have been no toxicity trials in humans,[11] making it difficult to endorse its use.

VALERIAN

A systematic review of nine randomized controlled trials of this herbal remedy for insomnia, obtained from a relative of the teazel plant, found them to be of poor quality and to provide little evidence of effectiveness.[12] However, gastrointestinal disturbances and vivid dreams can occur.

KEY POINTS

- Insomnia is defined by the quality rather than quantity of sleep.
- A more dispersed pattern of sleep is normal in older people.
- Always check for reversible psychological, physical and dietary causes.
- Simple sleep hygiene measures may be helpful.
- Benzodiazepines are the safest hypnotic drugs, but select an agent with a short half-life and watch out for clinical signs of accumulation.
- There is evidence for the effectiveness of cognitive behavioural therapy for insomnia in both cancer patients and the elderly.
- Complementary therapies currently lack systematic review evidence of effectiveness for insomnia in people with advanced disease.

REFERENCES

1. World Health Organisation. *The tenth revision of the international classification of diseases and related health problems (ICD-10)*. Geneva: World Health Organisation, 1992.
2. Malone M, Harris AL, Luscombe DK. Assessment of the impact of cancer at work, recreation, home, management and sleep using a general health status measure. *J R Soc Med* 1994; **87**, 386–9.
3. Savard J, Morin C. Insomnia in the context of cancer: a review of a neglected problem. *J Clin Oncol* 2001; **19**, 895–908.
4. Ayas NT, White DP, Manson JA *et al.* A prospective study of sleep duration and coronary heart disease in women. *Arch Intern Med* 2003; **163**, 205–9.
5. Holbrook AM, Crowther R, Lotter A, Cheng C, King D. The diagnosis and management of insomnia in clinical practice: a practical evidence-based approach. *Can Med Assoc J* 2000; **162**, 216–20.
6. Cannici J, Malcolm R, Peek LA. Treatment of insomnia in cancer patients using muscle relaxation training. *J Behav Ther Exp Psychiatry* 1983; **14**, 251–6.
7. Montgomery P, Dennis J. Cognitive behavioural interventions for sleep problems in adults aged 60+ (*Cochrane Review*). In: *The Cochrane Library*, Issue 1. Chichester: John Wiley & Sons, 2003.
8. Derogatis LR, Feldstein M, Morrow G. A survey of psychotropic drug prescriptions in an oncology population. *Cancer* 1979; **44**, 1919–29.
9. Holbrook AM, Crowther R, Lotter A, Cheng C, King D. Meta-analysis of benzodiazepine use in the treatment of insomnia. *Can Med Assoc J* 2000; **162**, 225–33.
10. Hirst A, Sloan R. Benzodiazepines and related drugs for insomnia in palliative care (*Cochrane Review*). In: *The Cochrane Library*, Issue 1. Chichester: John Wiley & Sons, 2003.
11. Herxheimer A, Petrie KJ. Melatonin for the prevention and treatment of jet lag (*Cochrane Review*). In: *The Cochrane Library*, Issue 1. Chichester: John Wiley & Sons, 2003.
12. Stevinson C, Ernst E. Valerian for insomnia: a systematic review of randomised clinical trials. *Sleep Med* 2000; **1**, 91–9.

NAUSEA AND VOMITING

Victor Pace

INTRODUCTION

Nausea and vomiting are frequent, troublesome symptoms in patients with advanced illness (Table 4.14.1). While mild emesis may only be a nuisance, severe nausea and vomiting totally disable patients, making their life miserable and isolating them from social interaction. In a recent survey, cancer patients rated emesis as their second most troublesome symptom. Whereas in many cases they are relatively easy to control, nausea and vomiting can tax the professional's skills and ingenuity to the limit. There are a number of reasons for this.

- Nausea is a very deep-seated sensation. Control of nausea is located in the medulla, the most primitive part of the brain, together with the control of all the most basic functions of life – breathing, control of heart rate and blood pressure, for example. It is also one of the most potent aversive stimuli known. One is far more likely to avoid re-exposure to a stimulus causing severe nausea than one that causes severe pain. A single exposure is likely to set up a lifelong aversion, which is unusual for other aversive stimuli. These facts suggest that nausea and vomiting are essential protective mechanisms, probably evolved in animals to avoid poisoning from ingesting dangerous materials.

- The physiology of nausea and vomiting, still being unravelled, is extremely complex.

- The interplay of physical and emotional causes is very significant.

Table 4.14.1 Frequency of nausea and vomiting in advanced disease

---

- Nausea found in 6–44% of cancer patients, vomiting in 4–25%
- Commoner in gynaecological, gastrointestinal and breast malignancies; nausea also frequent in leukaemias and lymphomas
- Probably slightly more common in AIDS
- Bereaved relatives report slightly less prevalence in the last year of life in patients dying from non-malignant illness than from cancer, but more likely to have been present for more than 6 months or to have been very distressing

---

PHYSIOLOGY OF NAUSEA AND VOMITING

Our picture of the physiology of nausea and vomiting, and therefore our management, has altered in recent years.

NAUSEA

Physiologically, nausea is poorly understood. It is known that the hypothalamus and the inferior frontal gyrus in the cerebral cortex are involved in its production, that antidiuretic hormone (ADH) levels rise and that there are electrical rhythm disturbances in the stomach. Whether these are cause or effect, or simply epiphenomena, is as yet uncertain, though the latter appears less likely. However, experimental models of nausea exist which produce no change in ADH or in the electrogastrogram. The situation is obviously complex.

VOMITING

Before stomach contents are expelled in vomiting, a series of preparatory events takes place. The mouth fills with saliva, air is swallowed and retching occurs. A powerful feeling of nausea is experienced, together with symptoms of intense sympathetic stimulation such as dizziness, skin colour changes and sweating. Peristalsis is reversed and the stomach becomes flaccid, filling with food from the small bowel. The epiglottis closes off the trachea and breath is held mid-inspiration; these actions prevent aspiration of vomited food. The muscles of thorax and abdomen then contract strongly, often at first against a closed glottis, until the glottis finally opens and the contents of the stomach are pushed out forcibly.

This very complicated sequence of events demands exact co-ordination. Delayed closure of the glottis could result in aspiration pneumonia or the very dangerous Mendelson's syndrome from aspiration of gastric acid, especially in altered consciousness. Strong contraction of the abdominal and chest muscles against a glottis that does not open results in huge pressure rises in the oesophagus, leading to tears of the mucosa at the gastro-oesophageal junction (Mallory–Weiss tears), which can bleed heavily, or even oesophageal rupture – the Boerhave syndrome. Thus fine co-ordination is vital. This is the function of the *vomiting pattern generator* (VPG), a complex system of neuronal networks in the brainstem, mainly in the lateral medullary reticular formation and possibly the midline medulla. Neurones in the VPG communicate with each other through a number of neurotransmitters, the most important being muscarinic cholinergic, histamine H_1, μ-opioid and 5-hydroxytryptamine-2 ($5HT_2$) receptors and neurokinins such as substance P. Drugs that block these neurotransmitters will prevent nausea and vomiting mediated by the VPG (Tables 4.14.2 and 4.14.3). These anti-emetics therefore tend to be useful in a variety of settings.

The VPG has two roles. It receives inputs from a wide array of structures involved in the production and modulation of the vomiting response, and it co-ordinates the events in vomiting alluded to above. Centres for the control of salivation,

A–Z OF SYMPTOMS

Table 4.14.2 Choosing an anti-emetic[a]

Area and receptors involved	Common causes	Recommended drugs
Vomiting pattern generator ACh(M), H_1, μ-opioid, $5HT_2$, NK-1	Final common pathway for all causes of vomiting	Anticholinergics: hyoscine Levomepromazine (methotrimeprazine) Antihistamines: cyclizine
Area postrema $5HT_3$, D_2, ACh(M)$_1$, α_2	Renal failure Hypercalcaemia Hyponatraemia Drugs: opioids (also effect on gut motility) NSAIDs SSRIs antibiotics, e.g. erythromycin digoxin theophylline dopaminergic drugs anticonvulsants, e.g. carbamazepine emetogenic chemotherapy agents, e.g. cisplatin: act mainly on gut chemoreceptors interleukins, interferon Radiation	Phenothiazines: prochlorperazine, levomepromazine Butyrophenones: haloperidol $5HT_3$ antagonists: ondansetron, granisetron, tropisetron
Nucleus of tractus solitarius $5HT_3$, D_2, ACh(M), H_1, ?NMDA	Taste aversions (with higher centre involvement) Pharynx: gagging, sputum in throat Bowel obstruction	Anticholinergics: hyoscine Butyrophenones: haloperidol Antihistamines: cyclizine $5HT_3$ antagonists: ondansetron

Site / receptors	Cause / example	Drugs
Gastrointestinal motility D_2, $5HT_3$ reduce motility, usually via ACh-dependent mechanism	Slow gastric emptying and intestinal motility problems: pyloric tumour/scarring pancreatic tumour innervation damage autonomic failure drugs: opioids, anticholinergics	Metoclopramide Domperidone Erythromycin
$5HT_4$, motilin: stimulate motility		
Gut wall chemoreceptors $5HT_3$, NK-1, NK-3	Chemotherapy, e.g. cisplatin dacarbazine streptozotocin nitrogen mustard	$5HT_3$ antagonists: ondansetron
Vestibular nuclei H_1, ACh(M)	Motion Cerebellopontine angle tumours Aminoglycosides	Phenothiazines: prochlorperazine levomepromazine Antihistamines: cyclizine
Cerebral cortex, limbic system 5HT, GABA	Anxiety Fear Chemotherapy-associated anticipatory vomiting Pain Smell Sight	Benzodiazepines: lorazepam

Read in conjunction with Table 4.14.3.
Ach(M), cholinergic muscarinic; D, dopamine; H, histamine; NK, neurokinin, e.g. substance P; NMDA, N-methyl-D-aspartate; 5HT, 5-hydroxytryptamine; α_2, alpha-2 adrenergic; SSRIs, serotonin selective reuptake inhibitors.

Table 4.14.3 Anti-emetics and the receptors they act upon[a]

Drug type and examples	Receptors involved
Anticholinergics Hyoscine hydrobromide Atropine	Antagonize ACh(M)
Phenothiazines Prochlorperazine Levomepromazine	Antagonizes D_2, H_1 Antagonizes $5HT_2$, H_1, D_2, ACh(M)
Antihistamines Cyclizine Meclozine Dimenhydrinate	Antagonize H_1, ACh(M)
Butyrophenones Haloperidol	Antagonize D_2
5HT$_3$ antagonists Ondansetron Granisetron Tropisetron	Antagonize $5HT_3$
Antidopaminergic prokinetics Metoclopramide Domperidone	Antagonizes D_2 peripherally and centrally Antagonizes $5HT_3$ at high doses Stimulates $5HT_4$ Antagonizes D_2 peripherally
Prokinetics Erythromycin	Stimulates motilin receptors
Benzodiazepines Lorazepam	GABA agonists plus other mechanisms

Read in conjunction with Table 4.14.2.
Ach(M), cholinergic muscarinic; D, dopamine; H, histamine; 5HT, 5-hydroxytryptamine; GABA, gamma-aminobutyric acid.

spasmodic breathing patterns and components of the vomiting response lie close to the VPG, so that stimuli overflow from one to the other. Thus the VPG can be thought of as a web of inputs and outputs.

Inputs into the vomiting centre
The chemoreceptor trigger zones   Emesis is often chemically induced (see Table 4.14.2). These chemical stimuli are picked up by specialized chemoreceptor trigger zones (CTZs) in the brain and elsewhere, which then feed into the vomiting centre to produce nausea and vomiting. The main CTZ lies in the *area postrema* in the floor of the fourth ventricle, outside the blood–brain barrier, so that it can pick up changes in the composition of the blood and cerebrospinal fluid. The important neurotransmitters regulating impulse traffic in the area postrema are $5HT_3$,

dopamine (D_2), anticholinergic muscarinic, and α_2 receptors. Useful anti-emetics are listed in Table 4.14.2. Metoclopramide has some activity here through its effect on dopamine receptors, and at very high doses it becomes a significant $5HT_3$ antagonist; but at normal clinical doses its main action is on the gut.

The gastrointestinal tract   Many events in the gastrointestinal tract (slow gastric emptying, bowel obstruction, gastritis, gastroenteritis) will provoke nausea and vomiting, through various pathways. Vomiting from chemotherapy is mainly mediated through local activity at $5HT_3$ receptors in the gut wall itself rather than any action on the area postrema. Vomiting can also be the product of a foul taste, pharyngeal stimulation (for example by phlegm in the throat), slow gastric emptying or bowel obstruction. In each of these the impulses travel to the *nucleus of the tractus solitarius* (NTS) in the brain, which forms part of the VPG complex. Taste impulses reach the NTS through the chorda tympani component of the facial nerve, stimuli from the pharynx act through the glossopharyngeal nerve, and stimuli from the stomach and intestine run to the NTS via the vagus. Interestingly, vagotomy blocks vomiting due to a large number of causes interrupting cholinergic input into the brainstem. Neurotransmitters in the NTS include $5HT_3$, dopamine D_2, muscarinic cholinergic (ACh(M)), histamine H_1, and possibly N-methyl-D-aspartate (NMDA). In the gut, stimulation of dopamine D_2, cholinergic muscarinic and $5HT_3$ receptors inhibits motility, while $5HT_4$ and motilin receptors increase it. Various neurokinins are also important.

The cerebral cortex   Cortical influences on vomiting and nausea are strong. Unpleasant sights, anxiety and fear all produce vomiting. Learned behaviour is very potent. After experiencing chemotherapy-induced vomiting, even meeting someone associated with the chemotherapy unit can set off severe nausea. Behavioural techniques and prophylactic benzodiazepines are useful here; antiemetics are often strangely powerless.

Thalamus   Severe pain can lead to vomiting; this is distinct from the reflex vomiting that accompanies strong colic.

Vestibular system   This is exemplified by motion sickness, or damage to the vestibular apparatus by tumours or drugs (see Table 4.14.2). Histamine H_1 and muscarinic cholinergic receptors are involved; thus antihistamines and anticholinergics are the treatments of choice. However, control can be difficult if the patient is severely afflicted; even in motion sickness, anti-emetics are much more effective if given prophylactically. There are close links between vestibular nuclei and cerebellum.

Inhibitory inputs   Some inputs via the vagus nerve, possibly arising from lung or airway receptors, may actually inhibit vomiting.

CLINICAL PICTURE

It is crucial precisely to define what is meant by vomiting. One sometimes sees terrible adverse effects from heavy doses of anti-emetics given to control what is

A–Z OF SYMPTOMS

actually not vomiting at all but regurgitation from an oesophageal carcinoma, for which anti-emetics are of no use at all. Treat the underlying cause when possible: treat colic not vomiting; loosen pharyngeal sputum rather than prescribe (usually ineffective) anti-emetics.

Some key questions to ask include:

- *Is the vomiting preceded by nausea?* This is one of the most useful questions. Vomiting occurring without warning is usually due either to slow gastric emptying or to raised intracranial pressure. In the former, the vomit is often large volume at first (the stomach acting as a massive reservoir of fluid), may contain identifiable food eaten a half day or more previously (as it is not passing into the small bowel for digestion), may be brought on by movement, can produce heartburn (as the lower gastro-oesophageal sphincter leaks easily when the stomach is full) and hiccups (from pressure on the diaphragm). A succussion splash can also be elicited. A large liver squashing the stomach gives similar symptoms, but the vomiting is frequent and small volume. Accompanying features of raised intracranial pressure are, of course, the early morning headache that is worse on straining and the presence of focal neurological signs or fits.
- *What is the nature of the vomit?* Faeculent vomiting is diagnostic of bowel obstruction. Vomit free from bile suggests total gastric outlet obstruction.
- *What drugs is the patient taking?* (See Table 4.14.2.)
- *What other treatments has the patient had recently?* Radiotherapy to the upper abdomen, large doses to the head, and hemibody radiation can all produce vomiting and nausea for a few days.
- *How are the bowels working?* Constipation may worsen vomiting; severe constipation can cause bowel obstruction, especially in someone weak and frail who lacks expulsive effort. Diarrhoea can point to partial bowel obstruction or to gastroenteritis.
- *What other conditions does the patient suffer from?* Concurrent illnesses can cause vomiting too.

One common misconception is that vomiting that is brought on by movement is necessarily of vestibular origin. It certainly happens commonly with delayed gastric emptying, for example.

MANAGEMENT

INVESTIGATIONS

Electrolytes and tests of renal function may be quite informative. Potassium may be low in repeated vomiting, sometimes producing paralytic ileus. A high sodium and urea may indicate dehydration. Addison's disease from adrenal infiltration may be suspected or hypercalcaemia confirmed. Plain abdominal films confirm bowel obstruction; contrast radiology and endoscopy show up gastric outlet obstruction. However, most patients are too frail for extensive investigations, and good decisions can usually be made on clinical grounds; investigations are reserved for those who do not respond to what seems like sensible management.

TREATMENT

Non-pharmacological

Strong smells or tastes that precipitate nausea and vomiting need to be avoided. Cold food is often more bland and more acceptable. Anxiety management techniques help in some situations. Acupuncture or transcutaneous electrical nerve stimulation at the P6 point at the wrist is effective for a very broad range of mechanisms of emesis. Some more esoteric methods have been described, for example placing neurosurgical lesions in the area postrema when vomiting has been truly intractable.

Pharmacological

This depends on deducing the mechanism of emesis for that particular patient if possible. Knowing the likely receptors allows us to predict which anti-emetics are likely to be most helpful. (See Tables 4.14.2 and 4.14.3).

Individual anti-emetics
Centrally acting drugs

- *Anticholinergics* (hyoscine hydrobromide, atropine) are potent general-purpose anti-emetics, acting mainly through the VPG but also via the gastrointestinal tract. Obviously, only anticholinergics that penetrate the blood–brain barrier have an effect on the VPG (therefore not hyoscine butylbromide or glycopyrronium to any great extent). However, this also means that they produce central effects, usually sedation for hyoscine and excitation for atropine, and lower seizure threshold. They produce anticholinergic adverse effects – dry mouth, constipation, blurred vision – and may precipitate retention of urine or acute closed-angle glaucoma in predisposed patients.

- *Phenothiazines* (prochlorperazine, levomepromazine (methotrimeprazine)) and *butyrophenones* (haloperidol) are all potent D_2 inhibitors apart from thioridazine, which has no anti-emetic activity. Levomepromazine even at low doses is a powerful anti-emetic, partly because it covers a broad spectrum of receptor types. However, it produces serious sedation and hypotension at high doses. Haloperidol has these adverse effects to a much lesser degree, but is more likely to produce Parkinsonism or dystonias.

- *Antihistamines* (cyclizine, dimenhydrinate, meclozine) act on the VPG. Like phenothiazines, they also have anticholinergic effects.

- *$5HT_3$ inhibitors* (ondansetron, granisetron) work on both the area postrema and on the chemoreceptor zones in the gut itself. They have a wide spectrum of activity but are particularly useful in early vomiting from highly emetogenic chemotherapy such as cisplatin.

Prokinetic agents

- *Metoclopramide* works centrally and peripherally as a D_2 blocker, though it is less potent than haloperidol. It liberates acetylcholine in the stomach and upper small bowel, and at very high doses inhibits $5HT_3$ receptors.

A–Z OF SYMPTOMS

It increases the rate of gastric emptying and motility in the upper small bowel and closes the lower gastro oesophageal sphincter.

- *Domperidone* has similar D_2 activity, but does not cross the blood–brain barrier, which robs it of central effects but also of central adverse effects such as dystonias, fairly common with metoclopramide. It has poor bioavailability by mouth but works very effectively by injection or suppository.

- *Erythromycin* is a motilin agonist, producing extensive waves of motility in the bowel. At low doses it is an effective prokinetic, though the effect is so strong at higher doses that it produces colic and vomiting. It is particularly useful in denervation states: oesophagectomy, diabetic and other autonomic gastrointestinal neuropathy, and intestinal pseudobstruction. However, it is often poorly tolerated, its effects may not last very long, and widespread use is discouraged for fear of promoting resistant bacteria. On the right occasion, however, it can work very effectively where nothing else has.

Less commonly used anti-emetics

- *Cannabinoids* such as dronabinol and nabilone are moderately effective anti-emetics in chemotherapy, but cause dysphoria (said to be reduced by concomitant prochlorperazine administration), dizziness, hallucinations and paranoia, tachycardia and hypotension.

- Prophylactic *lorazepam* reduces anticipatory vomiting with chemotherapy.

- *Corticosteroids* have some intrinsic and as yet unexplained anti-emetic activity and potentiate ondansetron in chemotherapy.

MANAGEMENT OF PARTICULAR FORMS OF VOMITING

Delayed gastric emptying is due to:

- gastric outlet obstruction (pyloric or pancreatic tumour, stricture from ulceration, functional through denervation); or

- slow exit of stomach contents (opioids, anticholinergic drugs, denervation).

Partial or functional obstruction often responds to prokinetic drugs. Tumour at the gastric outlet may be stented. However, vomiting from total or near-total gastric outlet obstruction can be almost impossible to treat. Surgical bypass through a gastrojejunostomy is best – not a major operation but one which some terminally ill patients cannot tolerate. Octreotide is sometimes used, although studies suggest it is of little use in such high obstruction. A nasogastric tube or a gastrostomy acting as a vent is another possibility, which, though too interventionist for some, can at times be the only way to make a patient comfortable.

Chemotherapy-associated and radiotherapy-associated emesis

Three forms of emesis are associated with chemotherapy: early, which occurs within a few hours of chemotherapy, delayed, i.e. more than 24 hours later, and anticipatory vomiting. Acute vomiting is especially severe with cisplatin, dacarbazine, streptozotocin and the nitrogen mustards, but can occur with most chemotherapy agents. $5HT_3$ inhibitors, usually given with steroids, have transformed the management of acute emesis. Delayed emesis occurs in up to 80 per cent of patients receiving high doses of highly emetogenic chemotherapy. $5HT_3$ inhibitors are less successful in delayed emesis, but some studies show that in combination with steroids their success rate can be good, up to almost 70 per cent, though other studies give much lower response rates. Anticipatory nausea and vomiting are commoner in younger patients, depressed patients and patients who expect to feel sick after chemotherapy. They respond best to behavioural techniques and possibly prophylactic benzodiazepines, but not to anti-emetics. Emesis after radiotherapy responds well to $5HT_3$ inhibitors.

Opioid-induced emesis
This is usually mediated via the CTZs and is therefore best treated with drugs such as haloperidol. Opioids also slow stomach and gut motility, and this too can contribute, so that on rare occasions prokinetics are a better choice.

ROUTE OF ADMINISTRATION OF DRUGS

In someone with frequent vomiting, drugs need to be given by injection or syringe driver to ensure they are absorbed. Hyoscine can also be given transdermally by a patch. Only once one ensures proper drug delivery can one judge how effective a particular medicine is. Cyclizine and levomepromazine are both likely to precipitate in a syringe driver and it may be necessary to dilute them further or to change to another drug if this occurs.

MANAGEMENT OF INTRACTABLE NAUSEA AND VOMITING

Although nausea and vomiting sometimes respond readily to treatment, at other times they can be extraordinarily difficult to control, in which case, try the following.

- Reconsider your working formulation of the cause, by retaking the history and re-examining the patient – another diagnosis may suggest another drug that works better.

- Always consider non-oral administration of drugs in severe cases to bypass the vomiting and ensure drug absorption.

- Do not celebrate too soon! In cases of emesis that prove difficult to control, introducing a new drug often leads to a day or two of respite from vomiting, only for it to return the next day, no less severe than previously.

- Rehydration, often with potassium supplementation, should be considered in severe prolonged cases, and the benefits balanced against the burden for that patient.

- If emesis does not improve after trying a number of different anti-emetics in a logical order, go for an incremental approach, adding anti-emetics to the ones the patient is already taking rather than changing them. Try progressively to block the various receptors involved in mediating nausea and vomiting.

- Check for drug interactions that can reduce the effectiveness of anti-emetics.

THE FUTURE

A number of newly investigated receptor antagonist types hold great promise. Drugs aimed at different 5HT receptors are being evolved, in particular the $5HT_{1a}$ receptor antagonists are very broad spectrum. Unfortunately, the latter also seem to induce anxiety, which at present limits the scope for clinical use. Tachykinin antagonists, especially against neurokinin-1, are also being investigated. They are broad spectrum, work against delayed as well as early post-chemotherapy vomiting and are well tolerated. They have other roles in the gut, particularly in inhibiting giant migrating contractions which can be associated with cramping and diarrhoea. At the time of writing, aprepitant, the first NK-1 antagonist to become clinically available, is starting to be used in the USA. Other techniques such as pacemakers for the gut are being looked into. There has been tremendous progress in the control of nausea and vomiting in the last 20 years, and the next 20 may well be equally momentous.

KEY POINTS

- Nausea and vomiting are common symptoms in palliative care and oncology that can be difficult to control.
- Understanding the physiology, receptors and structures involved and the clinical picture allows clinicians to choose anti-emetics appropriately.
- It is essential to elicit a detailed history to discover the most likely cause of emesis, although in some patients this remains unclear.
- Drugs acting on the VPG, such as cyclizine and hyoscine, are good general purpose anti-emetics.
- A revolution in our control of emesis occurred with the introduction of $5HT_3$ inhibitors; a similar one is likely to result from the introduction of other 5HT-subtype inhibitors and NK-1 antagonists.

FURTHER READING

Detailed referencing of this extensive subject would be cumbersome, but the following reviews are recommended for a deeper exploration of the management of nausea and vomiting.

NAUSEA AND VOMITING IN THE CONTEXT OF PALLIATIVE CARE

Morrow GR, Roscoe JA, Kirshner JJ, Hynes HE, Rosenbluth RJ. Anticipatory nausea and vomiting in the era of $5HT_3$ antiemetics. *Support Care Cancer* 1998; **6**, 244–7.

Pascoe JA, Morrow GR, Hickok JT, Stern RM. Nausea and vomiting remain a significant clinical problem: trends over time in controlling chemotherapy-induced nausea and vomiting in 1413 patients treated in community clinical practices. *J Pain Symptom Manage* 2000; **20**(2), 113–21.

Ripamonti C, Bruera E. Chronic nausea and vomiting. In: Ripamonti C, Bruera E (eds), *Gastrointestinal symptoms in advanced cancer patients*. Oxford: Oxford University Press, 2002, 169–92.

THE PHYSIOLOGY OF NAUSEA AND VOMITING

Andrews PLR, Naylor RJ, Joss RA. Neuropharmacology of emesis and its relevance to anti-emetic therapy: consensus and controversies. *Support Care Cancer* 1998; **6**, 197–203.

Koch KL. A noxious trio: nausea, gastric dysrhythmias and vasopressin. *Neurogastroenterol Motil* 1997; **9**, 141–2.

Miller A. Central mechanisms of vomiting. *Dig Dis Sci* 1999; **44**(8, Suppl.), 39S–43S.

Morrow GR, Roscoe JA, Hickok JT, Andrews PR, Matteson S. Nausea and emesis: evidence for a biobehavioral perspective. *Support Care Cancer* 2002; **10**(2), 96–105.

Peroutka SJ, Snyder SH. Antiemetics, neurotransmitter receptor binding predicts therapeutic actions. *Lancet* 1982; **1**(8273), 658–9.

Sarna SK. Tachykinins and in vivo gut motility. *Dig Dis Sci* 1999; **44**(8 Suppl.), 114S–18S.

DEVELOPMENT OF ANTI-EMETICS

Bleiberg H. A new class of antiemetics: the NK-1 receptor antagonists. *Curr Opin Oncol* 2000; **12**(4), 284–8.

Catnach SM, Fairclough PD. Erythromycin and the gut. *Gut* 1992; **33**, 397–401.

Diemunsch P, Grelot L. Potential of substance P antagonists as antiemetics. *Drugs* 2000; **60**(3), 533–46.

Ladabaum U, Hasler WL. Novel approaches to the treatment of nausea and vomiting. *Dig Dis* 1999; **17**, 125–32.

Loewen PS. Anti-emetics in development. *Expert Opin Investig Drugs* 2002; **11**(6), 801–5.

Rizk AN, Hesketh PJ. Antiemetics for cancer chemotherapy-induced nausea and vomiting: a review of agents in development. *Drugs* 1999; **2**(4), 229–35.

Roila F, Donati D, Tamberi S, Margutti G. Delayed emesis: incidence, pattern, prognostic factors and optimal treatment. *Support Care Cancer* 2002; **10**(2), 88–95.

A–Z OF SYMPTOMS

ORAL SYMPTOMS

Andrew N. Davies

XEROSTOMIA

DEFINITION

Xerostomia is defined as the subjective sensation of dryness of the mouth.

PREVALENCE

This symptom is one of the most common in patients with advanced cancer. The prevalence of xerostomia is affected by the patient's performance status. For example, in one study, 61 per cent of the patients complained of a dry mouth on their first assessment by a palliative care team, whilst 70 per cent of the patients complained of this symptom in their last week of life.[1]

PATHOPHYSIOLOGY

Xerostomia is usually the result of a reduction in the amount of saliva secreted. Patients normally complain of a dry mouth when their resting salivary flow rate falls by 50 per cent. However, xerostomia may also result from a change in the composition of the saliva secreted.

There are a number of potential causes of xerostomia in patients with cancer:

- *Disease of/damage to salivary glands*:
  related to cancer – tumour infiltration,
  related to cancer treatment – surgery, radiotherapy, chemotherapy, graft versus host disease,
  unrelated to cancer – e.g. Sjogren's syndrome.

- *Damage to/interference with nerve supply of salivary glands*:
  related to cancer – tumour infiltration,
  related to cancer treatment – surgery, radiotherapy,
  unrelated to cancer – e.g. dementia.

- *Interference with productive capacity of salivary glands*:
  dehydration,
  malnutrition.

- *Miscellaneous*:
  decreased oral intake,
  decreased mastication,
  anxiety,
  depression.

The most common cause of xerostomia in patients with cancer is drug treatment. There are a number of drugs that can cause this side effect, including many of the drugs used for symptom control in palliative care (e.g. analgesics, co-analgesics, anti-emetics, sedatives).[2]

INVESTIGATIONS AND EXAMINATION

Xerostomia may be associated with a number of local symptoms and signs. These clinical features reflect the various functions of saliva. However, xerostomia may also result in a more generalized deterioration in the patient's physical and psychological condition.

The symptoms associated with xerostomia include oral discomfort, impairment of taste, difficulty chewing, difficulty swallowing, difficulty speaking, and problems wearing dentures. The signs associated with xerostomia include dryness of oral mucous membranes, dental caries, oral candidosis and other oral infections. It should be noted that patients with xerostomia might exhibit no abnormal signs, including objective dryness of the mucous membranes.

Patients with xerostomia usually have a low resting salivary flow rate; however, some have a normal resting salivary flow rate. There is generally no indication for measuring salivary flow rates in patients with cancer.

MANAGEMENT

The management of xerostomia requires a multi-professional approach. In particular, patients may benefit from referral to a dentist or other dental-related professional (e.g. dental hygienist).

The management of xerostomia includes:

- treatment of the underlying causes of xerostomia, e.g. discontinuation of xerostomic drugs,

- symptomatic management of xerostomia.

A–Z OF SYMPTOMS

Symptomatic management

The symptomatic management of xerostomia involves the use of both saliva substitutes and saliva stimulants.

- Saliva substitutes:
  water
  artificial salivas
    mucin based
    carboxymethylcellulose based
  other substances, e.g. milk, vegetable oils.

- Saliva stimulants:
  organic acids, e.g. ascorbic acid, malic acid
  chewing gum (sugar free)
  parasympathomimetics
    choline esters, e.g. pilocarpine, bethanechol
    anticholinesterases, e.g. distigmine, pyridostigmine
  other substances, e.g. sugar-free mints, nicotinamide
  non-pharmacological methods, e.g. acupuncture, electrostimulation.

The choice of symptomatic treatment will depend on a number of factors, including the aetiology of the xerostomia, the patient's general condition and prognosis, the presence or absence of teeth and, most importantly, the patient's preference. For example, patients with radiation-induced xerostomia should be treated with pilocarpine. Also, dentate patients with xerostomia should not be treated with acidic products, e.g. some of the carboxymethylcellulose-based artificial salivas, all of the organic acids. (Acidic products cause demineralization of the teeth, and other oral problems.)

There are good theoretical reasons for prescribing saliva stimulants rather than saliva substitutes. The saliva stimulants cause an increase in secretion of normal saliva, and so will ameliorate both xerostomia and the other complications of hyposalivation. In contrast, the saliva substitutes will generally only ameliorate xerostomia. Furthermore, in studies that have compared salivary stimulants with saliva substitutes, patients have generally preferred the salivary stimulants.[3]

It should be noted that some patients do not respond to saliva stimulants. Furthermore, some patients will benefit from a combination of a saliva substitute and a saliva stimulant. Studies have shown that the mucin-based artificial saliva is more effective, and causes fewer side effects, than the carboxymethylcellulose-based artificial salivas.[4]

There have been a few studies of these treatments for patients with advanced disease. The results of the studies involving saliva substitutes (i.e. mucin-based artificial saliva) are shown in Table 4.15.1,[5–7] and those of the studies involving saliva stimulants (i.e. chewing gum, pilocarpine) in Table 4.15.2.[6,7] In general, patients have found the saliva stimulants more effective than the saliva substitutes.

Further studies are needed to determine the role of many of the aforementioned treatments for patients with advanced cancer.

Table 4.15.1 Trials of saliva substitutes in palliative care setting

Study	Treatment	Effectiveness of treatment	Side effects of treatment	Other comments
Sweeney et al. (1997)[5]	Mucin-based artificial saliva p.r.n.	Improvement in xerostomia: 60% of subjects	None reported	RCT: mucin-based artificial saliva vs 'placebo' spray – 93% of patients wanted to continue with artificial saliva
Davies et al. (1998)[6]	Mucin-based artificial saliva q.d.s.	Improvement in xerostomia: 73% of subjects	31% of subjects Nausea, diarrhoea, irritation of mouth	RCT: mucin-based artificial saliva vs pilocarpine – 64% of patients wanted to continue with artificial saliva
Davies (2000)[7]	Mucin-based artificial saliva q.d.s.	Improvement in xerostomia: 89% of subjects	19% of subjects Nausea, unpleasant taste, irritation of mouth	RCT: mucin-based artificial saliva vs chewing gum – 74% of patients wanted to continue with artificial saliva

p.r.n., as required; q.d.s., four times a day; RCT, randomized controlled trial.

Table 4.15.2 Trials of saliva stimulants in palliative care setting

Study	Treatment	Effectiveness of treatment	Side effects of treatment	Other comments
Davies et al. (1998)[6]	Pilocarpine 5 mg t.d.s.	Improvement in xerostomia: 90% of subjects	84% of subjects Sweating, dizziness, lacrimation	RCT: mucin-based artificial saliva vs pilocarpine – 76% of patients wanted to continue with pilocarpine. Pilocarpine more effective than mucin-based artificial saliva
Davies (2000)[7]	Chewing gum 1–2 pieces q.d.s.	Improvement in xerostomia: 90% of subjects	22% of subjects Irritation of mouth, nausea, unpleasant taste	RCT: mucin-based artificial saliva vs chewing gum – 86% of patients wanted to continue with chewing gum. Chewing gum as effective as mucin-based artificial saliva (Patients preferred chewing gum)

t.d.s., three times a day; q.d.s., four times a day.

TASTE DISTURBANCE

DEFINITIONS

There are three types of taste disturbance:

- ageusia – an absence of taste,
- hypogeusia – a reduction in taste,
- dysgeusia – a distortion of taste.

PREVALENCE

This symptom is relatively common in patients with advanced cancer. For example, in one study 40 per cent of patients admitted to a hospice complained of taste disturbance.[8]

PATHOPHYSIOLOGY

There are a number of potential causes of taste disturbance in patients with advanced cancer.

- *Related to cancer*:
  direct effect, i.e. tumour infiltration
  indirect effect, i.e. paraneoplastic syndrome.

- *Related to cancer treatment*:
  local surgery
  local radiotherapy
  systemic chemotherapy, e.g. platinum-based compounds (carboplatin, cisplatin), 5-fluorouracil
  local drug treatment, e.g. local anaesthetics (benzocaine, lignocaine)
  systemic drug treatment, e.g. angiotensin-converting enzyme inhibitors (captopril, enalapril), tricyclic antidepressants (amitriptyline, nortriptyline), allopurinol, metronidazole.

- *Related to other oral problems*:
  xerostomia
  poor oral hygiene
  oral infections.

- *Miscellaneous causes*:
  malnutrition
  zinc deficiency
  diabetes mellitus
  renal disease
  neurological disease.

INVESTIGATIONS AND EXAMINATION

Dysgeusia appears to be the most common type of taste disturbance in patients with advanced cancer.[8] In some cases, it is associated with hypogeusia (i.e. some foods taste different from normal, whilst some foods taste less intense than normal).

Taste disturbance may be associated with anorexia and weight loss.

MANAGEMENT

The management of taste disturbance requires a multi-professional approach. In particular, patients may benefit from referral to a dietician.

The management of taste disturbance involves:

- treatment of the underlying cause of taste disturbance, e.g. treatment of xerostomia,
- symptomatic management of taste disturbance.

Symptomatic management

The symptomatic management of taste disturbance primarily involves dietary modification, which aims to ensure an adequate intake of food. Strategies that may be useful include the use of strong flavours, texture (i.e. firm rather than soft) and temperature (i.e. hot rather than cold).[9]

Oral zinc supplements have been reported to be effective in some patients with cancer.[10] However, there appear to have been no studies of this treatment in patients with advanced cancer.

Oral corticosteroids have been reported to be effective in patients with advanced cancer,[9] although the response rate appears to be relatively small.

It should be noted that an improvement in the underlying malignant disease is sometimes associated with an improvement in the taste disturbance.

Studies are needed to determine the role of the aforementioned treatments for patients with advanced cancer.

> **KEY POINTS**
>
> - Oral symptoms cause significant morbidity in patients with advanced cancer.
> - Saliva substitutes (i.e. mucin-based artificial saliva) have been shown to be effective in treating xerostomia in palliative care patients.
> - Saliva stimulants (i.e. chewing gum, pilocarpine) have also been shown to be effective in treating xerostomia in palliative care patients.
> - Saliva stimulants have therapeutic advantages over saliva substitutes.

A–Z OF SYMPTOMS

REFERENCES

1. Conill C, Verger E, Henriquez I *et al*. Symptom prevalence in the last week of life. *J Pain Symptom Manage* 1997; **14**, 328–31.

2. Sreebny LM, Schwartz SS. A reference guide to drugs and dry mouth, 2nd edition. *Gerodontology* 1997; **14**, 33–47.

3. Bjornstrom M, Axell T, Birkhed D. Comparison between saliva stimulants and saliva substitutes in patients with symptoms related to dry mouth. A multi-centre study. *Swed Dent J* 1990; **14**, 153–61.

4. Visch LL, 's-Gravenmade EJ, Schaub RM, Van Putten WL, Vissink A. A double-blind crossover trial of CMC- and mucin-containing saliva substitutes. *Int J Oral Maxillofac Surg* 1986; **15**, 395–400.

5. Sweeney MP, Bagg J, Baxter WP, Aitchison TC. Clinical trial of a mucin-containing oral spray for treatment of xerostomia in hospice patients. *Palliat Med* 1997; **11**, 225–32.

6. Davies AN, Daniels C, Pugh R, Sharma K. A comparison of artificial saliva and pilocarpine in the management of xerostomia in patients with advanced cancer. *Palliat Med* 1998; **12**, 105–11.

7. Davies AN. A comparison of artificial saliva and chewing gum in the management of xerostomia in patients with advanced cancer. *Palliat Med* 2000; **14**, 197–203.

8. Davies AN, Kaur K. Taste problems in patients with advanced cancer. *Palliat Med* 1998; **12**, 482–3.

9. Twycross RG, Lack SA. Taste changes. In: Twycross RG, Lack SA (eds), *Control of alimentary symptoms in far advanced cancer.* Edinburgh: Churchill Livingstone, 1986, 57–64.

10. Ripamonti C, Fulfaro F. Taste alterations in cancer patients. *J Pain Symptom Manage* 1998; **16**, 349–51.

FURTHER READING

Davies AN. The management of xerostomia: a review. *Eur J Cancer Care* 1997; **6**, 209–14.

Edgar WM, O'Mullane DM (eds). *Saliva and oral health*, 2nd edn. London: British Dental Association, 1996.

MANAGEMENT OF PAIN

John Wiles, Dag Rutter, Louise Exton, Irene Carey, Polly Edmonds and Nigel Sykes

INTRODUCTION

Pain is popularly associated with cancer. However, around 30 per cent of cancer patients have little or no pain and a variety of progressive non-malignant conditions produce it frequently.[1] The International Association for the Study of Pain (IASP) defines pain as 'an unpleasant sensory and emotional experience associated with actual or potential tissue damage or described in terms of such damage'.[2]

However, pain is not merely the result of, or proportional to, tissue damage. Instead, it is a psychosomatic phenomenon, i.e. the overall result of a physical sensation modulated by the emotions. To express this, Saunders introduced the concept of 'total pain', in which pain has physical, psychological, social and spiritual dimensions.[3] Any assessment of pain must therefore move beyond the physical and encompass these other influences.

ASSESSMENT OF PAIN

Pain being a subjective experience, the patient's own report is fundamental in its assessment. A structured approach to pain assessment is likely to improve the quality of analgesia, and here is one framework that covers the essential steps.

- Believe the patient's complaint.

- Take a careful history.

- List and prioritize the pains (most patients have more than one).

- Assess each individual pain.

- Clarify the time pattern of the pain, both as a clue to diagnosis and because incident pain is more difficult to control with drugs.

- Evaluate response to previous treatment.

- Evaluate the psychological state of the patient.

- Evaluate the patient's social situation and level of support from family and friends.

- Enquire about religious or other beliefs and practices that are helpful.

- Ask about an alcohol or drug dependence history.

- Perform a medical and neurological examination, including a check for sensory distortions in the area of pain.

- Use appropriate diagnostic procedures.

- Treat the pain.

- Evaluate and monitor progress.

(Adapted from Foley.[4])

It is important to recognize that this assessment is not solely focused on the physical contribution to pain. For instance, mental impairment that prevents patients describing or remembering their pain is a severe handicap to effective pain management and needs to be assessed. A history of drug or alcohol abuse is one of a number of factors that have been shown to be indicators of poor prognosis for the analgesic control of pain. Others include pain with neuropathic or incident characteristics and a tendency for a patient to present emotional disturbances in the guise of a physical complaint.[5] Careful attention has to be paid to the psychological and social influences impacting on patients and the resources of the entire multi-professional team enlisted in their management, because these are factors that can influence the severity of pain from any cause.

The pain threshold may be lowered (that is the pain is exacerbated) by:

- insomnia

- fatigue

- anxiety

- fear

- anger

- boredom

- depression

- isolation

- social abandonment

- sadness.

The pain threshold may be raised (that is the pain is eased) by:

- relief of other symptoms
- sleep
- rest
- sympathy
- understanding
- companionship
- relief of anxiety
- mood elevation
- use of analgesics, anxiolytics, antidepressants and co-analgesics.

PAIN ASSESSMENT TOOLS

Simple, reliable and validated methods of recording pain intensity have been available for many years. These include verbal rating scales, numerical rating scales and visual analogue scales. They are easy to use and minimally intrusive, but have the shortcoming that they assume pain intensity to be one-dimensional. Other more sophisticated tools have been developed that look at pain more comprehensively or examine a specific type of pain. The multi-dimensional tools include the McGill Pain Questionnaire[6] (Fig. 4.16.1) and the Brief Pain Inventory.[7] A consequence of their broader and more detailed assessment is that they are more time-consuming to use than the simpler one-dimensional scales. A specific pain scale is the Leeds Assessment of Neuropathic Symptoms and Signs, aimed at assisting the diagnosis of neuropathic pain.[8]

DRUG MANAGEMENT OF PAIN

THE WORLD HEALTH ORGANISATION ANALGESIC LADDER

Nearly 20 years after its introduction, the World Health Organisation (WHO) three-step analgesic ladder[9] (Fig. 4.16.2) remains firmly established in clinical practice. Although evaluations have been based on case series without control groups, it is estimated that cancer pain will be well or moderately controlled in 80 per cent of cases with optimal use of guidelines. There remains, however, a population of more difficult pains that in addition to drugs may require the use of techniques such as radiotherapy or neural blockade, and possibly significant psychological or psychiatric input, for their control.

The ladder simply provides a rough categorization of general analgesics by potency, suggesting a place to start for those who have not needed pain relief before (non-opioids) and encouraging a move to a stronger agent if success is not

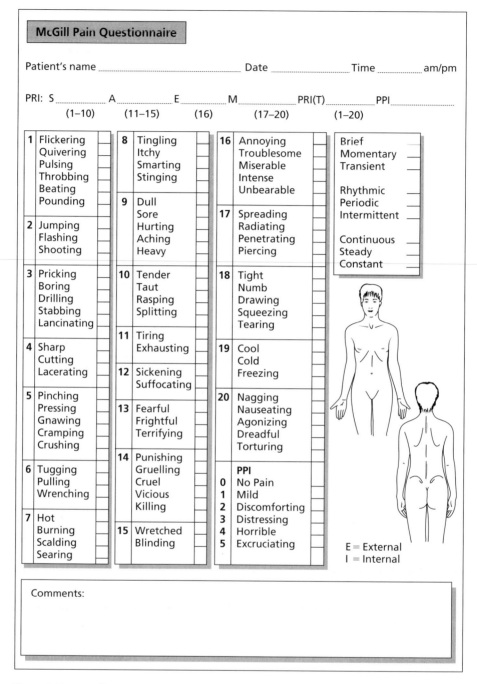

Figure 4.16.1 McGill Pain Questionnaire.

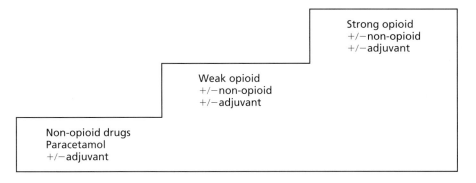

Figure 4.16.2 The WHO pain ladder. If side effects lead to a drug being withdrawn, an alternative on the step may be used. If a maximum tolerated dose is not effective, move up a step.

achieved. In practice, the highest rung of the ladder is used more often than the lower two, either of which may be missed entirely.[10]

Most pain associated with cancer and other progressive diseases is persistent. 'As-required' analgesia makes no sense in this context, as it simply sentences the patient to continue to experience pain repeatedly as the price for receiving another dose of medication. Therefore medicines should be provided regularly and orally if possible, as this maximizes the patient's control. The simple directive to use the right drug, in the right dose, at the right interval, by the right route maximizes the effectiveness of pain relief. The concept of regular review remains essential to managing pain. Lack of compliance is a major obstacle to good pain control, and whichever drug is used, it is essential that patients understand how to use it and feel safe with it.

Non-opioid analgesics

Paracetamol is the WHO analgesic ladder step 1 analgesic of choice; non-steroidal anti-inflammatory drugs (NSAIDs) are also step 1 analgesics and can also be used in conjunction with opioids in steps 2 and 3 for somatic, visceral and bone pain.[9]

Paracetamol Paracetamol has poorly understood mechanisms of action. Analgesic properties may stem from peripheral effects on the chemical mediators of pain or central non-opioid effects. Although antipyretic, it is not a significant anti-inflammatory agent. Adverse events, other than dose-dependent liver cell necrosis in overdose, are extremely rare.

Non-steroidal anti-inflammatory drugs The NSAIDs are a heterogeneous group of drugs that inhibit the enzyme cyclo-oxygenase (COX). The inhibition of COX prevents the conversion of arachidonic acid to prostaglandin G2. COX is now known to occur in two forms: COX-1, which is part of normal cells and serves several important physiological roles, and COX-2, which is induced in the inflammatory process. Inhibition of COX-2 is responsible for the anti-inflammatory properties of NSAIDs, whilst COX-1 inhibition causes many of the adverse effects associated with NSAID use.[11] Conventional NSAIDs inhibit both isoenzymes. Current interest lies in the development and use of selective COX-2 inhibitors to minimize toxicity. NSAIDs also inhibit the release of inflammatory mediators by

A–Z OF SYMPTOMS

acting on the cell membranes of neutrophils. Both these mechanisms reduce inflammation in tissues. However, there is only weak correlation between anti-inflammatory and analgesic efficacy of various NSAIDs[12] and it has therefore been proposed that NSAIDs may also have central effects by acting as N-methyl-D-aspartate (NMDA) inhibitors.[13]

Pharmacokinetics   The NSAIDs are well absorbed following oral administration and are highly protein bound. They are extensively metabolized and undergo variable renal clearance.

Efficacy   The NSAIDs are effective single-dose analgesics in acute postoperative pain and have been demonstrated to be effective single-agent analgesics in cancer pain in single and chronic dosing studies. A meta-analysis of 25 randomized control trials involving 1545 patients showed NSAIDs had analgesic efficacy roughly equivalent to 5–10 mg of intramuscular morphine and demonstrated a ceiling effect.[14] There is marked variation in patients' responses to NSAIDs. A crucial factor in NSAID choice is adverse effect profile.

Adverse effects   The common adverse effects attributed to NSAIDs are listed in Table 4.16.1. Gastrointestinal toxicity is the most common and important in clinical practice; the spectrum of adverse effects ranges from dyspepsia, nausea and vomiting to ulceration, haemorrhage and perforation. The overall risk of gastrointestinal ulceration is increased fourfold for patients taking NSAIDs as compared to the general population; factors that increase the risk further include age >60 years, past history of peptic ulcer disease and concomitant steroid, anticoagulant or aspirin use.[15] Patients with these risk factors should therefore receive concurrent gastro-protective prophylaxis with misoprostol or a proton pump inhibitor.[15] Patients should also be educated about potential gastrointestinal toxicity.[16]

Individual NSAIDs vary considerably in terms of gastrointestinal toxicity and there is an additional dose–response effect (Table 4.16.2).

Choice of drug   New-generation NSAIDs, including highly selective COX-2 inhibitors and nitric oxide-releasing NSAIDs, are promising in the search for safer drugs; however, further long-term data and specific studies in cancer pain are needed. In a systematic review, the COX-2 inhibitor celecoxib was as effective as other NSAIDs for the relief of symptoms of osteoarthritis and rheumatoid arthritis,

Table 4.16.1 Common adverse effects of non-steroidal anti-inflammatory drugs (NSAIDs)

Adverse effect	Mechanism	Comments
Renal	Fluid and water retention Interstitial nephritis Papillary necrosis	Patients with reduced circulatory volume are at particular risk of renal failure
Haemostasis	Inhibit platelet aggregation Increase bleeding time	
Hypersensitivity reactions	Bronchospasm in susceptible patients	Incomplete cross-tolerance between NSAIDS

but had significantly improved gastrointestinal safety and tolerability.[17] The long-term safety of the COX-2 inhibitors and the likelihood of serious non-gastrointestinal adverse effects compared to other NSAIDs remain controversial. At present in the UK, the National Institute for Clinical Excellence (NICE) recommends the use of COX-2 inhibitors only in high-risk patients.[18]

Opioid analgesics

Opioids comprise a diverse group of analgesic drugs with variable routes of administration, receptor affinities, pharmacokinetics and adverse effects. Opioids produce their effects by combining with endogenous opioid receptors. These effects are antagonised by naloxone. The International Union of Pharmacology (IUPHAR)[19] has recently re-classified the main groups of opioid receptor (Table 4.16.3). The relationship between opioid receptor subtypes and individual patient variations in responsiveness to opioid analgesics has yet to be established.

Opioids for mild to moderate pain

In the UK, patients with moderate pain have been traditionally treated with codeine, dihydrocodeine, dextropropoxyphene (either alone or in combination with paracetamol) and tramadol.[20] Dihydrocodeine and tramadol are available in modified-release (MR) preparations, which may be more convenient for patients; some may also find it more acceptable to be treated with a drug that is not morphine. The

Table 4.16.2 NSAID gastrointestinal toxicity

Least safe	Azapropazone
	Ketoprofen
	Piroxicam
⇓	Indomethacin
	Naproxen
	Diclofenac
Most safe	Ibuprofen

Table 4.16.3 NC-IUPHAR proposal for opioid receptor nomenclature

Current proposal	Previous proposal	Endogenous ligands
μ, mu or MOP	OP3	β-endorphin (not selective)
		Enkephalins (not selective)
		Endomorphin-1
		Endomorphine-2
δ, delta or DOP	OP1	Enkephalins (not selective)
		β-endorphin (not selective)
κ, kappa or KOP	OP2	Dynorphin A
		Dynorphine B
		α-neoendorphin
NOP	OP4	Nociceptin/orphanin FQ (N/OFQ)

titration of these opioids is limited by increasing adverse effects, which outweigh any increase in effectiveness at higher doses.

Codeine is a naturally occurring opium alkaloid whose analgesic effects may be attributable to variable biotransformation to morphine as well as the parent compound. Fixed combination tablets with 8 mg codeine + 500 mg paracetamol should be avoided in cancer pain due to sub-therapeutic opioid levels even at maximum paracetamol intake.

Dihydrocodeine is probably equipotent to codeine, although the higher dose range of dihydrocodeine may unacceptably increase adverse effects.[21]

Dextropropoxyphene generally has an elimination half-life of 15 hours, but this may be over 50 hours in the elderly.[22] Its efficacy has been questioned, but its dose-dependent first-pass metabolism leads to increasing systemic availability of the active principle metabolite norpropoxyphene with repeated dosing. This is thought to increase potency.[23]

Tramadol has a modest mu affinity with weaker delta and kappa affinity. It may also affect serotonin and noradrenaline pain pathways,[24] potentially broadening its spectrum of clinical activity.

Opioids for moderate to severe pain

Morphine-like agonist drugs are widely used to treat cancer pain. An increasing variety of opioids allows more individualization of pain management, although there is a lack of good-quality comparative data demonstrating significant differences between available compounds. In the UK, morphine remains the drug of choice for severe pain due to its wide availability and familiarity with its use. The relative potencies of opioid analgesics are shown in the appendix at the end of this chapter. These must be interpreted with caution, as relatively few studies have explored opioid equianalgesic dose ratios in the context of chronic pain management and repeated opioid dosing.[25,26]

Morphine is the main naturally occurring opium alkaloid. It exerts predominantly mu opioid effects. In the UK, it is available in immediate-release (IR) and MR forms, as elixirs, tablets, capsules and suspensions.

Absorption is almost complete in the upper small bowel, but extensive first-pass metabolism – both in passage across the bowel wall and through the liver – results in an oral bioavailability of 20–30 per cent,[27] with wide inter-individual variability. Following predominantly hepatic metabolism (to morphine-3-glucuronide and morphine-6-glucuronide), it is renally excreted. With normal renal function, morphine has a plasma half-life of 2–3 hours and 4–6-hour duration of analgesia; these lengthen with deteriorating renal function, with the potential for opioid toxicity (which may be linked to accumulation of toxic metabolites).[28] While dose reduction is therefore often necessary in renal failure, it is, in practice, less important in hepatic failure.

Starting oral morphine   Oral IR morphine is the drug of choice for patients with severe pain, uncontrolled by step 2 analgesics. An Expert Working Group of the European Association for Palliative Care (EAPC) has produced guidelines for the use of morphine in cancer pain.[29] Initial dose titration with IR morphine is usually required to determine the optimal dose for the patient.

For example:

- prescribe IR morphine 4-hourly;

- the starting dose is usually 5–10 mg every 4 hours, but depends on the severity of pain, previous analgesic requirements and age – reduced dose (e.g. half) in frail and/or elderly patients;

- prescribe the same (4-hourly) dose for breakthrough pain; this rescue dose can be given as often as required;

- adjust the regular dose according to how many rescue doses have been given in the previous 24 hours;

- The EAPC[29] recommends using a double dose of IR morphine at night for ease of administration. However one study has suggested that pain scores and some opioid-related side effects are worse in patients receiving a double dose at night rather than the 4-hourly schedule.[30]

Once the pain is controlled and the patient's analgesic requirements are stable, he or she should be converted to the equivalent dose of a modified morphine preparation (currently available as 12-hourly or 24-hourly preparations in the UK). Appropriate breakthrough doses of IR morphine must be prescribed and should be equivalent to the 4-hourly dose.

Oral to parenteral relative potency   Morphine has limited solubility. Single-dose studies in postoperative cancer pain patients demonstrated an oral to parenteral potency ratio of 1:6. However, current clinical practice suggests that, in the context of chronic dosing, parenteral morphine is only two to three times more potent than when given orally. This is supported by a recent study in advanced cancer patients receiving chronic administration of oral morphine, which suggested an oral to intravenous equianalgesic ratio of 1:2 to 1:3.[31] In the UK, parenteral opioids are usually given by the subcutaneous route of administration. This avoids the need for intravenous cannulae and is as effective as the intravenous route.[32] Other opioids are often preferred to morphine for parenteral use because of their greater solubility: diamorphine in the UK and hydromorphone in other parts of Europe and North America.

Alternative opioids for moderate to severe pain

Diamorphine (diacetylmorphine) is a semi-synthetic analogue of morphine. It is a pro-drug that is transformed to 6-acetylmorphine and morphine to produce analgesic effects.

Methadone is a synthetic opioid. It is active at mu and delta opioid receptors[33] and has been shown to be an inhibitor of NMDA receptors,[34] broadening its potential spectrum of activity. Methadone has an oral bioavailability that ranges from 41 to 99 per cent, which is greater and less variable[35] than that of morphine. It undergoes hepatic biotransformation to inactive metabolites, which are excreted in the urine and faeces. Due to its basic and lipophilic nature, methadone undergoes extensive tissue distribution, forming a peripheral reservoir, which releases the drug back to the systemic circulation. This sustains plasma concentration in multiple dosing. Chronic dosing, therefore, leads to an increasing half-life and the potential for accumulation and toxicity.[36,37]

Methadone is cheap and widely available, but care must be taken when converting a patient from oral morphine to methadone as the dose ratio varies markedly (in the range of 1:3 to 1:10) depending on the extent of previous exposure to opioids. The mechanisms for this are unclear but may relate to:[38]

- decreased cross-tolerance of opioid receptors,

- NMDA receptor antagonism,

- elimination of active opioid metabolites.

Several different schedules have been proposed for converting from oral morphine to methadone;[36] it is our practice to use the schedule outlined in the box below.

Methadone conversion schedule (adapted from Morley and Makin[39])

- Stop morphine abruptly, i.e. do *not* reduce gradually over several days.
- Prescribe a dose of methadone that is one-tenth total daily (24-hour) oral morphine dose (up to a maximum of 30 mg).
- Allow the patient to take the fixed dose, preferably 3-hourly, as required.
- A non-opioid analgesic may be used for breakthrough pain.
- On day 6, the amount of methadone taken over the previous 2 days is noted and converted into a regular 12-hourly dose, with provision for a similar or smaller dose 3-hourly as required.
- If as-required medication is still needed, increase the dose of methadone by one-half to one-third every 4–6 days.

Hydromorphone is a semi-synthetic mu opioid agonist. Its oral bioavailability varies from 30 to 40 per cent and its metabolites are renally excreted; it is not known whether these contribute to significant analgesic or toxic effects. Its safety in renal failure is unknown. A systematic review suggested that there is little difference between hydromorphone and other opioids in terms of analgesic efficacy, adverse effect profile and patient preference, but the review was limited by the limited quality and number of studies available.[40] Hydromorphone is used in the same way as morphine: either 4-hourly or 12-hourly if using a MR preparation. In the UK, the standard capsule size reflects the potency ratio of hydromorphone to morphine (×7.5); hence hydromorphone 1.3 mg = morphine 10 mg. Hydromorphone is also available in high-potency ampoules containing 10 mg/mL, 20 mg/mL and 50 mg/mL to facilitate use by continuous subcutaneous infusion (unlicensed in the UK). When converting from oral to subcutaneous, divide the dose of hydromorphone by 6.

Oxycodone is a synthetic opioid that may bind preferentially to kappa rather than mu opioid receptors.[41] It does not undergo extensive first-pass metabolism in the liver and has a higher and less variable oral bioavailability than morphine (60–87 per cent).[42] It may therefore be more predictable in its effects. It is predominantly renally excreted and has no clinically significant active metabolites. It provides as effective analgesia and has a similar side effect profile to morphine in the treatment of patients with cancer pain.[43]

Oral oxycodone is twice as potent as oral morphine.[44] IR oxycodone is used in the same way as morphine. The delivery system of the MR preparation allows biphasic absorption. Onset of analgesia may therefore be within 1 hour, leading to successful initiation of treatment with the MR formulation.[45] Oxycodone is also now available in a parenteral formulation in the UK. The manufacturers recommend an oral to subcutaneous conversion ratio of 2:1, although based on oral to subcutaneous bioavailability, a conversion factor of 1.5:1 would also be reasonable.

Fentanyl is a very potent and lipophilic mu agonist. For these reasons, it is very suited to a non-invasive transdermal delivery system. Fentanyl patches are available in four strengths: 25 mcg/h, 50 mcg/h, 75 mcg/h and 100 mcg/h. Application of a fentanyl patch results in formation of a subcutaneous depot which sustains serum concentrations, avoiding peaks and troughs. Patches are changed every 72 (occasionally 48) hours, which is convenient for patients and avoids the need for oral medication in cases of swallowing difficulties or poor compliance. Fentanyl may also cause less constipation than morphine.[46]

Fentanyl patches are slow and unpredictable in reaching analgesia and steady state. It is therefore vital to provide alternative analgesia for at least the first 12 hours after commencing therapy.

- If converting from 4-hourly morphine, continue to give regular dose for 12 hours.

- If converting from 12-hourly morphine, apply the fentanyl patch at the same time as giving the final 12-hourly dose.

- If converting from 24-hourly morphine, apply the first fentanyl patch approximately 12 hours after the last 24-hourly dose.

- If converting from a syringe driver, maintain the subcutaneous infusion for about 12 hours after applying the first patch.

Patients should use opioid rescue doses equivalent to a dose of 4-hourly morphine; where a patient continues to need two or more rescue doses in 24 hours, the patch strength should be increased by 25 mcg/h. About 10 per cent of patients experience opioid withdrawal symptoms when changing to fentanyl from morphine; patients should be warned that they may experience symptoms 'like gastric flu', which should resolve with rescue doses of morphine.

The presence of the skin depot for many hours after removal of a fentanyl patch means that serum concentration may not fall to 50 per cent until up to 24 hours later.[47] It is important to remember this reservoir when converting to an alternative opioid. This lack of flexibility means that patches are not generally suitable for unstable pain.

The manufacturers' recommendations regarding equianalgesic doses are reasonable, but it is worth noting the wide range of morphine doses equivalent to each patch size, and care should be taken in any opioid conversion. Simple dose conversions are as follows.

- Patients with inadequate pain relief from maximum therapeutic doses of codeine, dextropropoxyphene, dihydrocodeine or tramadol should start on the 25 mcg/h patch. Care should be taken in view of the large dose range covered by this patch.

- Patients on oral morphine: divide 24-hour dose in mg by 3 and choose nearest patch strength in mcg/h.

- Patients on subcutaneous diamorphine: choose nearest patch strength in mcg/h to mg/24 h diamorphine.

Transmucosal fentanyl: recent work on transmucosal[48] and intranasal fentanyl[49] suggests these novel routes of administration have a role for episodic (breakthrough) pain for patients on regular strong opioid therapy.

Oral transmucosal fentanyl citrate (OTFC) is a 'lozenge on a stick' containing fentanyl in a hard sweet matrix, available in 200–1600 μg preparations. About 25 per cent of the dose is absorbed rapidly through the buccal mucosa into the systemic circulation, leading to onset of pain relief within 5–10 minutes. The remainder is swallowed and absorbed more slowly, undergoing intestinal and hepatic first-pass metabolism; only one-third of this amount (25 per cent of the total dose) is available systemically.

The optimal dose is determined by titration, and cannot be predicted by a patient's regular dose of opioid. Pain relief is achieved more quickly than with oral morphine and it is generally well tolerated. About 25 per cent of patients fail to obtain relief at the highest dose, i.e. 1600 μg, or have unacceptable undesirable effects.

Alfentanil is a synthetic opioid that is dependent on hepatic metabolism. It is used mostly for patients in renal failure in whom there is evidence of morphine neuro-excitability.

The following are approximate dose conversion ratios:

- subcutaneous diamorphine to subcutaneous alfentanil, give one-tenth of the 24-hour dose,

- oral morphine to subcutaneous alfentanil, give one-thirtieth of the 24-hour dose.

Pethidine (meperidine) is not recommended in palliative care due to its short action and potential central nervous system excitation.

Common opioid adverse effects

- Daytime drowsiness, dizziness or mental clouding is common on commencing therapy but generally resolves within days; where it persists and is troublesome, consideration may be given to the prescription of a central stimulant such as dextroamphetamine or methylphenidate – this practice is more common in North America than in the UK.

- Nausea occurs initially in about a half of patients and often resolves; prophylactic anti-emetics should be given to patients commencing opioid therapy to use if required.

- Constipation is a troublesome, ongoing side effect, which affects compliance in many; concurrent laxative therapy is vital.

- Dry mouth.

- Difficulty with micturition or retention.

   Toxic effects of opioid excess/accumulation include the following.

- Confusion.

- Sedation.

- Visual hallucinations.

- Pinpoint pupils.

- Myoclonic jerks.

- Clinically significant respiratory depression is rarely a feature with chronic opioid use, where the dose has been titrated against the patient's pain; the use of naloxone is almost never indicated.

- Psychological dependence on opioids is rarely a problem with appropriate use and dose titration; opioids can be reduced and withdrawn without difficulty if alternative manoeuvres (such as radiotherapy or nerve block) reduce opioid requirements.

- Rarely, patients experience bronchospasm or urticaria secondary to histamine release.

- Chronic pruritus occurs in 2–10 per cent of patients (see Chapter 16 for management options).

Management of opioid adverse effects

Optimal pain management enables patients to achieve adequate pain control with minimal adverse effects. However, a substantial minority of patients do not achieve adequate pain control because of:[50]

- excessive adverse effects,

- inadequate analgesia,

- excessive adverse effects along with inadequate analgesia.

   An Expert Working Group of the EAPC has identified several strategies for the management of opioid adverse effects to optimize pain control.[51]

1 Symptomatic management of the adverse effect – see above.
2 Dose reduction of systemic opioid – accompanied by an evaluation of the role for adjuvant analgesics, therapy targeted at managing the underlying cause of the pain and/or non-drug or anaesthetic interventions, where appropriate.
3 Opioid rotation (or switching) – see below.
4 Changing route of administration, e.g. to transdermal or subcutaneous route.

The guidelines highlight the need to carefully evaluate individual patients, to identify factors likely to increase susceptibility to opioid adverse effects, e.g. co-morbidities such as the effect of age and impaired renal or liver function, dehydration and drug interactions. In these cases, an initial dose reduction is often appropriate.

Opioid switching or rotation

In recent years there have been numerous reports of the successful reduction in intolerable opioid side effects by switching from the currently administered opioid to an alternative opioid. This approach has been termed opioid switching/substitution.[52] In North America, planned rotation of opioids is sometimes undertaken to limit toxic adverse effects; this practice is unusual in the UK or Europe, although opioid substitution is commonplace.

The aetiology for the observed inter-individual variability in sensitivity to opioid analgesia and adverse effects is multi-factorial.[52,53] The factors that are thought to play a role include the following.

- *Receptor factors.* Opioids can act on different receptors or receptor sub-types and there is likely to be genetic variation between individuals. This may affect responsiveness in terms of both analgesic efficacy and adverse effects. The differential activation of non-opioid excitatory central nervous system receptors may also be important.[54]

- *Tolerance.* The repeated administration of opioids leads to tolerance; this can be favourable with respect to adverse effects. The development of tolerance for adverse effects usually occurs more rapidly than for analgesic effects, thereby leading to a potential widening of the therapeutic window. The variability in analgesic or adverse effect response to different opioid analgesics is common and is probably due to an incomplete cross-tolerance between opioids,[52] which may be caused by differential opioid receptor affinities.

- *NMDA activation.* In animal models, morphine tolerance is associated with NMDA receptor activation and the development of hyperalgesia.

- *Opioid efficacy.* Differences in receptor efficacy may also influence incomplete cross-tolerance. The number of receptors occupied by an opioid is inversely proportional to the intrinsic activity of the drug – hence a low intrinsic affinity agonist, such as morphine, will occupy a greater number of receptors and produce a greater tolerance effect than high-efficacy agonists such as methadone and fentanyl. This may contribute to a loss of efficacy with increasing doses of morphine (as there is a low receptor reserve).

- *Metabolite production.* Analgesic response in individuals may depend on their opioid/metabolite ratio. The role of morphine metabolites in developing adverse effects is controversial.[55] If the accumulation of toxic metabolites during chronic opioid therapy does lead to adverse effects, switching to an alternative opioid may allow for the elimination of these metabolites.[54]

Opioid switching requires familiarity with a range of opioid analgesics and of dose conversions. Cross-tolerance may lead to an unanticipated potency when switching from one opioid to another. To this end, the EAPC has produced helpful guidelines for switching and rotating opioids (see box below).

Guidelines for switching and rotating opioids (adapted from EAPC[51])

1. *Use dose conversion tables.* When switching from one opioid to another in naive patients, chronic pain opioid dose conversion tables should be used to calculate the dose of the new opioid. In tolerant patients, the possibility of incomplete cross-tolerance makes the use of a simple conversion on the basis of dose conversion tables potentially hazardous.
2. *Dose conversion tables are guidelines only.* There exists large inter-individual variability in response to various opioids and this variability cannot be captured in these tables. Recent studies indicate a wide range of dose ratios in relation to morphine, although current literature does not clarify the exact ranges. Caution should therefore be exercised in conversion, perhaps by decreasing the dose by an additional 30–50 per cent. This would accommodate the variability in most cases and address the phenomenon of a lack of complete cross-tolerance when switching from one opioid to another.
3. *Dosing with the new opioid.* The initial goal when switching opioids is to convert the patient to a new drug safely. As noted above, incomplete cross-tolerance may result in some patients being far more sensitive to the new agent than anticipated. Thus, it is suggested that clinicians be conservative in their calculations when switching between opioids. It is advisable to start at doses of the new opioid lower than those predicted by dose conversion tables, to monitor patients closely during the switch-over period and to titrate to clinical effect. If pain is not well controlled, the dose can be increased, whereas if the patient experiences adverse effects such as excessive somnolence, the dose may need to be reduced. It is always better to start at a lower dose and then titrate upward than to start with a dose that is too high. Close monitoring of patients during the switch is crucial.

Other factors associated with opioid use

- *'Morphine phobia'.* Many patients and families remain anxious regarding the use of opioid analgesics, specifically morphine, as they perceive the use of opioids as 'the end of the road'. An acknowledgement of the reality of these thoughts and an explanation of the use of opioids as effective strong painkillers will help patients. A full understanding by patients of the cause of their pain and the use of drugs and how they work will aid compliance and relieve anxiety regarding opioid use. Prescribing general practitioners, whose use of strong opioids is less common than those working in palliative care, will need support and guidance in using these drugs, especially with the heightened anxiety following the Shipman case in the UK.

- *Driving.* Patients often ask if they should be driving whilst receiving opioid analgesics. Drowsiness and cognitive effects are more likely to occur with starting medication, or on altering the dose, and it is generally recommended that driving is not safe until stable doses have been taken for at least 72 hours. Psychometric test scores in chronic pain patients improve after starting opioids for pain, suggesting that cognitive ability and psychomotor function are not impaired.[56] In practice, weakness or uncontrolled pain is likely to have a greater impact on a patient's ability to drive than either controlled pain or medication.

ADJUVANT/CO-ANALGESICS

Adjuvant or co-analgesic describes any drug that has a primary indication other than pain but is analgesic in some painful conditions. The WHO advocates the use of adjuvant analgesics at all three stages of the analgesic ladder. They may have an analgesic sparing effect and are therefore useful in the treatment of pain that is only partly responsive to opioids, e.g. neuropathic pain.

Antidepressants
There is considerable evidence for the analgesic properties of the older, mixed receptor-activity tricyclic antidepressants such as amitriptyline. Antidepressants with more receptor-specific properties such as selective serotonin reuptake inhibitors (SSRIs) may be less effective.[57]

Antidepressants are postulated to produce their analgesic effect by interacting with a variety of receptors (serotonin, acetylcholine and histamine) that modulate pain pathways. Controlled studies demonstrate that pain relief is more rapid and achieved at lower doses than antidepressant action. Analgesic response usually occurs within 1 week. Non-depressed patients experience analgesia and depressed patients report pain relief independent of change in mood.[58]

Tricyclic antidepressants are associated with several dose-limiting side effects, including somnolence, dry mouth, constipation, retention of urine, blurred vision, cardiac arrhythmias and orthostatic hypotension. SSRIs are better tolerated but can cause gastrointestinal toxicity and agitation.

A systematic review of antidepressants in neuropathic pain syndromes, including painful diabetic neuropathy, post-herpetic neuralgia and atypical facial pain, demonstrated an overall number needed to treat (NNT) of 2.9. The NNT for minor adverse effects was 3.7. The NNT for a major adverse effect was 22.[57]

Anticonvulsants
Several anticonvulsants, including carbamazepine, phenytoin, lamotrigine and gabapentin, have been studied in neuropathic pain models, predominantly in a non-cancer setting. Sodium valproate and clonazepam are also used in clinical practice.

The precise analgesic mechanism of this heterogeneous group of drugs is unknown, but probably relates to their anticonvulsant actions. These include blocking sodium and calcium channels and enhancing gamma-aminobutyric acid (GABA) activity to reduce neuronal excitability.

Serious haematological adverse effects have been reported with anticonvulsants, although the commonest adverse effects are sedation, dizziness, nausea and anorexia. Sodium valproate and gabapentin have a more favourable adverse effect profile.

A Cochrane systematic review concluded that although anticonvulsants are widely used in chronic pain management, few trials actually demonstrate analgesic effectiveness, with the exception of carbamazepine in trigeminal neuralgia. There was, however, no statistically significant risk of major harm. Whilst gabapentin is becoming increasingly popular, evidence to date suggests it is not superior to carbamazepine.[59,60]

Corticosteroids

Corticosteroids have been used as adjuvant analgesics for cancer pain of bone, visceral and neuropathic origin, especially in the setting of spinal cord compression and brain metastases. Their main analgesic action is probably related to their anti-inflammatory effect and reduction in peri-tumour oedema.[61,62] Some animal studies also point to a possible central analgesic effect. Steroids may also be used spinally (see below).

Dexamethasone is the corticosteroid most frequently used, due to its minimal salt-retaining properties and relative potency. The dose employed for pain is usually 8–16 mg daily. Steroids are associated with a wide range of side effects, including candidiasis, hyperglycaemia, hypertension, immunosupression, proximal myopathy and psychosis. Steroids should therefore be carefully monitored and reduced to the lowest dose and subsequently discontinued if possible.

Prednisolone may also be used, but has approximately one-seventh the potency of dexamethasone and more mineralocorticoid effects.

Anti-arrhythmics

Lidocaine (lignocaine) and related local anaesthetic-type drugs which block sodium channels have been used in the management of various chronic pain syndromes. A systematic review found that local anaesthetic-type agents were effective in non-malignant neuropathic pain but less clearly so in cancer-related pain.[63]

Muscle relaxants

Benzodiazepines and baclofen are thought to exert their effects by enhancing the inhibitory effects of the neurotransmitter GABA.[64] Dantrolene works at muscle level to prevent a contractile response to nerve stimulation by impeding calcium release. Tizanidine is an alpha-2 adrenergic agonist and, as well as its antispasticity effects, may have intrinsic analgesic efficacy. All these drugs can be used for acute painful muscle spasm, which can be a significant source of pain in neurological conditions such as motor neurone disease/amyotrophic lateral sclerosis. They all have sedative effects and it should be noted that relief of lower limb spasticity may abolish weight-bearing and hence the ability to transfer.

Diazepam is also used in combined pain and anxiety syndromes, but there is a lack of good trial evidence for any direct nociceptive effect separate from the drug's psychotropic actions.[65] Important considerations include the long-term risk of physical dependence/abuse and the potential for systemic accumulation leading to adverse events such as cognitive impairment.

Hyoscine butylbromide and other anticholinergics are smooth muscle relaxants and are used for the relief of painful colic in intestinal obstruction and of bladder spasm.

NON-PHARMACOLOGICAL APPROACHES TO PAIN MANAGEMENT

Despite appropriate use of the WHO guidelines for pain management, some patients will have inadequately controlled pain. For these patients, a variety of non-pharmacological and anaesthetic techniques is often employed.

ACUPUNCTURE

Acupuncture is an ancient therapeutic technique of Traditional Chinese Medicine that has been used for thousands of years. It has been reported to be beneficial in a variety of pain syndromes, with symptomatic improvement seen in 40–86 per cent of patients.[66] However, a recent systematic literature review concluded that there was limited evidence that acupuncture was more effective than no treatment for chronic pain, and inconclusive evidence that it is more effective than placebo, sham acupuncture or standard care. The heterogeneity of the studies precluded meta-analysis.[67] Infection, pneumothorax and bleeding have all been reported with acupuncture and it should not be used without training.

TRANSCUTANEOUS ELECTRICAL NERVE STIMULATION

Transcutaneous electrical nerve stimulation (TENS) was developed as a method of pain control, based on the 'gate theory' of pain, whereby selective stimulation of nerve fibres could block signals carrying pain impulses to the brain. TENS is available in three common forms: continuous (or conventional), pulsed (burst) and acupuncture-like (high-intensity pulsed). It has been reported to be beneficial for a variety of chronic pain syndromes,[68] but a systematic review of 38 randomized controlled trials in chronic pain found no objective evidence to support this.[69] This lack of evidence does not necessarily equate to a lack of effectiveness; small numbers, heterogeneity and difficulties in blinding all hamper the interpretation of studies.

Despite the paucity of controlled trials to support its use, clinical experience suggests that a trial of TENS is usually worthwhile for localized pain when other therapeutic interventions have not resulted in adequate pain relief. Specific pains that have been reported to respond well to TENS include:[70]

- painful bone metastases,
- painful vertebral collapse,
- liver capsule pain,
- nerve root compression pain,
- painful post-herpetic neuralgia,
- pain due to nerve infiltration, e.g. brachial plexopathy,
- post-chemotherapy painful neuropathy.

A detailed discussion of the techniques employed when utilizing TENS is outside the scope of this book. Generally, continuous TENS may be beneficial for skeletal, paravertebral or visceral pain, whereas pulsed or acupuncture-like TENS may be helpful for neuropathic pain states, especially where hyperaesthesia or dysaesthesia is a predominant feature.[70]

COMPLEMENTARY THERAPIES

The use of alternative and complementary therapies is increasingly common, and patients have increasing access to a variety of forms of therapies.

Herbal medicine

Many patients use herbal medicine or vitamin supplementation either instead of or alongside traditional medicine. There is no controlled evidence to support their use for pain relief in cancer.

Aromatherapy and massage without oils are widely used in palliative care. A systematic review concluded that aromatherapy massage had a mild, transient anxiolytic effect, but there is currently limited evidence to support its use for other indications.[71] However, uncontrolled trials and patient experience suggest that many patients value the positive psychological impact of aromatherapy or massage and, as such, it may be a useful adjunct to conventional treatment for some patients.

Relaxation and hypnotherapy

There are reports of improvements in cancer pain with hypnotherapy, but critical reviews of the literature are hampered by the heterogeneity of hypnotherapy techniques, patient populations and outcome measures. The techniques most often employed involve physical relaxation coupled with imagery that provides a substitute focus of attention to the painful sensation. One study of 54 women with metastatic breast cancer reported significant reductions in pain and suffering compared to controls.[72] Relaxation or distraction techniques can be used independently of hypnosis; as with other complementary therapies, there is limited controlled trial evidence to support their use, but these techniques may be helpful alongside conventional treatment for some patients.

ANAESTHETIC INTERVENTIONS

Anaesthetic interventions will be required for less than 10 per cent of cancer patients. They should be considered where pain does not respond to conventional measures or where there are unacceptable side effects by alternative routes. Anaesthetic techniques include:

- blockade of peripheral axonal transmission, e.g. brachial plexus or intercostal nerve block,

- blockade of the sympathetic nervous system, e.g. lumbar sympathectomy, coeliac plexus block,

- centrally acting agents, e.g. spinal drug administration.

Decisions regarding anaesthetic interventions for pain will depend on the patient's performance status and prognosis and the degree of pain and/or side effects despite systemic analgesia.

SPINAL ANAESTHESIA

Several groups of drugs, specifically local anaesthetics and opioids, can produce analgesia by the spinal route – this includes epidural and intrathecal administration. Spinal drug administration may be particularly helpful where there is:[73]

- movement-related (incident) pain,

- neuropathic pain.

Long-term drug administration via the spinal route is now feasible, either by the siting of percutaneous epidural catheters with micropore filters connected to infusion pumps or by totally implanted systems. Complications include catheter displacement, infection, leakage and blockage.

Spinal opioids

Opioids applied to the spinal cord have an analgesic effect but there are few trials evaluating their use in chronic cancer pain. Epidural opioids can cause any of the common opioid side effects but do not cause any motor block. The low opioid doses administered spinally may reduce intolerable opioid-related side effects with other routes.

Spinal local anaesthetics

In the management of cancer pain, local anaesthetics, e.g. bupivicaine, are usually combined with opioids to optimize pain relief. Local anaesthetics produce a dose-dependent motor block and can cause hypotension (because of sympathetic blockade).

Combinations of local anaesthetic and opioids

The combination of local anaesthetics and opioid analgesics has been found to provide effective postoperative analgesia.[73] Experimental studies have demonstrated synergism, and clinically low doses of local anaesthetic and opioid in combination can provide good analgesia without a loss of mobility. The mechanism of the synergy is unclear, but it has been postulated that chronic infusion of the combination can produce selective blockade, blocking pain fibres while leaving other sensory input and motor function intact.[73]

Other drugs

- *Alpha-2 adrenergic agonists* such as clonidine have an anti-nociceptive effect and are synergistic with spinal opioid and local anaesthetic. In one study, clonidine was shown to provide effective analgesia in cancer-related neuropathic pain.[73]

- Epidural *corticosteroids* are thought to provide analgesia by blocking peripheral pain input. They have been shown to provide statistically significant improvements in pain control compared to control for patients with sciatica.[74]

PERIPHERAL AND SYMPATHETIC NERVE BLOCKS

These can be undertaken with either local anaesthetic (effect lasting days) or neurolytic agents for a prolonged effect, such as alcohol or phenol. Sympathetic blockade is useful where characteristic signs of sympathetic nerve dysfunction (alterations in skin colour, temperature and sweating) are present in the presence of uncontrolled pain.

Coeliac plexus block

- Any pain originating from viscera innervated by the coeliac plexus can be alleviated by blockade of the plexus, e.g. pancreatic pain, pain from liver or splenic capsular distension, retroperitoneal or other upper gastrointestinal malignancies.

- A meta-analysis of 24 studies for the treatment of cancer pain reported that good to excellent pain relief was reported in 89 per cent of patients during the first 2 weeks; partial to complete pain relief was maintained in 70–90 per cent for several months until death.[75]

- Complications include temporary postural hypotension, motor or sensory block at T10–L1, failure of ejaculation, urinary retention and diarrhoea. Paraplegia occurs in less than 1 per cent, but patients should be warned of this possibility during the consent process.

SPECIFIC PAIN SYNDROMES

Specific pain syndromes should always be managed using the framework provided by the WHO analgesic ladder. Table 4.16.4 outlines pain-specific management options. Neuropathic pain is dealt with separately below.

A–Z OF SYMPTOMS

Table 4.16.4 Management of specific pain syndromes

Type of pain	Specific clinical features	Specific management options	Comments
Headache – raised intracranial pressure	Headache worse in the mornings, associated with nausea and vomiting ± neurological sequelae	High-dose corticosteroids, e.g. dexamethasone 16 mg/day NSAIDs or opioid analgesics may also be required	Treatment of underlying cause, e.g. radiotherapy for brain metastases; treatment of infection if brain abscess
Bone pain	Ache at rest; incident pain; local tenderness	Precise role of NSAIDs needs evaluation, although clinical practice supports use Radiotherapy: over 40% achieve at least 50% pain relief at 1 month; single fractions may be as effective as fractionated courses[81,82] Bisphosphonates reduce bone pain in 40–60%, sustained for 4–8 weeks[83]	Incident pain may cause specific management problems as attempts to give sufficient analgesia to cover episodic exacerbations can result in excess toxicity at rest
Incident pain	Pain directly occurring on movement, e.g. associated with bone metastases, changing dressings	Consider short-acting analgesics, e.g. oral transmucosal fentanyl or Entonox (50% oxygen, 50% nitric oxide) to cover movement/procedure Anaesthetic procedures may be required	Optimize management of underlying cause
Tenesmus	Painful sensation of rectal fullness arising from pressure from a tumour mass within or outside the rectum, or direct involvement of pre-sacral plexus and pelvic floor muscles	Calcium-channel blockers and nitrates to reduce pelvic floor muscle spasm Anxiolytics Local application of steroid foam, lidocaine (lignocaine), diamorphine Anaesthetic techniques, e.g. lumbar sympathectomy, epidural or intrathecal block	Treatment of local tumour, e.g. radiotherapy, laser [or] endoscopic resection

Type of pain	Clinical features	Management	Additional notes
Liver capsule pain	Aching in nature, may be worse on inspiration due to stretching of capsule. Localized to right subcostal region and/or referred to right scapula/shoulder	NSAID analgesics for anti-inflammatory effect; Corticosteroids	Treatment of underlying cause where appropriate
Intestinal colic	Differentiate between constipation and bowel obstruction	Antispasmodic agents, e.g. hyoscine butylbromide, should be given parenterally due to variable oral absorption; Octreotide should be considered in bowel obstruction[84]	Withdraw stimulant laxatives and/or prokinetic agents
Smooth muscle spasm	Intermittent griping pain in visceral distribution, e.g. oesophagus, ureter, bladder or urethra	May respond to antispasmodics, calcium-channel blockers or nitrates; Bladder washouts may be useful	
Limb spasm	Associated with contractures, e.g. post brain metastasis, cord compression, CVA, multiple sclerosis	May respond to dantrolene, baclofen or tizanidine[85]	Titrate versus sedative effects
Musculoskeletal and chest wall pain	Consider locally invasive lung cancer or mesothelioma. Usually severe ache ± neuropathic features	Benzodiazepines may reduce myotonic activity TENS or anaesthetic procedures may be required	
Cutaneous pain	Local pain in pressure sores or severe ulcers	Studies support use of topical morphine/diamorphine applied in a gel formulation, e.g. Intrasite gel[86]	
Ischaemic pain	Rest pain or pain on movement (claudication)	Regional anaesthetic blockade may be required if strong opioid analgesics ± neuropathic agents ineffective	Optimize medical management, e.g. vasodilators, and consider surgical options in appropriate patients

NSAIDs, non-steroidal anti-inflammatory drugs; CVA, cerebrovascular accident; TENS, transcutaneous electric nerve stimulation.

NEUROPATHIC PAIN

Neuropathic pain is defined as pain in an area of abnormal or altered sensation, and results from dysfunction of, or injury to, the peripheral or central nervous system. It is a complex and diverse syndrome and a difficult management problem, as pharmacological treatments are often only partially effective and associated with troublesome side effects. Central sensitization (or 'wind-up') as a result of NMDA receptor activation is thought to be important in maintaining neuropathic pain states, even after removal of the painful stimulus.

Patients may describe neuropathic pain as burning, numbing, stabbing, shooting or stinging. It can also be dull, aching or throbbing. On examination, sensory disturbance should be present; allodynia, hyperalgesia, hyperpathia or other evidence of neurological damage, e.g. autonomic changes or motor signs, may also be present.

A neuropathic component is present in up to 36 per cent of patients with cancer-related pain[76] and can be due to direct tumour infiltration, anti-cancer therapies or, rarely, paraneoplastic syndromes. In a non-cancer setting, it is most commonly metabolic, infective or inflammatory in origin.

The vast majority of clinical trials investigating the effectiveness of analgesic agents in neuropathic pain have recruited patients with non-cancer pain. The role of opioid analgesics in the management of neuropathic pain is controversial, but there is now limited evidence that neuropathic pain can respond to opioids.[77] It has been suggested that opioids with additional NMDA receptor activity such as methadone and tramadol have a specific role. A trial of opioid analgesia to efficacy or tolerance is advised.

Adjuvant analgesics are crucial in the management of neuropathic pain (Table 4.16.5). Systematic reviews of the literature have demonstrated similar efficacy for antidepressants[57] and anticonvulsants.[60]

NMDA receptor antagonists such as ketamine have been reported to be effective in non-malignant neuropathic pain, but adverse effects restrict their widespread use.[78] A recent Cochrane systematic review on the role of ketamine as an adjunct to opioids for cancer pain identified only four randomized controlled trials, of which two were excluded due to their poor quality. Meta-analysis was not possible, but both studies concluded that ketamine improved the effectiveness of opioid treatment in cancer pain.[79]

Topical agents such as *capsaicin*, an alkaloid derived from chillies which depletes the neurotransmitter substance P, have been applied to limited areas of hyperalgesia or allodynia. Topical antidepressants and *lidocaine (lignocaine)* patches are also currently being investigated.

Neuropathic pain is difficult to manage and pharmacological means alone may not be effective. Non-pharmacological options include the use of TENS, though there is a lack of good evidence to support this. Greatest pain relief is achieved if the nerve trunk proximal to the site of injury is stimulated.

CONCLUSION

There is a lack of robust evidence from randomized controlled trials in cancer or palliative care patients for many pharmacological and non-pharmacological

Table 4.16.5 Commonly used adjuvant analgesics in the management of neuropathic pain

Drug	NNT[a]	Starting dose	Maintenance dose	Comment
Antidepressants[57]				
Non-selective tricyclic antidepressants	2.1	Amitriptyline 10–25 mg nocte	Amitriptyline 25–150 mg daily	First-line adjuvant Proven benefit in non-cancer setting Side effects limit use, especially in the elderly
Selective serotonin reuptake inhibitors	6.7	Paroxetine 20 mg	Paroxetine 40 mg	Not commonly used for pain
Anticonvulsants[60]				
Carbamezepine	3.3	100 mg b.d.	200–800 mg/day in divided doses	Treatment of choice for trigeminal neuralgia
Phenytoin	2.1	100–300 mg	300 mg	Not commonly used for pain
Gabapentin	3.7	100–300 mg	900–3600 mg in divided doses	Useful for patients unable to tolerate amitriptyline Complex dosing schedule
Sodium valproate	N/A	100 mg b.d.	400–1000 mg in divided doses	No trial data
Clonazepam	N/A	0.5–1 mg	1–4 mg	No trial data May be useful if co-existing anxiety
Dexamethasone	N/A	8–16 mg daily	Reduce to lowest effective dose	May be useful whilst awaiting effect of another intervention, e.g. radiotherapy
Anti-arrhythmics[80]				
Mexiletine	10.0	50 mg t.d.s.	Up to 10 mg/kg	No evidence of efficacy in cancer pain
Flecainide	N/A	100 mg t.d.s.	100 mg t.d.s.	Little evidence of efficacy in cancer pain
Topical drugs				
Capsaicin	5.9	Topical application to affected area	0.075% q.d.s.	Initially causes skin burning May take 2 weeks to work

[a] Number needed to treat in painful neuropathy.
N/A, not available.

treatments for pain, and much evidence needs to be extrapolated from chronic pain populations. Despite this, the majority of patients will have their pain controlled with non-opioid and opioid analgesics according to the WHO guidelines.

KEY POINTS

- Remember the concept of 'total pain'.
- Accurate assessment will aid management.
- Following the WHO guidelines will enable pain to be controlled in the majority of patients.
- Opioid switching may alleviate persistent opioid adverse effects.
- Judicious use of adjuvant analgesics can enhance analgesia and limit adverse effects.
- A minority of patients will require anaesthetic interventions.
- Radiotherapy should be considered for bone and nerve compression pain.

REFERENCES

1. Bruera E, Neumann CM. The management of chronic pain in palliative non-cancer patients. In: Addington-Hall JM, Higginson IJ (eds), *Palliative care for non-cancer patients*. Oxford: Oxford University Press, 2001, 66–81.
2. IASP Subcommittee on Taxonomy. Pain terms: a list with definitions and notes on usage. *Pain* 1980; 8, 249–52.
3. Saunders C. The symptomatic treatment of incurable malignant disease. *Prescibers J* 1964; 4, 68–73.
4. Foley KM. Clinical assessment of cancer pain. *Acta Anaesthesiol Scand Suppl* 1982; 74, 91–6.
5. Bruera E, Neumann CM. History and clinical assessment of the cancer pain patient: assessment and measurement. In: Sykes N, Fallon MT, Patt RB (eds), *Cancer pain*. London: Arnold, 2003, 63–71.
6. Melzack R. The McGill Pain Questionnaire: the main properties and scoring methods. *Pain* 1975; 1, 277–99.
7. Daut RL, Cleeland CS, Flanery RC. Development of the Wisconsin Brief Pain Questionnaire to assess pain in cancer and other diseases. *Pain* 1983; 17, 197–210.
8. Bennett M. The LANSS Pain Scale: the Leeds assessment of neuropathic symptoms and signs. *Pain* 2001; 92, 147–57.
9. World Health Organisation. *Cancer pain relief*, 2nd edn. Geneva: World Health Organisation, 1996, 74.
10. Zech DF, Grond S, Lynch J, Hertel D, Lehmann KA. Validation of World Health Organisation guidelines for cancer pain relief: a 10-year prospective study. *Pain* 1995; 63, 65–76.
11. Cashan JN. The mechanism of action of non-steroidal anti-inflammatory drugs in analgesia. *Drugs* 1996; 52(Suppl. 5), 13–23.
12. McCormack K, Brune K. Dissociation between the antinociceptive and anti-inflammatory effects of the non-steroidal anti-inflammatory drugs. A survey of their analgesic efficacy. *Drugs* 1991; 41, 533–47.

13. Yalsh TL, Dirig DM, Malmberg AB. Mechanism of action of non-steroidal anti-inflammatory drugs. *Cancer Invest* 1998; **16**, 509–27.

14. Eisenberg E, Berkey CS, Carr DB, Mosteller F, Chalmers TC. Efficacy and safety of non-steroidal anti-inflammatory drugs for cancer pain: a meta-analysis. *J Clin Oncol* 1994; **12**, 2756–65.

15. Hawkins C, Hanks GW. The gastroduodenal toxicity of non-steroidal anti-inflammatory drugs. A review of the literature. *J Pain Symptom Manage* 2000; **2**, 140–51.

16. Herxheimer A. Many non-steroidal anti-inflammatory drug users who bleed don't know when to stop. *BMJ* 1998; **316**, 492.

17. Deeks JJ, Smith LA, Bradley MD. Efficacy, tolerability and upper gastrointestinal safety of celecoxib for treatment of osteoarthritis and rheumatoid arthritis: systematic review of randomised controlled trials. *BMJ* 2002; **325**, 619–23.

18. National Institute for Clinical Excellence (NICE). *Guidance on the use of cyclooxygenase II selective inhibitors, celecoxib, meloxicam and etodalac for osteoarthritis and rheumatoid arthritis.* London: NHS Executive, July 2001.

19. http://iuphar-db.org/iuphar-rd/query?type=link&lType=chapter&id=1295

20. McQuay HJ, Carroll D, Guest PG, Robson S, Wiffen PJ, Juniper RP. A multiple dose comparison of ibuprofen and dihydrocodeine after third molar surgery. *Br J Oral Maxillofacial Surg* 1993; **31**, 95–100.

21. Crome P, Gain R, Ghurye R, Flanagan RJ. Pharmacokinetics of dextropropoxyphene and nordextropropoxyphene in elderly hospital patients after single and multiple doses of distalgesic. Preliminary analysis of results. *Hum Toxicol* 1984; 3, 41–8S.

22. Perrier D, Gibaldi M. Influence of first-pass effect on the systemic availability of propoxyphene. *J Clin Pharmacol* 1972; **12**, 449–52.

23. Raffa RB, Friderichs E, Reimann W, Shank RP, Codd EE, Vaught JL. Opioid and non-opioid components independently contribute to the mechanism of action of tramadol, an 'atypical' opioid analgesic. *J Pharmacol Exp Ther* 1992; **260**, 275–85.

24. McQuay H, Moore A. *An evidence-based resource for pain relief.* Oxford: Oxford University Press, 1998.

25. Pereira J, Lawlor P, Vigano A, Dorgan M, Bruera E. Equianalgesic dose ratios for opioids: a critical review and proposals for long-term dosing. *J Pain Symptom Manage* 2001; **22**, 672–87.

26. Anderson R, Saiers JH, Abram S, Schlicht C. Accuracy in equianalgesic dosing: conversion dilemmas. *J Pain Symptom Manage* 2001; **21**, 397–406.

27. Hoskin PJ, Hanks GW, Aherne GW, Chapman D, Littleton P, Filshie J. The bioavailability and pharmacokinetics of morphine after intravenous, oral and buccal administration in healthy volunteers. *Br J Clin Pharmacol* 1989; **27**, 499–505.

28. Portenoy RK, Foley KM, Stulman J *et al.* Plasma morphine and morphine-6-glucuronide during chronic morphine therapy for cancer pain: plasma profiles, steady state concentrations and the consequences of renal failure. *Pain* 1991; **47**, 13–19.

29. Hanks GW, de Conno F, Cherny N *et al.* Morphine and alternative opioids in cancer pain: the EAPC recommendations. *Br J Cancer* 2001; **84**, 587–93.

30. Todd J, Rees E, Gwilliam B, Davies A. An assessment of the efficacy and tolerability of a 'double dose' of normal-release morphine sulphate at bedtime. *Palliat Med* 2002; **16**, 507–12.

31. Takahashi M, Ohara T, Yamanaka H, Shimada A, Nakaho T. The oral to intravenous equianalgesic ratio of morphine based on plasma concentrations of morphine and

metabolites in advanced cancer patients receiving chronic morphine treatment. *Palliat Med* 2003; **17**, 673–8.

32. Waldman CS, Eason JR, Rambohul, Hanson GC. Serum morphine levels. A comparison between continuous subcutaneous infusions and intravenous infusions in postoperative patients. *Anaesthesia* 1984; **39**, 768–71.

33. Traynor J. The mu-opioid receptor. *Pain Rev* 1996; **3**, 221–48.

34. Ebert B, Andersen S, Krogsgaard-Larsen P. Ketobemidone, methadone and pethidine are non-competitive N-methyl-D-aspartate (NMDA) antagonists in the rat cortex and spinal cord. *Neurosci Lett* 1995; **187**, 165–8.

35. Gourlay G, Cherry D, Cousins M. A comparative study of the efficacy and pharmacokinetics of oral methadone and morphine in the treatment of severe pain in patients with cancer. *Pain* 1986; **25**, 297–312.

36. Gannon C. The use of methadone in the care of the dying. *Eur J Palliat Care* 1997; **4**(5), 152–8.

37. Fainsinger R, Schoeller T, Bruera E. Methadone in the management of cancer pain: a review. *Pain* 1993; **52**, 137–47.

38. Sweeney C, Bruera E. New roles for old drugs: methadone. *Progr Palliat Care* 2001; **9**, 8–10.

39. Morley J, Makin M. The use of methadone in cancer pain poorly responsive to other opioids. *Pain Rev* 1998; **5**, 51–8.

40. Quigley C, Wiffen P. A systematic review of hydromorphone in acute and chronic pain. *J Pain Symptom Manage* 203; **25**, 169–78.

41. Ross FB, Smith MT. The intrinsic antinociceptive effects of oxycodone appear to be kappa-opioid receptor mediated. *Pain* 1997; **73**, 151–7.

42. Leow KP, Smith MT, Williams B, Cramond T. Single-dose and steady-state pharmacokinetics and pharmacodynamics of oxycodone in patients with cancer. *Clin Pharmacol Ther* 1992; **52**, 487–95.

43. Bruera E, Belzile M, Pituskin E *et al.* Randomised, double-blind, cross-over trial comparing safety and efficacy of oral controlled release oxycodone with controlled release morphine in patients with cancer pain. *J Clin Oncol* 1998; **16**, 3222–9.

44. Curtis GB, Johnson GH, Clark P *et al.* Relative potency of controlled-release oxycodone and controlled-release morphine in a postoperative pain model. *Eur J Clin Pharmacol* 1999; **55**, 425–9.

45. Kaplan R, Parris WC, Citron ML *et al.* Comparison of controlled-release and immediate-release oxycodone tablets in patients with cancer pain. *J Clin Oncol* 1998; **16**(10), 3230–7.

46. Radbruch L, Sabatowski R, Loick G *et al.* Constipation and the use of laxatives: a comparison between transdermal fentanyl and oral morphine. *Palliat Med* 2000; **14**, 111–19.

47. Portenoy RK, Southam MA, Gupta SK *et al.* Transdermal fentanyl for cancer pain. *Anaesthesiology* 1993; **78**, 36–43.

48. Portenoy RK, Payne R, Coluzzi P *et al.* Oral transmucosal fentanyl citrate (OTFC) for the treatment of breakthrough pain in cancer patients: a controlled dose titration study. *Pain* 1999; **79**, 303–12.

49. Zeppetella G. An assessment of the safety, efficacy and acceptability of intranasal fentanyl citrate in the management of cancer-related breakthrough pain: a pilot study. *J Pain Symptom Manage* 2000; **20**(4), 253–8.

50. EAPC. Morphine in cancer pain: modes of administration – Expert Working Group of the European Association for Palliative Care. *BMJ* 1996; **312**, 823–6.

51. Cherny N, Ripamonti C, Pereira J *et al.* for the Expert Working Group of the EAPC Network. Strategies to manage the adverse effects of oral morphine: an evidence-based report. *J Clin Oncol* 2001; **19**, 2542–54.

52. Bruera E, Pereira J, Watanabe S, Belzile M, Kuehn N, Hanson J. Opioid rotation in patients with cancer pain. *Cancer* 1996; **78**, 852–7.

53. Mercandante S. Opioid rotation for cancer pain. *Cancer* 1999; **86**, 1856–66.

54. Fallon M. Opioid rotation: does it have a role? *Palliat Med* 1997; **11**, 177–8.

55. Quigley C, Joel S, Patel N, Baksh A, Slevin M. Plasma concentrations of morphine, morphine-6-glucuronide and morphine-3-glucuronide and their relationship with analgesia and side effects in patients with cancer-related pain. *Palliat Med* 2003; **17**, 185–90.

56. Jamison RN, Schein JR, Vallow S, Ascher S, Vorsanger GJ, Katz NP. Neuropsychological effects of long term opioid use in chronic pain patients. *J Pain Symptom Manage* 2003; **26**, 913–21.

57. McQuay HJ, Tramer M, Nye BA, Carroll D, Wiffen PJ, Moore RA. A systematic review of antidepressants in neuropathic pain. *Pain* 1996; **68**, 217–27.

58. Max MB, Culnane M, Schafer SC *et al.* Amitriptyline relieves diabetic neuropathy pain in patients with normal or depressed mood. *Neurology* 1987; **37**, 589–96.

59. McQuay H, Carroll D, Jadad AR, Wiffen P, Moore A. Anticonvulsant drugs for management of pain: a systematic review. *BMJ* 1995; **311**, 1047–52.

60. Wiffen P, Collins S, McQuay H, Carroll D, Jadad A, Moore A. Anticonvulsants for acute and chronic pain (Cochrane Review). In: *The Cochrane Library*, Issue 1. Oxford: Update Software, 2001.

61. Haynes RC. Adrenocortical steroids. In: Gillman AG, Rall TW, Nies AS, Taylor P (eds), *The pharmacological basis of therapeutics*, 8th edn. New York: Pergamon, 1990, 1436–58.

62. Yamada K, Ushio Y, Hayakawa T, Arita N, Yamada N, Mogami H. Effects of methyl-prednisolone on peritumoral brain edema. *J Neurosurg* 1983; **59**, 612–19.

63. Kalso E, Tramer M, McQuay H. Systemic local-anaesthetic type drugs in chronic pain: a systematic review. *Eur J Pain* 1998; **2**, 3–14.

64. Skolnick P, Paul SM. Benzodiazepine receptors in the central nervous system. *Int Rev Neurobiol* 1982; **23**, 103–40.

65. Reddy S, Patt RB. The benzodiazepines as adjuvant analgesics. *J Pain Symptom Manage* 1994; **9**, 510–14.

66. Filshie J, Morrison PJ. Acupuncture for chronic pain: a review. *Palliat Med* 1988; **2**, 1–14.

67. Ezzo J, Berman B, Hadhazy VA, Jada AR, Lao L, Singh BB. Is acupuncture effective for the treatment of chronic pain? A systematic review. *Pain* 2000; **86**, 217–25.

68. Woolf CJ, Thompson JW. TENS, vibration and acupuncture. In: Wall PD, Melzak R (eds), *Textbook of pain*, 4th edn. Edinburgh: Churchill Livingstone, 1999, 1341–51.

69. McQuay H, Moore A. Transcutaneous electric nerve stimulation in chronic pain. In: *An evidence-based resource for pain relief*. Oxford: Oxford Medical Publications, 1998, 207–21.

70. Thompson JW, Filshie J. Transcutaneous electric nerve stimulation and acupuncture. In: Doyle D, Hanks G, MacDonald N (eds), *Oxford textbook of palliative medicine*, 2nd edn. Oxford: Oxford University Press, 1998, 421–37.

A – Z   O F   S Y M P T O M S

71. Cooke B, Ernst E. Aromatherapy: a systematic review. *Br J Gen Prac* 2000; **50**, 493–6.
72. Spiegel D, Bloom JR. Group therapy and hypnosis reduce metastatic breast carcinoma pain. *Pyschosom Med* 1983; **454**, 333–9.
73. McQuay HJ, Moore RA. Local anaesthetics and epidurals. In: Wall PD, Melzack R (eds), *Textbook of pain*. Edinburgh: Churchill Livingstone, 1999, 1215–31.
74. McQuay H, Moore A. Epidural corticosteroids for sciatica. In: *An evidence-based resource for pain relief*. Oxford: Oxford Medical Publications, 1998, 216–18.
75. Eisenberg E, Carr DB, Chalmers TC. Neurolytic celiac plexus block for treatment of cancer pain: a meta-analysis. *Anesth Analg* 1995; **80**, 290–5.
76. Grond S, Radbruch L, Meuser T *et al*. Assessment and treatment of neuropathic cancer pain following WHO guidelines. *Pain* 1999; **79**, 15–20.
77. Dellemijn P. Are opioids effective in relieving neuropathic pain? *Pain* 1999; **80**, 453–62.
78. Fisher K, Coderre TJ, Hagen NA. Targeting the N-methyl-D-aspartate receptor for chronic pain management: preclinical animal studies, recent clinical experience and future research directions. *J Pain Symptom Manage* 2000; **20**, 358–73.
79. Bell RF, Eccleston C, Kalso E. Ketamine as adjunct to opioids for cancer pain. A qualitative systematic review. *J Pain Symptom Manage* 2003; **26**, 867–75.
80. Sindrup S, Jensen T. Efficacy of pharmacological treatments of neuropathic pain: an update and effect related to mechanism of drug action. *Pain* 1999; **83**, 389–400.
81. McQuay HJ, Carroll D, Moore RA. Radiotherapy for painful bone metastases: a systematic review. *Clin Oncol* 1997; **9**, 150–4.
82. Barton R, Hoskin PJ, Yarnold JR *et al*. Radiotherapy for bone pains: is a single fraction good enough? *Clin Oncol* 1994; **6**, 354–5.
83. Mannix K, Ahmedzai SH, Anderson H, Bennett M, Lloyd Williams M, Wilcock A. Using bisphosphonates to control the pain of bone metastases: evidence based guidelines for palliative care. *Palliat Med* 2000; **14**, 455–61.
84. Feuer DJ, Broadley K. Systematic review and meta-analysis of corticosteroids for the resolution of malignant bowel obstruction in advanced gynaecological and gastrointestinal cancers. *Ann Oncol* 1999; **10**, 1035–41.
85. Smith HS, Barton AE. Tizanidine in the management of spasticity and muscular complaints in the palliative care population. *Am J Hosp Palliat Care* 2000; **17**(1), 50–8.
86. Flock P. Pilot study to determine the effectiveness of diamorphine gel to control pressure ulcer pain. *J Pain Symptom Manage* 2003; **25**, 547–54.

APPENDIX: ANALGESIC POTENCY TABLE

The relative analgesic potencies outlined in this table are only a guide; please see Chapter 4.16 for more information regarding use of alternative opioid analgesics.

Analgesic	Potency ratio to oral morphine	10 mg oral morphine equivalent (mg)	Duration of action (hours)
Buprenorphine (SL)	60	0.2	6–8
Codeine	1/12	120	3–5
Dextromoramide	2	5	2–3
Dextropropoxyphene	1/10	100	4–6
Diamorphine (SC)	3	3	3–4
Dihydrocodeine	1/10	100	4–6
Fentanyl (Patch)	150		72
Hydromorphone	7.5	1.3	4–6 (NR)
			12 (MR)
Methadone	5–10	1	8–12
Oxycodone	2	5	4–6 (NR)
			12 (MR)
Tramadol	1/4	40	4–5

NR, normal release; MR, modified release.
Handbook of Pain Management, 2001. Napp Pharmaceuticals.

PRURITUS

Andrew Thorns and Polly Edmonds

DEFINITION

Pruritus (or itch) is a skin sensation leading to a desire to scratch. The terms itch and pruritus are used interchangeably in this chapter.

PREVALENCE

Five per cent of patients with advanced cancer are reported to experience pruritus. It is more common in end-stage human immunodeficiency virus (HIV) and is reported in 70 per cent of patients with end-stage renal failure and in 80 per cent with cholestasis.

PATHOPHYSIOLOGY

The pathogenesis of pruritus is complex, with both local and central mechanisms involved.[1] Increased understanding of the roles of inflammatory mediators and endogenous opioids has enabled identification of new treatments. Most interest is currently focused on the role of histamine, opioid and 5-hydroxytryptamine-3 ($5HT_3$) receptors.

Itch was previously believed to be a low-threshold form of pain, but is now thought to be a distinct entity. Stimuli may be exogenous or endogenous. Exogenous stimuli can be either physical or chemical, and represent the only method with which to induce itch experimentally. Endogenous stimuli are poorly understood and may originate from the peripheral nervous system, the spinal cord or higher centres. A number of disease states cause pruritus by an endogenous route and the likely mediators involved include histamines, 5HT, opioids, tachykinins and interleukins.

MEDIATORS OF ITCH

- Four histamine receptor types (located mainly in mast cells) have been identified, of which the H_1 receptor is involved in itch. Experimentally, increased histamine concentrations are found in inflamed skin.

- Prostaglandin E_2 (PGE_2) is found in increased concentrations in itchy, inflamed skin. It appears to lower the itch threshold rather than being pruritogenic itself.

- Substance P, calcitonin gene-related peptide (CGRP) and vasoactive intestinal peptide (VIP) are the tachykinins involved in the propagation of itch. These are found in the free nerve endings responsible for sensations of both pain and itch.

- Mu opioid receptors play a central role in modulating itch and pain. There is also a possible peripheral role, as topical opioids worsen histamine-induced itch. This is not antagonized by naloxone and does not seem to depend on mu receptors.

- Interleukin-2 (IL-2) causes marked itching, and cyclosporin (a selective inhibitor of IL-2 biosynthesis) is effective in relieving the itch of atopic dermatitis.

NEURAL PATHWAYS

The neural pathways involved in the transmission of itch are not fully understood. Polymodal C-fibres appear most important in transmitting the sensation of itch. No specific itch receptors have been identified and it is thought that free nerve endings are responsible for the detection of this sensation. The central nervous system (CNS) does appear to play a part, as shown by the fact that just the suggestion of itch causes the sensation.

The exact method by which we perceive itch is not clear. It is suggested that surround inhibition, which normally permits accurate localization of skin stimuli, is not possible for very light sensations and so results in the more vague sensation of tickle or prickle. Rubbing or scratching the area returns the surround inhibition, which overcomes the more delicate itch sensation. Generalized itch results from alterations in the central inhibitory circuits.

INVESTIGATIONS AND EXAMINATION

The following scheme may be helpful in establishing a diagnosis.

The history should include:

- associated conditions,

- medication,

A–Z OF SYMPTOMS

- distinguish generalized from local pruritus,

- distinguish pruritus from other similar sensations that could indicate different pathology, e.g. neuropathic pain.

An assessment of total symptomatology should also be made, including:

- other physical symptoms,

- psychosocial and spiritual aspects,

- think of 'total itch'.

Examination of the patient should include:

- skin signs,

- damage to skin from scratching,

- jaundice.

Pruritus is a subjective symptom that is complex to assess. The following objective methods of assessment have been reported:[2]

- visual analogue scales,

- verbal rating scales,

- behaviour rating scales,

- frequency and length of scratching bouts measured by infrared camera at night triggered by movement,

- vibration (scratch) transducer to measure frequency of scratching.

MANAGEMENT

Pruritus is a distressing symptom that can result in psychological as well as physical morbidity: one-third of patients with generalized pruritus exhibit depressive symptomatology.[3] Management should be focused on the underlying cause as well as on symptomatic relief.

GENERAL

Skin diseases commonly causing itch and their management are shown in Table 4.17.1. Other systemic diseases that should be considered include:

- metabolic disease: hypothyroidism and hyperthyroidism, carcinoid syndrome, diabetes mellitus and insipidus;

Table 4.17.1 Skin conditions associated with pruritus

Condition	General management	Specific management
Contact dermatitis	Avoidance of allergen	Topical or systemic corticosteroids
Atopic dermatitis	Antihistamines, emollients	Topical corticosteroids
Xerotic dermatitis	Humidifier and emollients	Topical corticosteroids
Psoriasis	Emollients and keratolytic agents	Topical corticosteroids, coal tar, PUVA
Scabies	Lindane	Malathion, crotamiton
Lichen planus	Topical and systemic corticosteroids	Griseofulvin, retinoids
Dermatitis herpetiformis	Dapsone, sulfapyridine (sulphapyridine)	Gluten-free diet, prednisolone

- malignant disease: chronic lymphocytic leukaemia, lymphoma, cutaneous T-cell lymphoma, multiple myeloma, paraneoplastic syndrome with other carcinomas;

- haematological disease: polycythaemia vera;

- renal disease: renal failure with uraemia;

- liver disease: cholestasis;

- infections: HIV, syphilis;

- neurological conditions: stroke, multiple sclerosis, brain abscess/tumours;

- senile pruritus;

- drug induced: opioids, amphetamine, aspirin, quinidine, other cholestasis-inducing drugs, e.g. hormones, erythromycin, phenothiazines;

- psychogenic.

NON-PHARMACOLOGICAL SYMPTOMATIC MEASURES

Non-pharmacological symptomatic measures, although largely based on anecdote, can be useful.

- Exclude factors exacerbating pruritus: anxiety, boredom, dehydration (causing dry skin), heat.

- Avoid scratching, keep nails short, wear cotton gloves, allow gentle rubbing.

- Avoid soap (drying action).

- Use emulsifying ointment or aqueous cream as soap substitute and when bathing.

- Avoid hot baths and dry skin by gentle patting.

- Apply emollient and possibly menthol after bathing.

- Wear loose clothing, preferably cotton, to avoid irritation, heat retention and sweating.

- Avoid overheating and sweating.

- Topical corticosteroids for inflamed areas.

- Transcutaneous-electrical nerve stimulation (TENS).

- Acupuncture.

- Hypnotherapy.

- Behavioural therapy.

Conventional sedative medications such as benzodiazepines do not have any specific anti-pruritic action, but may be useful in alleviating associated anxiety.

PHARMACOLOGICAL GENERAL MEASURES

Pharmacological general measures can be divided into topical and parenteral treatments.

Topical treatments can be inconvenient to apply to the whole body so are more often used for localized or severe pruritus. They include the following options.

- *Phenol (0.5–2 per cent)*: acts by anaesthetizing cutaneous nerve endings but can be potentially hepatotoxic and ototoxic.

- *Menthol (0.25–2 per cent)* and *camphor (1–3 per cent)*: counterirritant and anaesthetic properties.

- *Zinc oxide, coal tar, calamine, glycerine* and *salicylates*: all suggested to work, but mechanism uncertain.

- *Crotamiton (Eurax)*: has been shown in a double-blind controlled trial to be ineffective.

- Topical local anaesthetics can be used for localized areas of itch.

- *Doxepin*: a tricyclic antidepressant with potent antihistaminic action (H_1 and H_2). It is available in a 5 per cent cream or as an oral preparation. Its side effects are similar to those of other tricyclics and can result from absorption of the topical formulation.

- *Capsaicin*: depletes substance P from sensory nerves and blocks C-fibre conduction. There is evidence for its use in uraemic pruritus and histamine-induced itch. Initial burning may be alleviated by the use of topical local anaesthetics.

Parenteral treatments are more convenient for generalized pruritus.

- *Antihistamines*: mainly effective for histamine-mediated pruritus; the effect may be augmented by concomitant use of H_2 antagonists. Itch from uraemia, cholestasis or lymphoma is rarely relieved by antihistamines. Sedating antihistamines are believed to be more effective, possibly because of a central action. A trial of antihistamines is usually worthwhile at standard doses.

- *$5HT_3$ antagonists*: have proven efficacy in cholestasis, uraemia and opioid-induced itch. The dose is the same as for standard anti-emetic therapy and, although constipation can be a problem, no major toxicity has been reported.[4] The selective serotonin reuptake inhibitor paroxetine has been reported to have an anti-pruritic effect.[5]

- *Opioid antagonists* (e.g. naloxone, nalbuphine, butorphanol): have been investigated for efficacy in treating itch and appear to offer some promise. However, two factors may limit their use: the oral preparations are expensive, and there is a risk of precipitating an opioid withdrawal effect – this has been noted in opioid-naive patients with cholestatic pruritus, and is thought to result from high levels of endogenous opioids. Withdrawal reactions are more likely in patients taking opioids, as physical dependence on mu agonists develops with prolonged use. Studies assessing opioid antagonists for postoperative opioid-induced pruritus suggest that naloxone is more likely than nalbuphine or butorphanol to impair pain control.

- *Thalidomide*: antagonizes the action of tumour necrosis factor. At a dose of 100 mg/day, there is evidence of its effectiveness in primary biliary cirrhosis and uraemia. Sedation and fatigue can be troublesome.

SPECIFIC TREATMENTS

Uraemic pruritus
Optimizing dialysis and the use of phosphate-binding agents such as aluminium hydroxide may improve pruritus. Other therapies that have also been considered are ultraviolet B photochemotherapy, colestyramine (cholestyramine), erythropoietin and parathyroidectomy.[6]

Cholestatic pruritus
Resolution of the biliary obstruction, e.g. by stent or biliary diversion, should always be considered.

There is evidence available to support the efficacy of several therapies:[7]

- cholestyramine: use may be limited by the side effects of nausea, diarrhoea and constipation, and the unpalatable nature of the medication;

- rifampicin: side effects of haemolytic anaemia, renal failure and nausea could limit use;

- S-adenosylmethionine (SAMe): can cause mild gastrointestinal side effects;

- prednisolone.

Other treatments with less evidence for efficacy include methyltestosterone, levomepromazine (methotrimeprazine) and heparin.

HIV-related pruritus
Indometacin (indomethacin) is thought to be effective by modulating immune dysfunction by its action on prostaglandins.

Opioid-induced pruritus
One case report commented on resolution of pruritus when switching a patient from morphine to hydromorphone.

FUTURE DEVELOPMENTS

Further investigation is required to assess the effectiveness of some of these treatments, particularly in patients with advanced disease. It is likely that increasing knowledge of the neurotransmitters and pathways will lead to the discovery of new treatment options, especially from the opioid and serotonergic systems.

KEY POINTS

- Itch is a distressing symptom with unpleasant physical and psychological consequences.
- Common causes include cholestasis, uraemia, HIV and opioids.
- The exact mechanism behind the sensation of itch remains unclear; however, there is increased understanding of the receptors involved.
- New developments reflect this increased understanding of the neurotransmission, but there is a need for controlled trials to confirm their efficacy, especially in palliative care patients.

REFERENCES

1. Greaves M, Wall PD. Pathophysiology of itching. *Lancet* 1996; **348**, 938–40.
2. Wahlgren C-F. Measurement of itch. *Semin Dermatol* 1995; **14**(4), 277–84.
3. Sheehan-Dare RA, Henderson MJ, Cotterill JA. Anxiety and depression in patients with chronic urticaria and generalised pruritus. *Br J Dermatol* 1990; **123**(6), 769–74.
4. Muller C, Pongratz S, Pidlich J *et al*. Treatment of pruritus in chronic liver disease with the 5HT$_3$ receptor antagonist ondansetron: a randomised placebo controlled, double blind crossover trial. *Eur J Gastroenterol Hepatol* 1998; **10**(10), 865–70.
5. Zylicz Z, Smits C, Chem D, Krajnik M. Paroxetine for pruritus in advanced cancer. *J Pain Symptom Manage* 1998; **16**, 121–4.

6. Tan JK, Haberman HF, Coldman AJ. Identifying effective treatments for uremic pruritus. *J Am Acad Dermatol* 1991; **25**(5:1), 811–18.
7. Connolly CS, Kantor GR, Menduke H. Hepatobiliary pruritus: what are effective treatments? *J Am Acad Dermatol* 1995; **33**, 801–5.

FURTHER READING

Pittelkow MR, Loprinzi CL. Pruritus and sweating in palliative medicine. In: Doyle D, Hanks G, Cherny N, Calman K (eds), *Oxford textbook of palliative medicine*, 3rd edn. Oxford: Oxford Medical Publications, 2004, 573–87.
Twycross R, Greaves MW, Handwerker H, Jones EA, Libretto SE, Szepietowski JC, Zylicz Z. Itch: Scratching more than the surface. *Q J Med* 2003; **96**, 7–26.

A–Z OF SYMPTOMS

chapter 4.18

SWEATING

Debra Swann and Polly Edmonds

DEFINITION

Sweating (perspiration, diaphoresis, hydrosis) is a normal physiological mechanism by which the skin regulates body temperature, causing cooling by evaporative heat loss.[1]

In certain pathological states, sweating may be troublesome or excessive. It may occur as a physiological response to fear and anxiety, which needs to be addressed separately in our patient group.

PREVALENCE

The prevalence of abnormal sweating in advanced cancer varies between 16 and 28 per cent. A higher incidence of night sweats has been reported in metastatic adenocarcinoma.[1]

PATHOPHYSIOLOGY OF ABNORMAL SWEATING

The precise mechanism of sweating in advanced cancer is poorly understood and it is often regarded as a paraneoplastic phenomenon.

Theories previously suggested have involved pyrogen release by leukocyte infiltration of tumour cells, necrosis of the tumour causing release of pyrogens and secretion of cytokines by the tumour that have a direct effect on the hypothalamus or act as endogenous pyrogens: tumour necrosis factor (TNF), interleukins 1 and 6 and interferons have been implicated.[2]

For some of our patients, a heightened emotional state such as fear and anxiety may cause sweating due to increased adrenergic stimuli.

INVESTIGATIONS AND EXAMINATION

Eliciting a careful history from the patient will establish the frequency, degree of discomfort and pattern of sweating for that individual.

A simple descriptive scale of the patient's symptoms, as detailed in the box below, may be useful in assessing the degree of severity of the sweating and the response to therapeutic interventions.[3]

Descriptive scale for sweating

Mild sweating
No changes of clothing necessary; sweating only reported after specific questioning.

Moderate
No change of clothing necessary; washing of affected areas required; sweating volunteered by patients as a specific problem.

Severe
Volunteered by patient as drenching sweats requiring a change of clothing or bed linen, or both.

Investigations and examinations should be aimed at identifying and treating the underlying cause (Table 4.18.1). Relevant investigations may include the following.

Table 4.18.1 Pathological causes of sweating

Infective	Viral
	Bacterial
	Fungal
Endocrine	Iatrogenic menopause/androgen depletion
	Thyrotoxicosis
	Diabetic autonomic neuropathy
	Hypoglycaemia
	Acromegaly
Malignancy	Lymphoma, leukaemia
	Renal cell carcinoma
	Carcinoid
	Solid metastatic tumours (liver metastases)
	Atrial myxoma
	Phaeochromocytoma
Drugs	Alcohol
	Opioids
	Amitriptyline
	Tamoxifen
	Immune-modulating agents: interferon, interleukins, granulocyte macrophage-colony stimulating factor (GM-CSF)
	Drug withdrawal, e.g. alcohol, opioids
Neurological lesions	Infiltration/injury of sympathetic nervous system, cortex, basal ganglia, spinal cord

Adapted from Hami and Trotman (1999).[1]

A–Z OF SYMPTOMS

- To exclude infection:
  full blood count (FBC)
  erythrocyte sedimentation rate (ESR)
  midstream urine for culture (MSU)
  blood cultures
  chest X-ray.

- Hormone profile.

- Drug history.

Temperature charts may be of use in helping to delineate the pattern and severity of the symptoms.

Tests that quantify the degree of sweating are usually not appropriate in the palliative care setting. These include quantitative sudomotor axon reflex tests (QSARTs) and thermoregulatory sweat tests.

MANAGEMENT

GENERAL

The aim of management is to try to treat any identifiable cause and to offer symptomatic relief where no obvious cause is found.

- Reassurance and explanation should be offered where appropriate.

- Cool ambient temperatures help to lower the body's core temperature.

- Side rooms are ideal, where windows and doors can be opened without distressing other patients.

- Fans may help to accelerate evaporation of sweat from the body's surface.

- Overcrowding should be avoided around the patient.

- Lightweight bedding, ideally cool cotton sheets, should be used, and heavy blankets and duvets avoided.

- Bed cradles may be of some use in lifting the bedding, thus aiding the circulation of air to help with cooling.

- An evaluation of the bed mattress used can also help to provide a cooler environment; air mattresses and low air loss mattresses can be temperature regulated.

- Clothing should also be cool, lightweight and made from natural fibres.

- Clothes should be changed as regularly as needed.

- Facilities should be available for cooling baths or showers.

SPECIFIC

Non-pharmacological

- Topical therapies such as formalin 1% soaks and glutaraldehyde 10% in a buffered solution can be used for feet but not hands.

- Topical preparations of aluminium chloride can be applied to the axillae.

- Acupuncture has been used to relieve excessive sweating, with varying success.[1]

Pharmacological

Antipyretics   If the patient is pyrexial when the sweating attack occurs, an antipyretic such as paracetamol (which is thought to act on the pre-optic anterior hypothalamus) may be of benefit.[4] Other antipyretics include the non-steroidal anti-inflammatory drugs (NSAIDs), which have been used with some effect in hyperhydrosis, e.g. naproxen at doses of up to 1500 mg/day. Where one NSAID has been ineffective, a trial of an alternative may be indicated.

Corticosteroids   High-dose steroids have been used with differing degrees of success in treating the B-cell tumours such as chronic lymphocytic leukaemia. They are thought to act by suppressing cytokine activity.

Anticholinergics   The use of anticholinergic agents in the treatment of excessive sweating has been the subject of clinical trails. Thioridazine, a phenothiazine with potent antimuscarinic effects, has been reported to improve symptoms in 50–88 per cent of cases.[5] In one uncontrolled series, 15 (88 per cent) of 17 patients reported an improvement in sweating at doses of 10–30 mg at night. Thioridazine has recently been withdrawn from the market, except for the treatment of adult-type schizophrenia, but is available for the treatment of sweating as a non-licensed indication. Patients need to be observed for signs of the potential interactions and side effects. Other anticholinergics, including hyoscine butylbromide and hyoscine hydrobromide, have also been used with good effect.[1] Propantheline tends to cause intolerable side effects, as high doses are needed to produce symptomatic benefit.

Beta-blockers   Where increased adrenergic activity is the cause of sweating, for example in thyrotoxocosis, beta-blockers such as propranolol 10 mg may be of benefit. Caution is needed in patients who are hypotensive and/or have the usual contraindications for the use of beta-blockers such as asthma, peripheral vascular disease and heart block.

Other drugs   Anecdotal reports suggest that cimetidine has been tried with some effect at doses of 400–800 mg daily.

FUTURE DEVELOPMENTS

Thalidomide at a dose of 100 mg at night for 10 days was found to be effective for 4 out of 7 patients in a short case series. Side effects (nausea and drowsiness) prevented two patients completing the study, and one further patient achieved a reduction in the interim assessment of distress but died before completing the study.[6]

Thalidomide has been shown to suppress TNFα production by monocytes *in vitro*. Excess TNFα production in tuberculosis causes fevers, night sweats, necrosis and progressive weight loss. Thalidomide has also been shown to reduce TNFα production and enhance weight gain in tuberculosis. It has also been used to treat immunologically related disorders such as chronic graft versus host disease, erythema nodosum leprosum, Behçet's syndrome, rheumatoid arthritis and aphthous ulceration in human immunodeficiency virus (HIV)-positive patients.

The side effects of drowsiness, skin rashes, dry mouth, nausea and peripheral neuropathy may limit its use in the palliative care population. The well-reported side effect of teratogenicity is unlikely to be relevant in our patient population.

Botulinum toxin injected locally has been used with some success in the management of hyperhydrosis. It blocks the release of acetylcholine in the neuromuscular junction and inhibits cholinergic transmission in postganglionic sympathetic cholinergic fibres to sweat glands, as seen in botulism and shown experimentally. It has a good cosmetic effect, but needs expert supervision when administered.

KEY POINTS

- Sweating has a multifactorial aetiology.
- Non-pharmacological symptomatic measures should be tried.
- No drug treatment has any proven efficacy.

REFERENCES

1. Hami F, Trotman I. The treatment of sweating. *Eur J Palliat Care* 1999; **6**(6), 184–7.
2. Johnson M. Neoplastic fever. *Palliat Med* 1996; **10**, 217–24.
3. Quigley CS, Baines M. Descriptive epidemiology of sweating in a hospice population. *J Palliat Care* 1997; **13**(1), 22–6.
4. Twycross R. *Symptom management in advanced cancer*, 2nd edn. Abingdon: Radcliffe Medical Press, 1997, 254–8.
5. Cowap J, Hardy J. Thioridazine in the management of cancer-related sweating. *J Pain Symptom Manage* 1998; **15**(5), 266.
6. Deaner P. The use of thalidomide in the management of severe sweating in patients with advanced malignancy. *Palliat Med* 2000; **14**(5), 429–31.

THE MANAGEMENT OF URINARY SYMPTOMS

Debra Swann and Polly Edmonds

Satisfactory voiding requires an unobstructed passage of urine from the bladder to the urethral meatus. Mechanisms that interfere with this flow of urine are dealt with in this chapter.

PREVALENCE

Up to 53 per cent of cancer patients develop urinary problems during the last 48 hours of life.[1] In one specialist palliative care unit, the need for urinary collecting devices was reported to be 74 per cent in patients admitted for terminal care.[2] Common causes are shown in Table 4.19.1.

PATHOPHYSIOLOGY

Unobstructed passage of urine from the bladder to the urethral meatus is necessary for satisfactory voiding to occur. It requires a functioning detrusor muscle, intact bladder wall and integrity of the nerves initiating and co-ordinating detrusor and sphincteric activity. Parasympathetic system stimulation of the nerves supplying the bladder results in contraction of the detrusor muscle and relaxation of the bladder neck sphincter. Sympathetic system stimulation has the reverse effect. A combination of bladder tone and the effect of the external sphincters maintains continence. All these factors are co-ordinated by higher centres to initiate or inhibit bladder emptying.[3]

Any component of the voiding pathway can be affected, resulting in urinary problems for the patient.

INVESTIGATIONS AND EXAMINATION

Obtaining a careful history from the patient about the nature of the problem is essential. Patients are often embarrassed to mention urological-related problems,

Table 4.19.1 Common urinary problems and related causes

Retention	Obstruction
	Enlarged prostate
	Impacted faeces in rectum
	Generalized weakness
	Depression
	Lack of awareness/delirium
	Drugs
	Tricyclic antidepressants
	Morphine (especially epidural)
	Spinal cord compression
Incontinence	
Total	Local tumour involvement
	Overflow due to urethral or catheter obstruction
	Confusion leading to inappropriate voiding
Stress	Weak pelvic floor, hypotonic bladder
Neurological	Hypotonic (neuropathic) bladder due to sacral plexus or spinal cord compression below T11
Other causes	Fistulae (vesicovaginal/vesicoenteric)
	Infection
	Diabetes
	Faecal impaction
Pain	Renal colic
	Obstructive bladder pain
	Irritative bladder pain
Discoloured urine	Blood
	Drugs
	Dantron
	Senna
	Rifampicin
	Chemotherapy
	Adriamycin
	Mitoxantrone
	Food dyes
	Beetroot
	Rhubarb
	Bile
Increased urine output	Drugs
	Diuretics
	Endocrine
	Diabetes mellitus
	Hypercalcaemia

(continued)

A–Z OF SYMPTOMS

Table 4.19.1 (continued)

	Chronic renal failure
	Diabetes insipidus
	Anxiety and excessive drinking
Decreased urine output	Dehydration
	Bilateral ureteric obstruction
	Urethral obstruction
	Catheter blocked
	Endocrine (SIADH)
Frequency of urine	Causes of increased urine output
	Infection
	Unstable bladder
	Anxiety
	Obstruction with overflow
	Small capacity bladder due to tumour/post-radiotherapy
Decreased frequency	Above causes of decreased urine output
	Anti-muscarinic drugs
	Hyoscine
	Tricyclic antidepressants
	Neurological problems
Catheter-related problems	Blocked catheter
	Bypassing of urine
	Infection
	Urethritis
	Encrustation
Bladder spasms	Consider retention
	Clot retention
	Balloon in urethra

SIADH, syndrome of inappropriate antidiuretic hormone secretion.

A–Z OF SYMPTOMS

so direct questioning might be necessary. Reassurance and understanding are imperative.

A history of retention should include whether or not it was associated with gradual onset of dribbling, difficulty initiating voiding or poor stream of urine, especially in elderly male patients. A history of sudden-onset inability to pass urine should raise the possibility of spinal cord obstruction, and neurological examination should be performed to ensure that the peripheral nervous system is intact.

In the elderly, bladder outlet obstruction may be masked and manifest itself instead as confusion or agitation, especially in patients taking neuroleptic or opioid drugs.

In the examination of bladder dysfunction, the anatomical and functional integrity of the bladder and urethra should be considered, spinal cord compression excluded and the drug history of the patient obtained to ensure that a drug-related cause of retention is not responsible. A rectal examination should be performed to exclude rectal impaction from faeces and an enlarged prostate in men.

Appropriate tests include:

- exclude biochemical causes that may cause increased urine flow, e.g. hyperglycaemia, hypercalcaemia, diabetes insipidus, chronic renal failure;

- midstream urine to exclude infection after dipsticking the urine to test for sugar, protein, blood and white cells.

MANAGEMENT

GENERAL

- Regular toileting.

- Incontinence pads/disposable underpants.

- Decrease nocturnal fluid intake.

SPECIFIC

- Treat infections with antibiotics if the patient is symptomatic (not for asymptomatic bacteriuria).

- Hypoglycaemic drugs if the blood glucose is high.

- Bladder washouts for blocked catheters.

- Reduce balloon volume or change the catheter if urine is bypassing the catheter.

- Supply continence aids, e.g. urine bottles, commodes, where weakness/ shortness of breath impairs the patient's ability to get to the toilet.

- Review drugs that may cause retention.

- Stop chemotherapy/non-steroidal anti-inflammatory drugs if the patient is developing cystitis.

Obstructive uropathy
Percutaneous nephrostomy tubes and urethral stents may be appropriate in patients with locally advanced pelvic disease and a good overall prognosis. Ethical considerations need to balance the benefits of improved life expectancy over quality of remaining life after the procedure, versus death from renal impairment. These decisions need to be individualized.

Vesicoenteric fistulae
Surgical correction may be appropriate.

- Segment of affected bowel and bladder removed and bowel and bladder integrity restored – this is only relevant in fit patients with small-volume disease.

- Colostomy or ileostomy formation for intestinal diversion of faeces – to help reduce the urinary symptoms.

- Urinary diversion via ileal conduit, or temporarily via percutaneous nephrostomies.

Non-pharmacological measures
- Vaginal pessaries for urethral prolapse due to laxity of the pelvic floor (if appropriate).

- Urethral convenes for men.

- Penis pouches (for small retractile penises).

- Intermittent self-catheterization (for neurological bladder problems, e.g. spinal cord compression, multiple sclerosis).

- Urethral or suprapubic catheters.

PHARMACOLOGICAL MEASURES

- Simple analgesia as per World Health Organisation analgesic ladder.

- Imipramine 10–50 mg nocte – useful in nocturnal urinary frequency or urge incontinence.

- Dienestrol (dienoestrol) cream – for stress incontinence in postmenopausal women with vaginal atrophy.

- Oxybutynin 5 mg t.d.s. – reduces bladder spasms and urgency.

- Bupivacaine 0.25% via urethral catheter (place 20 mL in the bladder and leave for 15 minutes, repeat every 12 hours) – can help relieve pain due to direct infiltration of bladder tumour.

- Diclofenac and hyoscine butylbromide (Buscopan) – useful for renal colic.

- Desmopressin 100–200 mcg nocte – a synthetic analogue of vasopressin, antidiuretic hormone (ADH), reduces urinary output overnight and can help in intractable nocturnal incontinence.

- Ketamine or spinal analgesia for intractable persistent pain.

KEY POINTS

- Urinary problems are common in the palliative care population.
- A sensitive approach is required to obtain accurate information.
- Accurate assessment and treatment of the underlying cause are important.
- Continence assessment is paramount to skin integrity.

REFERENCES

1. Lichter I, Hunt E. The last 48 hours of life. *J Palliat Care* 1990; **6**, 7–15.
2. Fainsinger RL, MacEachern T, Hanson J, Bruera E. The use of urinary catheters in terminally ill cancer patients. *J Pain Symptom Manage* 1992; 7(6), 333–8.
3. Norman RW. Genitourinary disorders. In: Doyle D, Hanks G, Cherny N, Calman K (eds), *Oxford textbook of palliative medicine*, 3rd edn. Oxford: Oxford University Press, 2004, 647–58.

CLINICAL CHALLENGES IN MALIGNANT DISEASE

FRACTURES AND IMPENDING FRACTURES

Anthony M. Smith and Luc Louette

Fractures occur in some 5–10 per cent of patients with advanced malignancy.[1] In a series of 500 consecutive patients admitted to hospice under the care of one of the authors, 31 had sustained fractures. Fractures arise as a consequence of:

- metastases from the original tumour,

- other pathological causes (e.g. osteoporosis, osteomalacia, disuse osteoporosis, osteoporosis due to steroid use, bone infection),

- trauma (commonly, falls).

The commonest cause is metastasis. Almost any malignant tumour may metastasize to bone, except the primary brain tumours. In one study, radionuclide imaging demonstrated bone metastases in 63 per cent of 933 patients with a primary adenocarcinoma.[1] Fifty per cent of bony secondaries are from breast primaries, with lung, prostate and kidney being the next commonest.[2] Prostatic carcinoma secondaries, unlike those from breast, lung, kidney and thyroid, tend to be sclerotic (or osteoblastic) and are much less likely to fracture than the lytic metastases of most other carcinomas: a survey of 150 pathological fractures showed that only 3 per cent were due to prostatic adenocarcinoma.[1]

Since the incidence of neoplasia is commonest in the elderly, there will also be a proportionately increased incidence of osteoporosis and other non-malignant pathological conditions in these patients. Falls are common in the elderly, particularly in association with the weakness and instability of advanced malignancy, and in these cases fracture does not necessarily relate to bone metastasis.

Secondaries in bone occur most commonly in the axial skeleton (skull, vertebrae, ribs, scapulae and pelvis) and proximal limb bones. However, any bone may be implicated – as, for example, a patient seen by one of the authors with a rectal carcinoma who presented with a pathological fracture in the foot.

DIAGNOSIS OF FRACTURE

Fractures present with a history of some or all of the following:

- pain
- deformity
- local swelling
- sudden incident (see below)
- loss of function (e.g. paraparesis, loss of sphincter control).

The pain may have been present for a long time, slowly getting worse, with or without recent exacerbation. It may be felt at the site of fracture or at a distance (e.g. in the hip or leg from spinal fractures, or in the thigh or knee from a femoral neck fracture). Long-standing pain, worse on activity but often also present at rest, may indicate bony metastasis before fracture has occurred. On the other hand, an incident such as turning in bed may result in fracture through a previously symptomless bone metastasis.

X-ray will confirm the diagnosis. Bone scan can help to identify bone metastases not yet large enough to be visualized on X-ray (and before fracture), thus identifying sites at risk and the extent of bony secondary spread.

Back pain associated with sensory changes in the legs and weakness in one or both legs is an important presentation of spinal cord compression due to vertebral pathological fracture and requires urgent diagnosis and treatment (see page 251 onwards). However, recent studies have shown that persistent severe back pain or spinal nerve root pain, even without neurological signs, in a patient who has had cancer should be investigated urgently with magnetic resonance imaging (MRI) scanning.[3] Only in this way can spinal cord compression be prevented.

PREVENTION OF FRACTURE

Preventive treatment with bisphosphonates (see Chapter 6.2) has been shown to reduce bone pain, and may decrease the risk of subsequent fracture.[1] Bone metastases found at bone scan, and part of disseminated malignancy, require special treatment if they cause pain or are at risk of fracture.

Identification of bone metastases that are at risk of fracture and would benefit from operative measures has led to various scoring systems based on site, radiographic appearance, severity of symptoms, and MRI scanning. Mirels in Johannesburg has developed a simple scoring system based on clinical examination (regarding site and pain severity) and plain radiographs (with respect to the nature and size of the lesion, Table 5.1.1).[4] This system is well validated and does not require an MRI scan.

The *nature* of the lesion is clear on X-ray: blastic or sclerotic metastases look denser than the surrounding bone; lytic metastases show as a hole in the structure of the bone. The *size* of the lesion refers to comparison with the diameter of the bone.

Table 5.1.1 The Mirels scoring system

	Score		
Variable	1	2	3
Site	Upper limb	Lower limb	Peritrochanteric
Pain	Mild	Moderate	Functional (i.e. incident)
Lesion	Blastic	Mixed	Lytic
Size	<1/3	1/3–2/3	>2/3

Thus a *lytic* lesion occupying *half the diameter* of the shaft of the *femur*, and causing *moderate pain*, would score 3 + 2 + 2 + 2 = 9. Bony secondaries with a score from 4 to 8 are at low risk of impending fracture and are best treated with bisphosphonates and radiotherapy for pain relief, generally by a single fraction.[5] Those with a Mirels score of 9–12 have a high risk of subsequent fracture, and prophylactic surgery or fixation should be considered if the patient is fit for surgery. Adjuvant radiotherapy is normally given a few weeks after surgery once the surgical wounds are healed.

Bone secondaries in the shaft of long bones are treated with intramedullary nail fixation or plate and screw fixation, plus curettage of the bony lesion and augmentation with bone cement. Bony secondaries close to joints are treated with cemented hemiarthroplasty or cemented total joint replacement surgery.

When a patient is known to have bone metastases, even though relatively symptom free, there is a natural tendency to restrict activity lest fracture occur. This happens especially with secondaries in the femora and in cervical vertebrae. It is important to remember the stage of the underlying malignancy and not to prevent activities that would give the patient pleasure during his or her last weeks or months, in the hope of preventing a fracture or disability that may never occur.

In this respect, too, it is worth remembering the nature of the metastasis because, as already noted, blastic bone metastases are less likely to fracture than lytic ones.

IMMEDIATE TREATMENT OF FRACTURE

When a fracture occurs in a patient with advanced malignancy, the urgent considerations are:

- analgesia,

- emergency action to make the patient comfortable,

- confirmation of diagnosis,

- arrangements for definitive treatment.

Appropriate analgesia will be provided by an injection of diamorphine or morphine (dose as indicated by the size and age of the patient and current opioid medication) with an anti-emetic and anxiolytic (such as haloperidol 3–5 mg). Injected midazolam (2.5–10 mg) at the same time has useful amnesiant and muscle relaxant actions.

If the fracture is of a limb bone, after the analgesic has had time to act, the limb may be straightened by gentle, firm pulling out. It should then be immobilized with a splint or by being tied to the side of the body (for an arm) or to the other limb in the case of a leg. Even if traction is not performed, the limb should be splinted to prevent painful movement at the fracture site.

It may be useful to obtain a portable X-ray of a suspected long bone fracture if the facilities are available without transfer to hospital, especially if there is doubt about the fracture and if the patient is very unwell.

In most cases, however, the patient should be transferred to the local hospital for X-ray confirmation of the fracture and definitive treatment. A full note of the patient's condition and current medication should be sent, and the promise made to take the patient back to a palliative care bed (if at all possible) after treatment as soon as convenient to the hospital.

DEFINITIVE TREATMENT OF LIMB FRACTURES

The best treatment for limb fractures is internal fixation with subsequent radiotherapy or (where internal fixation is not possible) immobilization or support for the fracture with radiotherapy.

Appropriate analgesia will be needed. Non-steroidal anti-inflammatory drugs act at the site of pain production in the limb, but do not provide total pain relief. They are complemented by opioids, but adequate analgesia with opioids is difficult to titrate in the case of fractures because the amount needed varies rapidly with rest or movement.

Hence the importance of surgical internal fixation whenever possible. We have seen such relief from pain gained by internal fixation of a fractured humerus or femur, and such recovery of hope from the simple ability to get up or move freely in bed after such a procedure, that we strongly commend surgery for long bone fractures, even in very sick patients. The anaesthetist will guide as to whether the patient will withstand anaesthetic, but fixation of a fracture, even in the last few days of life, gives best pain relief.

In fractures after trauma, healing may be expected; unfortunately, in pathological fractures through metastases, healing does not occur spontaneously but requires (after immobilization) radiotherapy to halt bone destruction and to stimulate repair processes. Radiotherapy can be given as soon as wound healing has occurred, or through plaster if the limb fracture is immobilized. A single treatment generally suffices and rarely causes systemic upset, as it is given so peripherally.[5]

DEFINITIVE TREATMENT OF LIMB FRACTURES IN THE VERY ILL

Where the patient is too ill to travel and to undergo surgical or radiotherapy procedures, relief of pain from the fracture may be obtained with immobilization, traction or an anaesthetic block. A portable X-ray, if possible, will confirm (or refute) the diagnosis, and an orthopaedic opinion can be gained by a visit from the local specialist.

For arm and wrist fractures or lower leg fractures, immobilization is achieved with plaster of Paris or a lightweight cast. The limb should be well padded before application of the plaster. Lightness in weight is an advantage for frail and elderly people. Manipulation may be performed under local anaesthetic if necessary.

For the shaft or neck of femur, plaster is unsatisfactory, as the joint proximal (i.e. the hip) cannot be immobilized. For these fractures, the simplest of traction systems – a straight pull over the end of the bed (Fig. 5.1.1) – will ease pain and allow better control with analgesics. Traction should not be used where it is envisaged that it will be needed for several weeks; instead, operation should be considered – time is too valuable at this stage of a patient's life to waste it on traction!

Another option is an anaesthetic block: an epidural, psoas or lumbar plexus block with bupivacaine can provide long-term pain relief. The block is performed with a single injection of bupivacaine 0.25% with or without steroids, and the pain relief can be prolonged by inserting an indwelling catheter for regular top-ups or by continuous infusion from a syringe driver. Total pain relief for a femoral neck or shaft fracture can be continued for days or even weeks, at the cost of a numb leg – a price generally well accepted if explained beforehand. It should be noted here that pressure area care will be even more important than usual, as one of the consequences of a long-term epidural will be sacral area numbness.

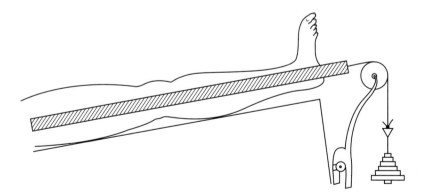

Figure 5.1.1 Simple straight traction. (1) The leg is gently and firmly straightened and pulled. (2). Tinct. Benz. Co. is applied to the sides of the leg. (3) An extension plaster strapping is applied. (4) The leg is crepe bandaged from ankle to top of the thigh. (5) The extension cord is taken over a pulley attached to the foot of the bed. (6) A weight of 5–7 lb is attached (this can be a plastic bottle containing 7 lb of water). (7) The foot of the bed is raised to provide countertraction (as shown in figure).

FRACTURES OF THE AXIAL SKELETON

Vertebral compression fracture without long tract signs is best treated with rest and analgesia – opioids plus non-steroidal anti-inflammatory drugs – and radiotherapy. The same is true for pathological fractures of clavicle or scapula. Where there is suspicion of spinal cord compression, urgent diagnosis and treatment are essential: this is discussed later (Chapter 5.4, p. 251).

Fractures of the pelvis may require simple traction as well as analgesia for a few days until the acute pain of the incident has subsided, and then radiotherapy. In this instance, mobilization will need to be delayed until pain is eased, and may then be started using crutches or a Zimmer frame.

Sometimes, a wheelchair enables the patient to begin to get around when the pelvis is not stable enough for weight-bearing. It is surprising how these fractures through metastases in the pelvis sometimes lead to very little pain. Where pain is a feature, however, an epidural injection of bupivacaine and steroid provides valuable relief.

KEY POINTS

- Bone pain? Remember the possibility of fracture and use the Mirels scoring system.
- Fracture of long bone? Think internal fixation and radiotherapy.
- Metastasis but no fracture? Think prophylactic fixation and radiotherapy.
- Managing bone pain? Remember immobilization, opioids, non-steroidal anti-inflammatory drugs, radiotherapy, bisphosphonates.
- Orthopaedic referral? Offer to take the patient back as soon as treatment is completed!

REFERENCES

1. Aaron AD. Current concepts review: Treatment of metastatic adenocarcinoma of the pelvis and the extremities. *Am J Bone Joint Surg* 1997; **79a**(6), 917–29.
2. Bates TD, Chalmers J, Mannix KA, Rawlins MD. The management of bone metastases (radiotherapy, orthopaedic procedures and non-steroidal anti-inflammatory drugs). *Palliat Med* 1987; **1**, 117–31.
3. Levack P, Graham J, Collie D *et al. Don't wait for a sensory level – listen to the symptoms.* Scottish Cord Compression Study Group report. *Clin Oncol (R Coll Radiol)* 2002; **14**(6), 472–80.
4. Mirels H. Metastatic disease in long bones; a proposed scoring system for diagnosing impending pathologic fractures. *Clin Orthopaed Related Res* 1989; **249**, 256–64.
5. Price P, Hoskin PJ, Easton D *et al.* Prospective randomised trial of single and multifraction radiotherapy schedules in the treatment of painful bony metastases. *Radiother Oncol* 1986; **6**(4), 247–55.

HAEMORRHAGE

Katie M. Emmitt

INTRODUCTION

Haemorrhage occurs in approximately 10 per cent of advanced cancer patients.[1] There may be a single episode with no cardiovascular consequence, recurrent episodes producing symptomatic anaemia, or a massive haemorrhage with rapid cardiovascular compromise and death. Bleeding causes distress for patients, carers and healthcare professionals alike. Management requires advanced planning and an individualized approach to care.

PATHOPHYSIOLOGY

Haemostasis is a process involving interactions between the vessel wall, platelets and coagulation factors. Damage to the vessel wall endothelium results in vasoconstriction, reducing blood flow to the area, and activation of platelets and the coagulation pathway. Platelets adhere to the damaged endothelium and release their contents, which results in the formation of a platelet plug. Coagulation involves a series of enzymatic reactions leading to the conversion of soluble plasma fibrinogen to fibrin, which binds platelets and red cells to form a haemostatic plug. The presence of fibrin also precipitates fibrinolysis, which limits coagulation to the site of injury and helps to restore vessel patency by causing the breakdown of fibrin and fibrinogen.

Abnormalities of clotting and fibrinolysis are detectable in 50 per cent of cancer patients.[2] Haemorrhage can occur due to abnormalities of any part of haemostasis (Table 5.2.1). Vascular invasion by primary or secondary tumours causes local bleeding which, if involving a large vessel, can be massive. Thrombocytopenia or abnormal platelet function is characterized by spontaneous generalized bleeding from small vessels. This usually presents as easy bruising (purpura, petechiae and echymoses) and bleeding from mucous membranes (mouth and nose). Coagulation disorders are typically associated with haemarthroses and muscle haematomas.

Table 5.2.1 Causes of bleeding in patients with advanced cancer

Vessel damage
- Primary tumour invasion
  - Head and neck tumours
  - Fungating breast carcinoma
  - Bronchial carcinoma – haemoptysis
  - Gastrointestinal tumour – haematemesis, melaena, fresh rectal bleeding
  - Genitourinary tumour – haematuria, vaginal bleeding
- Secondary tumour invasion
  - Lung metastases – haemoptysis
- Indirect effect or unrelated to tumour
  - Drugs – peptic ulceration due to NSAIDs and corticosteroids
  - Radiotherapy – radiation proctitis, oesophagitis
  - Co-morbidity

Thrombocytopenia or abnormal platelet function
- Haematological malignancies
- Bone marrow infiltration from non-haematological malignancies
- Drugs – chemotherapy, anticonvulsants, aspirin
- Radiotherapy – bone marrow suppression
- Co-morbidity

Coagulation abnormalities
- Impaired hepatic function
  - Primary hepatocellular carcinoma
  - Liver metastases
  - Biliary obstruction of any cause
- Disseminated intravascular coagulation
- Drugs – anticoagulants (warfarin, heparin, low-molecular-weight heparins)
- Co-morbidity

Mixed
Any combination of the above

NSAIDs, non-steroidal anti-inflammatory drugs.

CLINICAL FEATURES AND INVESTIGATIONS

Identifying the cause of bleeding will help to guide management. The extent of assessment will depend on the individual clinical situation. No examination or investigation would be appropriate in a patient imminently dying from massive haemoptysis due to advanced bronchial carcinoma, whereas a patient having recurrent smaller episodes may warrant bronchoscopy.

HISTORY

- Cancer history including site(s) of disease and management.
- Site(s) and pattern of bleeding.

- Drug history.

- Past medical history (co-morbid conditions).

- Family history (inherited disorders).

EXAMINATION

- Pulse and blood pressure to assess for cardiovascular compromise.

- Site(s) of bleeding – fungating tumour, purpura, echymoses, haematomas.

- Rectal examination – gastrointestinal bleeding.

INVESTIGATIONS

- Full blood count and film.

- Bleeding time (measure of platelet function).

- Coagulation tests.

- Liver function tests.

- Endoscopy – upper or lower gastrointestinal, bronchoscopy, cystoscopy.

- Angiography.

MANAGEMENT (Table 5.2.2)

PREVENTION

Identify those patients most at risk of bleeding, as in some cases this may be preventable. Patients who have had minor bleeds may go on to have more major episodes. Massive haemorrhage is rare, but may be predicted in patients with fungating tumours arising close to major vessels, such as proximal bronchial tumours and those of the head and neck. In these situations, prevention is not usually possible, but formulating a management plan may reduce the trauma for patients and their carers should it occur.

Appropriate oncological management may prevent bleeding, including surgery, hormone therapy, chemotherapy and radiotherapy. For example, all these treatment modalities may prevent disease progression and fungation with subsequent bleeding of a breast carcinoma.[2]

Medications that may cause or aggravate bleeding should be closely monitored in all patients with advanced malignancy, but particularly those at increased risk of bleeding. Non-steroidal anti-inflammatory drugs (NSAIDs) and corticosteroids are commonly used in the palliative care setting and are frequently co-prescribed, when the risk of intestinal bleeding is substantially greater than when either drug is used alone. Limiting the use of such combinations to where absolutely necessary

Table 5.2.2 Management of a non-massive haemorrhage

Prevention
- Identify patients at risk of bleeding or following a minor bleed
- Treat the underlying cause – appropriate oncological management including surgery, hormone therapy, chemotherapy, radiotherapy
- Review drugs – anticoagulants, NSAIDS, corticosteroids

In the event of haemorrhage consider appropriateness of acute medical management

Local treatments
- Direct pressure
- Pressure dressings/packing
- Haemostatic dressings
- Topical medications
- Radiotherapy
- Endoscopic techniques
- Interventional radiological techniques
- Surgical techniques

Systemic treatments
- Systemic medications
    Antifibrinolytic agents – tranexamic acid
    Haemostatic agents – etamsylate (ethamsylate)
    Vitamin K
- Blood products
    Red cells
    Platelets
    Fresh frozen plasma

Psychosocial support
- Explanation
- Reassurance
- Dark towels/basins
- Physical presence

NSAIDs, non-steroidal anti-inflammatory drugs.

and the appropriate use of proton pump inhibitors should minimize associated upper gastrointestinal bleeding. In addition, the risk:benefit ratio of therapeutic anticoagulation should be assessed on an individual basis. Where anticoagulation is considered to be indicated, the use of a low-molecular-weight heparin rather than warfarin may be safer.[3,4]

ACUTE MEDICAL MANAGEMENT

In patients with advanced incurable disease, acute medical management is rarely appropriate in the event of a life-threatening haemorrhage. However, in the setting of a reversible cause of bleeding, good quality of life and slowly progressive disease, this may need to be considered. Where possible, management decisions should be sensitively discussed with the patient and family.

LOCAL TREATMENTS

Direct pressure and pressure dressings should be applied to surface haemorrhages. Bleeding cavities, such as the nose or vagina, can be packed. Some specialist dressings contain haemostatic compounds such as calcium alginate (Kaltostat and Sorbsan) and thromboplastin (Thrombostat). Topical medications including adrenaline (epinephrine) or cocaine can be applied to produce vasoconstriction. Sucralfate, administered orally, has a topical effect in reducing upper gastrointestinal bleeding and has also been administered rectally and applied to surface wounds.

Palliative radiotherapy is well established to control haemorrhage, including haemoptysis, haematuria, vaginal or uterine bleeding, and surface bleeding from fungating tumours. Both external beam radiation and brachytherapy have a role. Small doses in single fractions or short courses are frequently effective.

In selected patients, more interventional treatments may be considered. Endoscopy in conjunction with the use of vasoconstrictor drugs or cauterization may be useful in gastrointestinal, genitourinary and bronchial haemorrhage. Alum and other chemical cauterizing agents administered intravesically and intrarectally have been used to treat bleeding from the bladder and rectum. Transcatheter arterial embolization has been effective in controlling bleeding from head and neck, abdominal and pelvic tumours, amongst others.[5] Occasionally, surgical procedures such as ligation or cauterization of a bleeding vessel are indicated.

SYSTEMIC TREATMENTS

The antifibrinolytic agent tranexamic acid has been used to control cancer-related bleeding from various sites, including the skin, bladder, bronchi and gastro-intestinal tract.[6] In patients with haematuria, there is a risk of ureteric obstruction and its use is contraindicated in thromboembolic disease. Etamsylate (ethamsylate) has haemostatic properties through correction of abnormal platelet adhesion. Vitamin K is necessary for the hepatic production of a number of coagulation factors and is often deficient in the presence of hepatic disease. It can be administered orally or intravenously, but intravenous use has been associated with anaphylactoid reactions.

BLOOD PRODUCTS

Transfusion of blood products in the palliative care setting is aimed at symptom management. Red-cell transfusions can improve weakness, dyspnoea and sense of well-being in palliative care patients with anaemia.[7] Spontaneous bleeding with thrombocytopenia is usually associated with platelet counts below 20 000/uL. Platelets have a short lifespan, and prophylactic transfusion is not routinely indicated in this group of patients. Fresh frozen plasma has a very limited role in palliative care. It may be used to reverse warfarin anticoagulation in a patient who is actively bleeding and temporarily to correct coagulation for an invasive procedure.

Table 5.2.3 Management of massive acute haemorrhage

- Prevention
- Psychosocial support
- Sedation

PSYCHOSOCIAL SUPPORT

Even small bleeds can be very frightening for patients and their carers. Massive haemorrhage can generate panic. If small bleeds have occurred, it is important to reassure that large ones are unusual. If a massive haemorrhage is predictable, it is usually appropriate to inform the family and healthcare professionals involved with the patient to allow advance planning for this event. Discussions need to include the likely irreversible nature of the situation, the inappropriateness of hospitalization and resuscitation and the importance of remaining with the patient to provide support. Dark towels and basins should be available to mask the colour of the blood. In the event of massive haemoptysis or haematemesis, placing the patient in the left lateral position reduces the risk of suffocation (Table 5.2.3).

SEDATION

In a massive haemorrhage resulting in death within seconds to a few minutes, sedation is not indicated, as by the time any medication is prepared and administered, it will not have time to take effect. Sedation may be indicated in a large haemorrhage that is prolonged enough for the patient to be aware and distressed. Midazolam 5–10 mg administered subcutaneously or intramuscularly should reduce awareness and may be repeated if necessary.

KEY POINTS

- Try to foresee the risk of haemorrhage and reduce it, e.g. by local radiotherapy to fungating tumours.
- The approach to investigation and management varies considerably depending on the size of the haemorrhage and the health of the patient.
- Topical vasoconstrictors and superficial radiotherapy can reduce surface bleeding.
- Tranexamic acid and etamsylate (ethamsylate) stabilize clots and may reduce bleeding, at the potential risk of causing clot obstruction.
- Platelets have a short lifespan, and prophylactic transfusion is not routinely indicated in palliative care patients with thrombocytopenia.
- Large haemorrhages are frightening. Patients' families and carers need preparation, and provision should be made for patients to be sedated if they are aware of the bleeding.

REFERENCES

1. Smith AM. Emergencies in palliative care. *Ann Acad Med Singapore* 1992; **23**(2), 186–90.
2. Hoskin P, Makin W. *Oncology for palliative medicine*, 2nd edn. Oxford: Oxford University Press, 2003; 367, 100–1.
3. Johnson MJ. Problems of anticoagulation within a palliative care setting: an audit of hospice patients taking warfarin. *Palliat Med* 1997; **11**, 306–12.
4. Johnson MJ. Problems of anticoagulation within a palliative care setting: correction. *Palliat Med* 1998; **12**, 463.
5. Broadley KE, Kurowska A, Dick R *et al*. The role of embolization in palliative care. *Palliat Med* 1995; **9**, 331–5.
6. Dean A, Tuffin P. Fibrinolytic inhibitors for cancer-associated bleeding problems. *J Pain Symptom Manage* 1997; **13**(1), 20–4.
7. Gleeson C, Spencer D. Blood transfusion and its benefits in palliative care. *Palliat Med* 1995; **9**, 307–13.

FITS

Jeremy Rees

INTRODUCTION

The occurrence of epileptic seizures in a patient with a malignant disease is distressing for the patient, relatives and carers. The seizures themselves may be so dramatic that witnesses often think patients are about to die, and this is compounded by the unpredictability and loss of control caused by these events. In this group of patients, the presence of fits usually indicates either a structural brain lesion or severe metabolic derangement. The key principles in the management of fits are to maintain a safe environment while the patient is fitting, institute effective anticonvulsant medication to prevent further seizure activity, and establish the underlying cause. Fits may be part of the dying process, but there is no reason why they cannot be effectively controlled.

This chapter reviews the principles of diagnosis and therapy of seizures due mainly to primary and metastatic brain tumours. In treating seizures, certain key principles will be emphasized that are as applicable to the patient dying of a brain tumour as to the patient with chronic idiopathic epilepsy. Special considerations applicable to the dying patient, in particular the use of benzodiazepine and phenobarbitone infusions, are discussed.

DEFINITION OF SEIZURES

Seizures can be defined as the clinical manifestation of paroxysmal electrical activity in the brain. The commonest form of seizure in a patient with malignant disease is a generalized tonic–clonic seizure that is associated with epileptiform activity arising synchronously from both cerebral hemispheres. The clinical manifestations are well known to all health professionals and are unmistakable when witnessed: there is sudden loss of consciousness followed by a tonic phase of muscle rigidity and cyanosis culminating in clonic jerking of all four limbs, often associated with urinary incontinence. The seizure is usually self-terminating and the patient may be unrousable for several minutes afterwards, waking up in a confused state and frequently complaining of headache. There is variable amnesia for the events immediately leading up to the seizure and the patient may wake up with soft tissue injuries, scalp lacerations, limb fractures and a bleeding tongue. Postictally there is confusion and sometimes behaviour change, including psychosis.

How focal seizures present is dependent on the localization and lateralization of the seizure focus. Typical examples include:

- focal motor seizures causing jerking and spasms of the contralateral limb,

- focal sensory seizures characterized by paraesthesiae in the contralateral limb,

- complex partial seizures characterized by altered consciousness and automatisms such as lip smacking.

Some focal seizures, such as those arising from medial temporal lobes, give rise to olfactory or gustatory hallucinations, usually described as a fleeting smell or taste associated with a feeling of unease. Seizures occasionally arise from the occipital lobes and are described as colourful visual hallucinations, usually of circular images.

AETIOLOGY

The main causes of fits in patients with malignant disease are structural lesions and metabolic derangements (Table 5.3.1). A combination of causes is frequently seen in the palliative care setting.

Table 5.3.1 Causes of fits in patients with malignant disease

Structural lesions	Primary brain tumours
	Low-grade gliomas
	astrocytoma
	oligodendroglioma
	mixed glioma
	Malignant gliomas
	anaplastic astrocytoma
	anaplastic oligodendroglioma
	glioblastoma multiforme
	Meningiomas
	Secondary brain tumours
	Cerebral metastases
	Leptomeningeal metastases
	Dural metastases
	Brain abscesses (immunocompromised patients)
Metabolic derangements	Hypercalcaemia
	Hyponatraemia
Other	Uraemia
	Vascular events, e.g. cortical vein thrombosis
	Chemotherapy, e.g. ifosfamide, methotrexate
	Paraneoplastic, e.g. encephalomyelitis

STRUCTURAL LESIONS

Brain tumours account for about 5 per cent of epilepsy cases seen by neurologists, although they are over-represented in cases of intractable epilepsy. The incidence of tumour-associated epilepsy varies from 35 to 70 per cent depending on two main factors, location and histology. Slow-growing lesions, e.g. low-grade gliomas (Fig. 5.3.1), are associated with a higher incidence of seizures, probably because of the longer natural history and the time necessary for the development of focal cellular changes responsible for seizure generation. In general, seizures associated with malignant tumours, such as glioblastoma multiforme (Fig. 5.3.2) or metastases (Fig. 5.3.3), do not cause the same management difficulties as those due to slower-growing tumours. Survival is limited and so seizure intractability is rarely a consideration.

The pathophysiology of tumour-related epilepsy is probably multifactorial. Mechanical changes related to mass effect, metabolic changes in the internal milieu of the cortex associated with vasogenic oedema and/or hypervascularity, alterations in neurotransmitter levels and impairment of inhibitory mechanisms from remote epileptogenic foci have all been postulated as possible causes.

Location
Supratentorial tumours, and in particular lesions near the surface of the cortex, have a propensity to cause epilepsy. The dysfunctional cortex may be adjacent to

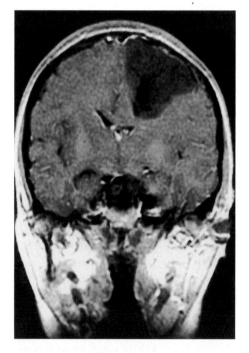

Figure 5.3.1 Coronal T1W MRI scan post-gadolinium showing non-enhancing low-signal lesion in the left frontal lobe which caused intractable focal motor seizures and occasional secondary generalized fits. The histology was an oligodendroglioma.

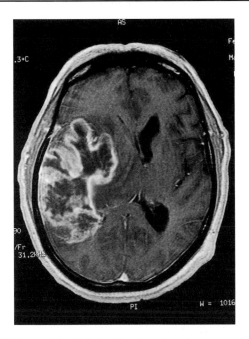

Figure 5.3.2 Axial T1W MRI scan with gadolinium showing a large, heterogeneous, irregular mass lesion with contrast enhancement in the right parietal lobe presenting as a progressive left hemiparesis. The lesion was debulked and histology revealed a glioblastoma multiforme.

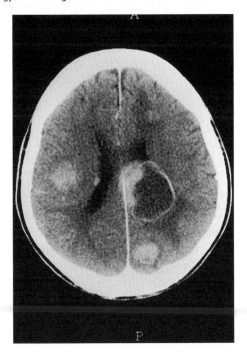

Figure 5.3.3 Contrast-enhanced CT brain scan showing multiple enhancing lesions which were metastases from a small cell lung cancer. The patient died shortly after this scan and never had seizures.

or remote from the tumour. Furthermore, the location of the tumour within the cerebral cortex is an important determinant of the likelihood of epilepsy developing. In a study of 337 cases of cerebral glioma, seizures occurred in 78 per cent of temporal lobe tumours, 62 per cent of parietal lobe tumours and 49 per cent of frontal lobe tumours.[1] Occipital epilepsy is, in comparison, very uncommon.

Histology
Gliomas are the most common type of brain tumour and account for 80 per cent of tumour-associated epilepsy. Nearly 40 per cent of patients with glioma present with a seizure as their initial symptom and seizures are a good prognostic factor.[2] The prevalence of epilepsy in patients with gliomas is inversely related to the histological grade. In a series of more than 1000 patients with gliomas, the frequency of epilepsy in glioblastomas (grade IV), anaplastic astrocytomas (grade III) and low-grade gliomas (grade II) was 49 per cent, 69 per cent and 85 per cent respectively.[3]

The incidence of seizures is lower (15–20 per cent) in patients with cerebral metastases, probably because they are more commonly located deep in the subcortical white matter where blood-borne seedlings deposit.[4]

METABOLIC DERANGEMENTS

The two major metabolic causes of seizures in patients with malignant disease are hypercalcaemia and hyponatraemia. Rapid identification and treatment of the biochemical abnormality will prevent further seizures. In this group of patients, anticonvulsants are ineffective until the metabolic derangement has been corrected.

Hypercalcaemia
This is the most common metabolic emergency in oncology and is discussed in detail in the chapter on metabolic problems (Chapter 6.2). Neurological symptoms consist initially of muscle weakness, fatigue and lethargy. These may progress to mental state changes, including psychotic behaviour, and seizures. Treatment consists of rehydration, effective anti-tumour therapy and bisphosphonate therapy with either clodronate or pamidronate. The mental state changes and seizures respond to correction of the hypercalcaemia.

Hyponatraemia
Hyponatraemia occurs in patients with the syndrome of inappropriate antidiuretic hormone secretion (SIADH), usually in association with small cell lung cancer. SIADH also occurs with pulmonary or cerebral metastases. Mild hyponatraemia is usually asymptomatic, but when the sodium concentration falls rapidly, patients develop mental state changes, seizures and psychosis. Treatment depends on the underlying cause, e.g. chemotherapy for small cell lung cancer, fluid restriction to between 500 mL and 1000 mL daily and, if this is ineffective, demeclocycline, which antagonizes the action of ADH in the distal convoluted tubules and collecting ducts. Patients in a coma or fitting because of hyponatraemia should receive 3 per cent hypertonic saline or isotonic saline with intravenous frusemide at a dose of 1 mg/kg.

EXAMINATION AND INVESTIGATIONS

As in all aspects of clinical care, a thorough history and examination will lead to the correct diagnosis in over 90 per cent of cases. It may be said that the most useful investigation in a patient with a possible seizure is a detailed history of the event from an observer. This is critical for both the diagnosis and classification of the seizure. In cases of doubt, the physician should avoid treatment and keep an open mind until further events occur. In particular, care must be taken to distinguish a seizure from a faint or a rigor. Key points in the history include the presence or absence of a warning, what the patient was doing at the time of the attack, the early manifestations of the seizure, what actually happened during the seizure, and the rapidity of recovery. Patients who have structural brain lesions causing seizures will often describe a focal onset or a postictal focal deficit (Todd's paresis). There may be an interictal deficit or symptoms and signs of raised intracranial pressure.

The main investigation for the diagnosis of a brain tumour is computerized tomography (CT) or magnetic resonance imaging (MRI) scanning with contrast. This will reveal a space-occupying lesion, which may or may not be exerting mass effect. In general, malignant brain tumours are surrounded by vasogenic white matter oedema and are associated with contrast enhancement due to breakdown of the blood–brain barrier. Low-grade intrinsic tumours rarely enhance and do not usually cause vasogenic oedema, although they may be associated with considerable mass effect.

TREATMENT

A person who has had a single seizure does not necessarily have to be started on anticonvulsant medication. The decision about whether or not to start treatment should be based on an analysis of the chances and consequences of another seizure for that person and an analysis of how the risks and benefits of treatment compare to remaining free of medication.

The treatment of tumour-associated epilepsy can be divided into treatment of the underlying tumour and treatment of the seizures.

TREATMENT OF THE UNDERLYING TUMOUR

The three conventional modalities of tumour treatment – surgery, radiotherapy and chemotherapy – all have some use in brain tumours, although only surgery is likely to be curative and then only for very low-grade tumours, e.g. juvenile pilocytic astrocytoma. Radiotherapy is the only treatment to have proven prognostic benefit for malignant gliomas, but even then the median survival still remains less than 1 year. Chemotherapy has some role, in the adjuvant setting, and may be particularly useful in the treatment of oligodendroglioma[5] and primary central nervous system lymphomas, especially in older patients for whom the risk of radiation-induced dementia is high.[6]

The treatment of low-grade gliomas, which frequently present with epilepsy as their only manifestation, is controversial.[7] The role of surgery on prognostic grounds alone has not been clearly established as there have been no prospective randomized clinical trials and so they can only be recommended if the tumour is causing symptoms of raised intracranial pressure or an evolving focal deficit. The majority of low-grade gliomas do eventually transform into higher-grade tumours and these need to be treated on their own merits. Radiotherapy has been shown to prolong progression-free survival but not overall survival.[8]

TREATMENT OF SEIZURES

The treatment of tumour-associated epilepsy does not differ from that of any other type of epilepsy (Tables 5.3.2 and 5.3.3). There are some basic principles that should be adhered to when considering the anticonvulsant of choice.

- The anticonvulsant selected should be the one most effective for that seizure type, should have the fewest side-effects and should be the least expensive.

- The dosage should be the lowest that controls seizures.

- Monotherapy is preferable to polytherapy.

Table 5.3.2 Principles of seizure treatment

Single seizure	Diazepam suppository if more than 5 minutes
Recurrent seizures	*First line* Phenytoin, carbamazepine, sodium valproate, lamotrigine *Second line* Gabapentin, topiramate, tiagabine, levetiracetam
Clusters of seizures	Clobazam
Status epilepticus	*First line* Lorazepam (i.v.) or diazepam (i.v. or p.r.) Phenytoin (i.v. loading dose) *Second line* Phenobarbital Paraldehyde *Third line* Propofol (i.v.) Midazolam (i.v.) Pentobarbital (pentobarbitone) (i.v.) Thiopental (thiopentone) (i.v.)
The dying patient	Midazolam (s.c.) Clonazepam (s.c.) Phenobarbital (phenobarbitone) (s.c.) Diazepam (p.r.)

i.v., intravenous; p.r., per rectum; s.c., subcutaneous.

There are four anticonvulsants – phenytoin, carbamazepine, sodium valproate and lamotrigine – that are generally regarded as first-line therapy. A number of newer anti-epileptic drugs, e.g., gabapentin, topiramate, tiagabine and levetiracetam, have become available for the adjunctive treatment of partial seizures, but they are all considerably more expensive than the older drugs. The efficacy of these drugs is uncertain and it is not yet known whether they cause less sedation and have fewer adverse systemic effects than the standard first-line drugs. The reader is referred to two excellent reviews for more detailed discussions of anti-epileptic drugs.[9,10]

The choice of first-line drug is influenced by many different factors. Carbamazepine, lamotrigine and phenytoin are equally effective in reducing the frequency of seizures, although carbamazepine and lamotrigine are preferred, particularly for young women. Both can be prescribed in a twice-daily formulation to aid compliance and smooth out plasma levels. Phenytoin has the advantage of once-daily dosing but has difficult (saturation) pharmacokinetics and multiple side effects. In addition there may be a significant drug interaction with dexamethasone (see below). Sodium valproate is said to be better for primary generalized epilepsy but this is rarely a consideration in patients with brain tumours. Furthermore, because of the greater risk of cognitive defects and teratogenicity, valproate is to be avoided in women of childbearing age.

In general, patients should be maintained on one drug if possible and on the lowest dose compatible with seizure control. An adequate trial consists of a systematic

Table 5.3.3 Dosages of commonly used anticonvulsants

Drug	Adult dosage	Frequency	Optimal plasma levels
Carbamazepine	400–2000 mg/day	t.d.s. or b.d. (Retard)	4–10 g/mL
Clobazam	10–60 mg/day	b.d. or t.d.s.	
Clonazepam	0.5–2 mg /day	o.d.	
	2–10 mg/day	cont. s.c. infusion	
Diazepam	10–30 mg (p.r.)	p.r.n. (max. 30 mg)	
Gabapentin	900–4800 mg/day	t.d.s.	
Lamotrigine	100–800 mg/day	b.d.	
Levetiracetam	500–3000 mg/day	b.d.	
Midazolam	10–20 mg (status)		
	0.75–10 μ/kg per min	Cont. i.v. or s.c. infusion	
Phenobarbital	60–200 mg/day	o.d./b.d.	15–35 μg/mL
(phenobarbitone)	600–2400 mg/day	s.c. infusion	
	15–20 mg/kg (status)	Loading dose	
Phenytoin	200–600 mg/day	o.d.	10–20 μg/mL
	15–20 mg/kg (status)	Loading dose	
Propofol	2–10 mg/kg per h (status)	Cont. i.v. infusion	
Tiagabine	15–60 mg/day	b.d.	
Topiramate	100–800 mg/day	t.d.s.	
Valproate (sodium)	400–3000 mg/day	t.d.s. or b.d. (Chrono)	No value

t.d.s., three times a day; b.d., twice a day; o.d., once daily; s.c., subcutaneous; p.r.n., as required; i.v., intravenous.

increase in the dosage and plasma drug levels until the seizures are controlled or intolerable side effects supervene. If the seizures remain uncontrolled, or the drug is poorly tolerated, it is likely that an inappropriate drug was chosen or the medication was introduced too rapidly. About 20 per cent of patients with epilepsy have seizures that are refractory to treatment with a single anti-epileptic drug, although this figure may be higher for patients with brain tumours. However, only about 10 per cent of patients will gain complete seizure control by the addition of other drugs.

Before long-term treatment with two or more drugs is undertaken, all reasonable options for monotherapy should be exhausted. A second drug should then be introduced gradually and if there is an apparent response, attempts should be made to withdraw the original drug slowly. There are no controlled trials that have identified the best second drug or combination of drugs. The likelihood of limiting side effects increases with the number of drugs prescribed, and so the patient and doctor may have to accept the persistence of some seizures if daily functioning is otherwise compromised. In this respect, it is important to achieve a balance between the adequacy of seizure control and quality of life. Gradual dosage increments and reductions are preferable to minimize side effects and/or seizure deterioration.

Drug monitoring should only be done to prove compliance, to confirm the clinical suspicion of toxicity or where there is a possibility of drug interactions or pharmocokinetic alterations. Specific instances of the latter relevant to dying patients include hypoalbuminaemia or uraemia. In all cases, it is more important to treat the patient than the drug level.[11] Phenytoin has saturation kinetics and therefore needs to be monitored more closely than the other anticonvulsants.

Occasionally, patients with brain tumours have clusters of seizures that do not amount to status epilepticus but that need urgent treatment. This may occur during radiotherapy or due to chemotherapy-induced vomiting. In these circumstances, where a short-term treatment is indicated, clobazam should be used at a starting dose of 10–20 mg nocte increasing up to 60 mg daily. However, tolerance develops within 3–4 weeks and so the drug is rarely useful as a long-term treatment.

DRUG INTERACTIONS

All the older anti-epileptic drugs interact with each other, with phenytoin and carbamazepine inducing and sodium valproate inhibiting liver enzymes. Thus phenytoin and carbamazepine reduce all other drug levels, whereas valproate increases levels. Clinically important interactions occur with a number of other drugs. Of particular importance is the interaction with dexamethasone, a corticosteroid frequently used in the treatment of patients with brain tumours. Phenytoin, phenobarbital (phenobarbitone) and perhaps carbamazepine increase the metabolic clearance of steroids and thereby reduce their therapeutic effect. In one study, the bioavailability of oral dexamethasone in patients taking phenytoin was only 33 per cent, compared to 84 per cent in patients not receiving phenytoin.[12] This may cause patients with raised intracranial pressure to become more symptomatic when they are started on phenytoin, and to require larger doses if already on phenytoin. Conversely, concurrent dexamethasone therapy may increase serum phenytoin levels.[13] In one case, a patient receiving dexamethasone required a daily dose of phenytoin greater than 10 mg/kg to maintain drug levels within the therapeutic range. When the steroid was discontinued, the concentration of phenytoin increased by nearly 300 per cent,[14] suggesting that caution is required when weaning patients off dexamethasone when they are also taking phenytoin.

Other drugs used in the treatment of brain tumours that may interact with anticonvulsants include BCNU and carboplatin, both of which reduce phenytoin levels and are cleared more rapidly in patients taking phenytoin. However these interactions are rarely of clinical significance. Finally, it should be borne in mind that certain drugs used in palliative care, e.g. tricyclics, phenothiazines and anticholinergics, may lower seizure threshold, but the effect is unpredictable and should not lead to prophylactic prescription of anticonvulsants.

TREATMENT IN THE DYING PATIENT

Seizures in the dying patient require urgent control. The considerations for the slow introduction of first-line anticonvulsants no longer apply. Intravenous phenytoin may be given as a loading dose (15–20 mg/kg) and works rapidly. In the palliative care setting it is preferable to administer rectal diazepam (10–30 mg) or subcutaneous/buccal midazolam (10–20 mg) as an emergency treatment.[15] Maintenance treatment can then be set up using a subcutaneous infusion of either midazolam (30–60 mg/day)[16] or clonazepam (2–10 mg/day). Occasionally, a twice-daily diazepam (20 mg) suppository may be preferable. Phenobarbital (phenobarbitone) is also useful in this setting, particularly in agitated patients,[17] and has the advantage that it can be given as a subcutaneous infusion (0.6–2.4 g/day).

KEY POINTS

- Epileptic seizures in patients with malignant disease are usually due to structural brain lesions or metabolic derangements.
- Seizures should be treated with effective first-line anticonvulsants and the underlying cause established.
- Monotherapy, a slow introduction and the use of slow-release formulations will minimize side effects and enhance patient compliance.
- Subcutaneous midazolam or phenobarbital infusions are useful in controlling seizures in the dying patient.

REFERENCES

1. McKeran RO, Thomas DGT. The clinical study of gliomas. In: Thomas DGT, Graham DI (eds), *Brain tumours: scientific basis, clinical investigations and current therapy.* London: Butterworths, 1980, 194–230.

2. Vertosick FT, Selker RG, Arena VC. Survival of patients with well-differentiated astrocytomas in the era of computed tomography. *Neurosurgery* 1991; **28**, 496–501.
3. Lote K, Stenwig AE, Skullerud K, Hirschberg H. Prevalence and prognostic significance of epilepsy in patients with gliomas. *Eur J Cancer* 1998; **34**, 98–102.
4. Delattre JY, Krol G, Thaler HT, Posner JB. Distribution of brain metastases. *Arch Neurol* 1988; **45**, 741–4.
5. Mason WP, Krol GS, DeAngelis LM. Low-grade oligodendroglioma responds to chemotherapy. *Neurology* 1996; **46**, 203–7.
6. Freilich RJ, Delattre JY, Monjour A, DeAngelis LM. Chemotherapy without radiation therapy as initial treatment for primary CNS lymphoma in older patients. *Neurology* 1996; **46**, 435–9.
7. Shaw EG. Low-grade gliomas: to treat or not to treat. A radiation oncologist's viewpoint. *Neurology* 1990; **47**, 1138–9.
8. Karim ABMF, Afra D, Conu P *et al.* Randomized trial on the efficacy of radiotherapy for cerebral low grade glioma in the adult: European Organization for Research and Treatment of Cancer Study 22845 with the Medical Research Council: an interim analysis. *Int J Radiat Oncol Biol Phys* 2002; **52**, 316–24.
9. Marson AG, Kadir ZA, Chadwick DW. New antiepileptic drugs: a systematic review of their efficacy and tolerability. *BMJ* 1996; **313**, 1169–74.
10. Brodie MJ, Dichter MA. Antiepileptic drugs. *N Engl J Med* 1996; **334**, 167–75.
11. Dodson WE. Level off. *Neurology* 1989; **39**, 1009–10.
12. Chalk JB, Ridgeway K, Brophy T, Yelland JD, Eadie MJ. Phenytoin impairs the bioavailability of dexamethasone in neurological and neurosurgical patients. *J Neurol Neurosurg Psychiatry* 1984; **47**, 1087–90.
13. Lawson LA, Blouin RA, Smith RB, Rapp RP, Young AB. Phenytoin–dexamethasone interaction: a previously unreported observation. *Surg Neurol* 1981; **16**, 23–4.
14. Lackner TE. Interaction of dexamethasone with phenytoin. *Pharmacotherapy* 1991; **11**, 344–7.
15. McNamara P, Minton M, Twycross RG. Use of midazolam in palliative care. *Palliat Med* 1991; **5**, 244–9.
16. Bottomley DM, Hanks GW. Subcutaneous midazolam infusion in palliative care. *J Pain Symptom Manage* 1990; **5**, 259–61.
17. Stirling LC, Kurowska A, Tookman A. The use of phenobarbitone in the management of agitation and seizures at the end of life. *J Pain Symptom Manage* 1999; **17**, 363–8.

SUPERIOR VENA CAVA OBSTRUCTION AND SPINAL CORD COMPRESSION

Sarah Harris, Emma Brown, Allan Irvine and John O'Dowd

SUPERIOR VENA CAVA OBSTRUCTION

INTRODUCTION

Obstruction of the superior vena cava (SVCO) results in a distressing collection of symptoms and signs caused by the impairment of blood flow returning from the head, neck, thorax and arms to the right atrium.

AETIOLOGY

Two cases of SVCO were described by William Hunter in 1757 which were caused by tuberculosis and syphilitic aneurysms. Intrathoracic malignancy – either primary or secondary – now accounts for approximately 95 per cent of cases. The commonest malignant cause is small-cell carcinoma of the bronchus, followed by squamous cell and adenocarcinoma of the lung and non-Hodgkin's lymphoma.[1] SVCO occurs in 3–10 per cent of patients with bronchogenic carcinoma and lymphoma. Rarer malignant causes include metastatic breast and colon cancers, germ-cell tumours, Kaposi's sarcoma, Hodgkin's disease and oesophageal cancer.[2] Thrombosis associated with intracaval catheters (e.g. Hickman lines) used for the administration of cytotoxic chemotherapy may also result in SVCO. Benign causes now account for less than 1 per cent of cases and include granulomatous and idiopathic sclerosing mediastinitis and retrosternal goitre.

PATHOPHYSIOLOGY

The superior vena cava is a thin-walled structure, formed by the union of the two brachiocephalic veins, and is easily compressed as it passes through the right side of the mediastinum to drain into the right atrium. Obstruction to blood flow in the SVC is caused by extrinsic compression, often by a primary tumour mass or mediastinal lymphadenopathy, by intravascular thrombosis, or occasionally by direct infiltration. Thrombus formation may be secondary to extrinsic compression of the SVC and be exacerbated by the hypercoaguability associated with advanced malignancy.

The upper body venous return is re-routed to the heart via the inferior vena cava (IVC) through four main pathways. The major pathway is by the azygos and hemi-azygous venous systems with the connecting lumbar veins. Other collateral circulations include the internal mammary venous system with tributaries to the superior and inferior epigastric veins, the long thoracic system with its connection to the femoral vein via the saphenous system and the vertebral veins and tributaries. The development of these venous collaterals reduces the symptoms of upper body venous engorgement but is a gradual process; tumours that rapidly obstruct the SVC cause severe symptoms initially.

CLINICAL FEATURES

Obstruction of the SVC presents as swelling of the face and upper torso, with dilatation of the veins across the chest, upper arms and neck. Dyspnoea is present in 50–80 per cent of cases. Accompanying symptoms, including cough, hoarseness, chest pain, dysphagia and haemoptysis, may relate to the original underlying pathology. In severe cases, the obstruction may result in headache, dizziness and syncopal episodes, particularly on bending, probably due to decreased venous return to the heart.

INVESTIGATIONS

Radiological investigations are used to support the diagnosis of SVCO and to help identify the underlying cause. A chest X-ray may show widening of the upper mediastinum in 60 per cent of patients relating to a soft tissue mass around the SVC, a primary bronchial carcinoma or metastatic disease, including pleural effusion or lung nodules. However, the chest X-ray may be completely normal.

For patients presenting with SVCO of unknown cause, a tissue diagnosis may be obtained from a sputum sample assessed cytologically, a needle biopsy taken from any clinically or radiologically involved disease site, or by cytology or histology samples taken at bronchoscopy. The theoretical increase in the risk of haemorrhage and anaesthesia in patients with SVCO undergoing biopsy or surgery is not substantiated in clinical practice.

Computed tomography (CT) scanning of the thorax is the investigation of choice for the diagnosis of SVCO, demonstration of the site(s) and extent of compression and mediastinal disease. Venous patency and the presence of thrombi are assessed by using contrast and rapid scanning techniques (Figs 5.4.1 and 5.4.2).[3]

The extent of the SVC obstruction is assessed by bilateral upper limb venography. Bilateral and simultaneous injection of iodinated contrast material is made into both antecubital veins, with digital subtraction imaging providing the best detail

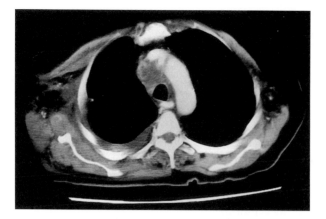

Figure 5.4.1 Axial computerized tomography showing a mass lying antero-laterally to the trachea causing superior vena cava obstruction.

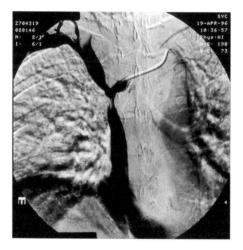

Figure 5.4.2 Venogram demonstrating superior vena cava obstruction.

of the location and extent of any obstruction. This method often overestimates the level of obstruction due to shunting into collateral vessels, and a more accurate assessment may require the introduction of a catheter through the antecubital veins into the subclavian vein, or actually through the obstruction via a femoral approach.

MANAGEMENT

Traditionally, SVCO was classified as a medical emergency that required prompt intervention, usually radiotherapy, to reduce its long-term consequences. However, SVCO itself is not commonly life threatening and as insertion of a stent by an interventional radiologist can provide rapid symptom relief, it is now more appropriate to establish the diagnosis first, to provide the information required to give an ever-increasing number and range of systemic treatments directed at the varied underlying pathologies.

Radiotherapy alone remains the correct treatment for some patients with poor performance status and significant co-morbidity who may not tolerate aggressive therapy. Approximately 3 per cent of patients presenting with SVCO will have a benign pathology.

Principles of treatment
The treatment of SVCO depends on:

- the aetiology of the obstruction,
- the severity of the symptoms,
- the patient's prognosis,
- the patient's own wishes.

It has two main objectives: palliation of distressing symptoms and treatment of the underlying cause.

Symptom control
Short-term palliation of symptoms may be achieved by:

- bed rest with head elevation, reducing venous pressure,
- oxygen and opioids to dampen the respiratory drive.

Corticosteroids (e.g. dexamethasone 4 mg q.d.s.) are usually administered to reduce tissue oedema around the SVC and optimize venous flow, although there have been no definitive studies to prove their efficacy. The role of diuretics and anticoagulants has not been proven.[4]

Stent placement
In patients in whom simple medical measures do not produce adequate symptomatic relief, insertion of a metallic stent may be undertaken by an interventional radiologist. Since the first publication on this subject in 1992, numerous case reports and papers have been published. Complete or partial relief of symptoms following stent placement is achieved in more than 90 per cent of cases.[5] As yet, no comparative series of stent placement versus chemotherapy or radiotherapy has been published. Venous access is usually from the femoral vein, allowing a pre-shaped catheter to be advanced up to the level of the occlusion or narrowing in the SVC under X-ray control and a guide wire to be manipulated through the abnormal area. The most commonly used stent nowadays is the Wall stent – a flexible stainless steel mesh that is self-expanding and pre-mounted. The pre-mounted stent is advanced over the guide wire and deployed under X-ray control (Fig. 5.4.3). Balloon angioplasty of the stent is used to ensure maximum opening of the stent, and the patient is maintained on heparin for 48 hours post-insertion to reduce the incidence of stent thrombosis. Lytic therapy via a catheter placed at the obstruction

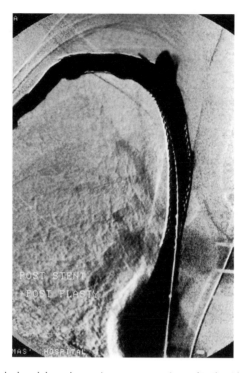

Figure 5.4.3 Wall stent deployed through superior vena cava stricture (SVC), with satisfactory opening of the narrowed SVC segment.

has been used to remove thrombus present prior to stent deployment. However, there is a risk of haemorrhagic complications, most seriously in the brain, and consideration should be given to exclude cerebral metastases by CT or magnetic resonance imaging (MRI) scan prior to lytic therapy. The role of long-term anti-coagulation after stent insertion is controversial.

Stent insertion is a straightforward procedure that is well tolerated by the patient, producing rapid symptomatic relief. Complication rates are low, with misplace-ment (10 per cent), stent migration (5 per cent) and cardiac arrhythmias being the most commonly reported.[4] As stent insertion becomes more accessible and less costly, it should perhaps be considered for symptomatic relief in all patients who have distressing symptoms from SVCO caused by an underlying malignancy.

Surgical bypass of an obstructed SVC is an uncommon procedure and more appropriate for patients with benign disease.

Treatment of the underlying malignancy

Treatment of the underlying malignancy depends on histological type and disease staging. Although previously patients presenting with SVCO were considered to have a poor prognosis and a mean survival of 3 months, with modern therapy, SVCO per se should not alter treatment intentions. SVCO has not been shown to be an independent poor prognostic indicator in small cell lung cancer (SCLC).[6,7]

Chemotherapy is the initial treatment of choice for chemosensitive tumours such as SCLC, lymphoma and, rarely, germ-cell tumours. Combination drug regimens have been shown to prolong survival and improve quality of life in SCLC. For patients with SVCO due to SCLC, combination chemotherapy produces complete or partial resolution of symptoms in 80 per cent.[8] Radiotherapy in addition to chemotherapy may reduce the local recurrence rate.

Radiotherapy was considered as the main treatment for SVCO, particularly for non-small cell lung cancer, occasionally with radical intent. Radiotherapy in combination with corticosteroids provides good symptom control, often within 72 hours, with 70–95 per cent of patients being symptom free by 2 weeks.[8] A range of doses and fractionations is used in the UK – from 8 Gy in one fraction to 30 Gy in ten fractions and, rarely, more radical treatment regimens. Side effects from radiotherapy are usually mild and include radiation oesophagitis and nausea.

SPINAL CORD COMPRESSION

INTRODUCTION

Metastatic spinal cord compression (MSCC) is found in approximately 7 per cent of patients with malignant disease. Defined as compression of the dural sac and its contents by an extradural mass, it is a major cause of morbidity, potentially rendering independent patients immobile with functional compromise of bowel and bladder sphincters such that they require long-term nursing care. The diagnosis is made on the basis of symptoms, clinical signs and radiological imaging. MSCC is treated as an emergency, using corticosteroids, surgery and radiotherapy to limit long-term neurological damage.

AETIOLOGY

Any metastatic malignancy, or occasionally a primary tumour, may result in spinal cord compression. Nearly two-thirds of patients with MSCC have breast, prostate or lung primary cancers. Less commonly, MSCC results from myeloma or metastatic renal cell, thyroid and bladder carcinomas, sarcoma or melanoma. It is rarely the patient's first presentation with malignant disease.

The compression may occur at any level in the spinal canal, with 60 per cent of lesions being in the thoracic, 10 per cent in the cervical and the remaining 30 per cent in the lumbosacral spine. The underlying pathological process is of mechanical compression of the spinal cord, or cauda equina, by an extradural mass in 75 per cent of patients, or structural bony collapse in the remainder. Rarely, intramedullary or meningeal disease also results in compression of the cord within the spinal canal. Continuing pressure on the cord increases the likelihood of permanent damage. At the time of treatment, approximately 80 per cent of patients who are ambulant (walking independently), 50 per cent of patients with paraparesis (not walking but some neurological function) and less than 10 per cent of paraplegic (paralysed) patients retain or regain enough function to walk.[9] For this reason, MSCC should be treated as a medical emergency and treatment started within 24 hours of presentation.

CLINICAL FEATURES

The clinical findings are variable and may not be pure in nature. The expected features include:

- lower motor neurone signs at the level of compression;

- upper motor neurone signs below the level of compression;

- a sensory level, present in 50 per cent of patients only, two to three segments below the compression;

- bowel and bladder sphincter compromise resulting in incontinence or retention.

A recent study correlating MRI results with the clinical level of compression showed that 25 per cent of patients had a sensory level more than four segments below or three segments above the radiologically demonstrated lesion.[10]

INVESTIGATIONS

The current investigation of choice is the MRI scan which, by imaging the whole spine, demonstrates the sites of disease (multiple in 20 per cent of patients) and the nature of the compression and excludes alternative diagnoses requiring different management (see Figs 5.4.4 and 5.4.5). In a series by Cook, 33 per cent of patients who underwent MRI scan with a clinical diagnosis of spinal cord compression had unrelated pathology, including spinal infarct, demyelination, radiation myelitis and brain metastases.[10]

For emergency 'out of hours' treatment, in the absence of MRI, X-ray findings combined with clinical signs may be used to initiate radiotherapy, but should be interpreted with caution, as epidural masses are not well visualized on X-ray, co-existing sites of compression may be missed and clinical findings may be misleading. Myelography and CT myelography have been superseded by MRI, which

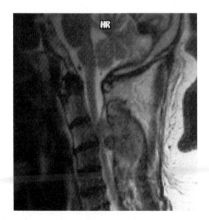

Figure 5.4.4 MRI demonstrating spinal cord compression with malignant mass at C2.

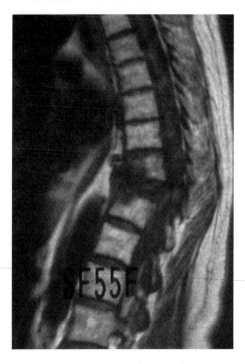

Figure 5.4.5 MRI demonstrating malignant infiltration of the spinal cord from bone metastasis.

is a more complete and less invasive form of spinal imaging and does not risk causing neurological deterioration.

X-ray-guided biopsy may be used to establish a tissue diagnosis for patients in whom the underlying diagnosis is unknown.

TREATMENT

The overwhelming concept of MSCC management is that paraplegia is a devastating consequence that shortens life expectancy: median survival 59 days for non-ambulant and 330 days for ambulant patients at the end of treatment.[9] Reducing the time between presentation and treatment is vital. Husband *et al.* have shown that of 300 patients with MSCC referred to their centre, only one-third were ambulant and one-half were catheter free at the time of their diagnosis – disappointingly similar figures to those for a series of patients managed between 1968 and 1982.[11]

Active treatment is aimed at rapidly reducing the cord compression by corticosteroids with surgery, radiotherapy or a combination of surgery followed by radiotherapy. There is a remarkable lack of evidence-based recommendations.[12]

Corticosteroids

For patients with suspected MSCC, the initial treatment is with corticosteroids – most commonly given in the UK as dexamethasone 16 mg in daily divided doses, possibly preceded by an intravenous bolus of 10 mg.

Decompressive and stabilization surgery

The main aims of treatment of MSCC are to control pain and disease and to treat salvageable neurological compression medically or surgically. The currently accepted indications for surgical intervention are for patients in whom there is:

- an unknown pathological diagnosis,

- a single site of compression,

- good performance status,

- a deterioration during radiotherapy or previous radiotherapy,

- mechanical disruption of the vertebral column causing spinal instability or bone extrusion into the spinal canal.

The majority of patients with vertebral skeletal metastatic disease are treated non-operatively. The decision to proceed with surgery must be made in conjunction with the treating oncologist, the multi-disciplinary team and the patient and his or her family.

Surgical complications are common, and most surgeons would consider surgery inappropriate if the estimated life expectancy was less than 3 months. In patients with very limited life expectancy, a better quality of life may be achieved with conservative management. The median life expectancy after surgery may be as little as 12 weeks in patients with MSCC from a primary lung cancer, but as long as 1 year in patients with breast or prostate cancers. Seventy-five per cent of patients who are ambulant at presentation will remain so, but only 50 per cent of paraparetics and less than 30 per cent of paraplegics will walk again after surgery.

In patients being considered for surgery, rapid neurological deterioration to paraplegia in less than 24 hours implies neurological injury secondary to thrombosis of the spinal arterial supply and a very small chance of improvement from surgical decompression. Conversely, decompression of the cord secondary to vertebral collapse or epidural tumour extension is likely to produce a good outcome. Contiguous multiple involved vertebral levels make spinal fixation technically difficult or impossible, whereas skip or non-contiguous lesions may allow surgery at two or, rarely, three non-adjacent levels.

Decompression of the spinal cord and stabilization of the spinal column has evolved from a posterior approach, first used in 1751, through an anterior technique in the 1980s and, latterly, the use of a pedicle screw implant system. Although laminectomy is the simplest procedure, the simultaneous reconstruction of the anterior column of the spine, via an anterior approach, prevents subsequent vertebral body collapse and neurological deterioration, but requires a thoracotomy or thoraco-abdominal procedure.[13,14] Many patients are unfit for major surgery but may benefit from the development of thoracoscopic spinal surgery in the future. The pedicle screw system allows satisfactory control of the anterior and posterior spinal columns by a posterior approach alone, but is technically demanding.[15] A staged surgical approach may be suitable for fit patients.

Postoperative radiotherapy and appropriate chemotherapy are given to prevent tumour re-growth, as the surgical clearance of tumour is usually incomplete in the spine.

Surgery may also be used for axial pain resistant to radiotherapy, chemotherapy and analgesia.

Radiotherapy

Radiotherapy fields are applied to areas of cord compression according to clinical and radiological findings. The dose delivered varies from 8 Gy as a single fraction to 40 Gy in 20 fractions – studies showing equivalent results.

Proceeding with emergency radiotherapy before obtaining an MRI scan risks missing the lesion wholly or partially, needing to modify radiotherapy fields during the course of treatment, or treating unrelated pathology.

Patients with epidural disease are more likely to improve with radiotherapy than those with bony collapse – 65 per cent versus 25 per cent.[9] The few patients receiving radiotherapy for asymptomatic MSCC found on radiological imaging have a better outcome than those with neurological impairment – 75 per cent remain ambulatory at the end of treatment and may not require concurrent steroids.

Further management

Following radiotherapy, the dose of steroids is gradually reduced, ideally to zero, to reduce the long-term side effects – in particular proximal myopathy, which also impairs mobility. A multi-disciplinary approach is needed, including nurses, physical and occupational therapists and social workers, to optimize mobility and increase the likelihood of the patient returning to the community.

CONCLUSIONS

Superior vena cava obstruction and MSCC are two medical emergencies whose functional outcome depends on the rapidity of starting treatment. In the past 5 years, the palliation of symptoms from SVCO has improved with the use of metallic stents. Identification of cord compression by MRI scan has facilitated the early delivery of treatment by surgery or radiotherapy.

KEY POINTS

SUPERIOR VENA CAVA OBSTRUCTION

- Rapid symptom relief from SVCO may be achieved by metallic stent insertion.
- This allows time to establish a pathological diagnosis and plan treatment.
- Radiotherapy provides symptom relief and may be combined with chemotherapy to treat the underlying tumour.

SPINAL CORD COMPRESSION

- Early diagnosis of spinal cord compression clinically and by MRI improves patient outcome.
- Treatment is with corticosteroids, decompressive or stabilization surgery and radiotherapy.
- Functional neurological outcome depends on ambulatory status at the time of treatment.

REFERENCES

1. Yellin A, Rosen A, Reichert N *et al*. Superior vena cava syndrome: the myth – the facts. *Am Rev Respir Dis* 1990; **141**(5), 1114–18.
2. Yahalom J. Superior vena cava syndrome. In: DeVita VT, Hellman S, Rosenberg SA (eds), *Principles and practice of oncology*, 4th edn. Philadelphia: JB Lippincott, 1993, 2111–18.
3. Taty WF, Winzelberg GG, Boller M. Computed tomographic evaluation of compression of the superior vena cava and its tributaries. *Cardiovasc Intervent Radiol* 1985; 8(2), 89–9.
4. Ostler PJ, Clarke DP, Watkinson AF, Gaze MN. Superior vena cava obstruction: a modern management strategy. *Clin Oncol* 1997; **9**, 83–9.
5. Thony F, Moro D, Witmeyer P *et al*. Endovascular treatment of superior vena cava obstruction in patients with malignancies. *Eur Radiol* 1999; **9**, 965–71.
6. Maddox AM, Valdivieso M, Lukeman J *et al*. Superior vena cava obstruction in small cell bronchogenic carcinoma: clinical parameters and survival. *Cancer* 1983; **52**, 2165–72.
7. Wurschmidt F, Bunemann H, Heilman HP. Small cell lung cancer with and without superior vena cava syndrome: a multi-variate analysis of prognostic factors in 408 cases. *Int J Radiat Oncol Biol Phys* 1995; **33**(1), 77–82.
8. Armstrong B, Perez C, Simpson J *et al*. Role of irradiation in the management of superior vena cava syndrome. *Int J Radiat Biol Oncol Phys* 1987; **13**, 531–9.
9. Piggott K, Baddeley H, Maher EJ. Patterns of disease in spinal cord compression on MRI scan and implications for treatment. *Clin Oncol* 1994; **6**, 7–10.
10. Cook A, Lau T, Tomlinson M *et al*. MRI of the whole spine in suspected malignant spinal cord compression: impact on management. *Clin Oncol* 1998; **10**, 39–43.
11. Husband DJ. Malignant spinal cord compression: prospective study of delays in referral and treatment. *BMJ* 1998; **317**, 18–21.
12. Loblaw D, Laperriere N. Emergency treatment of malignant extradural spinal cord: an evidence-based guideline. *J Clin Oncol* 1998; **16**, 1613–24.
13. Findlay G. Adverse effects of the management of malignant spinal cord compression. *J Neurol Neurosurg Psychiatry* 1984; **47**, 761–8.
14. Findlay G. The role of vertebral body collapse in the management of malignant spinal cord compression. *J Neurol Neurosurg Psychiatry* 1987; **50**, 151.
15. Jonsson B, Sjostrom L, Olerud C, Anderasson I, Bring J, Rauschning W. Outcome after limited posterior surgery for thoracic and lumbar spine metastases. *Eur Spine J* 1996; **5**, 36–44.

FURTHER READING

Loblaw D, Laperriere N. Emergency treatment of malignant extradural spinal cord compression: an evidence-based guideline. *J Clin Oncol* 1998; **16**, 1613–24.

Ostler PJ, Clarke DP, Watkinson AF, Gaze MN. Superior vena cava obstruction: a modern management strategy. *Clin Oncol* 1997; **9**, 83–9.

Yahalom J. Superior vena cava syndrome. In: DeVita VT, Hellman S, Rosenberg SA (eds), *Principles and practice of oncology*, 4th edn. Philadelphia: JB Lippincott, 1993, 2111–18.

DIABETES

Stephanie A. Amiel

INTRODUCTION

Diabetes mellitus is a group of diseases, characterized by hyperglycaemia and other metabolic and haematological disorders secondary to insufficient insulin action. 'Diabetes' encompasses conditions of total insulin deficiency (such as Type 1 diabetes mellitus, the result of beta-cell destruction) and conditions of insulin resistance, associated with insufficient insulin secretory reserve to combat it (as seen in many cases of Type 2 diabetes mellitus). The consequences of insulin deficiency include hyperglycaemia, lipolysis, ketogenesis and proteolysis. Chronic hyperglycaemia and insulin deficiency over years cause damage to small blood vessels, leading to retinopathy, nephropathy and neuropathy and accelerating large vessel atheroma, causing premature ischaemic heart disease, peripheral and cerebral arterial disease. Normally diabetes care is directed towards prevention – of acute symptoms from chronic hyperglycaemia or from side effects of its treatment, of long-term complications of diabetes by active management of hyperglycaemia and other vascular risk factors, and of disability, by active management of complications.

The prevention of symptomatic hyperglycaemia remains crucial in the management of the patient with diabetes who is terminally ill. Active management of symptomatic established complications is also important to ensure patient comfort and minimize distress for relatives and carers. It should be expected that diabetes control may be lost in patients who are terminally ill, because of the neuroendocrine responses to stress, which are hyperglycaemic; immobilization, which reduces peripheral tissue glucose consumption; drug effects, which may cause insulin resistance (classically steroid therapy); and the stress response to intercurrent infections. On the other hand, reduced appetite and anorexia may enhance the hypoglycaemic effects of any pharmacological therapy used for diabetes.

CONTROL OF BLOOD GLUCOSE

The healthy pancreas produces insulin constantly (background or basal) to control endogenous glucose production, lipolysis and proteolysis. At meals, prandial bursts of insulin create high but transient peaks of hyperinsulinaemia to switch off endogenous glucose production and stimulate glucose uptake and storage.

When insulin secretion and action are normal, blood glucose is maintained between very narrow levels despite wide fluctuations in glucose supply (e.g. in feeding) and utilization (e.g. by exercising muscle or other active tissue). While too high a blood glucose causes symptoms (see below), too low a blood glucose leads to failure of cerebral function, confusion and coma. The precise regulation of the blood glucose concentration is critical to survival. In opposition to insulin are ranged the hyperglycaemic hormones, specifically glucagon, adrenaline and noradrenaline, growth hormone and cortisol and also the sympathetic nervous system. When these counter-regulatory processes are activated by other systems and the patient is unable to secrete additional insulin in response, hyperglycaemia (loss of diabetic control) will result. Thus a sick patient or even a severely emotionally distressed patient is likely to be an insulin-resistant patient and, if dependent on medication to sustain his or her insulin levels, is likely to become symptomatically hyperglycaemic.

SYMPTOMS OF UNCONTROLLED DIABETES

Hyperglycaemia results in glycosuria, as the renal threshold for reabsorbing glucose from the urine (around 10 mmol/L) is exceeded. Glycosuria causes an osmotic diuresis resulting in polyuria. The heavy glucose content of the urine also makes it very prone to infection, both bacterial and candidal.

The polyuria leads to dehydration, creating thirst and excessive drinking (polydipsia). In severe insulin deficiency, as in Type 1 diabetes, or in the presence of very high levels of insulin antagonist hormones, there is insufficient insulin action to prevent lipolysis. Fat breakdown and raised circulating levels of non-esterified fatty acids result in ketogenesis; ketosis results in nausea and vomiting. In addition to the above, the acidosis causes hyperventilation – initially rapid, then the slow, sighing breathing of Kussmaul's respiration, as part of the symptoms of diabetic ketoacidosis. Untreated, this leads to confusion, coma and eventually death. Withdrawal of insulin from a Type 1 insulin-dependent diabetic patient will result in the patient's death; withdrawal of insulin from a non-insulin-dependent but insulin-treated patient is likely to worsen hyperglycaemic symptom control in the terminal phase.

The weight loss of uncontrolled diabetes is partly water loss, but later loss of fat and even muscle. In the terminally ill patient, who is already catabolic, this can increase muscle wasting and make preservation of skin surfaces more difficult.

However, intensified diabetes therapy, intended to maintain chronic near-normoglycaemia, is difficult and significantly increases the risk of severe hypoglycaemia. It is probably inappropriate for a patient with a short life expectancy.

MANAGEMENT OF CHRONIC COMPLICATIONS

RETINOPATHY

Laser therapy to the retinae can be sight saving for patients with pre-proliferative or proliferative retinopathy or macular oedema but cannot restore vision that has been lost already. Thus, in any except those with very short life expectancy, maintenance of the regular inspection of the optic retinae remains an important part of care.

DIABETIC NEPHROPATHY

In a patient with other advanced disease and a life expectancy of less than 5 years, prevention of nephropathy is unlikely to be important. However, nephrosis with marked oedema may require symptomatic management. Apart from improving glycaemic control, strict control of blood pressure is the only known retardant of urinary protein loss in this setting.

DIABETIC NEUROPATHIES

Peripheral neuropathy

Classical diabetic neuropathy is a symmetrical, peripheral, sensory and motor neuropathy resulting in an insensitive foot, with clawed toes and undue prominence of the metatarsal heads. Because of associated autonomic neuropathy, the skin is dry, its microcirculation is poor and it is prone to ulceration and infection. If there is also ischaemia due to macrovascular disease, infection can be difficult to treat and can lead to the need for amputation.

It is important to inspect the feet of diabetic patients with advanced disease regularly, and the heels are at very high risk in the bed-bound patient. The risk of heel ulceration is probably much greater than the risk of deep venous thrombosis. Vigilance to keep the heels out of contact with the mattress (even special mattresses) is essential. This may be aided by the use of sheepskin or placement of wedges under the Achilles tendon (and sometimes, in very immobile patients, water-filled latex gloves) or even the placement of the Achilles tendon and lower calf on a pillow.

Good routine foot care with the use of emollients to prevent cracking of otherwise dry skin is also recommended.

Autonomic neuropathy

Probably the most distressing symptoms of autonomic neuropathy are gastrointestinal, with intermittent diarrhoea and/or constipation and gastroparesis. These are managed symptomatically:

- diarrhoea: loperamide and codeine phosphate and intermittent courses of antibiotics such as tetracycline or erythromycin;

- gastroparesis (bloating or even vomiting): gastric motility agents such as domperidone and erythromycin, covered by H_2 antagonists.

Advanced diabetic neuropathy can be associated with anorexia and cachexia that may be difficult to distinguish from advancement of other disease.

SMALL AND LARGE VESSEL DISEASE

The prevention of stroke, myocardial infarction and the progression of peripheral vascular disease is a long-term aim, mostly appropriate to patients with a life expectancy of more than 5 years. However, silent myocardial ischaemic events can leave a patient in heart failure that may need active management.

MANAGEMENT OF BLOOD GLUCOSE

DIET

The appropriate management of diabetes in otherwise healthy individuals always includes the use of diet and exercise. The diabetic diet is not synonymous with a weight-reducing diet, but instead aims to provide food intakes that result in a gradual rise and fall of blood glucose levels rather than a very fast, short rise. Its principles are meals including complex carbohydrates spread evenly through the day and avoidance of the ingestion of large quantities of rapidly available carbohydrate (simple sugars) in isolation.

However, where anorexia is a major clinical problem, patients are encouraged to eat what seems tempting. This is reasonable unless it significantly compromises diabetes control to the extent that an asymptomatic patient becomes symptomatic of hyperglycaemia. Fluid food supplements that are high in simple carbohydrate are best administered slowly over hours rather than ingested as a single drink over a few minutes. It is more likely that therapy will have to be adjusted for a low carbohydrate intake, as discussed below.

DRUGS IN DIABETES

Great care needs to be exercised in the pharmacological management of diabetes in the context of other advanced disease, to achieve a balance between uncontrolled symptomatic hyperglycaemia and intermittent over-treatment and hypoglycaemia. There are very few published data on the optimal regimens to use, and the ensuing is based primarily on clinical experience.

Probably the greatest difficulty is the management of diabetes in a patient with anorexia. Patients with Type 2 diabetes that has been well controlled on diet and exercise with or without oral medication may remain normoglycaemic while not eating if they have adequate residual insulin secretory capacity. In such circumstances, monitoring the patient for symptoms and the urine for glucose to rule out excessive hyperglycaemia may be adequate.

Oral hypoglycaemic agents

Oral agents for diabetes take time to work and are inappropriately used to achieve glycaemic control over hours or days. Those agents that act primarily by increasing insulin sensitivity, such as metformin and the thiazolidinediones, carry a low risk of hypoglycaemia, as the patient is effectively still using endogenously secreted and therefore controlled insulin.

- *Metformin* (common side effects abdominal pain, flatulence and diarrhoea) may exacerbate anorexia, especially if taken on an empty stomach or re-started suddenly after a period of anorexia. It is not safe in the presence of elevated creatinine levels and impaired renal function where there is a risk of lactic acidosis.

- The *thiazolidinediones* are newer insulin-sensitizing agents that act at a cellular level. They may cause fluid retention and dilutional anaemias but appear to be well tolerated.[1] Although the manufacturers recommend 2-monthly checking of liver function with these new agents, this is unlikely to be important with currently available agents and not essential in the patient with advanced disease.[2]

- The *sulphonylureas* and the *meglitinides* act by artificial stimulation of insulin secretion. Longer-acting agents (e.g. chlorpropamide and glibenclamide) carry a significant risk of hypoglycaemia[3] and should not be used in anorexic patients. The hypoglycaemia can present as confusion rather than with autonomic symptoms.[4] Shorter-acting agents (e.g. tolbutamide and gliclazide) are also safer in patients with renal impairment. In theory, the meglitinides, designed to be taken before a meal and skipped if a meal is missed, may be of particular benefit for patients with advanced disease and of uncertain appetite, but no formal studies have been done.[5]

- *Other agents* that slow glucose absorption from the gut, such as the α-glucosidase inhibitors, are only really effective in early Type 2 diabetes, when there is a large residual insulin secretory capacity, and are unlikely to be of significant additional benefit to patients with advanced disease.

Insulin

Insulin is probably the least toxic of the artificial hypoglycaemic agents, as its only significant side effect, apart from very rare cases of allergy, is intermittent hypoglycaemia.

The only published work on insulin usage in the terminally ill advocated intermittent injections of soluble insulin when blood glucose was noted to be high on sporadic testing.[6] It should now be possible to maintain more stable glycaemic control with a mixture of insulins; overzealous attempts to minimize the number of insulin injections are rarely appropriate. Insulin injections are virtually painless – unlike the finger pricking required for capillary blood glucose monitoring.

A safe regimen in an anorexic patient with advanced disease is the use of twice-daily intermediate-acting insulins to replace basal insulin requirements, with fast-acting insulins at or just after meals when the patient eats. The intermediate insulin dose should be divided approximately equally between the morning and evening, and the latter injection should be given as late as possible to ensure adequate insulinization next morning without increasing the risk of hypoglycaemia in the night. Doses can be adjusted to achieve blood glucose levels of between 7 and 10 mmol/L before meals, and more than 5 mmol/L at 3 a.m. (this last to check for hypoglycaemia). These treatment goals minimize the risk of glycosuria, should avoid hypoglycaemia, and can be individually tailored to suit each patient. Higher levels may be acceptable in advanced disease, provided they are not associated with thirst or polyuria. The alternative use of the peakless insulin analogue insulin glargine (Lantus) probably offers the patient with advanced disease added advantage, as it usually lasts for about 24 hours and is therefore only given once a day and its peakless action profile minimizes the risk of hypoglycaemia at night. It is more expensive than conventional twice-daily intermediate-acting insulin but its advantages may outweigh this. In converting from twice-daily intermediate-acting insulin to once-daily Lantus in a well-controlled patient, it is usual to reduce the total dose by up to 20 per cent in the first instance and then adjust the dose every 2 to 3 days to achieve the fasting or pre-meal glucose targets. The use of the new fast-acting insulin analogues rather than conventional soluble insulins for meals allows administration of doses immediately after eating, with less risk of hypoglycaemia between meals (Table 6.1.1).

The use of more traditional regimens, such as twice-daily mixed insulins, depends on regular food intake for success and probably increases the risk of hypoglycaemia in anorexic patients. They may work in Type 2 patients, where the deficiencies of the regimen will be 'smoothed over' by residual pancreatic insulin secretion, but they do not provide optimal overnight glycaemic control. They are not appropriate once the patient has stopped eating meals, although they may have a role if formal nutritional supplementation is undertaken.

Glucose control for patients on supplemental liquid feeds can be difficult, but hyperglycaemia will negate the potential benefit of the supplement and lead to polyuria and dehydration. For patients requiring total enteral or parenteral nutrition, a dose of an intermediate-acting insulin given half an hour before the feed, with a much smaller dose given 12 hours later, can produce reasonable control. The addition of a small amount of soluble insulin in the first injection (sometimes conveniently given as a 30:70 pre-mixed) may be needed to obtain insulinization as soon as the liquid feed is started. Doses should be adjusted on the basis of 4-hourly glucose measurements, which can then be reduced to 6-hourly once a regimen is established.

Even with low-dose intermediate-acting insulin twice a day, the peak-trough pharmacokinetics may precipitate hypoglycaemia in anorexic patients. For these patients, the optimal regimen is a continuous subcutaneous infusion of fast-acting insulin, preferably one of the new analogues.[7] The basal rates and meal bolus

Table 6.1.1 Approximate pharmacodynamics of main classes of insulins given subcutaneously

Class	Onset of action	Peak action	Duration of action
Soluble, e.g. Human Actrapid, Humulin S	30 min	2–4 h	6–8 h
Intermediate-acting, e.g. Human Insulatard, Humulin I	2 h	4–8 h	12–18 h
Rapid-acting analogues, e.g. NovoRapid, Humalog	15 min	50 min	3–5 h

doses of the infusion are determined according to blood glucose measurements, which need to be done fairly frequently when such a regimen is initiated. The major disadvantage of pump therapy is that, should the insulin supply be interrupted, the patient has no insulin reservoir, and diabetic ketoacidosis can develop quite rapidly. In order to avoid this, it is usual for patients on pump therapy to perform approximately four blood tests a day (usually before meals and before bed). Although continuous subcutaneous insulin infusion may have its uses in the patient with advanced disease, the availability of Lantus insulin should make it less and less necessary.

MANAGEMENT OF THE DYING PHASE

NON-INSULIN-REQUIRING DIABETIC PATIENTS

As an expected part of the dying process, patients stop eating and drinking, and any oral hypoglycaemic medication can be discontinued. These patients are unlikely to require subcutaneous insulin.

INSULIN-REQUIRING DIABETIC PATIENTS

Insulin requirements in the dying phase may be unpredictable, the reduction in oral intake possibly being offset by a physiological stress response causing hyperglycaemia. For the majority of patients, the most appropriate regimen is likely to be replacement of background insulin with Lantus, twice-daily intermediate-acting or subcutaneous infusions of soluble insulin as outlined above. However, where patients' insulin requirements have become low in the pre-terminal phase (more likely in an insulin-requiring Type 2 diabetic), associated with a reduction in oral intake, intermittent injections of short-acting insulin or an insulin analogue may be safe and more appropriate. These may be administered in small doses when the blood glucose is high enough to be likely to cause distress to the patient. This necessitates blood glucose monitoring until a decision is made to withdraw all therapy if death is so imminent that diabetic ketoacidosis is unlikely to supervene or is regarded as acceptable by the carers involved.

KEY POINTS

- Good glycaemic control is required to prevent symptomatic hyperglycaemia or hypoglycaemia.
- Sulphonylureas should be avoided in anorexic patients.
- Metformin or the thiazolidenediones are the oral drugs of choice in anorexic Type 2 patients.
- Glycaemic control in advanced disease may be achieved in insulin-requiring patients with the use of basal insulin replacement by once-daily Lantus or twice-daily intermediate-acting insulin supplemented with rapid-acting analogues with meals where appetite is preserved.

REFERENCES

1. Krentz AJ, Bailey CJ, Melander A. Thiazolidinediones for Type 2 diabetes. New agents reduce insulin resistance but need long term clinical trials. *BMJ* 2000; **321**, 252–3.
2. Data sheet Rosiglitazone 2000.
3. Tessier G et al. [**other names**] Gibenclamide vs gliclazide in Type 2 diabetes of the elderly. *Diabet Med* 1994; **11**, 974–80.
4. Chan TY *et al.* Utilization of antidiabetic drugs in Hong Kong: relation to the common occurrence of antidiabetic drug induced hypoglycemia amongst acute medical admissions and the relative prevalence of NIDDM. *Int J Clin Pharmacol Ther* 1996; **34**, 43–6.
5. Landgraf R, Frank M, Bauer C, Dieken M. Prandial glucose regulation with repaglinide: its clinical and lifestyle impact in a large cohort of patients with Type 2 diabetes. *Int J Obes Relat Metab Disord* 2000; **24**(Suppl. 3), S38–44.
6. Boyd K. Diabetes mellitus in hospice patients: some guidelines. *Palliat Med* 1993; 7(2), 163–4.
7. Zinman B, Tildesley H, Chiasson JL, Tsui E, Strack T. Insulin lispro in CSII: results of a double-blind crossover study. *Diabetes* 1997; **46**(3), 440–3.

HYPERCALCAEMIA AND HYPONATRAEMIA

Andrew N. Davies

HYPERCALCAEMIA

EPIDEMIOLOGY

Hypercalcaemia is common in patients with cancer, with a reported incidence of about 10 per cent.[1] It usually occurs with advanced cancer and is particularly common in patients with multiple myeloma, breast cancer, lung cancer, and renal cancer.

AETIOLOGY

There are a variety of different causes of hypercalcaemia:

- primary hyperparathyroidism,
- malignant disease,
- other endocrine disorders, e.g. thyrotoxicosis, phaeochromocytoma,
- granulomatous disorders, e.g. sarcoidosis, tuberculosis,
- drugs, e.g. thiazide diuretics, lithium,
- diet, e.g. milk-alkali syndrome, vitamin D overdose,
- miscellaneous, e.g. renal disease, immobilization.

Primary hyperparathyroidism is the most common cause of hypercalcaemia in the general population, and is a relatively common cause in patients with cancer.[2] Malignant disease is the second most common cause of hypercalcaemia in the general population. The other causes of hypercalcaemia are relatively uncommon.

Malignant disease can cause two types of hypercalcaemia:

- humoral hypercalcaemia of malignancy,
- local osteolytic hypercalcaemia.

Humoral hypercalcaemia of malignancy

This is the most common type of malignancy-induced hypercalcaemia. It can occur in the presence or absence of bone metastases. The hypercalcaemia is usually due to the secretion into the systemic circulation of parathyroid hormone-related peptide by the tumour. This substance is structurally similar to parathyroid hormone and acts via the parathyroid hormone receptors. It causes an increase in osteoclast activity and mobilization of calcium from the bones. It also causes an increase in calcium reabsorption by the kidneys.

Humoral hypercalcaemia of malignancy may occasionally be related to the secretion into the systemic circulation of other substances by the tumour, such as 1,25-dihydroxycholecalciferol, and parathyroid hormone itself. (1,25-dihydroxycholecalciferol causes an increase in calcium absorption by the gastrointestinal tract).

Local osteolytic hypercalcaemia

Local osteolytic hypercalcaemia occurs only in the presence of bone metastases. The hypercalcaemia is usually due to secretion within the bone of cytokines by the tumour. A variety of different cytokines has been implicated in the process, including interleukin-1β, tumour necrosis factor α, tumour necrosis factor β, and interleukin-6. These substances cause an increase in osteoclast activity and mobilization of calcium from the bones.

Local osteolytic hypercalcaemia may also be related to the secretion within the bone of other substances by the tumour, such as prostaglandins and parathyroid hormone-related peptide.

In normal circumstances, osteolysis does not result in hypercalcaemia, because of the natural homeostatic mechanisms; however, in certain circumstances it does do so, e.g. renal dysfunction.

Hypercalcaemia causes a diuresis, which in turn leads to dehydration. Dehydration causes a decrease in renal blood flow, which in turn leads to a decrease in renal excretion of calcium (and an exacerbation of the hypercalcaemia).

CLINICAL FEATURES

The clinical features of hypercalcaemia include:

- general: polydipsia (thirst), polyuria, dehydration;
- gastrointestinal: anorexia, nausea, vomiting, constipation;
- neurological: fatigue, muscle weakness, decreased tendon reflexes, confusion, psychosis, seizures, coma;
- cardiovascular: bradycardia, arrhythmias. (Hypercalcaemia results in a prolonged PR interval, a shortened QT interval, and wide T waves on the electrocardiograph).

There is little correlation between the serum calcium level and the severity of the clinical features.[1]

Hypercalcaemia is associated with a poor prognosis, with median survival after the diagnosis of hypercalcaemia of about 3 months.[2]

INVESTIGATIONS

The diagnosis of hypercalcaemia is based on measurement of the 'protein-corrected' serum calcium:

$$\begin{bmatrix} \text{Protein corrected} \\ \text{calcium concentration} \end{bmatrix} = \begin{bmatrix} \text{measured total} \\ \text{serum calcium} \\ \text{concentration} \end{bmatrix} + 0.02 \times \begin{bmatrix} 40 - \begin{pmatrix} \text{total serum} \\ \text{albumin concentration} \end{pmatrix} \end{bmatrix}$$

The upper limit of normal varies from laboratory to laboratory, but is usually around 2.60 mmol/L. It should be noted that a spurious increase in serum calcium can occur with venous stasis (e.g. with the use of a tourniquet).

The serum phosphate is usually low in primary hyperparathyroidism and malignant disease. Measurement of plasma parathyroid hormone will usually differentiate between primary hyperparathyroidism (i.e. increased level) and malignant disease (i.e. decreased level). Plasma parathyroid hormone-related peptide measurements are available in some laboratories.

MANAGEMENT

The treatment of hypercalcaemia is usually associated with a significant improvement in the patient's quality of life. However, it is not necessarily associated with an improvement in the patient's overall prognosis.[2]

The management of hypercalcaemia involves treatment of the underlying cause (e.g. treatment of the malignant disease), correction of the dehydration, and correction of the hypercalcaemia. The following discussion concentrates on the management of hypercalcaemia associated with malignant disease. The bisphosphonates are the drugs of choice for treating this form of hypercalcaemia. However, there are a number of other drugs that can be used to treat hypercalcaemia of malignancy.

Correction of dehydration

Patients should be rehydrated with intravenous 0.9% normal saline. The rate of rehydration depends on a number of factors (e.g. severity of dehydration, presence of cardiac disease). However, the usual rate of rehydration is 2–3 L of fluid over 24 hours. Rehydration causes a fall in serum calcium, but usually does not lead to normocalcaemia. It may be associated with hyponatraemia and hypokalaemia. Therefore, it is important that plasma electrolytes are monitored during rehydration.

Correction of hypercalcaemia

Bisphosphonates The bisphosphonates inhibit bone resorption through various effects on osteoclasts. These effects include a direct inhibition of osteoclast function, an indirect inhibition of the osteoclast function (i.e. as a result of stimulation of osteoblast function), and a decrease in the number of osteoclasts (i.e. as a result of decreased recruitment of osteoclasts, or decreased survival of osteoclasts).

Table 6.2.1 Recommended dose of disodium pamidronate

Patient's serum calcium (mmol/L)	Dose of disodium pamidronate (mg)
<3.0	15–30
3.0–3.5	30–60
3.5–4.0	60–90
>4.0	90

The bisphosphonates are very successful in treating hypercalcaemia: for example, approximately 90 per cent of patients achieve normocalcaemia with disodium pamidronate.[3] Significant decreases in calcium occur within 2–3 days, whilst normocalcaemia occurs within 3–5 days. (Occasionally, the bisphosphonates cause mild hypocalcaemia.) The duration of the normocalcaemia is very variable, although it is usually less than 1 month.

Disodium pamidronate is given as a single, intravenous infusion; the manufacturers recommend that the dose should be based on the patient's serum calcium (Table 6.2.1). Nevertheless, there is an association between the dose of disodium pamidronate and the duration of normocalcaemia, i.e. the larger the dose, the longer the duration of normocalcaemia. This phenomenon has led some clinicians to ignore the manufacturers' recommendations and to treat all patients with relatively large doses of disodium pamidronate (i.e. 60–90 mg).

Sodium clodronate is given as a single, intravenous infusion; the recommended dose is 1500 mg. Oral sodium clodronate should not be used to treat hypercalcaemia, although it can be used as prophylaxis against hypercalcaemia (see below).

Zoledronic acid is a new, 'third-generation' bisphosphonate. It is given as a single, short (5-minute) intravenous infusion. The recommended dose is 4 mg. Nevertheless, there is an association between the dose of zoledronic acid and the duration of normocalcaemia, i.e. the larger the dose, the longer the duration of normocalcaemia.

Clinical studies suggest that zoledronic acid is more effective than disodium pamidronate,[4] which, in turn, is more effective than sodium clodronate.[5] Thus, zoledronic acid is associated with a greater response rate and with a longer duration of response. Zoledronic acid has a similar side-effect profile to disodium pamidronate. Sodium clodronate is contraindicated in patients with moderate to severe renal dysfunction.

The bisphosphonates are also used to prevent recurrences of hypercalcaemia; intravenous infusions can be given on an intermittent basis (e.g. 2–4 weekly). Alternatively, oral sodium clodronate can be given on a regular basis. Unfortunately, oral sodium clodronate is relatively ineffective in preventing recurrences of hypercalcaemia, because of its modest bioavailability. Furthermore, it is relatively poorly tolerated because of its gastrointestinal side effects (i.e. nausea, diarrhoea). Although the initial dose of bisphosphonate is usually very effective, subsequent doses tend to be less so.

Loop diuretics (e.g. furosemide [frusemide])

- Action: increases renal excretion of calcium.

- Effectiveness: produces small reductions in calcium; quick onset of action.

- Regimen: oral or parenteral administration (intravenous bolus); treatment given daily for several days.

- Comments: loop diuretics should only be used after rehydration.

Salcatonin [calcitonin (salmon)]

- Action: inhibits bone resorption through action on osteoclasts; increases renal excretion of calcium.

- Effectiveness: approximately 33 per cent of patients achieve normocalcaemia; quick onset of action (about 4 hours); tolerance develops after a few days of treatment.

- Regimen: parenteral administration (subcutaneous bolus, intramuscular bolus, intravenous infusion); treatment given daily for several days.

- Comments: calcitonin can be used in conjunction with bisphosphonates in the emergency situation.

Plicamycin [mithramycin]

- Action: inhibits bone resorption through action on osteoclasts.

- Effectiveness: approximately 80 per cent of patients achieve normocalcaemia; slow onset of action (about 24–48 hours).

- Regimen: parenteral administration (intravenous bolus, intravenous infusion); treatment given weekly.

- Comments: currently not available in the UK; causes significant toxicity.

Gallium nitrate

- Action: inhibits bone resorption through action on osteoclasts.

- Effectiveness: approximately 80 per cent of patients achieve normocalcaemia; slow onset of action (about 72 hours).

- Regimen: parenteral administration (continuous intravenous infusion); treatment given daily for 5 days.

- Comments: currently not available in the UK.

Other possible treatments

- Sodium cellulose phosphate.

- Intravenous phosphate.

- Intravenous trisodium edetate.

- Dialysis.

Immobility causes increased bone resorption, therefore patients with hypercalcaemia should be encouraged to mobilize as much as possible. It should be noted that a low calcium diet is usually inappropriate in patients with hypercalcaemia (gastrointestinal absorption of calcium is usually decreased in these patients).

Corticosteroids are generally not indicated in the management of hypercalcaemia. However, they may have a role in the treatment of hypercalcaemia secondary to 'steroid-responsive' tumours (e.g. myeloma, lymphoma) and to endocrine 'flare' reactions (e.g. breast carcinoma).

HYPONATRAEMIA

DEFINITION

Hyponatraemia is defined as a serum sodium of less than 130 mmol/L.

AETIOLOGY

There is a variety of different causes of hyponatraemia.

- *Pseudohyponatraemia*: misleadingly low serum sodium levels can occur in patients with elevated serum levels of lipids or proteins (pseudohyponatraemia). A compensatory hyponatraemia occurs in situations where there is an increase in plasma osmolality, e.g. significant hyperglycaemia.

- *Hyponatraemia associated with hypovolaemia*: examples of this type of hyponatraemia include renal disorders, vomiting, diarrhoea, severe sweating and diuretic therapy.

- *Hyponatraemia associated with normovolaemia*: this type of hyponatraemia is seen with the syndrome of inappropriate secretion of antidiuretic hormone (SIADH) and excessive intravenous therapy (i.e. fluid replacement with 5% dextrose solution).

- *Hyponatraemia associated with hypervolaemia*: examples of this type of hyponatraemia include renal disorders, cardiac failure, hepatic cirrhosis and excessive intravenous therapy (i.e. fluid replacement with 0.9% sodium chloride solution).

CLINICAL FEATURES

The clinical features of hyponatraemia are dependent on the absolute decrease in serum sodium and the rate of decrease in serum sodium. Patients may also present with clinical features of fluid depletion or fluid overload (see above).

The clinical features associated with mild hyponatraemia include anorexia, malaise, nausea, vomiting and headache. Moderate hyponatraemia may result in muscle cramps, muscle weakness, personality changes and confusion. The clinical features associated with severe hyponatraemia include drowsiness, convulsions and coma; indeed, severe hyponatraemia can be fatal.

MANAGEMENT

The management of this condition involves treatment of the underlying cause of the hyponatraemia and of the hyponatraemia itself.[6] In cases associated with hypovolaemia, the hyponatraemia may be corrected by fluid replacement (i.e. 0.9% sodium chloride solution). Similarly, in cases associated with hypervolaemia, this may be corrected by fluid restriction and the use of diuretics. The management of the SIADH is discussed below.

Rapid correction of hyponatraemia may lead to the development of central pontine myelinolysis, which may cause severe morbidity (e.g. quadriparesis) and mortality. It is therefore recommended that the serum sodium is increased slowly, i.e. by no more than 12 mmol/24 hours.[7]

SYNDROME OF INAPPROPRIATE SECRETION OF ANTIDIURETIC HORMONE

EPIDEMIOLOGY

This syndrome accounts for approximately 50 per cent of cases of hyponatraemia.[6]

AETIOLOGY

The SIADH is usually due to an inappropriate secretion of arginine vasopressin (antidiuretic hormone), although in some instances this does not appear to be the case (e.g. there is sometimes inappropriate secretion of atrial natiuretic peptide). This has led to the use of the alternative term syndrome of inappropriate antidiuresis (SIAD).

Arginine vasopressin is a polypeptide hormone that is secreted from the posterior lobe of the pituitary gland. It is involved in the control of water balance. Thus, its secretion is stimulated by a decrease in blood volume and/or an increase in plasma osmolality. Conversely, its secretion is inhibited by an increase in blood volume and/or a decrease in plasma osmolality. Physical and psychological stress may also affect the secretion of this hormone. Arginine vasopressin acts on the collecting tubules of the kidney, leading to increased absorption of water.

The SIADH has been reported as a complication of a number of diseases, and also of a number of drugs.

- *Malignant disease*: this is the most common underlying cause of the SIADH. A variety of different tumours have been associated with the SIADH, most commonly small-cell carcinoma of the bronchus (approximately 15 per cent of patients).[8]

- *Disorders of the central nervous system*, e.g. infection, trauma.

- *Disorders of the respiratory system*, e.g. infection, chronic obstructive airways disease.

- *Drugs*: a variety of different medications have been associated with the development of SIADH, including several drugs used in oncology (e.g. vinca alkaloids, cisplatin, cyclophosphamide) and in palliative care (e.g. opioid analgesics, thiazide diuretics, tricyclic antidepressants, carbamazepine).

CLINICAL FEATURES

The clinical features of the SIADH are related to the hyponatraemia (see above).

INVESTIGATIONS

The criteria for diagnosing the SIADH are:[8]

- hyponatraemia,

- hypo-osmolality of plasma,

- continued renal excretion of sodium in the absence of diuretics,

- absence of clinical evidence of fluid volume depletion,

- urinary osmolality greater than appropriate considering the plasma osmolality,

- normal renal function,

- normal adrenal function,

- normal thyroid function.

Thus the investigation of a patient with suspected SIADH should include estimation of plasma sodium, plasma osmolality, urine sodium and urine osmolality. The estimation of serum arginine vasopressin is not indicated in routine practice.

MANAGEMENT

The management of the SIADH involves treatment of the underlying cause and treatment of the hyponatraemia. In the emergency setting (e.g. coma, convulsions), the plasma sodium can be corrected by the use of intravenous 3% sodium chloride solution and intravenous furosemide (frusemide).[9] However, this method of treatment should be restricted to acute medical units, which have the ability to

monitor closely changes in plasma electrolytes. (Rapid correction of hyponatraemia may lead to the development of central pontine myelinolysis.)

In the non-emergency setting, the plasma sodium can be corrected initially by
the use of fluid restriction (i.e. 500 mL/24 hours), and subsequently by the use of
drugs that block the action of arginine vasopressin on the collecting tubules of the
kidney (i.e. demeclocycline, lithium). Demeclocycline is the drug of choice for
treating the SIADH. The recommended treatment dose is 300 mg t.d.s. or q.d.s.,
with a recommended maintenance dose of 300 mg b.d. or t.d.s.

KEY POINTS

- Severe hypercalcaemia is a medical emergency.
- Management of hypercalcaemia involves treatment of the underlying cause, correction of dehydration and correction of the hypercalcaemia itself.
- Intravenous bisphosphonates are the drugs of choice for correcting hypercalcaemia.
- Hypercalcaemia is associated with a poor prognosis.
- Hyponatraemia can cause a variety of different symptoms.
- Management of hyponatraemia involves treatment of the underlying cause and correction of the hyponatraemia itself.
- Rapid correction of hyponatraemia may lead to central pontine myelinolysis.

REFERENCES

1. Bower M, Cox S. Endocrine and metabolic complications of advanced cancer. In: Doyle D, Hanks G, Cherny N, Calman K (eds), Oxford textbook of palliative medicine, 3rd edn. Oxford: Oxford University Press, 2004, 687–702.
2. Kovacs CS, MacDonald SM, Chik CL, Bruera E. Hypercalcaemia of malignancy in the palliative care patient: a treatment strategy. J Pain Symptom Manage 1995; 10, 224–32.
3. Fleisch H. Bisphosphonates in bone disease. From the laboratory to the patient, 3rd edn. New York: Parthenon Publishing, 1997.
4. Major P, Lortholary A, Hon J et al. Zoledronic acid is superior to pamidronate in the treatment of hypercalcaemia of malignancy: a pooled analysis of two randomized, controlled clinical trials. J Clin Oncol 2001; 19, 558–67.
5. Purohit OP, Radstone CR, Anthony C, Kanis JA, Coleman RE. A randomised double-blind comparison of intravenous pamidronate and clodronate in the hypercalcaemia of malignancy. Br J Cancer 1995; 72, 1289–93.
6. Baylis PH. Water and sodium homeostasis and their disorders. In: Weatherall DJ, Ledingham JCG, Warrell DA (eds), Oxford textbook of medicine, 3rd edn. Oxford: Oxford University Press, 1996, 3116–26.
7. Sterns RH, Riggs JE, Schochet SS. Osmotic demyelination syndrome following correction of hyponatraemia. N Engl J Med 1986; 314, 1535–42.
8. Sorensen JB, Andersen MK, Hansen HH. Syndrome of inappropriate secretion of anti-diuretic hormone (SIADH) in malignant disease. J Intern Med 1995; 238, 97–110.

9. Hantman D, Rossier B, Zohlman R, Schrier R. Rapid correction of hyponatraemia in the syndrome of inappropriate secretion of antidiuretic hormone. An alternative treatment to hypertonic saline. *Ann Intern Med* 1973; **78**, 870–5.

FURTHER READING

Mayne PD. *Clinical chemistry in diagnosis and treatment*, 6th edn. London: Arnold, 1994.

Marshall WJ, Bangert SK (eds). *Clinical biochemistry. Metabolic and clinical aspects.* New York: Churchill Livingstone, 1995.

chapter 7

MALIGNANT ASCITES

Colin W. Campbell

INTRODUCTION

In a patient with cancer, the accumulation of ascitic fluid within the peritoneal cavity usually indicates an advanced stage of disease. Thus, with few exceptions, life expectancy is short and any intervention should palliate symptoms with the smallest possible burden for the patient. This chapter discusses the diagnosis of ascites and advises how to select the best management for the individual patient.

PREVALENCE

Malignant ascites is responsible for about 10 per cent of all cases of ascites.[1] Other common causes include:

- hepatic cirrhosis and portal hypertension

- cardiac failure

- nephrotic syndrome

- pancreatitis

- bacterial peritonitis, including tuberculosis.

  Ascites is present in more than 15 per cent of *all malignancies* at some stage.[2]

- In women with malignant ascites, 55–75 per cent of cases are due to a primary gynaecological malignancy, notably of the ovary, endometrium and cervix.[3]

- Of the women who die from ovarian cancer, 30–60 per cent develop ascites at some time.[4]

- In men with malignant ascites, more than 50 per cent are gastrointestinal in origin, colon, rectum and stomach being the commonest.[3]

- Unknown primary cancer is responsible for 6–20 per cent of cases in both sexes.

- Ascites is the first sign of cancer in around 50 per cent of cases of malignant ascites.[5]

PATHOGENESIS

In health, there is a continuous influx of fluid into the peritoneal cavity that is then reabsorbed at a rate of 5–6 mL/hour. About 50 mL of peritoneal fluid is normally present.[5] The predominant route for fluid reabsorption (efflux) is through the diaphragmatic lymphatics. In ascites, fluid influx is increased and efflux is impaired. Runyon et al.[1] have postulated four clinical entities in which malignant ascites is formed, although hepatic metastases can co-exist with peritoneal carcinomatosis (Table 7.1).

1 *Peritoneal carcinomatosis.* Cancer cells seed on to the visceral or parietal peritoneum, either by direct spread across the peritoneal cavity, or via lymphatic channels or the bloodstream. Tumour factors (such as vascular endothelial growth factor) increasing vascular permeability have been identified, which allow plasma proteins to pass through leaky venules. Leakage of protein-rich fluid causes *exudation* into the peritoneal cavity. At the same time, efflux may be impaired because of cancer cells obstructing the diaphragmatic lymphatics.
2 *Massive hepatic metastases.* Tumour may compress or encroach into hepatic or portal veins causing portal hypertension. Co-existing low plasma albumin secondary to cancer cachexia reduces the normal oncotic pressure in the vascular space. This, combined with the raised hydrostatic pressure in the portal venous system, causes an escape of fluid out of the vascular space into the peritoneal cavity, resulting in ascites production.
3 *Chylous ascites.* Lymphatics may be obstructed either by tumour invasion (commonly lymphoma) or secondary to radiotherapy or surgery. The resulting overspill of milky white chyle gives rise to the so-called chylous ascites.
4 *Hepatocellular carcinoma.* This is often superimposed on cirrhosis.

Table 7.1 Characteristics of malignant ascites according to aetiology

Aetiology of ascites	Malignant cytology in ascitic fluid[1]	Postulated response to diuretics
PC alone (≈50% of cases)	>95% positive	No[6]
PC and MHM	>95% positive	Possible
MHM alone	Negative	Yes[6]
Chylous ascites	Negative	No[6]
Hepatocellular carcinoma	Negative	Probable

PC, peritoneal carcinomatosis; MHM, massive hepatic metastases.

PROGNOSIS

Overall, malignant ascites is associated with a median survival of 6–20 weeks, but there are marked variations, depending on the primary malignancy (Table 7.2).

PRESENTATION

CLINICAL FEATURES

Table 7.3 outlines the common symptoms and signs associated with abdominal ascites.

Associated findings include:

- *umbilical hernia* because of increased intra-abdominal pressure,

- *pleural effusions* because of fluid passing through stomata in the diaphragm, or via lymphatic communications between the peritoneal and pleural cavities.

Table 7.2 Malignant ascites and survival

Type of cancer	Mean survival (weeks)
Lymphoma	58–78
Ovary	30–35
Gastrointestinal	12–20
Unknown primary	1–12

Adapted from Parsons et al.[5]

Table 7.3 Clinical diagnosis of ascites

Symptoms	Signs
Abdominal discomfort	Increased abdominal girth
Anorexia/early satiety	Bulging flanks
Nausea and vomiting	Shifting dullness on percussion
Gastro-oesophageal reflux	Fluid thrill (while an assistant presses firmly with
Dyspnoea due to diaphragmatic splinting	the medial edges of both hands in the vertical
or basal atelectasis	midline of the abdomen)
	Ankle oedema – men with no ankle swelling are
	unlikely to have ascites[7]

INVESTIGATION

- Ultrasound examination will detect as little as 100 mL of ascitic fluid.[5]

- Ultrasound may be used to guide the insertion of the paracentesis catheter in cases of fluid loculation within the peritoneal cavity or when bulky tumour masses are suspected within the abdomen.

- Cytology is positive in only 50 per cent of cases overall;[2] it is advised to submit 500 mL of ascitic fluid for cytology.[3]

- Microscopy with Gram and alcohol–acid-fast bacilli (AAFB) staining plus suitable culture methods are used to detect peritonitis.

TUMOUR MARKERS

Tumour markers do not alter the management, with the exception of carbohydrate antigen-125 (CA-125). A raised CA-125 is present in 80 per cent of women with ovarian cancer. However, it is not specific for this disease, as it is raised in several other cancers, specifically in the presence of intraperitoneal disease.[5]

MANAGEMENT

In all cases it is important to work closely with the referring specialist team. This is particularly so in cases of potential ovarian cancer and lymphoma, where appropriate oncological or surgical intervention may palliate symptoms and achieve disease remission. For symptomatic relief, the options are diuretics (Table 7.4), paracentesis or a peritoneovenous shunt (PVS).

DIURETICS

The response to diuretics is unpredictable in malignant ascites, with a limited evidence base. In a Canadian survey of 44 physicians who treat malignant ascites, only 20 (45 per cent) felt that diuretics were an effective treatment.[8]

Table 7.4 Drug profile of diuretics used in ascites

Diuretic	Dose (mg/day)
Spironolactone	100–400
Furosemide (frusemide)	40–80

In cirrhotic ascites, where there is activation of the renin–aldosterone system with sodium and water retention, diuretics plus a sodium-restricted diet may clear ascites in up to 90 per cent of cases. Ascites attributable to massive hepatic metastases may behave in a similar fashion, and diuretic therapy has been shown to mobilize peritoneal fluid effectively.[6]

Conversely, in those 50–60 per cent of cases of malignant ascites that are due to peritoneal carcinomatosis alone or chylous malignant ascites, the renin–aldosterone system is not activated. In these situations, diuretics do not remove ascitic fluid.[6]

However, in very ill cancer patients, it may be inappropriate to investigate the actual cause of ascites, and for this reason diuretics are often given on a trial basis.

- The onset of diuresis with spironolactone may take up to 2 weeks because of this drug's long half-life of 5 days.[9] The addition of furosemide (frusemide) will accelerate the onset of diuresis.

- Start with small doses and titrate upwards (see Table 7.4).

- Spironolactone has been associated with nausea and vomiting in 2–14 per cent of patients treated for ascites.[9]

- Potential adverse effects from diuretics may arise from hypovolaemia, and may include renal impairment and electrolyte disturbance.[10]

PARACENTESIS

Therapeutic paracentesis is the mainstay of treatment in symptomatic ascites. It is used by up to 98 per cent of physicians who treat patients with malignant ascites, and 89 per cent regard it as effective.[8]

- In almost 90 per cent of cases, there is improvement in symptoms after ascitic drainage.[11]

- The mean duration of symptom relief may be as short as 10 days.[11]

- It is necessary to remove 0.5 L or more to effect some relief of symptoms.[11]

- Limited-volume paracentesis may afford significant relief of discomfort, nausea and vomiting and dyspnoea.[12] Drainage to 'dryness' may extend the intervals between paracenteses.

- Paracentesis using vacuum assistance may allow drainage of more than 5 L in less than 30 minutes. However, it is customary in the UK to drain ascites by gravity into a collecting bag, typically limiting the rate to a maximum of 4 L in 24 hours to prevent hypovolaemia.

- Indwelling peritoneal drainage catheters are associated with a modest risk of sepsis, both in the abdominal wall and, more seriously, with peritonitis.

Safety profile of paracentesis

- *Hypovolaemia.* There is continuing debate as to whether rapid removal of ascitic fluid results in movement of plasma fluid volume out of the vascular space to rapidly refill the peritoneal cavity, with potential hypovolaemia, renal failure and hyponatraemia. In a study of 109 consecutive paracenteses for malignant ascites, there were 3 (2.8 per cent) serious complications from hypotension and 2 (1.8 per cent) were fatal.[11] However, other workers report no problems from hypovolaemia. It has been suggested that malignant ascites is produced at a constant rate independent of any fall in intra-abdominal pressure. In some studies, plasma renin is elevated following paracentesis, suggesting a fall in circulating plasma volume, but other studies measuring plasma volume with radioisotope dilution techniques have described constant plasma volumes. There is no consensus on whether plasma expanders are required in malignant ascites, although intravenous albumin has been shown to be no better than Dextran-70 or Haemaccel in cirrhotic ascites.

- *Haemorrhage.* There is a small risk of haemorrhage into the peritoneal cavity or into the abdominal wall.

- *Pulmonary emboli.* Pulmonary emboli have been reported, arising from compression and subsequent thrombosis of large intra-abdominal veins.

- *Peritonitis.* This may occur rarely, from intestinal perforation or prolonged placement of the catheter.

Clinical tips for paracentesis

- Choose a site avoiding the bladder, liver, palpable tumour masses or scars (which may have bowel adherent to their peritoneal surface).

- Consider seeking prior ultrasound guidance if there is uncertainty on clinical grounds.

PERITONEOVENOUS SHUNT

For patients needing repeated paracentesis, PVS offers a potential alternative in selected cases (Table 7.5). The procedure involves placing one end of the shunt into the peritoneal cavity and tunnelling it subcutaneously up into the neck, where it is inserted into the internal jugular vein.

Potential benefits

- Greater patient independence and preservation of serum albumin, compared to repeated paracentesis.

- Median survival after shunt insertion varies from just over 1 month to 5.5 months.

- Symptomatic relief is obtained in 60–75 per cent of cases.[13,14]

Table 7.5 Suggested symptomatic management of malignant ascites

Patient is not troubled by ascites *or* barely rousable and imminently dying	**No treatment**
Symptomatic but not requiring immediate relief and no renal impairment	**Spironolactone** 100–400 mg/day + **furosemide (frusemide)** 40–80 mg/day Monitor blood biochemistry regularly; stop if no response within 2 weeks
Symptomatic	**Paracentesis** repeated at intervals as required
Needs frequent large-volume paracentesis Refractory to diuretic therapy Prognosis more than 3 months Not gastrointestinal or unknown primary Ascites not loculated No significant liver impairment No history of bacterial peritonitis No heart or renal failure	**Peritoneovenous shunt**

Potential hazards

- In a study of 89 patients, 12 (13 per cent) died in the first month due to a complication of the shunt. In the same study, only 31 per cent of patients maintained a patent shunt and survived for more than 2 months.[13]

- Shunt blockages and other shunt complications occur in 25–50 per cent of cases.

- Disseminated intravascular coagulation (DIC) is common on laboratory evidence in the first few days, but is less likely to be troublesome clinically than in cirrhotic ascites.[14]

- Accelerated metastases are a theoretical risk by providing a conduit through which cancer cells may travel from the peritoneal cavity to other parts of the body. Recorded cases are rare, probably because of the short overall prognosis of patients with malignant ascites.

- Fluid overload, peritonitis and pulmonary emboli have also been reported.

ALTERNATIVE TREATMENTS

The appeal of injecting agents directly into the peritoneal space has resulted in a number of trials. Various agents, including mitomycin-C, ^{32}P, interferon-α and interferon-β, have been tried. A controlled trial of intraperitoneal versus intravenous cisplatin in ovarian cancer showed no difference between the two routes.[3] However, an intraperitoneal metalloproteinase inhibitor used in a trial involving

23 patients with malignant ascites prevented re-accumulation of ascites in 12 of these patients.[15] In a study of mice with ovarian cancer, the administration of an oral inhibitor of vascular endothelial growth factor significantly inhibited the formation of ascites and prolonged the animals' survival.[16]

FUTURE DEVELOPMENTS

For the limited number of patients who retain good performance status, more successful treatments for locoregional disease could result in potentially significant survival benefits. New biological treatments and gene therapies may yet fulfil expectations as oncological treatments, and become more widely available.

However, it is likely that for most patients palliative measures will still be the most appropriate option. A simple test to determine which patients would benefit from diuretics would be invaluable. Meantime, paracentesis remains the favoured management, and creative ways need to be explored of providing this treatment to frail patients, promptly and with the least disruption to their lives. The convenience of out-patient or domiciliary paracentesis may offer such a solution.

KEY POINTS

- Ascites indicates advanced disease and a short prognosis, although overall survival is notably better with ovarian cancer.
- Available treatments are often unsatisfactory, and may add to the patient's burden.
- The response to diuretics is unpredictable in malignant ascites, and evidence supporting their efficacy is limited.
- Paracentesis is the mainstay of treatment; peritoneovenous shunting remains an alternative in highly selected cases.

REFERENCES

1. Runyon BA, Hoefs JC, Morgan TR. Ascitic fluid analysis in malignancy-related ascites. *Hepatology*.1988; 8(5), 1104–9.
2. Kichian K, Bain VG. Jaundice, ascites, and hepatic encephalopathy. In: Doyle D, Hanks G, Cherny N, Calman K (eds), *Oxford textbook of palliative medicine*, 3rd edn. Oxford: Oxford University Press, 2004, 507–20.
3. Maringola FM, Schwartzentruber DJ. Malignant ascites. In: DeVita VT, Hellman S, Rosenberg SA (eds), *Cancer: principles and practice of oncology*, 5th edn. Philadelphia: Lippincott-Raven, 1997, 2598–606.
4. De Simone GG. Treatment of malignant ascites. *Progr Palliat Care* 1999, 7(1), 10–16.
5. Parsons SL, Watson SA, Steele RJC. Malignant ascites. *Br J Surg* 1996; 83, 6–14.
6. Pockros PJ, Esrason KT, Nguyen C, Duque J, Woods S. Mobilization of malignant ascites with diuretics is dependent on ascitic fluid characteristics. *Gastroenterology* 1992; 103, 1302–6.

7. Williams JW, Simel DL. Does this patient have ascites? How to divine fluid in the abdomen. *J Am Med Assoc* 1992; 267(19), 2645–8.
8. Lee CW, Bociek G, Faught W. A survey of practice in management of malignant ascites. *J Pain Symptom Manage* 1998; 16(2), 96–101.
9. Greenway B, Johnson PJ, Williams R. Control of malignant ascites with spironolactone. *Br J Surg* 1982; 69, 441–2.
10. Gines P, Arroyo V, Quintero E *et al*. Comparison of paracentesis and diuretics in the treatment of cirrhotics with tense ascites. *Gastroenterology* 1987; 93, 234–41.
11. Ross GJ, Kessler HB, Clair MR, Gatenby RA, Hartz WH, Ross LV. Sonographically guided paracentesis for palliation of symptomatic malignant ascites. *Am J Roentgenol* 1989; 153, 1309–11.
12. Macnamara P. Paracentesis – an effective method of symptom control in the palliative care setting? *Palliat Med* 2000; 14, 62–4.
13. Schumacher DL, Saclarides TJ, Staren ED. Peritoneovenous shunts for palliation of the patient with malignant ascites. *Ann Surg Oncol* 1994; 1(5), 378–81.
14. Wickremesekera SK, Stubbs RS. Peritoneovenous shunting for malignant ascites. *N Z Med J* 1997; 110, 33–5.
15. Beattie GJ, Smyth JF. Phase I study of intraperitoneal metalloproteinase inhibitor BB94 in patients with malignant ascites. *Clin Cancer Res* 1998; 4, 1899–902.
16. Xu L, Yoneda J, Herrera C *et al*. Inhibition of malignant ascites and growth of human ovarian carcinoma by oral administration of a potent inhibitor of the vascular endothelial growth factor receptor tyrosine kinase. *Int J Oncol* 2000; 16, 445–54.

FURTHER READING

Aslam N, Marino CR. Malignant ascites. New concepts in pathophysiology, diagnosis and management. *Arch Intern Med* 2001; 161, 2733–7.
Kichian K, Bain VG. Jaundice, ascites, and hepatic encephalopathy. In: Doyle D, Hanks G, Cherny N, Calman K (eds), *Oxford textbook of palliative medicine*, 3rd edn. Oxford, Oxford University Press, 2004, 507–20.
Parsons SL, Watson SA, Steele RJC. Malignant ascites. *Br J Surg* 1996; 83, 6–14.
Smith EM, Jayson GC. The current and future management of malignant ascites. *Clin Oncol* 2003; 15, 59–72.

chapter 8

PLEURAL EFFUSIONS

Polly Edmonds and John Wiles

INTRODUCTION

Cancer is the second most common cause of pleural effusion after heart failure in patients over 50 years old.[1] It is a common cause of morbidity for patients with advanced cancer, particularly patients with lung or breast cancer, who account for over 75 per cent of malignant pleural effusions (MPE).[2] This chapter concentrates on the management of MPE.

PATHOGENESIS

A pleural effusion is an abnormal volume of fluid that has collected between the visceral and parietal pleura. This may result from two mechanisms:

1 increased pleural fluid formation:
   tumour involving pleura,
   reduced serum albumin;
2 decreased pleural fluid resorption:
   tumour involving pleura,
   mediastinal lymphadenopathy,
   lymphangitis carcinomatosa.

ASSESSMENT

The majority of patients present with breathlessness, often associated with cough and/or chest pain. Clinical examination is useful to exclude non-malignant causes of pleural effusion, such as pneumonia and cardiac failure. The performance status of the patient should also be assessed to determine fitness for interventions (see box overleaf).

World Health Organisation performance status

0   Able to carry out all normal activity without restriction.
1   Restricted in physical strenuous activity but ambulatory and able to carry out light work.
2   Ambulatory and capable of self-care but unable to carry out any work; up and about more
    than 50 per cent of the working day.
3   Capable of only limited self-care; confined to bed or chair more than 50 per cent of waking
    hours.
4   Completely disabled; cannot carry out any self-care; totally confined to bed or chair.

Pleural effusions of greater than 500 mL can be diagnosed clinically. The typical findings are reduced chest expansion, stony dullness to percussion and reduced or absent air entry on the affected side. Bronchial breathing may be detectable at the upper limit of an effusion, and vocal resonance is reduced or absent. With a large effusion there may be clinical evidence of mediastinal shift away from the effusion; however, this may not be present if MPEs are associated with lobar collapse.

Pleural effusions can be detected on chest X-ray once there is more than 300 mL. The appearances range from obliteration of the costophrenic angle to dense opacification of some or all of the hemithorax associated with a meniscus (or curved upper edge).

MANAGEMENT

Where possible, the underlying cause of a pleural effusion should be treated. Some patients with MPE may benefit from palliative chemotherapy, but for the majority of patients the treatment is symptomatic.

A guide to the management of new and recurrent MPE is shown in Figure 8.1.

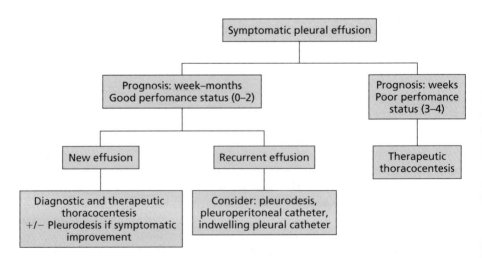

Figure 8.1 Guide to management of MPE.

THORACOCENTESIS

Thoracocentesis (or pleural tap) offers effective symptom relief in the majority of patients, but re-accumulation of pleural fluid occurs rapidly, and this is therefore only an effective short-term measure. Repeated thoracocentesis may result in loculated effusions and empyema, making further intervention difficult and minimizing effective symptom relief, and should therefore be avoided in fit patients (performance status 0–2 in the box above), who should be considered for definitive procedures. Unfit patients with a poor prognosis (performance status 3–4 in the box) may be managed by repeated thoracocentesis alone.

Healthcare professionals may have concerns regarding undertaking thoracocentesis where X-ray facilities are not available on site, specifically the risk of inducing a pneumothorax. For patients with far advanced disease and a large, symptomatic pleural effusion clinically, the benefits of thoracocentesis are likely to outweigh the risk of pneumothorax, particularly if the effusion is tapped to symptomatic relief rather than dryness.

PLEURODESIS

Pleurodesis aims to induce a chemical pleurisy by instillation of an irritant agent into the pleural cavity, the resolution of which results in adhesion of the pleural layers and obliteration of the pleural space. The commonest agents used for pleurodesis are talc, tetracycline and bleomycin. The factors that contribute to effective pleurodesis are drainage to dryness of MPE prior to instillation, completeness of lung expansion and adequate agent dispersal.[3] There is no consensus as to the most effective agent, although one study did suggest that bleomycin was superior to tetracycline in reducing recurrent MPE.[4] Surgical pleurodesis with talc has the advantages that the pleural space is visualized, adhesions can be divided and a definitive diagnosis made, but patients need to be fit enough to undergo a general anaesthetic.[5] However, a more recent report suggested that video-assisted talc pleurodesis can be performed safely under local anaesthesia, with an average length of hospital stay of approximately 4 days.[6] Only one study has compared medical and surgical pleurodesis, which demonstrated no difference in recurrence rates.[7]

RECURRENT MALIGNANT PLEURAL EFFUSION

A pleurodesis should be attempted on all patients fit enough to undergo a procedure. Where this has failed, the options include an indwelling pleural catheter[8] or pleuroperitoneal shunt.[9] The former is indicated for intermittent long-term drainage of recurrent MPE. The pleural catheter is tunnelled externally under local anaesthetic, and has a one-way valve attached to the external end. A drainage line and vacuum bottle are attached to drain the MPE, a procedure that can be undertaken in out-patients or the patient's home. Pleuroperitoneal shunt insertion requires a hospital stay of approximately 5 days, and patients need to be taught to use the pumping mechanism effectively.

FUTURE DEVELOPMENTS

- *Intrapleural streptokinase.* This has been shown to aid drainage of post-pneumonic effusions, empyema and haemothorax. It causes degradation of a variety of proteins, including fibrin, thereby possibly preventing the development of fibrinous septae or adhesions. One study included four patients with loculated MPE, three of whom achieved lysis of loci and subsequent pleurodesis following instillation of intrapleural streptokinase.[10]

- *Vascular endothelial growth factor inhibition.* Recent reports suggest that vascular endothelial growth factor (VEGF) plays a pivotal role in the accumulation of MPE.[11] Malignant effusions contain high levels of biologically active VEGF, resulting in increased vascular permeability. Experimental models suggest that inhibition of this factor may reduce recurrent MPE formation.

KEY POINTS

- Thoracocentesis may provide effective short-term symptom control, but recurrence is rapid.
- Repeated thoracocentesis may result in loculated effusions or empyema and should be avoided in fit patients.
- Pleurodesis should be considered in all patients, unless the prognosis is very poor.
- The outcomes following medical and surgical pleurodesis are similar.
- Strategies for managing recurrent MPE include pleuroperitoneal shunts and indwelling pleural catheters.

REFERENCES

1. Stretton F, Edmonds P, Marrinan M. Malignant pleural effusions. *Eur J Palliat Care* 1999; 6(1), 5–9.
2. Lynch TJ. Management of malignant pleural effusions. *Chest* 1993; 103, S385–9.
3. Petrou M, Kaplan D, Goldstraw P. Management of recurrent malignant pleural effusions. *Cancer* 1995; 75, 801–5.
4. Ruckdeschel JC, Moores D, Lee JY et al. Intrapleural therapy for malignant pleural effusions: a randomised comparison of bleomycin and tetracycline. *Chest* 1991; 100, 1528–35.
5. Webb WR, Ozmen V, Moulder PV, Shabahang B, Breaux J. Iodised talc pleurodesis for the treatment of pleural effusion. *J Thorax Cardiovasc Surg* 1992; 103, 881–6.
6. Danby CA, Adebonojo SA, Moritz DM. Video-assisted talc pleurodesis for malignant pleural effusions utilising local anaesthesia and IV sedation. *Chest* 1998; 113(3), 739–42.
7. Evans TRJ, Stein RC, Pepper JR et al. A randomised prospective trial of surgical against medical tetracycline pleurodesis in the management of malignant pleural effusions secondary to breast cancer. *Eur J Cancer* 1993; 29, 316–19.

8. Le-Van L, Parker LA, DeMars LR, MacKoul P, Fowler WC. Pleural effusions: out-patient management with pigtail catheter chest tubes. *Gynaecol Oncol* 1994; **54**, 215–17.

9. Lee KA, Harvey JC, Reich H, Beattie EJ. Management of malignant pleural effusions with pleuroperitoneal shunting. *J Am Coll Surg* 1994; **178**, 586–8.

10. Jerjes-Sanchez C, Ramirez-Reviera R, Elizalde A *et al*. Intrapleural fibrinolysis with streptokinase as an adjunctive treatment in haemothorax and empyema. *Chest* 1996; **109**, 1514–19.

11. Verheul HM, Hoekman K, Jorna AS, Smit EF, Pinedo HM. Targeting vascular endothelial growth factor blockade: ascites and pleural effusion formation. *Oncologist* 2000; **5**(Suppl. 1), 45–50.

chapter 9

MALIGNANT WOUNDS

Patricia Grocott

INTRODUCTION

Malignant wounds develop when tumour cells infiltrate the skin. The terms **ulcerating** and **fungating** are descriptive terms for the condition:

- fungating describes proliferative, fulminating growth,

- ulcerating describes necrotic craters.

Malignant wounds may present with both features. Ulceration occurs when there is a loss of blood supply to areas of the tumour through capillary rupture and occlusion of blood vessels by tumour infiltration or compression. The loss of vascularity is a major source of the problems associated with these wounds because of the loss of tissue viability and consequent necrosis. Anaerobic and aerobic bacteria proliferate in these conditions and may account for the characteristic symptoms of malodour and exudate.

Malignant wounds develop from primary or metastatic tumours. They may also be mistaken for, or closely linked with, radiation necrosis. A differentiating feature between the two conditions is the flattened margin of an ulcer caused by radiation, whereas malignant ulcers have raised and rolled margins.

Any uncontrolled tumour can result in a malignant wound. There is also a wide variation in their location, size and shape, as illustrated in Table 9.1. The variation reflects the progressive nature of the disease, which can result in massive

Table 9.1 Examples of the location and presentation of malignant wounds according to tumour type[1]

Tumour type	Description of malignant wound presentation
Carcinoma of the breast	• Extensive ulceration of the breast with satellite skin nodules, axillary and cervical nodes • Extensive cutaneous infiltration, anterior and posterior chest wall, axilla, upper and lower arm, induration, 'superficial' ulcerations • Extensive cutaneous infiltration, anterior and posterior chest wall, fungating and necrotic patches, fungating and necrotic breast

(continued)

Table 9.1 (*continued*)

Tumour type	Description of malignant wound presentation
	• Fungating breast nodule, glossy, blood capillaries visible to the naked eye; potential precursor to necrotic ulceration • Multiple, discoid, necrotic ulcers on large, hard, nodular breast • Multiple, fixed, raised nodules, telangiectasis, tissue turgor of surrounding skin, some wet necrotic ulcerations • Deep-seated wet necrosis of chest wall, satellite nodules, small exuding exit points (may include radiation necrosis)
Carcinoma of the nose, floor of the mouth, larynx and tongue	• Necrotic ulceration with proud, fungating, rolled margins located around the ear • Ulcerating and fungating lesion on the chin, communicating and non-communicating with the buccal cavity • Proud fungating nodule on the neck, progressive ulceration • Central ulceration of the nose and nasopharynx with rolled margins
Cancer of the parotid gland	• Necrotic ulceration with proud, fungating, rolled margins, located around ear and extended around the neck
Carcinomas of the vulva, ovary, caecum, colon and rectum with loco-regional infiltration of the anterior abdominal wall	• Multiple isolated, fungating and ulcerating nodules • Extensive fungating and necrotic masses on the abdomen which coalesce • Extensive fungating and necrotic masses on the abdomen which coalesce, with communicating sinus to the abdominal cavity • Extensive fungating and necrotic masses on the abdomen which coalesce, with communicating fistulae to the bowel and faecal leak
Carcinomas of the rectum, vulva, urethra and penis with loco-regional infiltration of the perineum and genitalia	• Necrotic and fungating vaginal and perineal mass • Necrotic and fungating vaginal and perineal mass, recto-vaginal and/or vesico-vaginal fistula • Necrotic erosion of the penis and scrotum with large perineal necrotic cavity • Fungating and ulcerating lesions along suture lines following penile amputation
Carcinoma of the skin	• Necrotic nodule on thumb extended to fungating and ulcerating nodules in the axilla • Ulcerated and necrotic scalp
Melanoma	• Multiple fungating and necrotic ulcers with dense tissue turgor of trunk and arms
Cutaneous T-cell lymphoma	• Multiple fungating and ulcerating lesions over whole body

destruction of the skin, distortion of the normal structure and function in and adjacent to the location of the wound, and erosion of organs. A clinical example of the physical impact of the disease is the patient with breast cancer, extensive destruction of the breast and the chest wall with adjacent limb lymphoedema. The psychological and social consequences of this disease to patients, their families and friends are obviously significant.[1]

INCIDENCE

The incidence of malignant wounds is not known, as these data are not collected alongside population-based cancer registries. A retrospective survey of UK oncology, hospice and community sites asked respondents how many malignant wounds had been seen over the previous 4 weeks and for an estimate of the number of wounds encountered during the previous year:[2] 114 respondents reported a monthly total of 295 wounds and an annual total of 2417. The conclusion was drawn that these figures reflect a significant incidence. However, given the fact that patients move between the sites surveyed during the course of their illness, it is impossible to tell whether the same patient was counted more than once.

TREATMENT

Diagnosis is based on histological assessment or knowledge of the primary tumour. The management aims are to arrest tumour growth and promote healing wherever possible. This may involve the use of conventional anti-cancer treatments, which can also be used palliatively to treat symptoms. Additional treatments are attempted in the face of intractable problems, for example embolization to arrest persistent fast bleeding from a vessel that can be isolated.

Because the presence of a malignant wound has a significant impact on patients and those who care for them, invasive palliative measures are used whenever they will avoid the unpleasant consequences of an open and deteriorating wound. For instance, excision of an advanced fungating breast tumour followed by closure with a myocutaneous flap can give the patient several months of life free from the problems of living with an open wound.[3] However, patients vary in their ability to accept anti-cancer treatments, and some refuse, in spite of factual descriptions of the consequences of allowing the tumour to go untreated. In addition, the tumour may be inoperable or resistant to anti-cancer therapies.

In the absence of effective treatment, the tumour cells extend along tissue planes, around and along blood and capillary systems, resulting in wounds that are continually enlarging, irregular in shape, necrotic and exuding. The management options include:

- systemic and topical symptom control measures,
- local wound dressings,
- supportive care to the individual and the family.

This chapter focuses on the symptomatic treatment of wound-related problems and local wound dressings. Effective management of both these dimensions of care can reduce the impact of the wound on day-to-day living, reduce the stigma associated with uncontrolled body fluids in particular, and enable the patient to maintain a social life.

SYMPTOMATIC TREATMENT

The evidence base for interventions in the palliative management of fungating wounds is sparse. Apart from the author's study,[1] the topic has not been researched clinically in the last 15 years. A number of discrete areas for future research are highlighted during the course of this chapter. In addition, relevant material from other disciplines that supports interventions for fungating wounds is referred to, for example chronic wound care and materials technology.

The major problems related to malignant wounds that require symptom management include:

- stinging and soreness

- pruritus

- soreness and irritation from excoriated skin conditions

- odour

- spontaneous bleeding and haemorrhage.

These problems may be interrelated, for example a superimposed infection may mimic the signs of accelerated tumour infiltration with pain, odour, bleeding and rapid extension of the wound. The differential diagnosis of the problems may not be straightforward, so that access to the multi-professional team for accurate diagnosis and choice of treatment is essential.

Cutaneous stinging and soreness
- The management of tumour pain requires identification of the nociceptors responsible for the pain so that appropriate systemic analgesia may be prescribed.

- Topical measures such as diamorphine in amorphous hydrogel can reduce the intensity of cutaneous stinging and soreness, with the potential for reducing the dose of systemic opioids.[4]

Pruritus
- The pruritus referred to is the creeping, intense itching sensation attributed to the activity of the tumour, particularly in inflammatory breast disease and where there is extensive, superficial cutaneous infiltration.

- Palliative chemotherapy can reduce this problem as it reduces the tumour infiltration. However, tumour resistance and unacceptable side effects may limit such treatment.

- A serotonin reuptake inhibitor, paroxetine, has been demonstrated to have a rapid and sustained antipruritic effect in patients with severe pruritus attributed to a number of causes, such as bullous skin lesions and as a side effect of morphine therapy.[5]

Soreness and irritation from excoriated skin conditions

- Excoriated skin conditions are the result of damage from exudate and effluent.

- Attention is needed to the selection of wound dressings and pads with a 'dry weave' layer to prevent the fluid from tracking back from the dressing to the skin.

- Alcohol-free topical agents provide a sustained barrier, a second skin in effect, to minimize excoriation.

- These measures must be implemented as soon as it is evident that the boundary of the skin has been broken and fluid is escaping, and then repeated scrupulously.

Odour

It is assumed that bacteria, particularly anaerobes, are the source of wound odour. However, a systematic literature review revealed significant gaps in knowledge about the actual causal mechanisms of odour that need to be addressed if interventions are to be targeted appropriately.[6] Accepting a bacterial source for odour, four main management options are generally adopted:

- systemic antibiotics

- topical metronidazole

- charcoal dressings

- debridement of necrotic tissue.

There are limitations to these approaches that are attributable to the size and eccentric shapes of malignant wounds, a lack of blood supply, the liquefaction of dead tissue and the management of exudate.

- Systemic antibiotics are used presumptively to manage bacterial colonization and the offensive odour that emanates from anaerobic bacteria in particular. The limitations to this approach include gastric side effects, which may be dose-related and avoided on low-dose regimens.

- The effectiveness of topical metronidazole is limited when the wounds are extensive and heavily necrotic because of a probable lack of penetration to bacteria located below the surface.

- The amount of gel and frequency of application needed to deodorize a given area of wound have not been quantified by the manufacturers. Given the high cost of the gels, there is a danger that insufficient quantity to achieve inhibition of the odour-producing bacteria will be applied in an effort to minimize costs.

- The efficacy of applying a topical gel to areas such as the perineum is questionable because the gel is lost to the absorbent dressings and pads.

- Activated charcoal dressings are said to act as filters to adsorb volatile malodorous chemicals from the wound before they pass into the air. Charcoal dressings are presented in pre-sized rectangular, square and oval shapes. However, they are redundant unless they can be fitted as a sealed unit. Airtight charcoal garments would be a more realistic approach to masking odour with charcoal filters.[7]

- Clearance of dead tissue by sharp or surgical debridement is not an option because of the potentially catastrophic haemorrhage that may occur if the tumour vasculature is damaged.

- However, dead necrotic tissue can be separated from the tumour bed via an autolytic process during which naturally occurring enzymes and colonizing bacteria liquefy the dead tissue and cause it to separate from the wound. This process occurs more quickly in a moist wound environment, and may therefore be facilitated with the use of dressings that add moisture to the wound (for example hydrogels) and those that prevent the wound from dehydrating (for example semi-occlusive foam dressings).[8] Other novel products, such as Manuka honey and krill enzymes, also speed up the process.[1,9]

- The clinical gains of autolytic debridement need to be assessed critically. Patients with extensive or multiple wounds covered in dry eschar and a life expectancy of weeks may not benefit from the mobilization of the eschar and the consequent wet necrosis and exudate.

- An endpoint of autolysis is exudate that has to be managed effectively if this approach to odour management is adopted. This topic is discussed further below.

Bleeding

Oral anti-fibrinolytics, radiotherapy and embolization are all used to control spontaneous bleeding from eroding blood vessels. The following topical measures are also applied as emergency measures.

- Adrenaline 1:1000 applied on a gauze pad with light pressure: adrenaline is vasoconstrictive and may result in ischaemic necrosis if used in large quantities.

- Sucralfate suspension is reported to be effective and simple to use.[10]

- Calcium alginate dressings are promoted as topical haemostats. Limitations to their use have been found which include:
rupture of surface capillaries through mechanical friction,

re-bleeding at the site of a previous bleed on removal of the dressing, particularly from the wound margins.

- Surgical haemostatic sponges are an effective alternative to the alginates, albeit more expensive on a unit cost basis. The natural collagen sponges, for example, have the advantage of not needing to be removed once haemostasis is achieved and are therefore less likely to be associated with the re-bleeding problem.

- Attention to the following issues at the change of a dressing can significantly reduce the incidence of bleeding:
  dressing application and removal techniques,
  maintenance of humidity at the wound and dressing interface,
  cleaning techniques,
  avoidance of fibrous materials (e.g. alginates and carboxymethylcellulose dressings) for friable tumours where the capillaries are visible to the naked eye.

LOCAL WOUND DRESSINGS

Local wound management is determined by the location, size and shape of the wound, not the cancer aetiology. Current practice in wound care, including the manufacturing focus for wound dressings, is still based on Winter's moist wound healing theory (MWHT).[11] Although MWHT explains the profound influence on epithelialization of restricting the evaporation of water from the wound surface, it does not adequately explain exudate management in malignant wounds. As a consequence, exudate may not be managed effectively with dressings that are designed to conserve moisture for epithelialization. Exudate leakage is a dominant problem,[1,12] whose essence is summarized below.

- The efficacy of dressings for the parameters of absorptive capacity, retention of fluid and/or venting of excess fluid across the back surface of the dressing is traditionally demonstrated according to defined laboratory protocols. This does not translate into clinical efficacy without the ability to ensure precise dressing fit, including methods of fixation. Key problems include:
  exudate leakage,
  soiling of personal clothes,
  a need to re-pad, re-fix or renew the dressings between planned changes.

- Absorption of exudate into gauze, alginate, gel and foam dressings is the principal method of managing exudate. However, this reliance on absorptive capacity may not be efficient. Standard and novel wound dressings are classified in systems (Table 9.2) according to the permeability of the material.[1] The materials for systems 1–4 range from permeable gauze and semi-occlusive foams to occlusive hydrocolloids and glycerine-based gel sheets.
  The permeable gauze systems were associated with variable dehydration of the primary wound contact layer, with adherence and trauma in apparently wet wounds.

Table 9.2 Local wound dressings

System 1: non-adherent wound contact layer with gauze pad and fixation material
System 2: absorbent fibrous alginate/methylcarboxycellulose wound contact layer with gauze pad and fixation method
System 3: semi-permeable foam and fixation method
System 4: occlusive gel sheets/hydrocolloids
System 5: sheet hydrogel and high moisture vapour loss (HMVL) polyurethane film
System 6: non-adherent wound contact layer, gauze pad and HMVL polyurethane film
System 7: fibrous and non-fibrous alginate and HMVL polyurethane film
System 8: incontinence products for perineal wounds

The semi-occlusive foam dressings were difficult to fit and needed additional absorbent dressings next to the wound and padding on top of the foam to improve the contact between the dressings and the exuding membranes. The occlusive hydrocolloids were also difficult to fit and had limited absorptive capacity. They were associated with the need to repeat the dressing or re-pad within 2 hours because of exudate leakage.

The gel sheets were more flexible and had a higher absorptive capacity. However, when they became heavy with exudate, the fixation methods did not tolerate the weight and the dressings failed.

- Systems 5–7 included novel materials in the form of non-fibrous alginates, hydrogel sheets and high moisture vapour loss (HMVL) polyurethane films. They comprised a fluid management system with the following components:
  a conformable primary wound contact layer which is non-adherent and in precise contact with the exuding wound surface;
  reservoir capacity in the primary wound contact layer;
  controlled venting capacity for excess exudate through the back surface of the secondary dressing over a range of $>3,000$ to $>10\,000\,g/m^2$ per 24 hours.

The dressings are not available through the normal supply chains at the time of writing. To accommodate the exudate management problems observed, including the potential for extensive loss of skin with this condition, the manufacturers have been approached to provide the above materials in their component parts and in metre rolls, in addition to the current convention of pre-sized composite dressings.

- System 8 incontinence products have not been evaluated against the unifying theory of moist wound healing. These patients need a careful choice of pad, which includes a top dry weave system across its full surface area, to prevent exudate and effluent from leeching back on to the skin. In conjunction with the alcohol-free barrier products mentioned earlier, excoriated skin conditions that are associated with the unrelieved presence of fluid on the skin may be minimized.

A glossary of wound care products and their modes of actions are displayed against malignant wound management goals in the appendix at the end of this chapter.

CONCLUSIONS

This chapter describes the variable presentation of malignant wounds. In the absence of effective treatment, either through patient choice or tumour resistance to conventional anti-cancer treatments, malignant infiltration of the skin progresses with the potential for massive damage to the skin, the supporting structures and organs local to the wound. The overall goal of the management of malignant wounds is to provide the least burdensome means of reducing the impact of the wound on patients and those around them.

Symptom control measures and local wound dressings are the mainstays of the management of these wounds. This chapter focuses on novel approaches to the management of intractable problems from malignant wounds, in particular the management of exudate. Limitations in the performance of wound care products for the management of exudate are identified, together with potential solutions.

KEY POINTS

- Dressing materials need to be supplied in component parts that can be assembled into systems according to patient need.
- Particular attention should be paid to the fit of primary wound contact dressings and secondary fixation material, together with high moisture vapour loss potential.
- High moisture vapour loss potential is crucial to vent exudate that is in excess to the moisture requirements at the wound/dressing interface, in order to prevent both leakage and adherence.

REFERENCES

1. Grocott P. An evaluation of the palliative management of fungating malignant wounds, within a multiple case study design. Unpublished PhD thesis. London: King's College, University of London, 2000.
2. Thomas S. *Current practices in the management of fungating lesions and radiation damaged skin*. Mid Glamorgan: Surgical Materials Testing Laboratory, 1992, 32.
3. Sainsbury R, Vaizey C, Pastarino U, Mould T, Emberton M. Surgical palliation. In: Doyle D, Hanks G, Cherny N, Calman K (eds), *Oxford textbook of palliative medicine*, 3rd edition. Oxford: Oxford University Press, 2004, 255–66.
4. Back IN, Finlay I. Analgesic effect of topical opioids on painful skin ulcers. *J Pain Symptom Manage* 1995; **10**, 493.
5. Zylicz Z, Smits C, Chem D, Krajnik M. Paroxetine for pruritus in advanced cancer. *J Pain Symptom Manag* 1995; **16**, 121–4.

6. Hampson JP. The use of metronidazole in the treatment of malodorous wounds. *J Wound Care* 1996; **5**, 421–6.

7. Suarez FL, Springfield J, Levitt MD. Identification of gases responsible for the odour of human flatus and evaluation of a device purported to reduce this odour. *Gut* 1998; **4**, 100–4.

8. Vowden K, Vowden P. Wound debridement. Part 1: Non-sharp techniques. *J Wound Care* 1999; **8**, 237–42.

9. Cooper R, Molan P. The use of honey as an antiseptic in managing *Pseudomonas* infection. *J Wound Care* 1999; **8**, 161–9.

10. Regnard C, Tempest S. *A guide to symptom relief in advanced disease*, 4th edn. London: Hague, Hochland & Hochland, 1998.

11. Winter GD. Formation of the scab and the rate of epithelialisation of superficial wounds in the skin of the young domestic pig. *Nature* 1962; **193**, 293–4.

12. Grocott P. The palliative management of fungating malignant wounds. *J Wound Care* 2000; **9**, 4–9.

FURTHER READING

Grocott P, Dealey C. Skin problems in palliative medicine: Nursing aspects. In: Doyle D, Hanks G, Cherny N, Calman K (eds), *Oxford textbook of palliative medicine*, 3rd edn. Oxford: Oxford University Press, 2004, 628–40.

APPENDIX: WOUND CARE PRODUCTS FOR LOCAL MANAGEMENT OF MALIGNANT WOUNDS

Individual patient assessment and management planning is crucial to the achievement of optimal outcomes. The following provides a list of generic products and their modes of action which may be considered for the management of key local symptoms and potential problems at the wound site. The product information sheets provided with the proprietary brands give detailed guidance for the use of individual products. See http://www.worldwidewounds.com for a continually updated resource on wound care products and their availability.

Management goal	Wound care product	Mode of action
Protection of the peri-wound skin	Alcohol-free barrier products: aerosols, wipes, sponge applicators, durable barrier creams	Providing protection, via a colourless barrier, to the peri-wound skin from irritation, excoriation and maceration from exudate and other body fluids
Control of wound odour	Option 1. Topical metronidazole gels	Inhibit the concentration of anaerobic bacteria within the wound bed
	Option 2. Topical medical grade honey dressings	Exert an antibacterial effect
	Option 3. Debriding agents: topical medical grade honey dressings, hydrogels, hydrocolloids, alginates, hydrofibres	Remove the dead tissue, which is an ideal environment for bacterial colonization. The products interact with devitalized tissue and exudate, promote autolysis and create a moist interface between the dressing and the wound, and painless removal

Control of bleeding	Option 1: Surgical haemostatic sponges Option 2: Adrenaline 1:1000 applied to the bleeding point via a pad and light pressure Option 3: Sucralfate suspension applied to bleeding point via a pad and light pressure	Promote haemostasis
Control of exudate	Option 1. Absorbent composite dressings with or without adhesive border: • An absorbent non-adherent composite dressing (e.g. foams, absorbent gel sheets) • Fixation tape, film, tapeless retention bandage/garment Option 2. A fluid handling system with the following core components: • Non-adherent primary wound contact layer (e.g. silicone/gel sheet layer, alginate, hydrofibre) • Absorbent secondary layer (e.g. dressing pad (omit if alginate/hydrofibre + film dressing handles exudate)) • Fixation tape, films, tapeless retention bandage/garment	Absorbs exudate and takes it into the dressing matrix, prevents it from tracking back to the peri-wound skin; the non-adherent layer between the wound and dressing prevents trauma and pain at removal The action is as for Option 1 but the systems approach may give more flexibility to fitting the dressings to eccentrically shaped wounds. The absorptive capacity of the system can be increased to manage heavily exuding wounds (i.e. the fibrous layer may be multi-layered and the absorbent pad added)

chapter 10

LYMPHOEDEMA

Ann Elfred

INTRODUCTION

Lymphoedema is a chronic swelling due primarily to a failure of lymph drainage.[1] It is most likely to affect a limb, because of limited drainage at the root of the limb, but may also extend into the adjacent trunk quadrant or occur in the midline, affecting the face or genitalia. As disease advances, oedema may become more widespread.

There are a number of reasons why oedema may occur in advanced disease, including:

- cardiac failure

- renal failure

- hypoproteinaemia, e.g. due to liver disease

- lymphatic obstruction

- venous obstruction, e.g. deep vein thrombosis, vena caval obstruction

- local infection or inflammation.

- related to medication, e.g. steroids

Frequently, a number of conditions may co-exist, producing an oedema of mixed origin, which is then exacerbated by immobility and limb dependency.

A number of classifications for lymphoedema have been put forward,[2] but it is generally classified as:

- primary lymphoedema – of congenital or idiopathic origin,

- secondary lymphoedema – resulting from acquired damage. Such secondary damage may result from:
  infection
  inflammation
  trauma
  malignancy or its treatment.

This chapter concentrates on the presentation and management of secondary lymphoedema resulting from cancer or its treatment.

PREVALENCE

Cancer-related lymphoedema is the most common form in the Western world and may be the direct result of the malignancy itself or due to surgery or radiotherapy. Lymphoedema may be associated with a number of tumours, including;

- breast cancer

- pelvic tumours (e.g. gynaecological, prostate, colon)

- melanomas

- sarcomas.

In a prospective study of referrals to 27 lymphoedema treatment units in the UK, 80 per cent had cancer-related lymphoedema and 86 per cent were female.[3]

Upper limb oedema is a common complication of breast cancer. One series of 1077 women treated for unilateral breast cancer showed a prevalence of 28 per cent[4] and identified significantly higher occurrence in patients treated with mastectomy compared to lumpectomy. Radiotherapy doubled the risk of arm swelling. Another study found a 25.5 per cent incidence of lymphoedema following treatment for operable breast cancer, rising to 38.3 per cent after axillary clearance plus radiotherapy.[5]

Few studies are available investigating incidence in the lower limbs, where a number of conditions may cause lymphoedema. One investigated the incidence of lymphoedema following groin dissection (the sample included melanoma, soft tissue sarcoma and squamous cell carcinoma) and found a 26 per cent incidence where the primary lesion was in the leg, compared with 6 per cent when in the lower trunk.[6] This rose to 45.8 per cent in patients who were non-compliant with a prophylactic regime of elevation and elastic hosiery.

PATHOPHYSIOLOGY

Lymphoedema occurs where there is imbalance between capillary filtration and lymphatic drainage, causing the accumulation of protein-rich fluid in the tissues.[7]

Fluid exchange between the capillaries and interstitium is governed by Starling's principle, involving the balance between a number of forces (filtration, hydrostatic and osmotic pressures).[8] The venous and lymphatic systems are responsible for the drainage of water, proteins, electrolytes and cell debris. In particular, the lymphatics receive protein and macromolecules too large to re-enter the blood vessels. Lymph is propelled from the initial lymphatics to the first vessels by external compression resulting from limb and tissue movements and blood vessel pulsation, and continues by active contraction of the lymph vessel walls.

Oedema will result either from excessive tissue fluid formation, which may, for example, be due to:

- increased venous pressure, causing increased filtration, e.g. due to cardiac failure,

- hypoproteinaemia, causing decreased plasma colloid osmotic pressure, e.g. due to liver or renal disease,

- inflammation,

or from a failure of drainage. This may result:

- directly from tumour obstruction,

- from surgical excision of nodes and vessels,

- from fibrosis due to radiotherapy.

Lymphoedema has traditionally been regarded as a 'high protein oedema' and is associated with the accumulation in the tissues of fibrous tissue and fat, giving the characteristic non-pitting presentation. More recent research casts some doubt upon this, suggesting a possible vascular or haemodynamic contribution, but study findings conflict.[9]

The development of lymphoedema is frequently associated with inflammatory processes caused by infections such as bacterial lymphangitis and cellulitis, resulting in further obliteration of vessels.[10]

CLINICAL FEATURES

The International Society of Lymphology has a graded classification of lymphoedema.

Grade 1:
    minimal or no fibrosis
    oedema pits on pressure
    oedema reduces on limb elevation.

Grade 2:
    substantial fibrosis
    oedema does not pit on pressure
    oedema does not reduce with limb elevation.

Grade 3:
    grade 2 plus trophic skin changes (elephantiasis).

Left untreated, lymphoedema will tend to increase in volume and grade with time.[11] Skin changes are important both clinically and diagnostically and develop over time. Features may include:

- inability to pick up a skinfold (at the base of the second toe, referred to as Stemmer's sign),

- increased skin thickness,

- deepening of skin creases,

- hyperkeratosis (scaly skin build-up).

This may eventually result in the build-up of nodules and produce a warty or 'cobblestone' appearance known as papillomatosis. These changes are frequently complicated and exacerbated by recurrent infections or acute inflammatory episodes.

PAIN

Pain or discomfort associated with lymphoedema was found to occur in 50 per cent of patients in one study.[12] An audit at St Christopher's Hospice found 82 per cent of lymphoedema patients to have pain at first assessment in 2003.

Pain may be directly due to the increase in volume, causing a heavy, aching sensation which may be associated with a feeling of tightness or bursting. It may also be due to associated factors, such as:

- inflammation

- musculoskeletal strain

- neuropathic pain, e.g. from tumour infiltration or due to fibrous entrapment by lymphoedema.

MUSCULOSKELETAL PROBLEMS

Reduced range of movement and muscle weakness may both be associated with lymphoedema, resulting in functional impairment and reduction of muscle pump activity, which will tend to exacerbate oedema formation, so establishing a vicious cycle. This may be particularly apparent if there is neurological impairment.

LYMPHORRHOEA

Lymphorrhoea is the leakage of lymph through the skin. It may be a particular problem in palliative care and can be difficult to manage.[13]

PSYCHOSOCIAL ISSUES

Lymphoedema may have considerable psychological impact[14] including poor body image, embarrassment, anxiety and depression.[15]

INVESTIGATIONS AND EXAMINATION

The diagnosis of lymphoedema is usually clinical, being made on the basis of history and examination findings. The term 'lymphoedema' is sometimes used in a rather general way. It is therefore important that other causes of oedema are excluded, as their management may differ. In particular, it is important that venous abnormalities such as deep vein thrombosis (DVT) are excluded – if this is considered a possible diagnosis, Doppler ultrasound should be considered.

In larger centres, techniques such as computed tomography (CT), magnetic resonance imaging (MRI) lymphography and lymphoscintigraphy may be available. These may assist in confirming malignant disease as the cause of lymphoedema, illustrating its extent and demonstrating a response to treatment.[16] However, they are seldom appropriate for patients with established advanced disease.

Clinical examination should include the following.

- Examination of the skin for:
  integrity
  quality
  signs of infection/inflammation.

- Measurement of limb volume: there is no standardized way of doing this; in the UK a commonly employed method is to measure the limb circumference at 4 cm intervals and calculate the volume using the formula:

$$\text{Volume per section} = \frac{\text{circumference}^2}{\pi}$$

These sections are then summated and may be compared to the unaffected limb, where swelling is unilateral.

In some centres, electronic measuring devices are available. Where disease is advanced, and volume reduction unlikely, such detailed measurements may be inappropriate if they serve only to highlight deterioration.

- Grade of swelling (see p. 308).

- Assessment for the presence of truncal or midline oedema and its extent. Genital oedema is a particularly distressing complication.

- Range of movement.

- Muscle power.

- Neurological integrity.

- Functional impairment.

It is also important to assess the impact that lymphoedema is having on the patient's life and his or her treatment priorities, including any psychosocial implications.

MANAGEMENT

The evidence base for lymphoedema treatments is generally poor, comprising mainly 'before and after' descriptive studies, with a lack of consensus on many aspects of care.[17] This is especially true in palliative care where there are particular difficulties in conducting research trials.[18]

Current consensus is that conservative methods are the most effective in the management of lymphoedema.[19] In the UK, this approach is based on the methods developed in the Foldi Clinic in Germany, termed complex decongestive physical therapy.[20] A number of terms have been used for this approach and various regimes adopted throughout the world, but all are based on the four cornerstones of:

- skin care

- compression

- exercise

- massage.

In this chapter, the term complex physical therapy (CPT) is used.

SKIN CARE

The aim is to maintain the skin in a healthy condition and thereby reduce the risk of infection and irritation.[21] Daily care of the affected region should include meticulous hygiene (including drying of the skin), particularly in skinfolds, and moisturization with an emollient.

Patients also need to be instructed in routine vigilance and precautions, for example:

- avoiding accidental injury (scratches, burns etc.),

- avoiding venepuncture/medical trauma,[22]

- avoiding insect bites where possible – if they occur, they should be cleaned promptly with antiseptic, adding antibiotics at any sign of infection.

Acute inflammatory episodes are a serious complication of lymphoedema, requiring prompt treatment.[23] They are characterized by:

- a general feeling of being unwell,

- heat, redness and increased swelling in the affected region,

- possibly pain, rash or pyrexia.

They will tend to recur, causing the lymphoedema to deteriorate. Treatment is rest and antibiotics.[23] Some patients may present with a chronic, low-grade infection, for which long-term antibiotics are necessary.

Complex physical therapy may give a sustained improvement in skin condition and reduction of acute inflammatory episodes.[24]

COMPRESSION

The aims of compression are twofold:

- to reduce new lymph formation,

- to enhance lymphatic drainage by improving muscle-pump efficiency.

Compression may be applied by the use of either hosiery or bandages.

MULTI-LAYER BANDAGING

Multi-layer bandaging (MLB) is used either as part of an intensive phase of treatment, or may be adopted for symptomatic relief in palliative situations where hosiery would be inappropriate. Indications include:

- severe lymphoedema (where hosiery cannot be fitted),

- fragile skin (where hosiery might cause damage),

- lymphorrhoea or ulceration,

- irregular or disproportionate limb shape,

- enhanced skinfolds,

- swollen digits,

- fibrosis.

Short-stretch bandages are used at low resting pressure, built up in layers with padding. The rationale is that sub-bandage pressure will rise as skeletal muscle contracts.

Multi-layer bandaging is a specialist skill, requiring training and supervised practice. It is contraindicated by arterial insufficiency, DVT and infection. It should not cause pain, discolouration or altered sensation.

Compression should be used only with caution where there is any degree of cardiac failure, and should be started gently and built up gradually.

HOSIERY

Elastic hosiery is used as part of the maintenance regime of lymphoedema. It may either be used following an intensive course of CPT (including MLB, where indicated), or applied at the start of therapy with smaller limbs or uncomplicated lymphoedemas. Careful prescription and monitoring are essential, especially when treatment is starting, to ensure that garments are properly fitting and comfortable and that patients (or carers) are able to apply and remove them.

EXERCISE

Active exercises are an integral part of lymphoedema management. They are prescribed to:

- enhance venous and lymphatic drainage[25] (most effective if performed with the limb contained in bandages or hosiery),

- to maintain or improve range of movement,

- to maintain or improve muscle strength,

- to improve posture,

- to maximize function.

Where voluntary active exercise is not possible, assisted or passive exercise should be substituted, using slow, rhythmical movements.

Advice should also be given regarding function and positioning.

MASSAGE

Various forms of massage have long been used to stimulate venous and lymphatic drainage.[26]

A specialist form of massage, manual lymphatic drainage (MLD), has been developed for the management of lymphoedema. This is a very gentle type of skin massage, using specific movements in certain directions, based on the anatomy and physiology of the lymphatic system.

Various 'schools' of MLD have developed (e.g. Vodder, Leduc, Casley-Smith), but all follow the same principles. MLD aims to:

- enhance the removal of protein from the tissues,

- increase lymphatic drainage without increasing capillary filtration.[27]

A modified form of MLD, simple lymphatic drainage (SLD), may be used by therapists or taught to patients and carers.

PNEUMATIC COMPRESSION THERAPY

Pneumatic compression therapy (PCT) is a form of therapy comprising an inflatable sleeve (single or multi-chambered) attached to an electrical pump, which encases the limb and is cyclically inflated and deflated. It has been used for a number of years in the management of lymphoedema.[28-30]

Concerns are now being expressed regarding the use of PCT, particularly with lower limb lymphoedema, where it may precipitate genital oedema,[31] also that pressures produced may be greater than that indicated on the unit's control device. It may be used with caution and supervision as part of the management of non-obstructive oedemas that do not involve the root of the limb or trunk and at low target pressures.

TREATMENT REGIMES

The successful management of lymphoedema requires a comprehensive approach. The above strategies are generally used in combination, and few data exist for the effectiveness of each element individually. Treatment regimes will vary in the detail of their protocols, for although evidence is published for the efficacy of this combined approach,[14,24,33-7] the quality of research evidence for treatment programmes is quite poor, being based mainly on descriptive studies.[17]

OEDEMA IN ADVANCED DISEASE

As disease advances, previously well-controlled lymphoedema may deteriorate or become complicated by other pathologies such as superior or inferior vena caval obstruction, hypoproteinaemia, neurological deficits and immobility.[38] Oedema may be localized or widespread, limiting management options.

Where tumour is rapidly extending, improvement in the oedema is unlikely, but modification of the techniques described may be used to ease discomfort and provide psychological support. The burden of treatment should not outweigh any expected benefit.

Therapy should concentrate on measures for comfort and quality of life, such as:

- skin care

- support and positioning, with elevation

- gentle exercise (passive or assisted where necessary)

- simple massage/MLD

- light garments or modified bandaging, where they improve comfort

- combined with other symptom control measures as required, e.g. appropriate analgesia, management of ulceration or fungating wounds.

In these ways, support can be given to both patients and carers to optimize comfort and quality of life until the end of life.

KEY POINTS

- Physical therapies for lymphoedema may have both symptomatic and psychosocial benefits.
- Benefits of combined therapy may include:
  volume reduction,
  improved skin condition,
  reduction in inflammatory episodes,
  decreased pain,
  improved strength,
  improved mobility,
  increased energy,
  psychological support.
- In palliative care, the burden of treatment should not outweigh benefit, the main aim being to improve quality of life.

REFERENCES

1. British Lymphology Society (BLS). *Strategy for lymphoedema care.* 1998. (Available from: BLS Administration Centre, PO Box 1059, Caterham, Surrey CR3 6ZU, England.)

2. Keeley V. Classification of lymphoedema. In: Twycross R, Jenns K, Todd J (eds), *Lymphoedema*. Abingdon: Radcliffe Medical Press, 2000, 22–43.

3. Sitzia J, Woods M, Hine P, Williams A, Eaton K, Green G. Characteristics of new referrals to twenty-seven lymphoedema treatment units. *Eur J Cancer Care* 1998; 7, 255–62.

4. Mortimer P, Bates D, Brassington H, Stanton A, Strachan D, Levick J. The prevalence of arm oedema following treatment for breast cancer. *Q J Med* 1996; **89**, 377–80.

5. Kissin M, Querci della Rovere G, Easton D, Westbury G. Risk of lymphoedema following the treatment of breast cancer. *Br J Surg* 1986; **73**, 580–4.

6. Karakousis C, Heiser M, Moore R. Lymphoedema after groin dissection. *Am J Surg* 1983; **145**, 205–8.

7. Mortimer P. Investigation and management of lymphoedema. *Vasc Med Rev* 1990; **1**, 1–20.

8. Stanton A. How does tissue swelling occur? The physiology and pathophysiology of interstitial fluid formation. In: Twycross R, Jenns K, Todd J (eds), *Lymphoedema*. Abingdon: Radcliffe Medical Press, 2000, 11–21.

9. Martin D. The pathophysiology of carcinoma related lymphoedema. *Newsletter of the British Lymphology Society* 2003; Issue 39(Sept/Oct), 3–5.

10. Mortimer P, Badger C, Hall J. Lymphoedema. In: Doyle D, Hanks G, Macdonald N (eds), *Oxford textbook of palliative medicine*, 2nd edn. Oxford: Oxford University Press, 1998, 657–65.

11. Casley-Smith JR. Alterations of untreated lymphoedema and its grades over time. *Lymphology* 1995; **28**, 174–85.

12. Carroll D, Rose K. Treatment leads to significant improvement. Effect of conservative treatment on pain in lymphoedema. *Professional Nurse* 1992; **8**(1), 32–6.

13. Ling J, Duncan A, Laverty D, Hardy J. Lymphorrhoea in palliative care. *Eur J Palliat Care* 1997; **4**(2), 50–2.

14. Sitzia J, Sobrido L. Measurement of health-related quality of life of patients receiving conservative treatment for limb lymphoedema using the Nottingham Health Profile. *Qual Life Res* 1997; **6**, 373–84.

15. Woods M. Patients' perception of breast cancer-related lymphoedema. *Eur J Cancer Care* 1993; **2**, 125–8.

16. Keeley V. Clinical features of lymphoedema. In: Twycross R, Jenns K, Todd J (eds), *Lymphoedema*. Abingdon: Radcliffe Medical Press, 2000, 44–67.

17. Sitzia J, Harlow W. Lymphoedema 4: research priorities in lymphoedema care. *Br J Nurs* 2002; **11**(8), 531–41.

18. Everett J. How strong is the evidence base underpinning present practice in lymphoedema management? *Newsletter of the British Lymphology Society* 2003; **38**, 3–8.

19. Jenns K. Management strategies. In: Twycross R, Jenns K, Todd J (eds), *Lymphoedema*. Abingdon: Radcliffe Medical Press, 2000, 97–117.

20. Foldi E, Foldi M, Weissleder H. Conservative treatment of lymphoedema of the limbs. *Angiology – J Vasc Dis* 1985; **36**, 171–80.

21. Ryan T. Caring for the skin, modern know-how adds urgency. *Newsletter of the British Lymphology Society* 2004; **41**, 6.

22. Smith J. The practice of venepuncture in lymphoedema. *Eur J Cancer Care* 1998; 7, 97–8.

23. Mortimer P. Acute inflammatory episodes. In: Twycross R, Jenns K, Todd J (eds), *Lymphoedema*. Abingdon: Radcliffe Medical Press, 2000; 130–9.

24. Todd J. A study of lymphoedema patients over their first six months of treatment. *Physiotherapy* 1999; **85**(2), 65–76.
25. Casley-Smith JR, Casley-Smith JR. *Modern treatment for lymphoedema.* Adelaide: Lymphoedema Association of Australia Inc., 1994.
26. Wood G, Becker P. *Beard's massage*, 3rd edn. Philadelphia: WB Saunders, 1981, 26–7.
27. British Lymphology Society (BLS). *Guidelines for the use of manual lymphatic drainage (MLD) and simple lymphatic drainage (SLD) in lymphoedema*, 2nd edn, 1999. (Available from the BLS Administration Centre – see reference 1 for address.)
28. Raines J, O'Donnell T, Kalisher L, Darling R. Selection of patients with lymphedema for compression therapy. *Am J Surg* 1997; **133**, 430–7.
29. Swedborg I. Effects of treatment with an elastic sleeve and intermittent pneumatic compression in post-mastectomy patients with lymphoedema of the arm. *Scand J Rehab Med* 1984; **16**, 35–41.
30. Newman G. Which patients with arm oedema are helped by intermittent external pneumatic compression therapy. *J R Soc Med* 1988; **81**, 377–9.
31. Boris M, Weindorf S, Lasinski B. The risk of genital oedema after external pump compression for lower limb lymphedema. *Lymphology* 1998; **31**, 15–20.
32. Segers P, Belgrado JP, Leduc A, Leduc O, Verdonck P. Excessive pressure in multi-chambered cuffs used for sequential compression therapy. *Physical Therapy* 2002; **84**(10), 1000–8.
33. Hutzschenreuter P, Wittlinger H, Wittlinger G, Kurz I. Post-mastectomy arm lymphoedema: treated by manual lymph drainage and compression bandage therapy. *Eur J Phys Med Rehab* 1991; **1**(6), 166–70.
34. Rose K. Volume reduction of arm lymphoedema. *Nurs Stand* 1993; **7**(35), 29–32.
35. Matthews K, Smith J. Effectiveness of modified complex physical therapy for lymphoedema treatment. *Aust Physiother* 1996; **42**(4), 323–7.
36. Boris M, Weindorf S, Lasinski B. Persistence of lymphoedema reduction after noninvasive complex lymphoedema therapy. *Oncology* 1997; **11**(1), 99–114.
37. Franzeck U, Spiegal I, Fischer M, Bortzler G, Stahel H, Bollinger A. Combined physical therapy for lymphoedema evaluated by fluorescence microlymphography and lymph capillary pressure measurements. *J Vasc Res* 1997; **34**, 306–11.
38. Keeley V. Oedema in advanced cancer. In: Twycross R, Jenns K, Todd J (eds), *Lymphoedema*. Abingdon: Radcliffe Medical Press, 2000, 338–58.

FURTHER READING

Twycross R, Jenns K, Todd J (eds). *Lymphoedema*. Abingdon: Radcliffe Medical Press, 2000.

SYSTEMATIC REVIEWS

Megens A, Harris S. Physical therapist management of lymphoedema following treatment for breast cancer: a critical review of its effectiveness. *Phys Ther* 1998; 78(12), 1302–11.

CLINICAL CHALLENGES IN NON-MALIGNANT DISEASE

chapter 11

CLINICAL CHALLENGES IN NON-MALIGNANT DISEASE: OVERVIEW

Julia M. Addington-Hall

INTRODUCTION

The development of the modern hospice movement, in the UK and the USA, challenged conventional thinking that symptoms could not be controlled and that death was failure. Although a small number of homes for the dying had existed for many years, the development by Dame Cicely Saunders of St Christopher's Hospice in South London in 1967 marks for many the beginning of a modern hospice movement. Dame Cicely did not just want to improve care for the patients admitted to St Christopher's; by combining research, education and clinical care, she sought to revolutionize the care received by all dying cancer patients.[1] Contemporary studies of the experiences of these patients show that such a revolution was badly needed: many terminally ill cancer patients suffered poorly controlled symptoms, received little psychological support, and were largely ignored by doctors.[2,3] As a result of the advances achieved within hospice and palliative care, dying from cancer need no longer be such a distressing and isolating experience.

Hospice care has continued to be focused almost entirely on cancer patient care. In 1994/5, more than 95 per cent of patients who received care from hospice or specialist palliative care services in the UK had a diagnosis of cancer.[4] The initial focus on cancer allowed rapid advances to be made in symptom control and in psychosocial support for patients and families. The continued focus of these services on cancer is, however, increasingly challenged.

CHALLENGES TO CANCER-ONLY PALLIATIVE CARE

ACQUIRED IMMUNE DEFICIENCY SYNDROME

The first major challenge came in the 1980s, when increasing numbers of people were dying from a new illness, acquired immune deficiency syndrome (AIDS).

They were mainly young and experienced considerable symptom distress, in addition to complex psychological and existential concerns heightened by the stigma associated with the diagnosis. Until the discovery of combination therapies in the 1990s, AIDS was always a terminal illness. However, although it had been recognized that the principles and philosophy of modern hospice care might also apply to patients dying from other causes, the emphasis has been on encouraging other areas of medicine to integrate terminal care into their own practice, rather than extending hospice care to these patients.

> ... many of the symptoms to be treated and much of the general management will be relevant to other situations ... Terminal care should not only be part of oncology but of geriatric medicine, neurology, general practice and throughout medicine.[5]

A debate therefore ensued as to whether hospices should extend their provision to include AIDS patients, or whether separate services should be developed. Some of those favouring separate services did so because they believed they should continue to focus on cancer; others were concerned about infection, and about the effects on fund-raising of caring for such a stigmatized group.[6] New AIDS-specific services were developed, partly due to the availability of ring-fenced National Health Service (NHS) monies for AIDS care. However, the pattern of provision has now shifted, with most people with AIDS who require palliative care being cared for by generic, rather than AIDS-specific, services. In part, this is due to changes in the number and characteristics of people dying from AIDS (from primarily being gay men to increasing numbers of heterosexuals, particularly from sub-Saharan Africa) and to changes in funding with the demise of ring-fenced monies. However, it also reflects a greater willingness on the part of generic hospices and palliative care services to care for these patients.

IMPACT OF HEALTH SERVICE REFORMS

The second major challenge to the focus of hospices and palliative care services in the UK on cancer came with the health reforms of the late 1980s. Prior to these, health authorities in England and Wales acted as line managers for local NHS services. The reforms instigated a purchaser/provider split, with health authorities now being responsible for assessing the health needs of their resident population and then purchasing services from community and hospital trusts. This led to a new emphasis on needs assessment when determining NHS funding for hospice and palliative care services. In 1992, an expert report to the Department of Health argued that 'all patients needing them should have access to palliative care services ... although often referred to as equating with terminal cancer care, it is important to recognise that similar services are appropriate for and should be developed for patients dying from other diseases'.[7] With its emphasis on the development of similar, but presumably separate, services, it was consistent with the approach to non-cancer patients adopted by the hospice movement since its inception.

However, the emphasis then changed. In 1994, a Scottish Office Management Executive Letter (MEL (1994) 104) said that 'palliative care is currently provided mainly for people suffering from cancer, but it is increasingly recognised that people with a range of life threatening diseases may also benefit from it'.[8] Similarly, in 1996, an Executive Letter from the NHS Executive on palliative care stated that 'purchasers are asked to ensure that provision of care with a palliative approach is included in all contracts of services for those with cancer and other life-threatening diseases ... although this letter is focused on services for cancer patients, it applies equally to patients with other life-threatening conditions, including AIDS, neurological conditions, and cardiac and respiratory failure'.[9] An epidemiologically-based needs assessment on palliative and terminal care provided guidance on the numbers of people within health authority populations with different diseases who may have needs for palliative care.[10]

These publications focus on providing care informed by the principles of palliative care for non-cancer patients, rather than arguing specifically that hospices and specialist palliative care services should care for non-cancer patients. These services primarily lie outside the NHS and at best are part-funded by it: the NHS does not, therefore, have the authority to insist on this. It is clear, however, that the view of the NHS is that palliative care should be provided on the basis of need, not diagnosis. This is reflected in the National Service Framework for cardiac disease, which has specified that patients with severe heart failure should have access to specialist palliative care services.[11]

In the UK at least, the rhetoric around palliative care provision has shifted from one primarily concerned with cancer patients to one that argues that it should be provided to all patients who need it. Of course, this need not necessarily lead to any significant shift in service provision. Educating other health professionals in the palliative care approach is essential. In addition, cancer patients may be in greater need of palliative care than other patients and may therefore continue to receive the bulk of hospice and palliative care provision.

PALLIATIVE CARE NEEDS OF NON-CANCER PATIENTS

There is, however, growing evidence that cancer patients do not necessarily have more palliative care needs than other patients with advanced or life-threatening illnesses. Patients who die from chronic conditions such as chronic heart failure (CHF) and chronic obstructive pulmonary disease (COPD) have also been reported to experience poor symptom control, a lack of psychological and social support, inadequate personal care, and a lack of open communication with health professionals in their last months of life.[12] Similar problems have been reported for patients with shorter dying trajectories, such as post-dialysis renal patients.[13] According to bereaved relatives' reports, one in six people who die from non-malignant disease have similar symptom severity to the most symptomatic half of hospice patients.[14] Cancer patients are clearly not alone in experiencing physical, psychological, social and existential distress at the end of life. Given that three out of four deaths are not from cancer, the number of non-cancer patients experiencing distress at the end of life may well exceed the number of cancer patients.

The available evidence therefore suggests that if access to hospice and palliative care services in the UK was determined solely on the basis of need, cancer patients would not make up more than 90 per cent of patients, as at present. The needs of non-cancer patients are increasingly recognized within palliative care – as evidenced by the addition of this section to the fourth edition of this textbook. However, there are a number of barriers (real and imagined) to the move beyond cancer,[15] which are discussed below.

BARRIERS TO THE PROVISION OF PALLIATIVE CARE FOR NON-CANCER PATIENTS

ARE SKILLS TRANSFERABLE?

Many health professionals currently working in hospice and specialist palliative care in the UK have a background in oncology, and have developed specialist knowledge in caring for terminally ill cancer patients. They are understandably concerned about the gaps in their own knowledge of, for example, CHF, COPD and AIDS. Palliative care clinicians already working with non-cancer patients emphasize the importance of joint working with the referring team, the patient's GP and district nurse, enabling an exchange of experience and expertise.

Specialists in palliative care may also be concerned about the extent to which their skills are relevant to the care of non-cancer patients. Subsequent chapters in this section demonstrate that palliative care skills do apply outside of cancer, albeit needing modification and re-working in conjunction with existing service providers for each patient.

CAN SUITABLE CANDIDATES BE IDENTIFIED?

Traditionally, hospice and palliative care services have cared for cancer patients for whom death is certain. Some non-cancer patients also have an identifiable, relatively predictable terminal phase – including patients with renal failure who have come off, or never started, dialysis and patients with end-stage liver disease. Judging prognosis is much more difficult in many other non-cancer patients. For example, one study found that CHF patients on the day before death were estimated to have an 80 per cent chance of surviving for two months.[16] Most palliative care services are geared to providing short-term support, rather than long-term care, and fear that services could become overloaded with non-cancer patients who have survived longer than predicted, and who then block access for other patients. This may result in few non-cancer patients being seen as suitable candidates for palliative care.

In cancer, it is increasingly recognized that palliative care may benefit patients throughout the 'cancer journey' – from diagnosis to death. One way of overcoming the difficulties caused by prognostic uncertainty for non-cancer patients might be to develop a similar model, with palliative care services contributing to the development and provision of symptom control, psychological support, family care and existential support throughout the disease trajectory. Taken to its logical conclusion, this could lead to patients receiving care from two teams – one concerned with the body and the other with the whole person. This would clearly be undesirable. It also overlooks the fact that palliative care is not alone in placing emphasis on the importance of holistic care – general practice, care of the elderly, and nursing all see this as important. Further research is therefore needed to enable a better understanding of the needs of non-cancer patients, of those that come within the remit of palliative care, and of appropriate models of service provision.[17]

TOO MUCH NEED, TOO FEW SERVICES?

Faced with growing evidence of unmet need amongst non-cancer patients at the end of life, palliative care professionals may fear their services being swamped with new referrals. Certainly, the number of non-cancer patients who experience distressing symptoms in the last year of life is at least as large as the number of cancer patients who currently receive care from hospice and palliative care services. However, there is no evidence to date that services are overwhelmed when they accept non-cancer patients; few appear to be referred to specialist palliative care services. Several factors may influence this, including the following.

- The difficulty of judging whether and when non-cancer patients are eligible for these services.

- The emphasis of much of medicine is on cure: this may result in a reluctance to recognize when no further treatment is warranted – or to be able to see that patients with an uncertain prognosis might benefit from palliative care support alongside active treatment.

- Non-cancer patients may not want to access services associated with cancer care – and terminal cancer care at that.

These factors are likely to change, especially if hospice and palliative care services are seen to benefit non-cancer patients. In the meantime, there is probably time for these services to move slowly into non-cancer care, building expertise and developing appropriate service models as they do so.

One team with particular experience in providing palliative care to non-cancer patients argues that it is important to recognize that not all non-cancer patients (and, indeed, not all cancer patients) require the full range of palliative care services. Three tiers of care may be provided:

- one-off consultation between the referring team and the palliative care team;

- short-term interventions, that is, specialist palliative care for a limited time period, with the expectation of discharge established from the beginning and with re-referral offered if required;

- a small number of non-cancer patients may require a continuing commitment from the palliative care team because of the complexity of their needs.[18]

Although the effectiveness of this model of care provision needs to be established, it does suggest one way to handle an increase in non-cancer referrals.

FUNDING

St Christopher's Hospice was set up outside the NHS, albeit with the expectation that the ideas and practices developed within it would then filter back into the NHS. Many hospices and specialist palliative care services remain independent of the NHS and raise most of their money through local fund-raising. It has been estimated that the independent hospice sector as a whole receives no more than a third of its funding from the NHS. Although additional state funding is currently being sought, many value their independent status, primarily because it enables them to develop the services they see as appropriate in their local setting. As outlined above, this means that the Department of Health has limited power to insist that independent hospices provide care on the basis of need, not diagnosis. It also means that services may be very cautious of changes that they fear will reduce support (and hence funding) in the local community. Cancer is still greatly feared in our society, and many people – particularly in the older generations – have powerful memories of appalling deaths from cancer. They are therefore often strongly motivated to support their local hospice. Some hospices fear that the local population will be less willing to support a service caring for non-cancer patients, particularly if, as a consequence, some cancer patients with less complex needs do not receive care. There is no evidence of this to date – and, despite initial fears, the move to include AIDS patients has apparently not adversely affected support for independent hospices. However, funding concerns may make hospices reluctant to take on non-cancer patients.

Outside the voluntary hospice sector, two charities have played important roles in developing and supporting palliative care services. Macmillan Cancer Relief provides 3 years' funding for posts that are subsequently taken over by the NHS. It is best known for funding clinical nurse specialist posts (often known as 'Macmillan nurses'), but it also funds medical and social work posts, and has provided capital funds for new in-patient services. Marie Curie Cancer Care is best known for its nursing service, which provides hands-on care for patients at home, and for its network of palliative care homes. Both are dedicated to the care of cancer patients and, although willing to provide some care to non-cancer patients, will not be able to play the same role in the extension of non-cancer palliative care as they have in cancer. Again, this raises questions of where the funding will come from to allow expansion beyond cancer.

The importance of adequate funding in motivating services to move into non-cancer palliative care is shown in the USA. The majority of patients who receive care from hospice programmes have cancer, but non-cancer patients make up a much higher proportion than in the UK. The National Hospice Organisation fact sheet for Spring 1999 stated that, in 1995, 60 per cent of hospice patients had cancer; 6 per cent had heart-related diagnoses; 4 per cent had AIDS; 1 per cent had renal diagnoses; 2 per cent had Alzheimer's disease; and 27 per cent had 'other' diagnoses. One reason for this is that the MEDICARE hospice programme enables hospices to access funding for non-cancer patients with a limited prognosis as well as for cancer patients. It is interesting to speculate what the greater availability of state funding for hospice and palliative care services in the UK would do to the proportion of non-cancer patients receiving care.

CONCLUSION

This chapter has sought to provide an overview of the reasons why there is increasing emphasis on the palliative care needs of non-cancer patients, and of some of the barriers to meeting these needs. With the exception of motor neurone disease and AIDS, the extension of palliative care beyond cancer is at an early stage and many questions remain to be answered. More research into the palliative care needs of these patients and into appropriate and effective services is needed.[17] Most importantly, hospice and palliative care services already providing care for these patients need to share their experiences. This section of this book is an important opportunity to share what we already know about meeting the palliative care needs of patients with diseases other than cancer. I hope it will encourage others to begin caring for these patients, so that all of us receive high-quality, appropriate care at the end of life, regardless of diagnosis.

KEY POINTS

- From its onset, modern hospice care has been focused almost entirely on the care of cancer patients. More than nine in every ten patients who receive hospice or palliative care in the UK have cancer.
- The focus on cancer has allowed rapid advances to be made in patient and family care.
- It is increasingly recognized, however, that:
  other non-cancer patients might also benefit from palliative care, and
  palliative care should be provided on the basis of need, not diagnosis.
- There is growing evidence that many non-cancer patients have unmet needs at the end of life for symptom control, psychological and social support, and open communication with health professionals.
- Three out of four deaths are not from cancer. The number of non-cancer patients with unmet needs at the end of life may well exceed the number of cancer patients.
- There are a number of barriers to palliative care services moving beyond cancer. These include:
  concerns about whether existing skills and knowledge are transferable,
  difficulties in identifying suitable candidates, given greater prognostic uncertainty outside cancer,
  fears that existing services will be overwhelmed by referrals, and
  anxieties over funding.
- More research is needed into the needs of non-cancer patients at the end of life, of those that come within the remit of palliative care, and of appropriate models of service provision.

REFERENCES

1. De Boulay S. *Cicely Saunders: the founder of the modern hospice movement.* London: Hodder & Stoughton, 1984.
2. Hinton JM. The physical and mental distress of the dying. *Q J Med* 1963; **32**, 1–21.
3. Glaser B, Strauss A. *Awareness of dying.* Chicago: Aldine, 1965.
4. Eve A, Smith AM, Tebbit P. Hospice and palliative care in the UK 1994–5, including a summary of trends 1990–5. *Palliat Med* 1997; **11**, 31–43.
5. Saunders C, Baines M. *Living with dying: the management of terminal disease.* Oxford: Oxford University Press, 1983.
6. Brogan G, George R. HIV/AIDS. In: Addington-Hall JM, Higginson IH (eds), *Palliative care for non-cancer patients.* Oxford: Oxford University Press, 2001, 137–46.
7. Standing Medical Advisory Committee, Standing Nursing and Midwifery Advisory Committee. *The principles and provision of palliative care.* London: Standing Medical Advisory Committee, Standing Nursing and Midwifery Advisory Committee, 1992.
8. Scottish Office. *Contracting for specialist palliative care.* MEL(1994)104. Edinburgh: Scottish Office, 1994.
9. NHS Executive. *A policy framework for commissioning cancer services: palliative care services.* EL(96)85. London: NHS Executive, 1996.
10. Higginson IJ. Health care needs assessment: palliative and terminal care. In: Stevens A, Raftery J (eds), *Health care needs assessment*, 2nd Series. Abingdon: Radcliffe Medical Press, 1997, 1–79.
11. Department of Health. *National Service Framework for coronary heart disease.* London: Department of Health, 2000.
12. Lynn J, Teno JM, Philips RS *et al.* Perceptions by family members of the dying experience of older and seriously ill patients. *Ann Intern Med* 1997; **126**, 97–106.
13. Cohen LM, Reiter G, Poppel DM, Germain MJ. Renal palliative care. In: Addington-Hall JM, Higginson IJ (eds), *Palliative care for non-cancer patients.* Oxford: Oxford University Press, 2001, 103–13.
14. Addington-Hall JM, Fakhoury W, McCarthy M. Specialist palliative care in non-malignant disease. *Palliat Med* 1998; **12**, 417–27.
15. Field D, Addington-Hall JM. Extending specialist palliative care to all? *Soc Sci Med* 1999; **48**, 1271–80.
16. Lynn J, Harrell F Jr, Cohn C, Wagner D, Connors AF Jr. Prognoses of seriously ill hospitalised patients on the day before death: implications for patient care and public policy. *New Horizons* 1997; **5**, 56–61.
17. Addington-Hall JM, Higginson IJ (eds). *Palliative care for non-cancer patients.* Oxford: Oxford University Press, 2001.
18. George RJ, Sykes J. Beyond cancer? In: Clark D, Ahmedzai S, Hockley J (eds), *New themes in palliative care.* Buckingham: Open University Press, 1997, 239–54.

chapter 12

HIV AND AIDS

Sarah Cox

INTRODUCTION

Human immunodeficiency virus (HIV) is a retrovirus and causes infection that is, as yet, incurable. The infection results in a variety of illnesses, which can be prevented by suppressing the virus. The illness experience of a patient with HIV therefore depends on access to and effectiveness of antiretroviral medication. In strong market economy countries, advanced disease is uncommon and problems relate more to the side effects of therapy. Here, symptom management is aimed at enabling individuals to tolerate their life-sustaining treatment. However, in situations in which resistance to treatment has developed or where adherence to therapy is poor, advanced disease can still occur. In these circumstances and in those parts of the world where access to drugs remains poor, devastating problems such as wasting, severe diarrhoea, overwhelming infections, tumours, blindness and dementia may occur.

The palliative care of this group of individuals has some differences from and some similarities to cancer palliative care. HIV-infected individuals are often younger than other patients with advanced disease. Children may also be infected and may lose their parents to infection. In the UK, many affected individuals are from minority groups such as asylum seekers from sub-Saharan Africa and homosexual men. Close adherence to disease-modifying treatment is appropriate, even in advanced illness, and death is difficult to plan for, as it more often occurs during active management. Symptoms are as prevalent in this group, although the profile of symptoms varies.

DEFINITIONS

Human immunodeficiency virus is an RNA virus, which causes predominantly cell-mediated immunodeficiency and is one of the ten major causes of death worldwide. There are two types of HIV that infect humans: HIV-1 and HIV-2. Worldwide, HIV-1 is the commonest virus to cause progressive disease; HIV-2 is found predominantly in West Africa, is less infectious and causes immunodeficiency more slowly than HIV-1.

Table 12.1 CDC AIDS indicator conditions for adolescents and adults[2]

Candidiasis of oesophagus, trachea, bronchi, or lungs
Cervical cancer, invasive
Coccidioidomycosis, extrapulmonary
Cryptococcosis, extrapulmonary
Cryptosporidiosis with diarrhoea for >1 month
Cytomegalovirus of any organ other than liver, spleen or lymph nodes
Herpes simplex with mucocutaneous ulcer for >1 month or bronchitis, pneumonitis, oesophagitis
Histoplasmosis, extrapulmonary
HIV-associated dementia; disabling cognitive and/or motor dysfunction interfering with occupation or
    activities of daily living
HIV-associated wasting; involuntary weight loss of >10% of baseline plus chronic diarrhoea (>2
    loose stools/day for >30 days) or chronic weakness and documented enigmatic fever for >30 days
Isosporiasis with diarrhoea for >1 month
Kaposi's sarcoma
Lymphoma of brain
Lymphoma, non-Hodgkin's of B-cell or unknown immunological phenotype and histology showing
    small, non-cleaved lymphoma or immunoblastic sarcoma
Mycobacterium avium or *M. kansasii*, disseminated
Mycobacterium tuberculosis, pulmonary or disseminated
Nocardiosis
Pneumocystis carinii pneumonia
Pneumonia, recurrent bacterial
Progressive multifocal leukoencephalopathy
Salmonella septicaemia (non-typhoid), recurrent
Strongylosis, extra-intestinal
Toxoplasmosis of internal organ

Acquired immune deficiency syndrome (AIDS) was first described in 1981 in the USA.[1] The immunodeficient state results in increased susceptibility to various conditions, including infections and malignant disease. Some of these conditions are AIDS-defining illnesses. The case definition for AIDS was developed for surveillance purposes and is not particularly useful clinically. Even after experiencing an AIDS-defining illness, an individual's prognosis depends on what options for antiretroviral treatment are left. If some degree of immunocompetence can be restored, the outlook is good (Table 12.1).[2]

Antiretroviral therapy is now given in combinations referred to as highly active antiretroviral therapy (HAART).

INCIDENCE AND PREVALENCE

Human immunodeficiency virus has caused a global epidemic that has exceeded the projections of 10 years ago. The World Health Organisation (WHO) estimates that at the end of the year 2003 there were 40 million people worldwide living with HIV or AIDS.[3] During the same year, 3 million individuals died from the disease. The incidence of HIV in different parts of the world is related to the pattern of spread and the implementation of prevention strategies. HIV prevalence has remained relatively steady in sub-Saharan Africa, with high levels of new infection balanced by high mortality. In Asia and the Pacific, 1 million people acquired HIV in 2003, mostly via injecting drug use and the commercial sex industry. The explosive epidemic in Vietnam demonstrates how rapidly HIV can spread wherever significant levels of injecting drug use occur. More than 2 million people are living with HIV in Latin America and the Caribbean. Stigma and discrimination remain obstacles to the prevention of further infections.

The news from the richer countries of the world is no less gloomy. The rate of new infection is rising because of the low priority placed on prevention. In the UK, the number of new HIV diagnoses reported in 2002 was double that in 1998. A large part of this increase is attributable to individuals infected heterosexually, and more than 70 per cent of these are recorded as acquiring infection abroad. The challenge will be to provide care and prevention programmes to those whose language, culture or immigrant status might otherwise limit their access to services.[4] The HIV-infected population is concentrated in large cities, with 54 per cent of individuals resident in London. It is a disease of younger adults: 76 per cent are aged 15–39 at diagnosis.

The prevalence of HIV infection is rising, as, with effective antiretroviral therapy, there are more individuals living with HIV.

PATHOPHYSIOLOGY

Human immunodeficiency virus infection generally occurs after transfer of bodily fluids from an infected person. The methods of transmission are sexual contact including oral sex; sharing infected needles; transmission from mother to baby before birth, during labour or via breast milk; and inoculation with infected blood and blood products. The virus becomes established in the lymph nodes, where T-helper lymphocytes (CD4 T-cells) and monocytes are infected. After entry to the cell, viral reverse transcriptase forms a DNA template that becomes incorporated into the host DNA before further transcription. Given the right conditions, viral replication can be rapid but is prone to transcriptional error, producing viral mutations.

Acute infection is followed some weeks later by the primed immune system producing neutralizing antibodies. At this time the virus is cleared from the blood and there is a rebound in CD4 T-cell numbers. The virus is not cleared from the body, however, and over subsequent years it replicates in lymph nodes, eventually spilling over into the peripheral blood once more. Progressive immunosuppression occurs partly as a result of viral proteins damaging cellular immune responses such as cytotoxic T lymphocytes.

There is a small group of individuals who have been infected with HIV but do not develop progressive disease. It is suggested that these individuals may have deficiencies in one of the receptors required for viral entry. Other individuals have been infected with defective virus.

Suppression of the virus with combination antiviral therapy can be associated with a rise in CD4 T-cell count. The degree to which the immune system can be reconstituted depends on the level of function prior to treatment.

CLINICAL FEATURES

The clinical consequences of HIV infection largely correlate with the degree of immunosuppression and therefore the CD4 T-cell count.

Seroconversion occurs some weeks after acute infection and 75 per cent of individuals can recognize a period of flu-like illness associated with their body's development of specific antibody responses.

At a CD4 T-cell count above 500×10^6/L, patients may experience generalized lymphadenopathy from the presence of virus in the lymphatic system. Less common features at this time include aseptic meningitis and Guillain–Barré syndrome resulting from the neurotrophic virus.

With more advanced immunological damage, as the CD4 T-cell count falls below 500×10^6/L, patients experience increased susceptibility to opportunistic infections, diseases of the central nervous system and malignancies. Oesophageal candida, recurrent bacterial pneumonia, Kaposi's sarcoma and non-Hodgkin's lymphoma are examples.

If the CD4 T-cell count falls below 200×10^6/L, prophylaxis against infection with *Pneumocystis carinii* pneumonia should be prescribed. At this level of immune dysfunction, patients are also at risk from cerebral toxoplasmosis, progressive multifocal leukoencephalopathy, dementia and wasting disease. Cytomegalovirus infection causing retinitis and colitis and disseminated non-tuberculous mycobacterial infection occur at CD4 T-cell counts less than 50×10^6/L.

STANDARD TREATMENT APPROACHES IN ADVANCED DISEASE

The principles of treatment in HIV/AIDS are:

- effective antiretroviral therapy can suppress HIV replication,

- CD4 T-cells recover, restoring immune function,

- at elevated CD4 T-cell levels, the patient experiences less illness.

But:

- HIV is prone to mutation because of rapid viral replication,

- some mutated virus will not be sensitive to individual drugs and will multiply, causing further immune damage,

- single or dual drug regimens result in the development of resistance more quickly than three or more,
- resistant HIV (treatment failure) is more likely to emerge if the virus is incompletely suppressed.

So:

- combinations of drugs are used that interfere with different stages of HIV replication,
- strict adherence (95 per cent of medication taken) to the regimen must be advised to suppress the virus completely,
- care must be taken with drug interactions and drug holidays.

Preventing the immunological consequences of HIV infection is the most effective way to improve quality of life as well as prognosis. As a result, complex antiretroviral regimens will be important in the care of even those with very advanced disease. Decisions about which drugs to use and in which order require knowledge of current research on drug combinations, their efficacy and likely cross-resistance. Manipulations in therapy, including drug holidays (structured drug interruptions), should therefore be supervised by the HIV unit overseeing the patient's care. The palliative care role in HIV/AIDS is in managing symptoms arising from disease or drug therapy, and providing psychological support and advice in terminal care.

ANTIRETROVIRAL THERAPY

Nucleoside analogues such as zidovudine (AZT), lamivudine (3TC) and, more recently, abacavir inhibit viral reverse transcriptase and were the first class of drugs to be developed. When used alone, resistance usually developed in 6–12 months (although a more sustained drop in viral load is produced by abacavir). Side effects are many and various and include bone marrow suppression (AZT), nausea and vomiting, diarrhoea or constipation, peripheral neuropathy, insomnia, headache, myalgia and lethargy. Abacavir can also cause an allergic reaction, with fatal results if the drug is stopped and restarted (Table 12.2).

Nucleotide analogues are a newer development and inhibit reverse transcriptase in a more direct way than nucleoside analogues. An example is tenofovir, which can cause headache, diarrhoea, nausea and vomiting and a skin rash.

Non-nucleoside reverse transcriptase inhibitors include nevirapine and efavirenz and produce a rash as a major side effect. Occasionally this can be severe and even life threatening. In addition, efavirenz causes unpleasant dysphoric symptoms, including nightmares and dizziness.

Protease inhibitors are highly active and can produce profound viral load drops, but adverse effects are common. In the short term, they produce nausea, vomiting, diarrhoea, headache and fatigue. Longer term, they can raise plasma lipids and cause a pattern of redistribution of body fat called lipodystrophy.

Table 12.2 Antiretroviral therapy

Group	Drug names
Nucleoside reverse transcriptase inhibitors (NRTIs)	Zidovudine (AZT), stavudine (d4T), didanosine (ddI), lamivudine (3TC), abacavir (ABC)
Nucleotide reverse transcriptase inhibitors	Tenofovir
Non-nucleoside reverse transcriptase inhibitors (NNRTIs)	Nevirapine, efavirenz, delavirdine
Protease inhibitors (PIs)	Ritonavir, indinavir, saquinavir, nelfinavir, amprenavir lopinavir, atazanavir, fosamprenavir

Table 12.3 Symptom incidence in the last 3 months of life[6]

Symptom	Incidence (%)
Anorexia	63.1
Fatigue	60.1
Pain	60.1
Fever	47.6
Cough	37.5

Some patients develop diabetes. In addition, indinavir crystals can precipitate in the renal tract, resulting in renal colic.

MANAGEMENT OF SYMPTOMS IN HIV AND AIDS

Patients with advanced HIV disease experience a burden of symptoms similar to that of their fellow-sufferers with advanced malignancy. In one series of patients referred to a specialist palliative care service, 95 per cent had problems with symptom control.[5] Table 12.3 shows the incidence of symptoms in a group of 168 patients with HIV in the last 3 months of life.[6]

Pain is experienced by 50–88 per cent of patients with advanced disease[5–8] and may be due to HIV itself (peripheral neuropathy, myalgia, arthropathy), disease related to immunosuppression (headache from cerebral tumours or toxoplasmosis, herpes infections) or treatment related (peripheral neuropathy from antiretroviral therapy, mucositis from chemotherapy). Analgesia follows the usual guidelines for acute and chronic pain, although care must be taken with drug interactions. Patients with a history of recreational drug use should be treated with the same compassion afforded all others and not have analgesia withheld in the mistaken fear that it will 'feed their drug habit' (Table 12.4).

Peripheral neuropathy has a multi-factorial aetiology in HIV disease. Neuropathy can be a result of damage by the virus itself, and also occurs in 10–20 per cent of

Table 12.4 Incidence of different pains in HIV hospice in-patients[7]

Pain	Incidence (%)
Visceral	25
Neuropathy	19
Oral	12
Headache	11
Musculoskeletal	11
Genital	8

patients taking nucleosides, especially stavudine (d4T). It presents as a distal symmetrical sensory neuropathy, usually in the feet but also in the hands. Patients describe numbness, paraesthesiae and pain, which may result in reduced mobility. Occasionally, a change in antiretroviral therapy is appropriate, but sufficient relief is often possible using tricyclic antidepressants and anti-epileptic medications. Some individuals find benefit from non-prescribed therapies such as acupuncture, massage, cannabis and magnetic insoles.

Nausea and vomiting occur commonly as a consequence of medication, including septrin and protease inhibitors, which may have to be discontinued as a consequence. Tolerance to this side effect does develop in some individuals, but anti-emetic medication is often required. Haloperidol is commonly used because of both its action at the chemoreceptor trigger zone and the convenience of its once-daily dosing.

Diarrhoea is another common side effect of antiretroviral treatment and occurs in 32 per cent of individuals on protease inhibitors. Treatment with calcium supplements (Calcichew) is effective in some, whereas others respond to dietary manipulation, bulking agents or anti-diarrhoeal medication. Parenteral opioids and octreotide are infrequently required.

Cachexia–anorexia is very common in advanced disease as a consequence of chronic infections and progressive malignancy arising in the immunocompromised host. Treatment of the underlying problem, for example suppression of atypical mycobacterial infection, is helpful. Symptomatic treatment with progestogens, particularly megestrol acetate, can produce weight gain but causes impotence in many and may not be tolerated. Anabolic steroids are also used but can cause aggression. Weight loss is treated more intensively in this group of patients where the potential for a life-prolonging response to antiretroviral medication exists. Enteral feeding via a nasogastric tube or gastrostomy should be considered if oral supplementation fails. The involvement of an experienced dietician is invaluable.

SURVIVAL AND PROGNOSIS DATA

Data are available from prospective epidemiological studies showing the rate of progression of HIV. Some untreated individuals will develop advanced disease within 2–3 years, although the median is 10 years. This information is longitudinal and, by necessity, does not reflect the impact of effective antiviral therapy, with which survival has been greatly prolonged.

In the UK, deaths from HIV and AIDS peaked with just over 1700 individuals dying in 1995. The rate has been falling steadily since, with 414 deaths reported in the year 2003.

Progression is more rapid in individuals infected through transfusion, adults over 35 years of age and those with acute symptoms at the time of infection (a seroconversion illness). Clinical predictors of progression include the CD4 T-cell count and viral load. Population-based studies in homosexual men show that the CD4 T-cell count begins at around 1000×10^6/L and falls to 670×10^6/L after the first year of infection. Subsequent years see a decrease of 40–80×10^6/L on average. An acceleration of this decline heralds progression of disease. Severe immunosuppression is defined as a CD4 T-cell count $<200 \times 10^6$/L and at this level opportunistic infections and tumours are more likely.

Plasma HIV RNA viral load correlates well with the extent of virus replication and is highest in acute infection and advanced disease. However, there can be marked variation and in clinical practice the changing viral load is interpreted together with the trend in the CD4 T-cell count. As a result, these tests are described as surrogate markers for HIV progression.

RESEARCH

In comparison to the advanced state of research into the active management of HIV, research into palliative care and HIV is very limited.

There are some data obtained from looking at symptom profiles and the experiences of different groups of affected individuals.[5–8] In a large review examining symptom data from 808 participants of a multi-centre trial, patient and provider agreement on the presence and severity of symptoms was poor.[9] A growing body of literature has demonstrated the under-treatment of pain in patients with AIDS. Ethnicity and gender have been shown to affect the experience of symptoms. Important differences exist in the prescription of analgesia to different groups. Intravenous drug users with HIV-related pain are significantly more likely to receive inadequate analgesia and experience greater psychological distress.[10]

Research at the end of life in patients with HIV and AIDS is difficult for the same reasons as in advanced cancer. More work needs to be done with this group to evaluate their needs and how they can best be met.

MODELS FOR PALLIATIVE CARE INVOLVEMENT

Specialist palliative care input may be needed at multiple points during an individual's illness (see Fig. 12.1).[11]

(A)

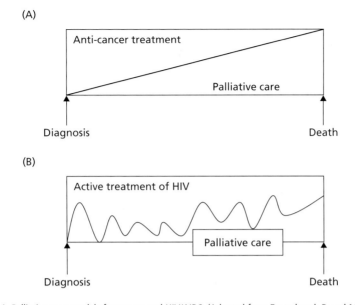

Figure 12.1 Palliative care models for cancer and HIV/AIDS. (Adapted from Easterbrook P. and Meadway J.)[11] (A) Current view of cancer palliative care. (B) Suggested model of HIV/AIDS palliative care.

Early in the disease, specialist advice about symptomatic management may enable a patient to adhere to antiretroviral treatment. This care can often be provided in an out-patient clinic and is appropriate at larger HIV centres. During acute illnesses, hospital palliative care teams need to provide symptom management alongside active care. In between these episodes, patients who are well will be discharged from the palliative care service.

Hospice in-patient care is appropriate for the small number of patients for whom active treatment is futile and death predicted. There is also a need for 1–2-week admissions for psychological respite. These patients are physically much less unwell than most hospice in-patients and may be uncomfortable among the dying, and considered a lower priority for admission. Special consideration must be given to the different needs of gay men, ethnic minorities and recreational drug users in in-patient units. Patients with HIV encephalopathy require long-term nursing care but are not comfortably placed in nursing homes. These issues suggest the need for units specializing in providing palliative care for HIV patients.

LIMITATIONS OF PALLIATIVE CARE IN HIV AND AIDS

Outside the major centres, only a very small number of patients with HIV disease will present to specialist palliative care services. In a retrospective review of

12 hospices in Yorkshire over a period of 6 years, only 39 individuals with HIV and AIDS accessed in-patient care.[12] This review was undertaken when AIDS diagnoses were three to four times more common; lower numbers might be expected to access hospice care today. Lack of exposure to affected individuals makes it difficult to keep updated with new developments in management. This may lead to palliative care teams lacking confidence in their ability to look after patients with HIV and AIDS.

CHALLENGES FOR PALLIATIVE CARE IN HIV AND AIDS

- Very small numbers of patients.

- Centralized care.

- Unpredictable disease trajectory.

- Problems with adherence to antiretroviral therapy.

- Drug interactions.

- Ethical issues.

- Dealing with chaotic behaviour and recreational drug use.

- Need for respite care for psychological support.

- Need for long-term admissions for cognitively disabled patients.

Care for HIV patients tends to be centralized at a few large specialist units. Patients may travel huge distances from their homes to these centres and may lose confidence in local community services. In some cases, at the patient's request, primary care teams are not kept informed about HIV care, or are unaware of the diagnosis.

The need for palliative care input in HIV disease fluctuates throughout the course of the infection. Individuals may present with apparently advanced disease, only to recover dramatically after some months on antiretroviral therapy. As a result, it is difficult to identify when active management becomes futile, and the period of acknowledged terminal care can be very short.

The potential effectiveness of HAART can only be achieved with strict adherence to drug regimens. Part of the palliative care for individuals may be to help them take their antiretroviral medications regularly and to control any adverse effects. A particular challenge is the possibility of drug interactions, usually as a result of potentiation or inhibition of drug metabolism via the cytochrome P450 enzymes. Even seemingly innocuous substances such as St John's wort have been shown to reduce the plasma concentration of protease inhibitors, efavirenz and nevirapine. Methadone metabolism may be enhanced and the dose may need to be increased in patients starting certain antiretroviral regimens. The list of potential interactions is enormous and too large to detail here. The reader is advised to check the details of such interactions in the *British National Formulary* or other appropriate source.

Ethical concerns are common in relation to HIV disease. There may be uncertainty about confidentiality within the multi-disciplinary team in in-patient units, especially in situations in which family members are unaware of the diagnosis. This can also be problematic when it comes to the writing of death certificates and handling of an HIV-infected body. The Birth and Death Registration Act 1953 requires that 'the registered medical practitioner ... state to the best of his knowledge and belief the cause of death'. However, at HIV centres, it is usual practice not to include HIV or AIDS on the certificate, but to indicate that further information will be made available and to inform the Office of Population and Census confidentially of the diagnosis. Funeral directors may need some guidance in the appropriate handling of HIV-infected bodies. Body bags may be necessary for situations in which leaking of body fluids presents a hazard. Coffins can be opened safely for viewing, however; indeed, refusal to do so may lead to unwanted disclosure of the diagnosis to friends or family.

Hospice units often find recreational drug use challenging. The use of contracts and boundaries is essential but may not come naturally in the hospice environment.

It may be that hospice in-patient care is not meeting the current needs of this group of patients. There is a need for respite care for psychological support for individuals living with HIV and AIDS. Some specialist units exist to provide such care, for instance Mildmay Hospital in London and Bethany in south-west England. Others have had funding removed and have closed. Individuals are finding it increasingly difficult to persuade their health authority to fund respite placements.

Another group that is difficult to provide for is that of patients with permanent cognitive disability. These individuals are often too young to be suitable for nursing home care and too vulnerable to be returned home. Admission guidelines for many hospices would exclude the prolonged admissions that these patients require. However, there are similarities between this group and the young patients who develop cerebral tumours. A small number of in-patient beds is needed for such individuals for longer-term in-patient stays.

KEY POINTS

- The progression of HIV disease can be postponed for long periods of time with highly active antiretroviral therapy (HAART).
- Advanced disease is still seen, and palliation needed, where treatment is unavailable, not tolerated, or options for treatment run out.
- Palliative care is also helpful to control symptoms caused by antiretroviral therapy.

REFERENCES

1. Gazzard B (ed.). *Chelsea and Westminster Hospital AIDS care handbook*. London: Mediscript, 1999.

2. Revised classification system for HIV infection and expanded surveillance case definition for AIDS among adolescents and adults. *Morbidity and Mortality Weekly Report* 1992; **41**(RR-17), 1–19.

3. World Health Organisation. *AIDS epidemic update: December 2003.* Joint United Nations Programme on HIV/AIDS (UNAIDS). Geneva: World Health Organisation, 2003.

4. HIV and AIDS in the United Kingdom quarterly update: data to end December 2003. Health Protection Agency, London. *CDR Weekly* 2004; **14**(7).

5. Cox S, Kite S, Broadley K, Johnson MA, Tookman A. Comparison of specialist palliative care needs of patients with HIV from 1994 to 1997. Poster presentation. BHIVA, Oxford, November 1998.

6. Fantoni M, Ricci F, Del Borgo C, Bevilacqua N, Damiano F, Marasca G. Symptom profile in terminally ill AIDS patients. *AIDS Patient Care and STDS* 1996; **10**(3), 171–3.

7. Kelleher P, Cox S, McKeogh M. HIV infection: the spectrum of symptoms and disease in male and female patients attending a London hospice. *Palliat Med* 1997; **11**, 152–8.

8. Frich LM, Borgbjerg FM. Pain and pain treatment in AIDS patients: a longitudinal study. *J Pain Symptom Manage* 2000; **19**(5), 339–47.

9. Justice AC, Rabeneck L, Hays R, Wu A, Bozzette S. Sensitivity, specificity, reliability, and clinical validity of provider-reported symptoms: a comparison with self-reported symptoms. *J Acquir Immune Defic Syndr* 1999; **21**(2), 126–33.

10. Breitbart W, Rosenfield B, Kaim M, Funesti-Esch J, Stein K. A comparison of pain report and adequacy of analgesic therapy in ambulatory AIDS patients with and without a history of substance abuse. *Pain* 1997; **72**(1–2), 235–43.

11. Easterbrook P, Meadway J. The changing epidemiology of HIV infection: new challenges for HIV palliative care. *J R Soc Med* 2001; **94**, 442–8.

12. Salt S, Wilson L, Edwards A. The use of specialist palliative care services by patients with human immunodeficiency virus-related illness in the Yorkshire Deanery of the northern and Yorkshire region. *Palliat Med* 1998; **12**(3), 152–60.

chapter 13

NEURODEGENERATIVE CONDITIONS INCLUDING DEMENTIA AND STROKE

David Oliver and Don Williams

INTRODUCTION

As patients with advanced neurological disease deteriorate, there is an increasing role for palliative care. The World Health Organisation (WHO) defines palliative care as:

> An approach that improves the quality of life of patients and their families facing problems associated with life-threatening illness, through the prevention and relief of suffering, early identification and impeccable assessment and treatment of pain and other problems, physical, psychosocial and spiritual.[1]

It is also stressed that palliative care:

- affirms life and regards dying as a normal process,

- intends neither to hasten nor postpone death,

- provides relief from pain and other distressing symptoms,

- integrates the psychological and spiritual aspects of patient care,

- offers a support system to help patients live as actively as possible until death,

- uses a team approach to address the needs of patients and their families, including counselling, if indicated,

- will enhance quality of life, and may also positively influence the course of the illness,

- offers a support system to help the family cope during the patient's illness and in their own bereavement.[1]

The aim of palliative care is to look at the 'whole patient' in the context of their social support system, which is often their family. The role of palliative care is to consider not only the physical aspects of the disease but also the psychological, social and spiritual aspects.

The extent of the involvement of palliative care will depend on the diagnosis and the individual patient. With some neurodegenerative diseases, such as motor neurone disease (MND), there is no cure and the aim of treatment will be palliative from the time of diagnosis. Other diseases may require intensive treatment early in the disease process, and only a proportion of patients deteriorate so that palliative care becomes appropriate. For instance, after a stroke most patients will receive active intervention and rehabilitation, but for some patients with severe cerebral involvement and damage, this active treatment may be inappropriate and palliative care is more appropriate from the time of the stroke. For others, deterioration may occur after an initial period of active treatment, and there is a change in emphasis of care to palliative care. In slowly deteriorating conditions, such as multiple sclerosis or dementia, there will be a need for palliative care as the disease advances, depending on the individual.

Patients with Alzheimer's disease and other dementias differ from most patients who receive palliative care in two ways.

- Although Alzheimer's disease is a terminal illness, it is impossible to predict the length of survival. The rate of progression is very variable: the time from onset of symptoms to death varies from 1 to 16 years, while the average length of the illness is 9 years.

- In advanced dementia there is severe mental deterioration and patients are unable to participate in decisions about their management.

The changing needs of patients can be seen in Figure 13.1, and there is the need for an integrated approach to the care of a patient with a potentially incurable disease. The diagram shows how these approaches to care are complementary and are not in competition.[2]

The approaches are:

- active treatment of the disease, if this is possible,

- active medical treatment of complications of the disease, e.g. treatment of infection,

- symptomatic and supportive palliative care.

The level of involvement will vary during the disease progression and with the individual and, for patients who lack mental capacity, sensitive discussion with substitute decision-makers is essential.

In all cases there is a need to ensure that the treatment offered to patients, and their families, is appropriate to the stage of the illness. Regular careful review does not always occur and as a result active treatments may continue, even though it seems that there is little benefit to the patient. For instance, there is clear evidence that cardiopulmonary resuscitation is of little benefit for people with advanced

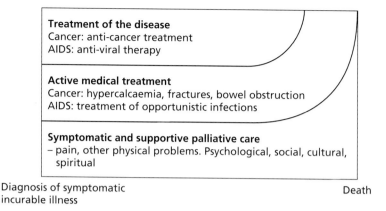

Figure 13.1 A modern view of palliative care. Symptomatic and supportive palliative care is complementary to, and seamlessly integrated with, active treatment of the underlying disease. (From Woodruff R. *Palliative medicine – symptomatic and supportive care for patients with advanced cancer and AIDS*, 3rd edn. Oxford: Oxford University Press, 1999.)

dementia, as fewer than 2 per cent of nursing home residents receiving it are successfully resuscitated and virtually no-one resuscitated in hospital survives to leave hospital.[3] However, the decision not to resuscitate is often not made.

Throughout the disease process, it is essential that the patient's needs are carefully assessed and addressed. The palliative care approach should be used for all patients, regardless of the stage of the disease, and in this way the appropriate treatment options may be chosen. The palliative care approach 'aims to promote both the physical and psychosocial well being and is a vital and integral part of all clinical practice, whatever the illness or its stage, informed by a knowledge and practice of palliative care principles'.[4]

This approach should be part of the everyday care given to all patients and encompasses:

- focus on quality of life, which includes good symptom control,

- a whole-person approach, taking into account the person's past life experience and current situation,

- care that encompasses both the dying person and those who matter to that person,

- respect for patient autonomy and choice (e.g. with regard to place of death, treatment options),

- emphasis on open and sensitive communication, which extends to patients, informal carers and professional colleagues.[4]

Thus palliative care should be part of the care of all patients, especially as the disease advances and death can be foreseen in the near future – this is usually in months or weeks, but the period may vary for each disease. For instance, the

National Hospice Organization in the USA has developed a Functional Assessment Staging (FAST) for determining prognosis in dementia,[5] and studies have shown that patients in the later stages of the disease, with a score of FAST 7C (inability to sit up without assistance) or greater had an average life expectancy of only 4.1 months.[6] Although these guidelines are helpful, it is extremely difficult to predict how long individual patients with dementia will live.

The care of any patient should be the most appropriate for their needs, and all patients should be carefully assessed, together with their family, but in advancing neurodegenerative disease this becomes even more crucial. Palliative care is essential for these patients to ensure that their quality of life is as good as possible and that the 'whole patient' is cared for in the context of their family. Detailed care planning is facilitated by the use of a problem-orientated approach[7] in which all the medical, psychological and social problems are addressed in turn.

THE PHYSICAL NEEDS

The physical needs of people with advancing neurodegenerative disease are many. Studies have shown that people with non-malignant disease suffer symptoms similar to those of advanced cancer: 94 per cent of patients with non-malignant disease reported pain in the last year of life, compared to 96 per cent of cancer patients; 56 per cent of patients with non-malignant disease reported having dysphagia for more than 6 months, compared to 37 per cent of cancer patients.[8] However, these symptoms may go undetected, as patients and their families may consider the problems to be part of the condition itself.[9] It is therefore important to assess the patient thoroughly to ensure that the various problems are elucidated and then treated appropriately.

PAIN

Pain may be experienced by many patients with advanced neurodegenerative disease: studies have shown that up to 76 per cent of patients with MND,[10] up to 82 per cent in patients with multiple sclerosis,[11] 2 per cent in patients with stroke,[11] and many patients with dementia experience pain.[12] There are specific pain syndromes related to certain disease progression, but there are common pains experienced by many patients:

- musculoskeletal pain from the abnormal tone around joints or abnormal or altered posture; non-steroidal anti-inflammatory medication may be of help;

- cramp pains from contracted or spastic muscles; muscle relaxants, such as baclofen or dantrolene, may be helpful, but they can often add to weakness and may reduce the patient's ability to walk, as this may be dependent on some spasticity;

- skin pressure pain due to immobility and ensuing discomfort; this may respond well to the use of opioid analgesics on a regular basis.[13]

Opioids may also be helpful for patients with dementia who seem uncomfortable and in pain but no clear cause can be found.[12]

Patients with multiple sclerosis may experience paroxysmal pains and often dysaesthetic pain as part of a central pain syndrome and myelopathy.[11] The control of this pain is difficult, but anticonvulsants and antidepressants may be helpful. Cannabinoids have also been suggested for the management of these pains.

One to two per cent of patients with stroke may experience a central post-stroke pain, which can be severe.[14] There may be hyperalgesia and the pain may be paroxysmal, starting with emotion or movement, and antidepressants may be helpful.

It is often difficult to assess pain in the person with advanced dementia. Possible causes of pain are constipation, lodged food, contractures, bedsores, urinary tract infection and gum disease. Careful examination is essential so that the pain can be treated appropriately. On rare occasions, new aggressive behaviour can be triggered by deep-seated pain. Often morphine is helpful in ensuring that any discomfort is eased.[12]

The assessment of the cause of the pain is essential before treatment in this patient group. Specific treatments may be possible, but the use of regular morphine, titrating to the pain, may be necessary. Carefully used morphine, or other opioids, can be very helpful. It may be necessary to consider not only the type and dose of medication, but also the route of administration. If swallowing becomes difficult, such as in motor neurone disease with bulbar involvement, or compliance is unsure, a transdermal patch or a continuous subcutaneous infusion using a portable syringe driver may be considered.[14,15]

DYSPNOEA

As neurological disease advances, respiratory muscle involvement may occur, for instance with advancing MND. This may lead to dyspnoea and evidence of respiratory insufficiency leading to hypoventilation – poor sleep, dreams, lethargy in the morning, morning headaches. Careful assessment is essential before starting treatment, and simple measures such as ensuring that the patient is positioned so that the chest can move freely and is not obstructed may be helpful.

Respiratory support may be helpful,[16] either as non-invasive ventilation[17] or as ventilation and tracheostomy.[18] However, these options need careful discussion, as there is a risk of the patient becoming 'locked in', with no movement and no means of communication, and there are profound ethical dilemmas.[19] Opioid medication may be helpful in relieving the distress of dyspnoea.[14]

DYSPHAGIA

The ability to swallow safely and effectively may be affected by advancing disease. Patients with dementia may be unable to control the pattern of their eating and may overfill their mouth, exacerbating any swallowing difficulty. The involvement of a speech and language therapist and a dietician allows a full assessment of the swallowing problems. Simple measures and advice to carers about feeding (both the technique of feeding and the consistency of foods) may be necessary. Augmentative feeding systems may be considered. The percutaneous endoscopic gastrostomy (PEG) can be inserted with minimal distress, allows feeding to continue[20] and is preferable to a nasogastric tube, which can stimulate secretions, cause discomfort, lead to aspiration and be easily dislodged by an agitated or confused person.

As the disease progresses, careful consideration is necessary before intervention. If the patient is in the terminal stages of the disease, it may be inappropriate to interfere, and the intervention could cause more distress to the person. For instance, the passing of a nasogastric tube in a severely confused patient can be very difficult, and not without risk, and the benefits of feeding may be short-lived and less than the problems that ensue. The key to the successful management of dysphagia and other eating problems in the confused patient is high-quality nursing by dedicated experienced staff. In units specializing in advanced dementia care, the use of a PEG or nasogastric tube is rarely contemplated.

If swallowing deteriorates, it may become difficult for the patient to cope with the control and swallowing of the normal saliva production, leading to drooling. This is a very distressing symptom and can be eased by the use of anticholinergic medication, such as hyoscine hydrobromide as a sublingual tablet, injection or continuous subcutaneous infusion by syringe driver, or a tricyclic antidepressant such as amitriptyline.[10]

INCONTINENCE

Most patients fear incontinence. Sphincter dysfunction may occur in neurological disease, particularly in multiple sclerosis or where there is spinal involvement. Patients may also become incontinent where there is a reduction in cortical control of the sphincters, as in dementia, or if mobility reduces so that they are unable to reach a toilet.

Urinary infection should always be excluded. Antimuscarinic medication, such as flavoxate, can be helpful. Regular toileting and the use of padding should be considered. The use of a condom catheter or urinary catheterization may need to be considered to reduce the risk of bedsores.

Faecal incontinence may be more difficult to treat. Faecal impaction should always be excluded and constipation avoided. Anti-diarrhoeal medication may be helpful.

CONSTIPATION

Constipation may occur in any patient with a reduced diet, reduced mobility and with certain medication, such as opioids, anticholinergics and antidepresssants. Constipation should be prevented, if possible, by aperients and local measures, including suppositories and enemata if necessary.

SPEECH AND COMMUNICATION

The ability to communicate may be reduced or lost completely as the disease progresses. This can be one of the most difficult losses to cope with, as communication is so basic to our roles as members of a family and other social organizations. A speech and language therapist can be very helpful in assessing and in the management of these problems so that some form of communication can be retained.

In dementia, communication may be lost because of mental changes, leading to expressive and/or receptive dysphasia and an alteration in the pragmatics of speech – the rhythm, intonation, prosody and gestures of speech may remain even if the content is altered.[3] Attention must be given to taking time to try to understand the underlying feelings as well as the content. Following a stroke, there may again be expressive and/or receptive dysphasia, and assessment by a speech and language therapist is essential in planning forms of communication.

In certain neuromuscular diseases, such as MND, there may be dysarthria, due to the dysfunction of the muscles of the head and neck. A speech and language therapist can again allow patients and their carers to continue to communicate. This may involve augmentative communication aids, such as the Lightwriter or computer systems.

DELIRIUM

Delirium is a common complication, particularly with dementia. There is a wide spectrum of severity and symptom pattern. Delirium usually presents with altered consciousness or new strange behaviour. Altered sleep pattern, delusions and visual hallucinations are usually present. After diagnosis, careful physical examination is made and investigation may be necessary to exclude common causes, such as urinary sepsis, upper and lower respiratory tract infections and new cardiac disease. The successful management of delirium depends on accurate diagnosis and effective treatment of the underlying cause. Skilled nursing is directed to maintaining fluid intake, gentle diet and good-quality sleep. Patients are invariably frightened, and a major tranquillizer, such as promazine, is very beneficial.

As patients with dementia are physically and mentally compromised, mild self-limiting disorders such as the common cold and constipation can precipitate delirium. A small stroke affecting higher centres, with complete sparing of the motor and sensory symptoms, may also cause similar effects.

ANXIETY AND DEPRESSION

In view of the nature of these illnesses, it is easy to understand how symptoms of anxiety and depression commonly occur – estimates of depression in dementia vary from 15 to 57 per cent,[21] and up to 60 per cent in patients with MND.[22] In dementia, they are particularly pronounced in the early stage of these illnesses but, as mental deterioration proceeds and insight is lost, the possibility of depression recedes and occasionally euphoria develops. Although anxiety and depression can be regarded as discrete entities, there is a pronounced overlap between these symptoms, and in routine clinical practice it is easier to consider the two states as a continuum. In addition, the causes of anxiety and depression are probably the same.

In terminal illness, a degree of anxiety and overwhelming sadness is a normal reaction to the realization that life is coming to an end. As a consequence, it can be difficult to be certain when this reaction becomes a pathological clinical state. There are a number of pointers to aid diagnosis:

- anxiety that is all pervasive and cannot be interrupted by positive interaction with relatives and staff;

- a markedly diminished interest or pleasure in all, or almost all, activities most of the day, with a lack of reactivity;

- anxiety that is so severe as to cause restlessness – this indicates that true agitation has emerged;

- a persisting poor sleep pattern, including onset and early waking insomnia;

- anorexia, persistent lack of interest and retardation, with brooding or feelings of self-pity and often social withdrawal;

- classical diurnal variation of mood – the hallmark of a true depressive illness;

- the advent of suicidal ideas;

- a past history of mental illness, a neurotic personality or fraught close interpersonal relationships.

If there is doubt about the development of a pathological state, psychotropic medication should be considered, although there is a risk of side effects. In the absence of severe symptoms and suicidal ideas, management with psychotropic medication should be straightforward. With effective treatment of anxiety and insomnia with benzodiazepines, early improvement will occur. If agitation or other psychotic symptoms are present, major tranquillizers must be used, starting with the milder ones such as promazine, resperidone or pericyazine in small doses.

The presence of depressive symptoms suggests the need to introduce an antidepressant. Tricyclic antidepressants, such as amitriptyline, may be sedative and have anticholinergic side effects, although these may be helpful if there is drooling. Selective serotonin reuptake inhibitors, such as fluoxetine or sertraline, may be helpful, and the slightly more sedative paroxetine may be useful if there is concomitant anxiety. If there is only a poor response after 2–3 weeks, expert psychiatric assessment is indicated.

PSYCHOSOCIAL CARE

Coping with the multiple losses of a deteriorating illness will cause many varied and varying emotions for both the patients and those close to them. Many of these reactions and concerns will be shared by patients and their families, but they will also have specific concerns, which may be different for different diseases.

A neurodegenerative disease will lead to many continual losses. The effect and depth of the losses will depend on the disease process, the individual and previous losses experienced by the individual. The losses may be:

- physical changes, such as reduced mobility or speech in MND, or mental deterioration in dementia;

- cognitive losses, especially in the early stages of dementia when patients may have insight into their deteriorating mental state and may become anxious as they face these losses;

- emotional losses, as patients feel unable to express themselves, for example the person with MND or stroke who is restricted in movement and speech and feels unable to communicate and express emotions effectively.

Many people with a deteriorating disease are fearful of the disease itself.[23] Whereas people with advancing cancer have often seen a family member or friend with cancer and know a little of the likely progression, someone with a rarer disease, such as MND, will be fearful as to the possible deterioration and may read about distressing events that could occur in the future – the cause of death in MND is often reported to be choking and severe distress, whereas with good palliative care death is rarely distressing and usually peaceful.[10] Fears of dying and death are common and need to be addressed. There is no easy answer, but fears and concerns can be heard, and simple explanations of the control of symptoms and distress can be reassuring.

Patients' families and other carers may also have their own fears and concerns. They will be facing multiple losses and changing roles within the family.

- Changes in roles as they have to make decisions, often on behalf of the patient, who is now unable to communicate clearly due to communication or cognitive deterioration.

- Loss of the patient's ability to undertake simple activities, such as washing or toileting, so that family members have to take on these extra roles, with the knowledge that the person feels the loss of dignity and control.

- Fears of the disease, similar to those of the patient, with the need to address these fears and myths: for instance, the carers of someone with MND may fear that the patient will choke to death or the family of someone with dementia may fear violent or aggressive behaviour.[3] There may be an imperative to provide information about the disease process for family members. The disease-specific societies and associations often provide information leaflets, a website and a helpline for the support of patients and families (see the list of useful contact details at the end of this chapter).

- They may have their own concerns and fears about dying and death. Many people, even in middle age, have little experience of someone dying and they may have various concerns, some of which may be unfounded, which they need the opportunity to express.

- Problems about how to approach the patient as the disease progresses. When someone has lost speech, as a result of either dysarthria (as in MND) or dysphasia (as in stroke), it is essential for carers to continue to speak to them normally and not to treat them as if they have lost their cognitive functions. Sensitivity and tact are always necessary, as even patients with progressive dementia may have brief lucid moments.

- Changes in sexuality and intimacy may be very important to both patients and their partners. In MND and stroke, there may be no change in the sexual drive or needs of the patient, but the physical changes and reduced mobility alter their ability to have sexual intercourse. Partners may fear that sexual activity could cause further harm and may need reassurance that they can take the lead and perhaps be prepared to alter the previous sexual behaviour. Sensitive discussion may be necessary to allow partners to discuss these matters. People with dementia may feel that their sexual needs are difficult to express, but there may also be a lack of inhibition and overt sexual activity, which may be difficult for the carers. Careful discussion and a clear plan to help reduce this disinhibited behaviour may be required.[3] Medication to decrease the sexual drive, such as cyproterone or benperidol, may be helpful.

- There may be financial concerns. Due to the disease progression, patients may have been forced to give up work and their family and carers may also have reduced their earnings. These practical issues need to be addressed, including ensuring that they are claiming their entitlement to benefits.

The support of both the patient and the family is crucial in the care plan. The family should be encouraged to be involved in the patient's care and to include all family members, including children. There are often fears that children will not be able to cope with the patient and the knowledge about the disease, but they will be aware that all is not well and usually it is more helpful to ensure that their questions are answered honestly and openly so that they feel involved.[24]

Carers may feel many differing emotions.

- Grief, as they face the losses associated with the disease.

- Anger – at the disease process, the professionals involved, the patient and the changes that have occurred. This may be more common when carers feel that they have been cheated of time together, or that the period of retirement has been shortened by the disease progression or dementia. These emotions may be difficult to express, or even acknowledge.

- Sadness, depression and demoralization, as the carers cope with the disease and the effects on the patient. These feelings may make it difficult to cope with the practical needs of the patient and may increase the problems faced by both patient and family.

- Guilt, particularly as carers see that they can continue with their activities without hindrance, whereas the patient feels trapped by the disease. In dementia, guilt is often experienced as family members are forced to take decisions on behalf of patients and, although the decisions may be to protect the patients, such as stopping them driving, they may blame the carers for these 'impositions' and increase the family's guilt.[3]

- Fatigue may ensue if insufficient help is accepted or provided, compromising the care of the patient.

Thus there is the need to provide support for families to enable them to cope not only with the practical issues of caring but also with the emotional aspects. This support should be offered from all the professionals within the multi-disciplinary team, but specialized psychosocial support may require the involvement of a social worker. Voluntary agencies, such as patient support organizations, which are usually disease specific, such as the Alzheimer's Society, MND Association or the Stroke Association, are able to offer information and support for patients and their families and their involvement can be very helpful (see the list of useful contact details at the end of the chapter).

DECISION-MAKING

Although with many neurodegenerative diseases patients remain cognitively intact, there may be occasions when these functions are reduced or lost. Patients with progressive dementia may have increasing loss of cognitive function and the capacity to make decisions about care. Patients with severe stroke may have lost awareness or consciousness and, again, decision-making ability is lost. For these patients, decision-making may be complex and other methods of coming to healthcare decisions will need to be found.

For patients with progressive dementia, it is necessary to assess the capacity to make decisions. This may be difficult for many patients, as the mental state can vary. However, it has been suggested that an assessment should include six questions to be asked of the patient.[3] Can the patient:

- identify the issue?

- state the major options to address this issue?

- understand the most likely outcomes of each option?

- state a choice from among the options?

- provide a reason that justifies that choice?

- show consistency over time?

If these questions cannot be answered clearly, there is doubt about the patient's capacity to make a decision, and other decision-making courses will need to be considered.

If a person is unable to make a decision because of their physical condition – unconsciousness or inability to communicate clearly – the decision may need to be taken by the clinician in charge of the patient's care, and in the best interests of the patient, although this may vary from country to country.[25] All care must be in the patient's best interests and it may be possible to take into account the past wishes, values and preferences of the patient when making decisions.[25] Another way of making decisions on behalf of patients is by means of an Enduring Power of Attorney or an Advance Directive.

POWERS OF ATTORNEY

In the UK, through an ordinary Power of Attorney, one person (the donor) gives another person (the attorney) legal authority to manage their affairs. However, an ordinary Power of Attorney becomes invalid if the donor becomes mentally incapable. An Enduring Power of Attorney (EPA) was created to meet these circumstances providing it has been registered with the Public Trust Office. Once the EPA form has been completed, it may be used as an ordinary Power of Attorney unless restricted by the donor. The EPA gives everyone the opportunity to plan ahead and select one or more people they trust to act for them should they become mentally incapable. It is particularly important to consider setting up this procedure in progressive neurological disease and dementing illness.

ADVANCE DIRECTIVES AND PROXY DECISION-MAKING

The nature of the doctor–patient relationship continues to evolve away from medical paternalism and into joint participatory decision-making between the patient and doctor. Many factors have fostered this change, particularly consumerism, a better-informed public and a tendency to challenge the professional view. Advance Directives are designed to set out people's preferences for treatment if they become mentally incapable or are unable to communicate their views to their carers. This legal instrument is becoming more widely used in North America and is beginning to be introduced into the UK, where it is not yet enshrined in statute law. As patients want to participate more fully in decisions about their medical care, particularly about the ethical decision to withhold treatment, the use of advance directives or the appointment of proxy decision makers to guide the decision-making process on their behalf is more likely to occur.

CARE IN THE TERMINAL STAGES

The terminal stages of a neurodegenerative disease are often difficult to define. In some diseases, the deterioration may occur over only a few days, and studies of MND patients have shown that many – up to 58 per cent – deteriorate and die within 24 hours.[26] The period of change may be much longer for someone with dementia, but if the patient is no longer walking, is immobile, unable to dress or bathe, has frequent urinary and faecal incontinence and is unable to communicate more than six words, death is likely.[3] For patients with stroke, there may have been active rehabilitation initially, and the continued deterioration and reduction in activity again show an increased risk of death.

Even if it is difficult to define clearly the terminal stage, it is important to ensure that preparations have been made – symptoms are controlled, medication is available and all carers are aware of the deterioration and the best ways of helping the person as death approaches.

SYMPTOM CONTROL

The control of symptoms in the final stages of the disease is very important, as the memories of this time live on for the bereaved family. The use of medication is as described above, considering in particular the following factors.

- Pain control. Pain may become commoner and more severe as the patient is less mobile, and opioid analgesics may be necessary. The dose should be titrated to the pain and, if carefully monitored, opioids can be used safely.[14] The method of administration should also be considered, as oral medication may no longer be possible. The use of suppositories, continuous subcutaneous infusions by means of a portable syringe driver, or transdermal preparations (such as fentanyl) should be considered so that analgesia is continued until death.

- Dyspnoea. The use of ventilatory support may need to reconsidered and, sometimes, patients and their families may request the cessation of treatment.[27] This may be very difficult for all involved and requires discussion among all members of the caring team and family. Opioids and sedation will be necessary to prevent any distress when the ventilator is switched off or reduced.[28] Opioids are also effective in reducing the distress of dyspnoea at other times and may be required, as described, for the control of pain.

- Choking. Choking is often feared by patients who have swallowing problems. With good control of pain, dyspnoea and secretions, choking should be rare.[26] Medication should be readily available to give if there is an episode of choking or other breathing problems.

- Salivation. This may become a problem if swallowing deteriorates, and anticholinergic medication such as hyoscine hydrobromide may be helpful, sublingually or as a continuous subcutaneous infusion.

- Chest secretions. These may be a problem in the very terminal stages, as the patient cannot clear them easily. Anticholinergic medication is helpful – injection or continuous subcutaneous infusion of hyoscine hydrobromide or glycopyrronium bromide. In the terminal phase, the use of antibiotics is often inappropriate.[29]

- Oral care. Good oral hygiene is essential to reduce the risk of discomfort.

- Bedsores. If possible, bedsores should be prevented by the use of appropriate pressure-relieving mattresses and skin care. With very cachectic patients, this is not always possible and careful dressing of the sores and pressure care can minimize the problems.

CRISIS PREVENTION

As it may be difficult to assess when the terminal stages are approaching, it is important to ensure that the communication amongst all involved in the patient's care is as good as possible. This includes not only the patient and family/close carers, but also the various professionals in the multi-disciplinary team involved in the care plan. When the deterioration has been very gradual, over a longer period of time, it can be difficult to decide when the terminal phase has been reached. Careful discussion amongst all involved in the patient's care – family, carers and healthcare professionals – is essential so that all are aware of the changes that are occurring. The professionals need to communicate regularly so that the changes in the care plan are clear to all. As the patient deteriorates, the aims of care change and the primary concerns become the control of symptoms and ensuring the patient is as comfortable and settled as possible. Regular meetings are helpful and patients and their families need to be closely involved in these discussions.

The medication that may be necessary as death approaches should be readily available. For instance, if continuation of oral medication is unlikely to be possible, injection medication should be provided so that it can be given without delay. The MND Association has produced the Breathing Space Programme, with the aim of providing information about the medication for the terminal stages of this disease and the box provided allows the medication to be stored in the patient's home.[30] In this way, the medication is available and everyone has been involved in discussion about its use.

There is also a need to look at the appropriateness of resuscitation. There is good evidence that cardiopulmonary resuscitation is usually futile for people with advanced disease.[3] This area of care should be discussed by the multi-disciplinary team and shared with the patient's family/close carers.

SEDATION

As advanced physical and mental deterioration occurs, the need for the sedation of patients with dementia often diminishes, as elderly patients frequently enter a calmer phase. This is often in contrast to younger dementia sufferers, who can remain agitated even when all functional ability has been lost. They can enter into periods of delirium that are difficult to manage and very thoughtful management is essential and neuroleptics, benzodiazepines and opioid drugs may be necessary.

For patients with increasing confusion, often with hallucinations and delusions, antipsychotic medication will be required. Many of these drugs will lead to sedation and other side effects, such as postural hypotension. Careful assessment of the patient's particular needs is necessary and the drugs to be considered include risperidone and haloperidol.[3] Great care is necessary with patients with Lewy body dementia, as they are particularly sensitive to phenothiazine drugs.

In the terminal stages of the disease progression, sedation may be particularly difficult. Patients may become terminally agitated and require sedation, but may not regain consciousness again and die within a few days. The aim of the sedation is to control a difficult symptom, terminal distress, and there is the possible 'double effect' of leading to death slightly earlier than if no sedation had been given. However, the aim of care should always be to help the patient, and in these circumstances the reduction in confusion is not only of direct help to the patient, but can also relieve their family of the distress of seeing them confused and agitated.

HYDRATION AND NUTRITION

As death approaches, there may be discussion about the need for the continuation of feeding and/or hydration. Families and carers often feel that it is very important to continue to try to feed the patient, as feeding and nurturing are such a basic instinct for all people. However, oral feeding may become difficult, if not hazardous, as there is a high risk of aspiration as death approaches. Other methods may be suggested, and the use of intravenous or subcutaneous fluid replacement may be considered. There is little evidence that fluids reduce the distress of dying, and studies have shown that homeostasis may maintain the blood biochemistry in the majority of patients without the need for replacement.[31] The use of intravenous fluids may, in fact, increase the risk of vomiting, incontinence and chest secretions. Moreover, if the patient is cachectic and confused or agitated, the continuation of an intravenous line may be very difficult, and not without hazard and discomfort.[32] Often, such therapy may require admission to hospital and thus removal of patients from their own surroundings at this crucial time. The main symptom of dehydration is a dry mouth and this can easily be helped by regular mouth care.

For a patient with advancing neuromuscular disease, stroke or dementia, the use of enteral or parenteral nutrition and hydration needs to be considered very carefully. The risks may outweigh the benefits, but these should be discussed with the family and carers so that all are aware of the decision process. There may be concerns that the removal of hydration is hastening death, but there are many arguments that the fundamental cause of death is the disease process and not the withdrawal of treatment.[33]

HOSPICE INVOLVEMENT

Many hospices are involved in the care and support of people with neurodegenerative disease. In particular, more than 75 per cent of specialist palliative care providers in the UK are involved with patients with MND.[34] However, the involvement with other disease is variable: in the UK less than 4 per cent of admissions to hospices are patients with non-malignant disease[35] and in the USA less than 1 per cent of hospice patients have dementia.[5] There is a development worldwide to provide palliative care for people with dementia, and palliative care services have been shown to be appropriate for this patient group.[36]

The experience of the Jacob Perlow Hospice in New York has shown that increased care at home with, on occasions, in-patient care can support patients at home. The average time on the hospice service was 155 days and the majority of patients (70 per cent) were able to die at home.[12] This experience will encourage further developments in the care for dementia patients. In the UK, most departments of old age psychiatry have continuing care beds for patients with advanced dementia with complex needs, and they are increasingly aware that the care of these patients should involve a similar approach to that of hospices.

The management of patients with advanced dementia presents many difficult ethical, legal and moral problems, for example in the decision about whether or not to treat a chest infection. No rigid, uniform approach can be adopted, but the emphasis is on building up a consistent policy that members of the multi-disciplinary team understand and are committed to. Van der Steen et al.[37] and Helme[38] have teased out some of the complex issues in this area. The need for closer liaison between old age psychiatry and palliative care in the management of these patients has been emphasized.[39] Progress has been slow, but joint meetings between the two disciplines are beginning to be organized.

Patients dying following a stroke will rarely be involved with specialist palliative care services. There are difficulties in defining the terminal stages, and the numbers of patients requiring care are large – in England and Wales, 100 000 people suffer a first stroke in a year and there are 60 000 deaths a year.[40] However, it is important that the palliative care approach, outlined above, is applied to the care of all patients, and particularly to this group, whose prognosis is variable and who have many needs.

EUTHANASIA AND END-OF-LIFE ISSUES

There has been increasing debate regarding voluntary euthanasia and physician-assisted suicide. In the Netherlands, where euthanasia is allowed under certain conditions – when the request is voluntary, there is unbearable suffering without any hope of improvement, and the doctor has sought the opinion of a colleague – people with MND have been one of the larger groups receiving it. It has been reported in one study that 4.1 per cent of MND deaths and 5.35 per cent of multiple sclerosis deaths were by euthanasia, compared to 0.82 per cent of all deaths.[41] It would appear that people with stroke and dementia were less likely to receive euthanasia.

Experience from the Netherlands has suggested that the main reasons for requests for euthanasia are fears of choking or pain, emotional burn-out due to the emotional stress/exhaustion of coping with the disease progression, the desire to retain control, depression and pain.[42] People with neurodegenerative disease may be at a higher risk of these factors developing, particularly if there is inadequate palliative care. People with dementia cannot usually give clear consent to a request for euthanasia, although there is evidence that some people are dying in this way without clear consent.[43]

The provision of good palliative care may reduce requests for an early death. The holistic care described above will enable patients to retain some control of their lives and allow their fears to be addressed. People with progressive disabling disease need help to enable them to cope with the changes, and do not need an early death.

KEY POINTS

- Palliative care should be provided for patients with neurodegenerative conditions.
- Although the prognosis may be unclear, the palliative care approach is applicable to patients with neurodegenerative disease.
- Symptoms must be assessed carefully and managed with the involvement of the multi-disciplinary team.
- Involvement of families and carers, both informal and professional, is essential in the care of patients with neurodegenerative disease and dementia.

REFERENCES

1. World Health Organisation. *WHO definition of palliative care.* World Health Organization: www.who.int/cancer/palliative/definition/en 1.1.04.
2. Woodruff R. *Palliative medicine*, 2nd edn. Melbourne: Asperula, 1996.
3. Rabins PV, Lyketsos CG, Steele CD. *Practical dementia care.* Oxford: Oxford University Press, 1999.
4. National Council for Hospice and Specialist Palliative Care Services. *Specialist palliative care: a statement of definitions.* London: National Council for Hospice and Specialist Palliative Care Services, 1995.
5. The National Hospice Organization. Medical guidelines for determining prognosis in selected non-cancer diseases. *Hospice J* 1996; **11**, 47–59.
6. Hanrahan P, Raymond M, McGowan E, Luchins DJ. Criteria for enrolling dementia patients in hospice; a replication. *Am J Hospice Palliat Care* 1999; **48**, 395–400.
7. Cherny N. The problem of suffering. In: Doyle D, Hanks G, Cherny N, Calman K (eds), *Oxford textbook of palliative medicine*, 3rd edn. Oxford: Oxford University Press, 2004, 7–14.
8. Addington-Hall J, Fakhoury W, McCarthy M. Specialist palliative care for non-malignant disease. *Palliat Med* 1999; **12**, 417–27.
9. Dunlop R. Wider applications of palliative care. In: Saunders C, Sykes N (eds). *The management of terminal malignant disease*, 3rd edn. London: Edward Arnold, 1993, 287–96.
10. Oliver D. The quality of care and symptom control – the effects on the terminal phase of ALS/MND. *J Neurol Sci* 1996; **139**(Suppl.), 134–6.
11. Borasio GD, Rogers A, Voltz R. Palliative medicine in non-malignant neurological disorders. In: Doyle D, Hanks G, Cherny N, Calman K (eds), *Oxford textbook of palliative medicine*, 3rd edn. Oxford: Oxford University Press, 2004, 924–34.

12. Brenner PR. The experience of Jacob Perlow Hospice: hospice care of patients with Alzheimer's disease. In: Volicer L, Hurley A (eds), *Hospice care for patients with advanced progressive dementia*. New York: Springer, 1998, 257–75.

13. Oliver D. Opioid medication in the palliative care of motor neurone disease. *Palliat Med* 1998; **12**, 113–15.

14. Payne R, Gonzales GR. Pathophysiology of pain in cancer and other terminal illnesses. In: Doyle D, Hanks G, Cherny N, Calman K (eds), *Oxford textbook of palliative medicine*, 3rd edn. Oxford; Oxford University Press, 2004, 288–98.

15. Oliver DJ. Syringe drivers in palliative care: a review. *Palliat Med* 1988; **2**, 21–6.

16. Aboussouan MD, Khan SU, Meeker DP, Stelmach RRT, Mitsumoto H. Effect of noninvasive positive-pressure ventilation on survival in amyotrophic lateral sclerosis. *Ann Intern Med* 1997; **127**, 450–3.

17. Meyer TJ, Hill NS. Noninvasive positive pressure ventilation to treat respiratory failure. *Ann Intern Med* 1994; **120**, 760–70.

18. Oppenheimer EA. Decision-making in the respiratory care of amyotrophic lateral sclerosis: should home mechanical ventilation be used? *Palliat Med* 1993; 7(Suppl. 2), 49–64.

19. Polkey MI, Lyall RA, Davidson AC, Leigh PN, Moxham J. Ethical and clinical issues in the use of home non-invasive ventilation for the palliation of breathlessness in motor neurone disease. *Thorax* 1999; **54**, 367–71.

20. Park RHR, Allison MC, Lang J, Morris AJ, Danesh BJZ. Randomised comparison of percutaneous endoscopic gastrostomy and nasogastric tube feeding in patients with persistent neurological dysphagia. *BMJ* 1992; **304**, 1406–9.

21. Lazarus LW, Newton N, Cohler B, Lesser J, Schwein C. Frequency and presentation of depressive symptoms in patients with primary degenerative dementia. *Am J Psychiatry* 1987; **144**, 41–5.

22. Hunter MD, Robinson IC, Neilson S. The functional and psychological status of patients with amyotrophic lateral sclerosis: some implications for rehabilitation. *Disabil Rehabil* 1993; **15**, 119–25.

23. Oliver D. Palliative care. In: Oliver DJ, Borasio GD, Walsh D (eds), *Palliative care of amyotrophic lateral sclerosis*. Oxford: Oxford University Press, 2000, 21–8.

24. Gallagher D, Monroe B. Psychosocial care. In: Oliver DJ, Borasio GD, Walsh D (eds), *Palliative care for amyotrophic lateral sclerosis*. Oxford: Oxford University Press, 2000, 83–103.

25. British Medical Association. *Witholding and withdrawing life-prolonging medical treatment: guidance for decision making*. London: BMJ Books, 1999.

26. O'Brien T, Kelly M, Saunders C. Motor neurone disease: a hospice perspective. *BMJ* 1992; **304**, 471–3.

27. Goldblatt D, Greenlaw J. Starting and stopping the ventilator for patients with amyotrophic lateral sclerosis. *Neurol Clin* 1989; **7**, 789–805.

28. Edwards MJ, Tolle SW. Disconnecting a ventilator at the request of a patient who knows he will then die: the doctor's anguish. *Ann Intern Med* 1992; **117**, 254–6.

29. Smith SJ. Providing palliative care for the terminal Alzheimer patient. In: Volicer L, Hurley A (eds), *Hospice care for patients with advanced progressive dementia*. New York: Springer, 1999, 247–56.

30. Oliver D. Ethical issues in palliative care – an overview. *Palliat Med* 1993; 7(Suppl. 2), 15–20.

31. Oliver D. Terminal dehydration. *Lancet* 1984; **ii**, 631.
32. Dunphy K, Finlay I, Rathbone G, Gilbert J, Hicks F. Rehydration in palliative and terminal care: if not – why not? *Palliat Med* 1995; **9**, 221–8.
33. Randall F, Downie RS. *Palliative care ethics*, 2nd edn. Oxford: Oxford Medical Publications, 1999, 271–3.
34. Oliver D, Webb S. The involvement of specialist palliative care in the care of people with motor neurone disease. *Palliat Med* 2000, **14**, 427–8.
35. Kite S, Jones K, Tookman A. Specialist palliative care and patients with noncancer diagnoses: the experience of a service. *Palliat Med* 1999; **13**, 477–84.
36. Luchins DJ, Hanrahan P, Litzenberg K. Acceptance of hospice care for dementia patients by health care professionals and family members. In: Volicer L, Hurley A (eds), *Hospice care for patients with advanced progressive dementia*. New York: Springer, 1998, 207–30.
37. Van der Steen JT, Muller MT, Ooms ME, Van de Wal G, Ribbe MW. Decisions to treat or not to treat pneumonia in demented psychogeriatric nursing home patients: development of a guideline. *J Med Ethics* 2000; **26**, 114–20.
38. Helme T. Editorial comment on euthanasia and other medical decisions in the terminal care of dementia patients. *Int J Geriatr Psychiatry* 1995; **10**, 727–33.
39. Black D, Jolley D. Slow euthanasia? The deaths of psychogeriatric patients. *BMJ* 1990; **300**, 1321–3.
40. Humphrey P. Stroke and subarachnoid haemorrhage. In: Williams AC (ed.), *Patient care in neurology*. Oxford: Oxford University Press, 1999, 179–95.
41. Van der Wal G, Onwuteaka-Philipsen BD. Cases of euthanasia and assisted suicide reported to the public prosecutor in North Holland over 10 years. *BMJ* 1996; **312**, 612–13.
42. Zylicz Z. Dealing with people who want to die – part II. *Palliat Care Today* 1998; **VI**(3), 54–6.
43. Post SG, Whitehead PJ. The moral basis for limiting treatment; hospice care and advanced progressive dementia. In: Volicer L, Hurley A (eds), *Hospice care for patients with advanced progressive dementia*. New York: Springer, 1998, 117–31.

Useful contact details

Alzheimer's Society
Gordon House
10 Greencoat Place
London SW1P 1PH
Tel.: 020 7306 0606
Helpline: 0845 300 0336
www.alzheimers.org.uk

Huntington's Disease Association
108 Battersea High Street
London SW11 3HP
Tel.: 020 7223 7000
www.hda.org.uk

Motor Neurone Disease Association
PO Box 246
Northampton NN1 2PR
Tel.: 01604 250505
Helpline: 08457 626262
www.mndassociation.org

Multiple Sclerosis Society
MS National Centre
372 Edgware Road
London NW2 6ND
Tel.: 020 8438 0700
Helpline: 0808 800 8000
www.mssociety.org.uk

Parkinson's Disease Society
215 Vauxhall Bridge Road
London SW1V 1EJ
Tel.: 020 7931 8080
Helpline: 0808 800 0303
www.parkinsons.org.uk

Stroke Association
Stroke House
123–127 Whitecross Street
London EC1Y 8JJ
Tel.: 020 7566 0300
www.stroke.org.uk

chapter 14

HEART, RENAL AND LIVER FAILURE

J. Simon R. Gibbs and Louise M.E. Gibbs

INTRODUCTION

The unmet palliative needs of those living with and dying from heart and renal failure were recognized 40 years ago. Hinton investigated the quality of care in dying patients on the wards of a London hospital and described high levels of physical and mental distress, which were more marked in patients dying from heart or renal failure than from cancer.[1]

In the last decade, these areas have attracted a well-deserved growing interest, both within the relevant specialties as well as in primary and palliative care. This chapter brings together three distinct clinical syndromes: heart, renal and liver failure. In all three, acute 'organ failure' may be encountered in any clinical setting, but their aggressive investigation and active management are likely to be most appropriate in acute medical settings. Joint management between acute and palliative clinicians may be required in hospital and the community, and a working knowledge of active management is important, even for palliative clinicians in in-patient units.

Palliative care texts have tended to concentrate on acute renal and liver failure in the scenario of advanced malignancy. Regardless of aetiology, chronic heart, renal and liver failure share a poor prognosis, a potentially high symptom burden and level of unmet psychological and social need that make them very pertinent to the principles and practice of palliative care. The degree to which this has been researched or applied to clinical practice varies, and this is reflected in the disparity in length and content of the three sections of this chapter.

HEART FAILURE

DEFINITION

Heart failure is a chronic progressive disease that constitutes the final common pathway of many cardiovascular diseases. It can be defined in many ways, such as acute or chronic, left-sided or right-sided and systolic or diastolic. For clinical purposes, heart failure is defined by the European Society of Cardiology(2) as the presence of symptoms of heart failure at rest or during exercise and objective evidence of cardiac dysfunction.[2] In addition, a favourable response to treatment of heart failure is further evidence for the diagnosis. The objective evidence of cardiac dysfunction is most commonly obtained by echocardiography. This evidence is important because heart failure is a clinical syndrome. The symptoms are non-specific and other conditions such as circulatory failure, renal failure, liver failure and myxoedema may present with the same clinical picture. A description of aetiology completes the diagnosis of heart failure, but may not be possible or appropriate to pursue, especially in the elderly.

This chapter covers both acute and chronic heart failure. The need for palliative care is in chronic heart failure. Acute heart failure is included because patients with chronic heart failure experience episodes of acute decompensation. Unless stated, the text refers to chronic heart failure.

INCIDENCE AND PREVALENCE

Heart failure is a serious health problem. It is the only major cardiovascular disease with increasing incidence. With age-adjusted mortality rates from cardiovascular disease declining and the size of the elderly population growing, the absolute number of individuals living with compromised cardiac function is expected to increase dramatically over the next few decades. Furthermore, the treatment of heart failure may prolong the time patients live with an impaired quality of life.

In the UK, the crude incidence rate is at least 1.3 cases per 1000 population per year for those aged 25 years or over.[3] The incidence rate increases from 0.02 cases per 1000 population per year in those aged 25–34 years to 11.6 in those aged 85 years and over. The incidence is higher in males than in females. The median age at presentation is 76 years. The number of deaths from heart failure in the UK is uncertain because the diagnosis of heart failure is not acceptable on a death certificate without qualification. The estimated number of deaths is between 30 000 and 60 000 per annum.

Hospital admissions and expenditure on heart failure have been increasing progressively for more than a decade,[4] and 0.2 per cent of the population is hospitalized for heart failure every year. Heart failure patients occupy up to 10 per cent of medical beds at any time and account for up to 2 per cent of National Health Service (NHS) costs.

PATHOPHYSIOLOGY

The pathophysiology of heart failure is a complex interaction of changes in circulatory haemodynamics with the neuroendocrine system which is activated in response to a reduced cardiac output. The disease has consequences for other organs, such as hypoperfusion of the kidneys and congestion of the liver. While mechanical pump failure is the cause of heart failure, the clinical syndrome is a result of these interactions, in particular the neuroendocrine activation. The commonest cause of heart failure is coronary artery disease.[5] Other causes include hypertension, valve disease, arrhythmias, dilated cardiomyopathy and alcohol abuse.

The cause of breathlessness and fatigue is not a direct result of poor cardiac function; the functional ability of patients with heart failure correlates poorly with left ventricular dysfunction. Instead, the pathophysiological explanation for breathlessness and fatigue may involve deconditioning, wasting and metabolic changes in skeletal muscle that activate ergoreflexes and chemoreflexes.

CLINICAL FEATURES

The clinical course of heart failure is characterized by progressively worsening symptoms and frequent acute episodes of deterioration requiring hospitalization.

The cardinal symptoms of heart failure are breathlessness and fatigue. Breathlessness occurs on exertion, and patients with heart failure overbreathe for a given level of exercise. Breathlessness may progress to being present at rest. Its severity is measured using the New York Heart Association (NYHA) classification (Table 14.1). Orthopnoea is the most sensitive and specific symptom of elevated left ventricular filling pressure, and it tends reliably to parallel filling pressures in a given patient.[6] Nocturnal or exertional cough is often a dyspnoea equivalent. In practice, fatigue also contributes to exercise limitation in some patients. Tiredness or fatigue may be severe in advanced disease.

Fluid retention is often evident at presentation or subsequently if deterioration occurs and is associated with breathlessness, cough, nocturia, swollen lower limbs/sacrum, anorexia, nausea, abdominal bloating and liver capsular pain.

Other important symptoms include pain, poor-quality sleep, feeling down or anxious, confusion, short-term memory loss, dizziness, nausea, vomiting, constipation, loss of appetite, weight loss and loss of libido.[7–10] Pain is a surprisingly common symptom in advanced disease. It may be caused by a variety of problems, including angina, liver capsular distension, ankle swelling and as a consequence of co-morbid disease such as arthritis. Whereas some patients have disturbed sleep, others with severe disease may develop sleep-disordered breathing.

Anxiety and depression are common and frequently go unrecognized. In hospitalized patients it has been shown that 38 per cent suffer major depression and 21 per cent minor depression.[11] The consequence of depression may be increased

Table 14.1 New York Heart Association functional classification

Class	Symptoms
I	No limitation: ordinary physical activity does not cause undue dyspnoea or fatigue.
II	Slight limitation of physical activity. Comfortable at rest. Ordinary physical activity results in dyspnoea, fatigue or palpitations.
III	Marked limitation of physical activity. Comfortable at rest. Less than ordinary physical activity causes symptoms.
IV	Inability to carry on any physical activity without discomfort. Symptoms of dyspnoea or fatigue may even be present at rest. If any physical activity is undertaken, discomfort is increased.

Table 14.2 Some clinical features of chronic heart failure

Poor peripheral perfusion
Cyanosis
Tachypnoea
Cachexia
Sinus tachycardia (although this may be absent in severe
  disease or in patients on beta-blockers)
Raised venous pressure
Third heart sound
Functional mitral regurgitation
Peripheral oedema
Hepatomegaly

Table 14.3 Investigation of chronic heart failure

Electrocardiogram
Chest radiograph
BNP (brain natriuretic peptide)
Echocardiogram
Urinalysis
Full blood count
Blood glucose
Liver, renal and thyroid function tests

hospital readmissions and mortality, both of which are related to severity of depression.[12]

Dizziness may be associated with over-zealous treatment with diuretics and vasodilators and is disabling in some patients. Mild weight loss is common, but profound cardiac cachexia has a particulary bad prognosis.

Clinical examination findings are shown in Table 14.2. In particular, raised venous pressure and a third heart sound carry a poor prognosis.[13]

Essential investigations are shown in Table 14.3. Coronary artery disease is under-diagnosed, and coronary angiography should be considered if it is thought that the patient might benefit from revascularization. Cardiac enzymes should be measured in acute exacerbations of heart failure to exclude myocardial infarction. Measurement of natriuretic peptides may be useful for screening for heart failure in primary care, but their role in monitoring disease progression once the diagnosis has been made is uncertain.

STANDARD TREATMENT APPROACHES IN ADVANCED HEART FAILURE

There is a rapidly increasing number of approaches to the treatment of heart failure, involving general measures, drugs, pacing to resynchronize the heart and surgery. (For a full review, see the published guidelines in the 'Further reading' section at

Table 14.4 Desirable components of patient and carer education in heart failure

Nature and cause of heart failure

Symptoms to expect

Prognosis of heart failure

Drug therapy
    Aims of therapy and side effects including written information
    Use of dosette box

Self-monitoring
    Weight recording
    Diuretic adjustment according to weight
    When to seek unplanned medical advice (e.g. weight gain, worsening symptoms)

Lifestyle advice
    Salt intake
    Fluid restriction
    Alcohol intake
    Diet
    Exercise

the end of this chapter.) At present, treatments for heart failure slow but do not arrest progression of the disease. Deterioration is inevitable, but the rate at which this occurs varies between patients.

Following diagnosis, the treatment of heart failure is aimed at treating any reversible causes and implementing standard medical therapy to obtain and maintain clinical stability. Thereafter patients require serial assessment, with appropriate changes to their drug regimen.

General measures

The complexity of the management of heart failure presents significant challenges to ensuring patients are adequately treated. There is clear evidence for the inadequate education of patients and carers and failure to commence or adequately uptitrate evidence-based treatments to obtain maximum benefit and manage concomitant co-morbid disease appropriately.[14,15] The implementation of guidelines is worst in women and the elderly. In addition, the elderly population presents particular difficulties because of co-morbid disease, cognitive limitations, inadequate social support and mental health problems.

There is increasing evidence that heart failure care is best provided by a multi-professional heart failure team working in hospital and in the community. This may reduce hospital readmission[16,17] and possibly mortality.[18]

Providing patients and their carers with training and education is essential to optimizing their management and well-being. The desirable components of this education are detailed in Table 14.4.

Exercise training regimes have improved breathlessness, fatigue, general well-being and exercise capacity.[19] A meta-analysis of exercise training trials has shown a reduction in mortality.[20] Strenuous exercise or weight lifting should be avoided.

Where patients are severely disabled, exercise training may commence with training small muscles before progressing to larger muscle groups. Controlled breathing techniques in selected heart failure patients may reduce breathlessness and improve oxygen saturation and exercise tolerance compared to controls.[21]

Drug therapy

Angiotensin-converting enzyme inhibitors There have been major advances in the pharmacological management of heart failure in the last 20 years which enable progression of the disease to be slowed and survival to be improved. Angiotensin-converting enzyme inhibitors (ACEIs) are the cornerstone of therapy[22] and should be used in all patients who do not have a contraindication such as significantly impaired renal function or hypotension. Patients with severe heart failure benefit most. The ACEIs may cause or contribute to renal failure, which is often detected late because of lack of judicious monitoring of renal function. Withdrawal of ACEI treatment should be considered if there are unexpected increases in serum creatinine concentration above the normal range or by 25 per cent of the baseline value, or both. The benefits of treatment to some patients outweigh renal dysfunction (for example those with severe heart failure), so that treatment should be continued, albeit with diligent monitoring.

The ACEIs produce a consistent improvement in symptoms and cardiac function and significantly reduce all-cause mortality (by 20–25 per cent) and recurrent hospital admissions for heart failure. Long-acting ACEIs are preferred and are normally started at a low dose and progressively uptitrated to reach doses that have been shown to be of benefit in clinical trials. The dose of ACEI in heart failure is greater than those used in routine practice.[23]

Beta-blockers Randomized trials of beta-blockers (carvedilol, metoprolol and bisoprolol) have shown that, when added to ACEI therapy, mortality and hospital readmissions are reduced and functional class is improved.[24] Cardiac function is improved and there is a significant reduction in both all-cause mortality (by 30–35 per cent across all NYHA classes) and recurrent hospital admissions for heart failure. Like ACEIs, beta-blockers are started at low dose and require progressive uptitration over multiple clinic visits. Care should be taken during initiation or uptitration in the presence of low systolic blood pressure or a serum creatinine >250 μmol/L. Beta-blockers may cause worsening of symptoms during uptitration; provided the symptoms are not severe (breathlessness at rest or orthopnoea), they should not be stopped. A transient increase in diuretic dose may resolve the deterioration.

Angiotensin-II antagonists The angiotensin-II antagonists valsartan and candesartan may be used in patients who are intolerant of ACEIs because of side effects. In combination with an ACEI, they may improve symptoms and reduce hospitalization for heart failure when beta-blockers cannot be used.

Aldosterone antagonists Spironolactone in low dose is indicated in severe heart failure (NYHA III and IV), in addition to the above regimen, and also improves symptoms and prognosis.[25] Particular care should be taken to monitor renal function in patients receiving spironolactone.

Diuretics Diuretics are used to control fluid overload. Most patients will be maintained on a loop diuretic and this will be most effective if the dose is spread over the day and not given as a single, large dose. Note that oral furosemide (frusemide) has variable intestinal absorption and in severe heart failure may be replaced with one of the newer loop diuretics such as torasemide. Where more than a moderate dose of loop diuretics is required, the addition of a thiazide diuretic such as bendroflumethiazide (bendrofluazide) may be more effective than increasing the dose of loop diuretic. Metolazone should be reserved for oral therapy in refractory oedema, but care should be taken to monitor electrolytes and renal function frequently. For severe oedema, a continuous intravenous infusion of diuretics is most effective.

Digoxin   Digoxin used in patients with sinus rhythm may improve symptoms and reduce hospitalization but does not improve prognosis.[26] It is indicated where patients remain symptomatic despite optimal therapy with ACEI, beta-blockers and diuretics. In atrial fibrillation, digoxin is indicated for any severity of heart failure and is best combined with a beta-blocker to control heart rate.

Other drugs
- Nitrates are beneficial to relieve acute dyspnoea and angina. Frequent dosing results in tolerance, although this is reduced in the presence of ACEI or hydralazine.

- Inotropes have been shown to increase mortality. Oral phosphodiesterase inhibitors have little effect on improving symptoms and are not used. Intravenous inotropes may be required in severely ill, hospitalized patients to improve acute episodes or as a bridge to transplantation.

- Anticoagulation with warfarin is used in the presence of atrial fibrillation. Aspirin should be used as secondary prophylaxis for coronary artery disease. Low-molecular-weight heparins should probably be used in patients with severe heart failure who require bed rest.

- Oxygen is not required in chronic heart failure, as patients are not usually hypoxaemic. Nevertheless, some patients derive symptomatic benefit and it is reasonable to administer oxygen on an as-required basis.

- Recent evidence has shown that in severe heart failure, exercise capacity may be improved by erythropoietin and/or iron when the haemoglobin is less than 12 g/dL. This requires confirmation in randomized trials.

A therapeutic approach to the management of symptoms in heart failure is shown in Table 14.5.

Management of related symptoms
- *Depression.* The management of depression in heart failure has not been investigated in research trials. Some major groups of drugs are relatively contraindicated and the safety of others is not well established. Tricyclic antidepressants mimic quinidine and affect cardiac conduction, cause orthostatic hypotension, may interact with concomitant drug therapy and cause lethal cardiotoxicity in overdose. Sertraline has no clinically relevant

Table 14.5 Symptomatic treatment of chronic heart failure

Symptom	Possible causes	Treatment
Breathlessness	Pulmonary oedema	Diuresis
	Pleural effusion	Diuresis ± pleural tap
	Ascites	Diuresis ± paracentesis
	Dehydration	Fluid replacement
	Pulmonary infarction	Anticoagulation
	Arrhythmias (e.g. atrial fibrillation)	Anti-arrhythmic drugs ± DC cardioversion
	Low cardiac output	Symptomatic support; discontinue negatively inotropic drugs (e.g. verapamil, diltiazem)
	Infection	Antibiotics
Fatigue	Low cardiac output	Symptomatic support
	Sleep disturbance	Night sedation
	Sodium depletion	Fluid restriction and reduction of diuretics
	Dehydration	Fluid replacement
	Beta-blockers	Therapy review
Nausea and vomiting	Gastric stasis	Metoclopramide
	Biochemical abnormality	Haloperidol
	Ascites	Diuresis ± paracentesis
	Digoxin toxicity	Discontinuation of digoxin and monitoring of levels

effects on cardiac conduction, is unlikely to cause orthostatic hypotension, has a wide margin of safety in overdose and has been used safely after myocardial infarction in a small number of patients.[27] Nevertheless, the risks of not treating depression must be weighed against the risk of cardiotoxic side effects. Non-pharmacological therapies for depression will be subject to clinical trials in the future.

- *Pain.* Analgesics should be prescribed according to the World Health Organisation (WHO) pain ladder, with the exception of non-steroidal anti-inflammatory drugs (NSAIDs), which should be avoided.

- *Breathlessness.* The use of opioids to manage uncontrolled breathlessness does not appear in guidelines for the management of heart failure. One pilot study of ten patients has been published, investigating the use of oral morphine for the relief of breathlessness in patients with chronic heart failure. This demonstrated clinically significant improvement in breathlessness, with few side effects and good tolerability of chronic dosing.[28] Low-dose opioids should be used with caution, since the pharmacokinetics are unknown in heart failure, and renal function is frequently impaired.

Table 14.6 Drugs to avoid in heart failure

Symptoms	Drugs	Cautions and contraindications
Pain	Non-steroidal anti-inflammatory drugs	Salt and water retention and worsen renal function
Depression	Tricyclic antidepressants	Cardiotoxic
	Lithium	Salt and water retention
Nausea/vomiting	Cyclizine	Cardiotoxic
Weakness/fatigue/anorexia	Steroids	Water retention
	Progestogens	Water retention
Neuropathic pain	Flecainide/mexiletine	Depress myocardial function
	Tricyclic antidepressants	Cardiotoxic

Some drugs commonly used in palliative care are contraindicated in heart failure and these are shown in Table 14.6.

Pacing
Multi-site pacing to synchronize ventricular contraction may improve the symptoms of selected patients, but more evidence about who benefits most is awaited. The role of internal cardioverter defibrillators is under investigation.

Surgery
Surgery is indicated where it may improve the underlying cause of heart failure (e.g. myocardial ischaemia or valve disease). Cardiomyoplasty and partial left ventriculotomy are not normally recommended. Heart transplantation is limited by organ availability and is for the minority of patients. The role of ventricular assist devices and artificial hearts remains to be determined.

ACUTE HEART FAILURE

Acute heart failure occurs most commonly in the setting of acute myocardial ischaemia. An acute rise in the filling pressure of the left ventricle results in raised pulmonary venous pressure which leads to fluid leak into the lungs. Breathlessness results from alveolar flooding, small airway obstruction and stiff lungs. The management involves sitting the patient up and administering oxygen. Intravenous diamorphine, metoclopramide and furosemide (frusemide) are first-line drug therapy; intravenous nitrates may help if the patient is not hypotensive. Respiratory support may be required in severe cases. The in-hospital mortality for these episodes is less than 10 per cent.

SURVIVAL AND PROGNOSIS

In the community, newly diagnosed cases of heart failure have a poor short-term survival:[29] mortality is 25 per cent at 3 months; at 1 year, 38 per cent have died.

In hospital-based studies, chronic heart failure has a mortality rate of 31–48 per cent at 1 year and 76 per cent at 3 years. The mean mortality rate is 10 per cent per annum. Half of the deaths occur suddenly and about one-quarter occur without any significant deterioration of the heart failure.

Poor prognosis in heart failure is predicted by poor left ventricular function, severe symptoms and metabolic markers.[30,31] Cachexia, low systolic blood pressure, low serum sodium, high serum creatinine and greater extent of crackles on auscultation of the lungs are independently predictive of cardiovascular mortality. Nevertheless, no prognostic models of heart failure are satisfactory and there is no accepted marker to determine which patients will die suddenly.

REVIEW OF RESEARCH INTO PALLIATIVE NEEDS

Much of the evidence for the palliative needs of heart failure patients comes from two large contemporary studies of dying. The first study to investigate symptoms in terminal heart disease in the UK was the Regional Study of Care for the Dying (RSCD).[7] This was a population-based, retrospective survey of a random sample of people dying in 20 English health districts in 1990, including 675 patients dying from heart disease of all causes. The Study to Understand Prognoses and Preferences for Outcomes and Risks of Treatment (SUPPORT) was a prospective study undertaken in the USA at five academic medical centres.[8] This study included nine diagnostic groups of hospitalized patients with an aggregate mortality rate of 50 per cent within 6 months. Out of a total of 9105 patients, 1404 had heart failure.

Symptom control

There is ample evidence for poor symptom control in patients with severe heart failure. In the RSCD, people who died from heart disease were reported to have experienced a wide range of symptoms, which were frequently distressing and often lasted for more than 6 months.[7] Pain was the most common symptom and was very distressing in 50 per cent of patients. Dyspnoea was the second most common symptom and was very distressing in 43 per cent. Low mood was reported in 59 per cent, and 45 per cent reported anxiety: these symptoms ranked with pain and urinary incontinence in their cause of distress. Management of these symptoms in hospital brought little or no relief in between a quarter and a third of the sample. At least one in six had symptom severity comparable to that of cancer patients managed by specialist palliative care services.

In SUPPORT, functional impairments, depression scores and percentage of patients reporting severe pain or dyspnoea increased as death approached, with 41 per cent of patient surrogates reporting that the patient was in severe pain and 63 per cent reporting that the patient was severely short of breath during the 3 days before death.[8]

Communication and information

The RSCD showed half the patients had been unable to obtain adequate information about their condition. Although many patients were thought to have known that they were dying, 82 per cent had worked this out for themselves.[32]

Healthcare professionals rarely discussed dying with their patients. In a qualitative study, patients with heart failure believed that doctors are reluctant to talk about death or dying, and some would have welcomed timely and frank discussion about prognosis.[33] Patients tended to attribute the symptoms of heart failure to advancing age and decreasing physical and mental capacities, and this may have reinforced their belief that nothing could be done about their symptoms. This lack of everyday knowledge of chronic heart failure serves to highlight the importance of patient education and information as well as public education. Patients report confusion, short-term memory loss, fatigue and reduced mobility, creating significant barriers to doctor–patient communication and making attendance at hospital out-patients difficult. A study which aimed to determine the main concerns of people with end-stage heart disease has shown that surveying concerns in this structured way prompted action in 71 per cent of patients. This action would not otherwise have taken place.[9]

Social support
There is good evidence of the impairment of activities of daily living and of social isolation.[34] Despite this, access to therapy and social services support is poor.[9]

Hospice management of heart failure patients has been shown to be feasible by applying the general principles of specialist palliative care learned from other diseases.[35] Physical symptoms and non-physical needs were similar to those seen with cancer patients. Non-physical needs predominated and included distress, exhaustion, communication and adjustment difficulties for patients and carers. Interventions included management of the psychological distress of family or carers, discontinuing unnecessary cardiac and non-cardiac drugs, early bereavement follow-up of family or carers at risk, mobilizing increased nursing, social or financial support, appropriate medication required for terminal care, and abdominal paracentesis for ascites. Adjustments to cardiac medication were made in consultation with the patients' physicians. The time spent under specialist palliative care was no greater than for patients with cancer. The majority of patients died in the hospice rather than in an acute hospital bed.

MODELS FOR PALLIATIVE CARE INVOLVEMENT IN ADVANCED HEART FAILURE

Barriers to developing approaches to palliative care in heart failure have been identified.[36,37] These barriers fall into three main areas: the organization of health care; the unpredictable course of heart failure and lack of clear terminal functional decline; and doctors' views of their colleagues' roles. Specific organizational barriers include poor community support, a lack of coordination between and within community and hospital, and a lack of planning of care for people dying with heart failure.

Models of palliative care are only starting to be developed at the time of writing. A group in Cleveland, USA, has published its screening criteria for identifying which patients in its heart failure programme should be assessed for palliative care.[38] There are no similar programmes yet reported on in the UK. New models of palliative care in heart failure should depend on research providing a definition of the palliative needs of patients, and a needs assessment tool that can direct patients to palliative interventions that are shown to improve outcomes. The implementation of palliative care without monitoring outcomes should be discouraged.

Specialist palliative care for patients with heart failure became part of government health policy in 2000 when the UK Department of Health published the National Service Framework for Coronary Heart Disease.[39] Specific recommendations with regard to palliative care included improving symptoms, improving the end-of-life experience for both patients and carers, and considering the potential to benefit from palliative care services. The *National clinical guideline on chronic heart failure* has expanded on this.[40] The issues of supporting patients and carers, communication, prognosis and management of anxiety and depression are given priority. There are three recommendations specific to end-of-life care.

1 Issues of sudden death and living with uncertainty are pertinent to all patients with heart failure. The opportunity to discuss these issues should be available at all stages of care.
2 The palliative needs of patients and carers should be identified, assessed and managed at the earliest opportunity.
3 Patients with heart failure and their carers should have access to professionals with palliative care skills within the heart failure team.

The increasing burden of heart failure on health care providers, the complexity of treatments and the demand for better care from patients and the government in the UK are driving changes in the management of this disease. The development of heart failure teams based both in hospital and in the community has been an important step forward. The heart failure team is multi-professional and should provide supportive care for all patients from the point of diagnosis, modelled on the palliative care approach. Where palliative needs are extraordinary and stretch beyond the ability of the heart failure team, advice from specialist palliative care should be sought. The timing of palliative care involvement will vary with individual cases and the experience and capabilities of the local heart failure, primary care and palliative care teams. Specialist palliative care involvement may only be transitory, and long-term follow-up is unlikely to be required in the majority of patients. Regrettably, most patients with heart failure do not yet have the benefit of receiving care from specialist teams.

Heart failure therapies are given continuously, and patients with heart failure want a physician who will manage their heart failure throughout the course of their illness. As a consequence, for most patients, aggressive medical management of heart failure will be concomitant with palliative care. This may mean that although a patient is receiving palliative care, he or she may still require emergency hospital admission for episodes of acute decompensation.

The difficulty in determining prognosis in heart failure should not be a barrier to palliative care. In the majority of cases of heart failure, the terminal phase is not currently recognized, even taking sudden death into account. Ongoing application of the palliative approach, close liaison with primary and specialist palliative care and the wider application of generic models such as the Liverpool Care of the Dying Pathway should help counteract this issue.

Often palliative care in diseases other than cancer is considered only at the end of life. Earlier intervention may enable patients (and their carers) to plan how they wish to be managed later in their disease. It also provides an opportunity to discuss prognosis and living with uncertainty. Since death may come without warning, an awareness of the risk of sudden death may be helpful for both patients and their carers. Although in the USA the Agency for Health Care Policy and Research guideline recommends training family members in basic life support and the use of an automatic defibrillator for patients who wish to be resuscitated,[41] this has found little following in the UK. It should only be employed where psychological support can be provided for the patient and carers.[42]

For patients who are severely ill and dying, good symptom control is imperative. The cause of the symptoms should be identified and treated appropriately. Some examples of the diverse causes of common symptoms are illustrated in Table 14.5, which is not intended to be exhaustive. Treatment of these causes will vary depending on individual patient circumstances and should be carried out after close liaison with the heart failure team.

LIMITATIONS OF PALLIATIVE CARE IN HEART FAILURE

Research into heart failure has concentrated on developing effective pharmaceutical and surgical therapies, but there is now a need to measure the effectiveness of appropriate palliative care interventions in properly controlled trials. Future planning for patients with heart failure should be conducted jointly by heart failure specialists, primary care and specialist palliative care to determine strategies for symptom control, the management of mental health and psychological support, communication and end-of-life issues. Local differences in service provision and expertise necessitate local negotiation between these agencies to plan where the wide variety of needs of heart failure patients are best managed. Only in this way can appropriate and acceptable services for these patients be developed.

KEY POINTS

- Heart failure is common and a disease of old age. The number of patients with heart failure is increasing.
- New therapies for heart failure are evolving rapidly and these are best delivered by multidisciplinary heart failure teams.
- In patients with advanced heart failure, symptom control is frequently poor.
- There is a high incidence of depression that goes unrecognized and untreated.
- Patients with heart failure have communication difficulties.
- The pharmacological treatments for heart failure that improve symptoms and prognosis are under-used.
- In the main, palliative care in heart failure will be managed concomitantly with active heart failure treatments.
- Heart failure can be managed using generic palliative care skills.

RENAL FAILURE

DEFINITIONS

Acute renal failure (ARF) is a rapid deterioration in renal function occurring over hours or days. It is usually detected by a rapidly rising plasma urea and creatinine and caused by a declining glomerular filtration rate. Chronic renal failure (CRF) is a permanent and usually progressive loss of renal function, shown by a rising creatinine and caused by end-stage renal disease (ESRD). Both ARF and CRF have particular relevance to palliative care. Although aggressive investigation and management are likely to be carried out by acute clinicians, ARF is a relatively common problem in palliative patients with a range of primary diagnoses. A working knowledge of the common causes and basic management of ARF and CRF is important in decision-making and in the joint management of these patients.

INCIDENCE/PREVALENCE

The UK incidence (per million population per annum) of ARF is around 172[43] and the prevalence of renal insufficiency (serum creatinine >150 μmol/L) is 2058.[44] The incidence of patients with ESRD requiring dialysis is 78 and the acceptance onto renal replacement programmes is 65 patients. The incidence of ESRD varies dramatically among different age, gender and race population subgroups, with higher rates in minority ethnic groups and the elderly.

PATHOPHYSIOLOGY

Acute renal failure

The commonest cause of ARF is acute tubular necrosis, accounting for more than 80 per cent of cases. The most common risk factors (both in acute and in palliative care) are hypotension/hypovolaemia, sepsis and drugs (such as NSAIDs). Less common risk factors include hypercalcaemia, rhabdomyolysis and tumour lysis. An increasing proportion of cases of ARF occur in the context of multi-system illness.

Urinary tract obstruction accounts for approximately 5 per cent of all cases of ARF. Tumour, fibrosis and calculae are frequent causes. Although uncommon, obstruction is an extremely important cause of ARF, as it is easily diagnosed and often treatable if identified early. Relief of obstruction may be appropriate, even in palliative situations.

Glomerulonephritis is a rare cause of ARF and early diagnosis and treatment are important for improving prognosis.

Chronic renal failure

In CRF, both kidneys are irreversibly damaged. The primary disease is most commonly diabetes or hypertension, which together account for over half of the cases. Heart failure and multi-system organ failure are also common. Some causes, such as glomerulonephritis, outflow obstruction and chronic pyelonephritis, are much

Table 14.7 Common symptoms and signs of uraemia

Anorexia
Nausea/vomiting
Lethargy/fatigue
Itching, scratch marks
Hiccups
Uraemic pigmentation
Decreased libido/sexual function

less common, but are important because they are potentially treatable. Rare causes include myeloma and systemic lupus erythematosis.

CLINICAL FEATURES

Distinguishing between ARF and CRF is important because of the very different management and prognosis of the two conditions. Clearly, there will be clinical features of any underlying cause.

The history in acute/acute-on-chronic renal failure may give clues as to the aetiology (as in the list of causes above). Signs of circulatory compromise suggest acute/acute-on-chronic renal failure. Urinary tract obstruction may present with a history suggestive of a risk factor such as renal stones, prostatism, previous malignancy or surgery. Signs may include a palpable bladder or prostatic, vaginal or abdominal mass.

Symptoms and signs suggesting a chronic history include previously abnormal blood biochemistry, a long history of ill-health or diseases predisposing to CRF, or the common symptoms and signs of uraemia (Table 14.7).

The investigation of patients must be directed at elucidating the cause and targeting specific treatments. Simple investigations such as blood and urine tests are not always helpful in distinguishing ARF and CRF. The metabolic changes such as anaemia, and abnormal calcium and phosphate levels, occur within days of the onset of renal failure and are unhelpful. Urinalysis may help diagnose specific causes such as urinary tract sepsis or glomerulonephritis (the presence of red or white blood cell casts).

The most important initial radiological investigation is ultrasonography; this can rapidly exclude obstruction. Small renal size and increased echogenicity may suggest chronic disease.

STANDARD TREATMENT APPROACHES IN ADVANCED RENAL FAILURE

Acute renal failure

The most important aspect of initial management is to identify and treat any reversible causes. Obstruction should be diagnosed by urgent ultrasound. In the context of palliative care, renal obstruction is usually only treated if specific options for disease management are still available. Rapidly progressive disease with no active treatment options should contraindicate intervention. Treatment options include general measures (percutaneous nephrostomy), ureteric stents (double j or expanding metal) and more specific treatments, such as chemotherapy, radiotherapy or high-dose steroids in malignancy. Poor prognostic factors in malignant disease include tumour type (e.g. breast cancer), tumour grade or stage, age and severity of renal failure.

Nephrotoxic drugs, particularly ACE inhibitors and NSAIDs, should be stopped. Specific causes such as glomerulonephritis, sepsis and hypercalcaemia need specific treatment.

The management options in the general management of ARF are summarized below. Treatment of hyperkalaemia and volume replacement may be undertaken in a palliative setting, but more invasive treatment is likely to be managed by acute clinicians.

- Hyperkalaemia is the potential killer. A level of >6.5 mmol/L will usually require treatment with intravenous calcium gluconate (to protect the heart), intravenous dextrose, insulin and oral/rectal Resonium resin to bring the serum potassium down.

- Volume depletion needs aggressive fluid replacement, but also frequent assessment of fluid status to avoid overload. Once rehydrated, output and input should be matched (allowing 500 mL per 24 hours for insensible losses).

- Diuretics may convert oliguria to polyuria, but they have not been shown to accelerate recovery of glomerular function in human ARF.

- Dopamine (given intravenously) increases renal blood flow in normal subjects. It is a potent diuretic and natriuretic. However, there are few controlled studies in acute tubular necrosis and those available show no demonstrable benefit.[45]

- Renal replacement therapy (see below): indications for dialysis include a rapidly rising urea, refractory hyperkalaemia, severe acidosis, pulmonary oedema, pericarditis, tamponade and severely symptomatic uraemia.

End-stage renal disease/chronic renal failure
Referral for a specialist renal opinion should be timely: a rough guide is at a creatinine level >250 μmol/L.

General measures include treating reversible causes such as obstruction and hypertension (tight control needed) and avoiding nephrotoxic drugs. Patients should be immunized against influenza and *Pneumococcus*. Associated risk factors such as hyperlipidaemia need effective management. Dietary advice is likely to include avoidance of high protein intake, low salt intake and ensuring adequate calories, vitamins and iron.

Anaemia and renal bone disease are specific related problems. Anaemia can have multiple causes, such as lack of erythropoietin, blood loss, haemolysis and hyperparathyroidism. Anaemia causes many of the symptoms experienced by those with ESRD. The UK guidelines (published by the Royal College of Physicians) state that the anaemia of CRF should be corrected by the administration of erythropoietin. The haemoglobin concentration has a major effect on the quality of life, exercise capacity and sexual function.[46] Erythropoietin corrects the chronic anaemia in more than 90 per cent of patients in controlled trials. Oral or intravenous iron is often also required. Renal bone disease (identified by a rise in parathormone) should be treated early: first by lowering phosphate (diet and phosphate binders), then with vitamin D and/or calcium supplements. This may also help the itch of hyperphosphataemia.

Renal replacement therapy

Most decisions regarding the appropriateness of long-term renal replacement therapy are likely to involve referral to a renal specialist or renal unit for assessment. The options include no renal replacement therapy, peritoneal dialysis, haemodialysis and renal transplantation. Dialysis is one of the best methods of control of symptoms related to uraemia. However, patients on long-term dialysis suffer from many symptoms such as tiredness, headaches, sleep disturbance, thirst, nausea, vomiting, low mood, anxiety, memory impairment, cramps, itching, joint pain and dyspnoea.[47,48] This high symptom burden is frequently poorly addressed. In addition there are specific dialysis issues such as the physical, psychological and emotional consequences of time-consuming and invasive treatments.

- *Peritoneal dialysis* involves using the peritoneum as a dialysate membrane. Dialysate is introduced into the peritoneum via a permanent subcutaneous catheter and intermittently replaced with fresh fluid up to five times a day (continuous ambulatory peritoneal dialysis, CAPD) or overnight using an automated peritoneal dialysis (APD) machine. The concentration gradient across the peritoneum performs the dialysis. Common complications are infection and catheter blockage. The technique of fluid exchange is not difficult and can be taught to relatives, and to non-specialist staff in hospices or nursing homes, if continuation of CAPD is appropriate once patients are unable to perform this themselves.

- *Haemodialysis* will be performed intermittently on a specialist unit or at home. Blood and dialysate, separated by a semipermeable membrane, flow in opposite directions. The concentration gradient across the membrane performs the dialysis. Common complications include infection and problems with vascular access. Very strict diet and fluid regimes are required.

- *Haemofiltration* is a continuous process used in emergency situations such as on an intensive care unit. Blood is filtered continuously across a semipermeable membrane that removes small molecules. Fluid lost is replaced.

- *Renal transplants* can be performed using the organs from live or cadaveric donors. The commonest problems are of acute and chronic rejection, complications of long-term immunosuppression (infection and malignancy) and cardiovascular complications such as atherosclerosis and hypertension. The median cadaveric graft survival is 8 years.

SURVIVAL/PROGNOSIS

The outcome in ARF depends on the cause. Overall, the mortality rate is about 40 per cent. There is a wide range of survival, from 90 per cent in uncomplicated ARF to 5–10 per cent in multiple organ failure. The major causes of death in patients with ESRD on dialysis are cardiovascular diseases (nearly half in most big series/large registries) and infection. Patients with asymptomatic cardiovascular disease also have increased mortality. The overall 5-year survival of patients on haemodialysis is 70 per cent. In transplanted patients, a smaller proportion of deaths are from cardiac causes. Renal registry data also include figures for discontinuation of dialysis treatment (see next section). There are few data on those not accepted onto renal replacement therapy programmes.

REVIEW OF RESEARCH INTO PALLIATIVE NEEDS

Multi-disciplinary renal teams have long been established, aiming to help manage the physical and non-physical problems associated with CRF and its treatment. The high symptom load of patients with end-stage renal disease receiving renal replacement therapy or just supportive treatment is well described. The specialist palliative care needs of those dying from renal failure have only recently been the subject of research.

Initiation of and withdrawal from dialysis

Renal registry data across the world report that dialysis discontinuation is a common factor leading to death from uraemia. The highest figures are from the USA, where in several published studies dialysis was discontinued in 9 per cent of patients and accounted for up to 22 per cent of deaths.[49,50] European figures are very much lower (less than 5 per cent of deaths). It is likely that this discrepancy is partly due to under-reporting in Europe of uraemia/dialysis withdrawal as the underlying cause of death, rather than the immediate cause, such as pneumonia. The USA also has the most liberal acceptance policies for acceptance on to renal replacement therapy programmes. Renal registry data give some evidence that the major patient risk factor for dialysis discontinuation is dissatisfaction with current lifestyle, particularly where patients are in pain (e.g. from diabetic neuropathy) or need surgery. These papers emphasize the need for the necessary training and mechanisms to manage the complexities of dialysis withdrawal to be in place in renal units.

Cohen and colleagues have published both a pilot study and a large multi-centre prospective cohort observational study of the terminal course and end-of-life care of patients after dialysis discontinuation in North America.[51,52] The decision to stop dialysis was generally prompted by progressive physical deterioration from chronic disease (66 per cent) or an acute intercurrent disorder (22 per cent). Significant multiple co-morbidity was common. Symptoms were common during the last day of life, particularly pain, agitation, myoclonus, dyspnoea and fever. The symptom prevalence was similar to generic palliative care data, but most symptoms were not severe. Pain medications were administered through the terminal phase in 87 per cent of patients. Symptom control in the last 24 hours was considered effective in 93 per cent of patients by professional and/or family caregivers. The mean survival time from the last dialysis session was 8.2 days (maximum 46 days).

Particular initiatives and guidelines have recently been reported from North America, including a clinical practice guideline, 'Shared decision-making in the appropriate initiation of and withdrawal from dialysis'.[53,54]

In the UK, debate in the literature about issues surrounding dialysis withdrawal and trials of treatment[55] concentrates on the need for multi-disciplinary renal unit teams to follow general principles that encourage open, sensitive communication and unrushed, explicit decision-making. The need for psychosocial and spiritual support is acknowledged. One renal unit has developed and reported its own standards of supportive and palliative care.[56] The development of these standards has been felt to be beneficial in a number of ways, including acknowledgement of the needs of staff for support when caring for dying patients. There are currently no data to show whether these standards have affected the care of dying patients.

Management of upper urinary tract obstruction

There are small series and case reports in the literature about the management of malignant upper urinary tract obstruction where anti-tumour therapy is not an option.[57,58] Whilst treatments such as high-dose steroids, nephrostomy and stenting are described, these are clearly going to be appropriate in only a minority of cases, and patients and relatives need to participate fully in the decision-making processes involved.

MODELS FOR PALLIATIVE CARE INVOLVEMENT IN ADVANCED RENAL FAILURE

In the mid-1990s, letters were published in the UK literature making it clear that mobilizing specialist palliative care for patients discontinuing or not embarking on renal replacement therapy was difficult. The obstacles to renal patients appeared to be those common to most patients with non-malignant disease, basically unfamiliarity. The situation is different in many areas now that most specialist palliative care services, both in hospital and in the community, will take patients with diseases other than cancer, motor neurone disease and acquired immunodeficiency syndrome (AIDS). Compared to other non-malignant diagnoses, the absolute numbers are tiny – in the latest Hospice Information Service data sets, renal failure did not specifically appear. Only the large series of patients with non-malignancy receiving specialist palliative care contain one or two patients, but with little renal-specific detail.[59] It is likely that they are being taken on by palliative care in small numbers, using the generic cancer model as the framework. One particular initiative, the Liverpool Care of the Dying Pathway, has been specifically adapted to those dying from renal failure.[60] Anecdotally, new renal services are developing dedicated to patients with a low creatinine clearance currently not receiving dialysis, which have an even greater emphasis on supportive and palliative care.

PRESCRIBING GUIDELINES FOR SYMPTOM CONTROL IN RENAL FAILURE

The principles of symptom control in renal disease are common to other areas of palliative care as described elsewhere in this book. Two specific issues in renal failure are the likely cause of a symptom in renal disease and the effect of poor renal function on drug handling. Increased sensitivity or toxicity can occur, for example by decreased drug excretion, metabolite accumulation, decreased protein binding or increased permeability of the blood–brain barrier. A creatinine >300 µmol/L is usually taken as defining *moderate* renal impairment and the need for caution in prescribing. *Severe* renal impairment is >700 µmol/L. (Urea is not as accurate an indicator as protein intake, tissue catabolism, surgery, infection and steroids influence it.)

The management of nausea and vomiting is a good example of symptom management needing to be adapted in the case of renal failure. The likely cause of nausea in renal failure is metabolic disturbance, so a drug such as haloperidol is an appropriate choice. In severe renal failure, care must be taken due to increased cerebral sensitivity to antipsychotics. The initial doses used should therefore be smaller than usual.

The *British National Formulary* contains specific guidance about drug usage in renal failure. One region has developed and published consensus-prescribing guidelines for analgesics in patients with renal failure.[61] This guideline has morphine as the first-line strong opioid of choice. Many clinicians would debate this point, since the problem of the accumulation of metabolites causing additional side effects is well known. The use of alternative opioids first line in patients with renal failure is widespread, with the fentanyl 'family' and methadone most commonly quoted in discussion fora. Care should also be taken with many drugs such as laxatives and bisphosphonates, not just analgesics and co-analgesics. Tables 14.8 and 14.9 summarize guidance on commonly used drugs in palliative care in the context of renal failure.[62–66]

LIMITATIONS OF PALLIATIVE CARE IN RENAL FAILURE

Most renal patients are likely to be emotionally attached to the renal units in which they have been treated. Even when renal replacement therapy is discontinued, it will frequently be appropriate for terminal care to be in those centres. Multi-disciplinary renal teams are well established and are already addressing some of the challenges of supportive care in CRF. Specialist renal services clearly also need ready access to specialist palliative care advice and support. Shared care with specialist palliative care services could also give patients and their families

Table 14.8 Symptom control drug guidance in renal failure: non-analgesics

Drug group	Comments
Laxatives and antacids	Avoid those with high sodium, magnesium or aluminium content in severe renal impairment, e.g. Gaviscon, magnesium hydroxide mixture, sucralfate Decrease dose of H_2 blockers such as ranitidine
Anti-emetics and antipsychotics	Antipsychotics (e.g. haloperidol, levomepromazine [methotrimeprazine]): increased cerebral sensitivity in severe renal impairment – reduce dose Metoclopramide: increased risk of extrapyramidal reactions in severe renal impairment – reduce dose $5HT_3$ antagonists and cyclizine: safe
Anxiolytics and hypnotics	Benzodiazepines (e.g. diazepam, midazolam): increased cerebral sensitivity, decreased protein binding in severe renal impairment – reduce dose
Anti-epileptics	Sodium valproate: reduce dose in mild or moderate renal impairment; alter dosage according to serum levels in severe Gabapentin: reduce dose even in mild renal impairment; in moderate or severe, decrease dosing frequency Carbamazepine: use with caution
Antidepressants	Tricyclics: possibility of increased anticholinergic side effects SSRIs: generally require reduction in dose and/or dosing frequency in moderate renal impairment Avoid fluoxetine in severe renal impairment Mirtazapine: use with caution
Corticosteroids	Beware increased risks of salt and water retention, peptic ulceration and impaired glucose tolerance
Glycopyrronium	Possibility of increased anticholinergic side effects
Bisphosphonates	Clodronate sodium: use half dose and monitor in mild/moderate renal impairment; avoid in severe Pamidronate: maximum infusion rate 20 mg/h in moderate/severe renal impairment Zoledronic acid: avoid if serum creatinine >400 μmol/L

$5HT_3$, 5-hydroxytryptamine-3; SSRI, selective serotonin reuptake inhibitor.

choice in their end-of-life care, with the mobilization of the necessary support to die at home or in a hospice. Most hospices are now likely to accept such patients, in contrast to the findings of a small survey in 1995.[67]

Key issues for the future are likely to lie in the dissemination of the kind of collaborative initiatives mentioned in the last section and their integration into all renal services.

Table 14.9 Symptom control drug guidance in renal failure: analgesics

Drug group	Prescribing comments
Non-opioids *Paracetamol* Generally safe	
	Consider decreasing dosing frequency to t.d.s. in severe renal failure
Non-steroidal anti-inflammatory drugs May worsen renal function further, cause fluid retention or increase risk of gastrointestinal bleeding	Always weigh-up risks and benefits before prescribing; COX-2 inhibitors may be safer Always prescribe a proton pump inhibitor for gastric protection
Weak opioids Active metabolites of *codeine* and *dihydrocodeine* accumulate and cause drowsiness	Dose reduce, e.g. maximum 120 mg/24 hours in moderate renal impairment, 60 mg/24 hours in severe
Effervescent *cocodamol* preparations have high sodium content	Avoid effervescent cocodamol in severe renal impairment
Dextropropoxyphene (*Coproxamol*) may cause cerebral/respiratory depression or cardiotoxicity	Avoid dextropropoxyphene
Tramadol Active metabolite renally excreted	Reduce dose and frequency in moderate renal impairment to maximum 50–100 mg every 12 hours Avoid in severe renal impairment
Strong opioids *Morphine* Consider alternative strong opioids with different pharmacological profiles	Avoid long-acting preparations
Toxicity results from metabolite accumulation, particularly in the cerebrospinal fluid	Dose reduce by 25% even at creatinine of 150 μmol/L; use smaller starting doses, e.g. 1.25–2.5 mg, in moderate/severe impairment Increase dose interval to 6–8 hourly if creatinine >300 μmol/L
Drowsiness and agitation may worsen terminal agitation	Consider reducing dose by 30% in terminal agitation unresponsive to sedatives

Diamorphine

Parenteral route may lead to lower metabolization than with oral morphine, causing less toxicity

Opioid levels fall significantly during haemodialysis; consider extra dose of immediate-release morphine before and/or after dialysis

As for morphine

Fentanyl

Metabolites are inactive; clearance of parent drug delayed, but no evidence of adverse clinical consequences

Patches for chronic dosing and lozenges for breakthrough pain

Watch carefully for toxicity during chronic dosing. Consider dose reduction of patches by 25% in moderate, 50% in severe renal impairment

Alfentanil

Metabolites inactive and very short half-life

Large volume of diluent required for intravenous/subcutaneous use can be a practical drawback

Intranasal/sublingual preparations for incident pain

Dose adjustments not necessary

Methadone

Metabolites inactive; gut excretion in renal failure

Oral strong opioid of choice for many clinicians

No dose adjustments required in mild/moderate renal impairment

Some authors suggest 50% dose reduction in severe renal impairment; most suggest no dose adjustment

Hydromorphone

Metabolites accumulate in similar way to morphine; these can cause agitation and confusion

Data from retrospective review showed improvement in side effects after rotation from morphine to hydromorphone

Reduce dose and dosing frequency and avoid long-acting preparations as for morphine

Oxycodone

Half-life prolonged in renal failure

Active metabolite excretion severely impaired in severe renal failure

Safe to use in mild renal failure but use with great caution in severe renal failure

COX-2, cyclo-oxygenase-2 inhibitor.

> **KEY POINTS**
>
> - Multi-professional renal teams are well established. Liaison between them and specialist palliative care teams is to be encouraged.
> - Palliative care can include patients with acute and chronic renal failure, not necessarily related to malignancy.
> - A basic knowledge of the management of acute and chronic renal failure is important for palliative clinicians.
> - Dialysis discontinuation is a scenario particularly pertinent to palliative care.
> - Specific guidance should be followed when prescribing in terminal renal failure.

LIVER FAILURE

DEFINITION

Liver failure can occur acutely in a previously healthy liver, or as decompensation in chronic liver disease. Acute failure in a previously healthy liver is unlikely to involve palliative care services, but patients with malignancy-related liver disease or reaching end-stage liver disease after a number of years of illness might be referred for palliative care.

INCIDENCE/PREVALENCE AND PATHOPHYSIOLOGY

End-stage liver disease is most commonly caused by cirrhosis secondary to alcohol or chronic viral hepatitis (hepatitis B and C). Worldwide there are large differences in the relative importance of alcohol and viral hepatitis. Other causes, such as haemachromatosis, primary biliary cirrhosis, autoimmune hepatitis and drugs, are rare. Many malignancies metastasize directly to the liver and can cause painful hepatomegaly, jaundice and encephalopathy. Primary hepatocellular carcinoma is rare.

CLINICAL FEATURES

The classic signs of chronic liver disease include finger clubbing, Dupuytren's contractures, palmar erythema, spider naevi, gynaecomastia and testicular atrophy. Fluid overload is primarily caused by hyperaldosteronism and renal sympathetic activity leading to renal tubular sodium retention. This can lead to ascites, pleural effusions and oedema. These in turn cause pain/discomfort, squashed stomach syndrome and dyspnoea and may affect mobility and independence. The ascites can become spontaneously infected.

Jaundice is common. It is usually classified as prehepatic (such as haemolysis), intrahepatic (such as hepatitis, metastases or chronic heart failure) or extrahepatic (such as malignant extrinsic bile duct compression). As in urinary tract obstruction, a combination of simple tests (urinary bilirubin without urobilinogen) and an ultrasound can help identify potentially treatable obstructive jaundice. Pruritus is commonly associated with jaundice. Porto-systemic venous shunting causes gastro-oesophageal varices, with consequent risks of gastrointestinal bleeding. Non-specific symptoms such as anorexia, fatigue and depression are common.

Hepatic encephalopathy is thought to be primarily due to the central nervous system toxicity of nitrogen degradation products from the gut. A healthy liver can remove them, but in liver disease a combination of liver cell failure and porto-systemic venous shunting bypassing the liver allows them into the general circulation. Encephalopathy is not a defined state, but a continuum from altered reaction times detectable only on special testing through drowsiness, behavioural changes and confusion to coma. Alcohol, infection, drugs, gastrointestinal haemorrhage and constipation can all precipitate hepatic decompensation and worsening encephalopathy. Hypoglycaemia should always be excluded and treated.

STANDARD TREATMENT APPROACHES IN ADVANCED LIVER FAILURE

The standard treatment approach to advanced liver disease is treatment of any underlying causes and avoidance of further damage by toxins such as alcohol. Herbal remedies may also be hepatotoxic.

The symptomatic treatment of end-stage disease is aimed at fluid overload, jaundice and encephalopathy. The management of squashed stomach syndrome, pain and general symptoms such as depression and fatigue is dealt with elsewhere in this book. Care should always be taken to prescribe drugs that are safe in severe liver impairment. Paracetamol at low dose is safe, as is the judicious use of opioids, but NSAIDs may exacerbate fluid retention or haemorrhage. All anti-hypnotics and sedatives can precipitate encephalopathy. Tricyclic antidepressants are thought to be safer than serotonin reuptake inhibitors.

Fluid overload

Fluid overload causing ascites, pleural effusions and oedema can be managed by a combination of paracentesis, salt restriction and diuretics. Therapeutic paracentesis followed by diuretics has been shown to be quicker and more effective with fewer side effects than diuretics alone. Often a combination of spironolactone and a loop diuretic such as furosemide (frusemide) is needed. Care must be taken not to over-diurese and worsen encephalopathy. There is no clear evidence that intravenous fluid replacement alongside paracentesis is beneficial. The practice of using shunts (Denver or LeVeen) in refractory ascites is now uncommon due to their high complication rates. Bacterial peritonitis can occur spontaneously or after paracentesis and is usually heralded by fever, abdominal pain and worsening encephalopathy. Ascitic fluid should be sent for culture, and treatment (if appropriate) is with broad-spectrum antibiotics.

Encephalopathy

Treatment is aimed at reducing precipitating factors such as infection, decreasing the absorption of gut toxins and increasing the excretion of nitrogenous waste. Dietary protein restriction and lactulose both help. The lactulose works not only as a laxative, but also specifically alters the metabolism of gut bacteria and ammonia absorption. Oral antibiotics such as neomycin to 'disinfect' the gut are not now used since trials have shown no additional benefit to lactulose alone. If treatment of the encephalopathy is inappropriate, terminal confusion and agitation may require sedation.

Jaundice

Jaundice may be improved in some circumstances. Extrinsic bile duct compression may be amenable to biliary stenting or extrahepatic biliary drainage. The pruritus that almost always accompanies prolonged jaundice can be very resistant to symptomatic treatment. Bile salts are deposited in the skin, causing the irritation. Topical agents such as emollients and calamine are often of little benefit. Systemic treatments such as antihistamines and phenothiazines seem to work by sedation, though some find that complete histamine blockade by a combination of 'anti-allergy' and 'anti-ulcer' antihistamines is effective. Colestyramine (cholestyramine) and stanozolol are commonly tried in resistant cases. There are case reports of the use of ondansetron. Rifampicin and ursodeoxycholic acid are specifically indicated in primary biliary cirrhosis.

Catastrophic gastrointestinal haemorrhage is frequently the immediate cause of death in these patients, so appropriate doses of parenteral opioids and benzodiazepines should always be prescribed on an as-needed basis.

SURVIVAL/PROGNOSIS

Worldwide, the prognosis from diagnosis is around 5 or 6 years. In countries with a liver transplant programme, this may be longer, but it is still only a minority who receive a transplant rather than die on the waiting list. Attempts to develop prognostic models on the basis of clinical features and metabolic markers have not been successful.

PALLIATIVE CARE IN LIVER FAILURE

Specific research into the palliative needs of patients dying from end-stage liver disease is even more in its infancy than that into either heart or renal failure. It has been aimed at the standard treatment approaches to advanced disease as outlined above. There are no published models for palliative care involvement. Specific relationships may exist locally between palliative care and liver teams, and collaborative partnerships may in the future lead to new developments in the areas of psychological and social support and symptomatic management in advanced liver disease.

KEY POINTS

- End-of-life care in liver failure has been less extensively researched than in heart or renal failure.
- Symptomatic treatment of end-stage disease is aimed at controlling fluid overload and managing jaundice and encephalopathy.
- Collaborative working between liver and specialist palliative care teams should be encouraged.

REFERENCES

1. Hinton JM. The physical and mental stress of dying. *Q J Med* 1963; **32**, 1–21.
2. Task Force for the Diagnosis and Treatment of Chronic Heart Failure, European Society of Cardiology. Guidelines for the diagnosis and treatment of chronic heart failure. *Eur Heart J* 2001; **22**, 1527–60.
3. Cowie MR, Wood DA, Coats AJ et al. Incidence and aetiology of heart failure; a population-based study. *Eur Heart J* 1999; **20**(6), 421–8.
4. McMurray JJ, Stewart S. Epidemiology, aetiology, and prognosis of heart failure. *Heart* 2000; **83**(5), 596–602.
5. Fox KF, Cowie MR, Wood DA et al. Coronary artery disease as the cause of incident heart failure in the population. *Eur Heart J* 2001; **22**(3), 228–36.
6. Stevenson LW, Perloff JK. The limited reliability of physical signs for estimating hemodynamics in chronic heart failure. *J Am Med Assoc* 1989; **261**(6), 884–8.
7. McCarthy M, Lay M, Addington HJ. Dying from heart disease. *J R Coll Physicians Lond* 1996; **30**(4), 325–8.
8. Levenson JW, McCarthy EP, Lynn J, Davis RB, Phillips RS. The last six months of life for patients with congestive heart failure. *J Am Geriatr Soc* 2000; **48**(5 Suppl.), S101–9.
9. Anderson H, Ward C, Eardley A et al. The concerns of patients under palliative care and a heart failure clinic are not being met. *Palliat Med* 2001; **15**, 279–86.
10. Norgren L, Sørensen S. Symptoms experienced in the last six months of life in patients with end-stage heart failure. *Eur J Cardiovasc Nurs* 2003; **2**, 213–17.
11. Koenig HG. Depression in hospitalized older patients with congestive heart failure. *Gen Hosp Psychiatry* 1998; **20**(1), 29–43.
12. Jiang W, Alexander J, Christopher E et al. Relationship of depression to increased risk of mortality and rehospitalization in patients with congestive heart failure. *Arch Intern Med* 2001; **161**(15), 1849–56.
13. Drazner MH, Rame JE, Stevenson LW, Dries DL. Prognostic importance of elevated jugular venous pressure and a third heart sound in patients with heart failure. *N Engl J Med* 2001; **345**(8), 574–81.
14. Chin MH, Goldman L. Correlates of early hospital readmission or death in patients with congestive heart failure. *Am J Cardiol* 1997; **79**(12), 1640–4.
15. Ashton CM. Care of patients with failing hearts: evidence for failures in clinical practice and health services research. *J Gen Intern Med* 1999; **14**(2), 138–40.
16. Blue L, Lang E, McMurray JJ et al. Randomised controlled trial of specialist nurse intervention in heart failure. *BMJ* 2001; **323**(7315), 715–18.
17. Rich MW, Beckham V, Wittenberg C, Leven CL, Freedland KE, Carney RM. A multidisciplinary intervention to prevent the readmission of elderly patients with congestive heart failure. *N Engl J Med* 1995; **333**(18), 1190–5.
18. Stewart S, Pearson S, Horowitz JD. Effects of a home-based intervention among patients with congestive heart failure discharged from acute hospital care. *Arch Intern Med* 1998; **158**(10), 1067–72.
19. Coats AJ, Adamopoulos S, Radaelli A et al. Controlled trial of physical training in chronic heart failure. Exercise performance, hemodynamics, ventilation, and autonomic function. *Circulation* 1992; **85**(6), 2119–31.

20. ExTraMATCH Collaborative. Exercise training meta-analysis of trials in patients with chronic heart failure. *BMJ* 2004; **328**, 189–95.
21. Bernardi L, Spadacini G, Bellwon J, Hajric R, Roskamm H, Frey AW. Effect of breathing rate on oxygen saturation and exercise performance in chronic heart failure. *Lancet* 1998; **351**(9112), 1308–11.
22. Flather MD, Yusuf S, Kober L *et al.* Long-term ACE-inhibitor therapy in patients with heart failure or left-ventricular dysfunction: a systematic overview of data from individual patients. ACE-Inhibitor Myocardial Infarction Collaborative Group. *Lancet* 2000; **355**(9215), 1575–81.
23. Packer M, Poole-Wilson PA, Armstrong PW *et al.* Comparative effects of low and high doses of the angiotensin converting enzyme inhibitor, lisinopril, on morbidity and mortality in chronic heart failure. ATLAS Study Group. *Circulation* 1999; **100**(23), 2312–18.
24. Shibata MC, Flather MD, Wang D. Systematic review of the impact of beta blockers on mortality and hospital admissions in heart failure. *Eur J Heart Fail* 2001; **3**(3), 351–7.
25. Pitt B, Zannad F, Remme WJ *et al.* The effect of spironolactone on morbidity and mortality in patients with severe heart failure. Randomized Aldactone Evaluation Study Investigators. *N Engl J Med* 1999; **341**(10), 709–17.
26. The Digitalis Investigation Group. The effect of digoxin on mortality and morbidity in patients with heart failure. *N Engl J Med* 1997; **336**, 525–33.
27. Shapiro PA, Lesperance F, Frasure-Smith N *et al.* An open-label preliminary trial of sertraline for treatment of major depression after acute myocardial infarction (the SADHAT Trial). Sertraline Anti-Depressant Heart Attack Trial. *Am Heart J* 1999; **137**(6), 1100–6.
28. Johnson MJ, McDonagh TA, Harkness A, McKay SE, Dargie HJ. Morphine for the relief of breathlessness in patients with chronic heart failure – a pilot study. *Eur J Heart Failure* 2002; **4**, 753–6.
29. Cowie MR, Wood DA, Coats AJ *et al.* Survival of patients with a new diagnosis of heart failure: a population-based study. *Heart* 2000; **83**(5), 505–10.
30. Swedberg K, Eneroth P, Kjekshus J, Wilhelmsen L. Hormones regulating cardiovascular function in patients with severe congestive heart failure and their relation to mortality. CONSENSUS Trial Study Group. *Circulation* 1990; **82**(5), 1730–6.
31. Cohn JN, Johnson GR, Shabetai R *et al.* Ejection fraction, peak exercise oxygen consumption, cardiothoracic ratio, ventricular arrhythmias, and plasma norepinephrine as determinants of prognosis in heart failure. The V-HeFT VA Cooperative Studies Group. *Circulation* 1993; **87**(6 Suppl.), VI5–16.
32. McCarthy M, Addington-Hall JM, Ley M. Communication and choice in dying from heart disease. *J R Soc Med* 1997; **90**, 128–31.
33. Rogers AE, Addington-Hall JM, Abery AJ *et al.* Knowledge and communication difficulties for patients with chronic heart failure: qualitative study. *BMJ* 2000; **321**(7261), 605–7.
34. Stewart AL, Greenfled S, Hays RD, Wells K, Rogers WH, Berry SD. Functional status and well-being of patients with chronic conditions. Results from the medical outcomes study. *J Am Med Assoc* 1989; **262**, 907–13.
35. Thorns AR, Gibbs LM, Gibbs JS. Management of severe heart failure by specialist palliative care. *Heart* 2001; **85**(1), 93.

36. Teno JM, Weitzen S, Fennell ML, Mor V. Dying trajectory in the last year of life: does cancer trajectory fit other diseases? *J Palliat Med* 2001; **4**, 457–64.

37. Hanratty B, Hibbert D, Mair F *et al*. Doctors' perceptions of palliative care for heart failure: focus group study. *BMJ* 2002; **325**, 581–5.

38. Albert NM, Davis M, Young J. Improving the care of patients dying of heart failure. *Cleve Clin J Med* 2002; **69**, 321–8.

39. *National Service Framework for Coronary Heart Disease*. London: Department of Health, 2000.

40. National Institute for Clinical Excellence. *Chronic heart failure: national clinical guideline for diagnosis and management in primary and secondary care*. London: NICE, 2003.

41. Agency for Health Care Policy and Research (AHCPR). Heart failure: evaluation and treatment of patients with left ventricular systolic dysfunction. *J Am Geriatr Soc* 1998; **46**(4), 525–9.

42. Dracup K, Guzy PM, Taylor SE, Barry J. Cardiopulmonary resuscitation (CPR) training. Consequences for family members of high-risk cardiac patients. *Arch Intern Med* 1986; **146**(9), 1757–61.

43. Feest TG, Round A, Hamad S. Incidence of severe acute renal failure in adults: results of a community-based study. *BMJ* 1993; **306**(6876), 481–3.

44. Feest TG, Mistry CD, Grimes DS, Mallick NP. Incidence of advanced chronic renal failure and the need for end stage renal replacement treatment. *BMJ* 1990; **301**(6757), 897–900.

45. Denton MD, Chertow GM, Brady HR. 'Renal-dose' dopamine for the treatment of acute renal failure: scientific rationale, experimental studies and clinical trials. *Kidney Int* 1996; **50**(1), 4–14.

46. The Renal Association. *Treatment of adult patients with renal failure: recommended standards and audit measures*. London: Royal College of Physicians of London, 1995.

47. Parfrey PS, Vavasour HM, Henry S, Bullock M, Gault MH. Clinical features and severity of nonspecific symptoms in dialysis patients. *Nephron* 1988; **50**(2), 121–8.

48. Fainsinger RL, Davison SN, Brennis C. A supportive care model for dialysis patients. *Palliat Med* 2003; **17**, 81–2.

49. Neu S, Kjellstrand CM. Stopping long-term dialysis. An empirical study of withdrawal of life-supporting treatment. *N Engl J Med* 1986; **314**(1), 14–20.

50. Mailloux LU, Bellucci AG, Napolitano B, Mossey RT, Wilkes BM, Bluestone PA. Death by withdrawal from dialysis: a 20-year clinical experience. *J Am Soc Nephrol* 1993; 3(9), 1631–7.

51. Cohen LM, McCue JD, Germain M, Kjellstrand CM. Dialysis discontinuation. A 'good' death? *Arch Intern Med* 1995; **155**(1), 42–7.

52. Cohen LM, Germain M, Poppel DM, Woods A, Kjellstrand CM. Dialysis discontinuation and palliative care. *Am J Kidney Dis* 2000; **36**(1), 140–4.

53. Moss AH for the Renal Physicians Association and American Society of Nephrology Working Group. A new clinical practice guideline on initiation and withdrawal of dialysis that makes explicit the role of palliative medicine. *J Palliat Med* 2000; 3(3), 253–60.

54. Poppel DM, Cohen LM, Germain MD. The renal palliative care initiative. *J Palliat Med* 2003; **6**(2), 321–6.

55. Auer J. Issues surrounding the withdrawal of dialysis treatment. *Nephrol Dial Transplant* 1998; **13**(5), 1149–51.

56. Hine J. Standards of palliative care in a renal care setting. *EDTNA ERCA J* 1998; **24**(4), 27–9, 35.

57. Pandian SS, Hussey JK, McClinton S. Metallic ureteric stents: early experience. *Br J Urol* 1998; **82**(6), 791–7.

58. Smith P, Bruera E. Management of malignant ureteral obstruction in the palliative care setting. *J Pain Symptom Manage* 1995; **10**(6), 481–6.

59. Kite S, Jones K, Tookman A. Specialist palliative care and patients with noncancer diagnoses: the experience of a service. *Palliat Med* 1999; **13**(6), 477–84.

60. Ellershaw J, Smith C, Overill S, Walker SE, Aldridge J. Care of the dying: setting standards for symptom control in the last 48 hours of life. *J Pain Symptom Manage* 2001; **21**(1), 12–17.

61. Farrell A, Rich A. Analgesic use in patients with renal failure. *Eur J Palliat Care* 2000; **7**(6), 201–5.

62. Mercadante S, Caligara M, Sapio M, Serretta R, Lodi F. Subcutaneous fentanyl infusion in a patient with bowel obstruction and renal failure. *J Pain Symptom Manage* 1997; **13**(4), 241–4.

63. Lee MA, Leng ME, Tiernan EJ. Retrospective study of the use of hydromorphone in palliative care patients with normal and abnormal urea and creatinine. *Palliat Med* 2001; **15**(1), 26–34.

64. Kirkham SR, Pugh R. Opioid analgesia in uraemic patients. *Lancet* 1995; **345**(8958), 1185.

65. Broadbent A, Khor K, Heaney A. Palliation and renal failure: common non-opioid medication dosage guidelines. *Prog Palliat Care* 2003; **11**, 59–65.

66. Broadbent A, Khor K, Heaney A. Palliation and chronic renal failure: opioid and other palliative medications – dosage guidelines. *Prog Palliat Care* 2003; **11**, 183–90.

67. Andrews PA. Palliative care for patients with terminal renal failure. *Lancet* 1995; **346**(8973), 506–7.

FURTHER READING

Addington-Hall JM, Higginson IJ (eds). *Palliative care for non-cancer patients*. Oxford: Oxford University Press, 2001.

Agency for Health Care Policy and Research (AHCPR). Heart failure: evaluation and treatment of patients with left ventricular systolic dysfunction. *J Am Geriatr Soc* 1998; **46**(4), 525–9.

National Institute for Clinical Excellence. *Chronic heart failure: national clinical guideline for diagnosis and management in primary and secondary care*. London: NICE, 2003.

Task Force for the Diagnosis and Treatment of Chronic Heart Failure, European Society of Cardiology. Guidelines for the diagnosis and treatment of chronic heart failure. *Eur Heart J* 2001; **22**, 1527–60.

chapter 15

RESPIRATORY DISEASE

Charles Shee

INTRODUCTION

This chapter concentrates on the management of chronic obstructive pulmonary disease (COPD) as this is much the commonest cause of severe chronic respiratory disability. Palliative medicine is concerned with the treatment of patients with disease that is progressive, active, far advanced and with a limited prognosis. Patients with severe COPD fall into this category. Most of those who have developed markedly low oxygen levels (hypoxia) will be dead within 3 years if not given long-term oxygen.[1]

The previous tendency to therapeutic nihilism with respect to the management of COPD patients is changing, with increasing interest in the management of the disease and the value of 'pulmonary rehabilitation'. There is also increasing awareness of the psychosocial problems associated with COPD. It is becoming apparent that there are unmet needs and that emphasis needs to shift from ad hoc management of acute exacerbations towards a more holistic and palliative approach to care.[2]

DEFINITION AND PREVALENCE

Chronic obstructive pulmonary disease includes chronic obstructive bronchitis and emphysema. It is a chronic, slowly progressive disorder characterized by airways obstruction that is largely fixed, although it may be possible to improve airflow obstruction to a minor degree with bronchodilator therapy. COPD predominantly affects older people, and mortality figures for England and Wales show approximately 250–300 deaths per 100 000 persons aged 65–84 years per annum.[3] Morbidity is considerable, with general practice consultation rates for older patients two to four times those for angina[4] and frequent use of hospital services.

Asthma (reversible airways obstruction) affects up to 4 per cent of the population at some time, but in most people is mild and does not cause long-term morbidity. There is a small group of non-steroid-responsive asthmatics with predominantly 'fixed' airways obstruction and chronic morbidity. Apart from a greater stress on the use of bronchodilators and oral steroids, the management of these patients is similar to that of those with COPD.

Cystic fibrosis affects about 1 in 2500 children. It causes recurrent pulmonary infection with or without pancreatic insufficiency, and the infection is associated with airways obstruction, lung damage and scarring. The basic defect involves the control of ion and water transport across epithelial cells. Survival has improved progressively over the last few decades and the median survival in developed countries now approaches 30 years. Treatment in specialist centres improves overall care and survival and some of these centres now have their own home support teams. The large number of complications and the management problems in cystic fibrosis are beyond the scope of this chapter.

Some patients with *severe fibrotic lung disease* (for instance due to fibrosing alveolitis or sarcoidosis) may enter a phase in which active treatment is no longer successful and palliative treatment is required. In comparison with the 26 000 deaths per year in England and Wales attributed to COPD, there are thought to be only a few thousand deaths per year in the whole of the UK from lung fibrosis.

Respiratory failure can occur from *respiratory muscle disorders* (e.g. muscular dystrophy or old poliomyelitis) or with *severe chest wall disease* (e.g. scoliosis). A variety of positive and negative pressure devices is available for domiciliary respiratory support, which can improve quality of life and reduce mortality.[5,6] In view of the major symptomatic improvement that can occur in some of these patients following ventilatory support, they should usually be referred to an appropriate specialist centre.

PATHOPHYSIOLOGY AND CLINICAL FEATURES OF COPD

The single most important cause of COPD is cigarette smoking. The mortality and most of the morbidity associated with COPD relate to the airways obstruction and not the chronic mucus hypersecretion (chronic bronchitis). Airflow obstruction is due to permanent narrowing of the large and medium-sized airways.

Emphysema is defined as destruction of the air spaces (alveoli) and terminal bronchioles. It is associated with loss of the normal elastic recoil of the lungs and destruction of the 'scaffold' that serves to keep small airways open during expiration.

A diagnosis of COPD in clinical practice requires a history of chronic progressive symptoms such as breathlessness, wheeze or cough associated with objective evidence of airways obstruction that does not return to normal with treatment. There is usually a cigarette-smoking history of more than 20 pack-years.

Airways obstruction is often measured as the volume expired during the first second of a forced expiration (FEV_1). Obstruction may be associated with 'gas trapping' (hyperinflation) and reduction in gas transfer in the lungs. In patients with mild disease, clinical examination is likely to be normal. In moderate disease, there may be wheeze or evidence of over-inflation. In severe disease, there may also be weight loss, central cyanosis, peripheral oedema or evidence of pulmonary hypertension.

Table 15.1 Some problems associated with severe chronic obstructive pulmonary disease

Respiratory
Cough
Breathlessness
Non-respiratory
Fatigue
Pain
Difficulty sleeping
Thirst
Frequent exacerbations and hospital admissions
Immobility and inactivity
Psychosocial
Uncertain prognosis
Isolation
Depression
Low self-esteem
Burden on carers
Poverty

Some of the symptoms associated with COPD are shown in Table 15.1. Patients with severe COPD are usually troubled by progressive disabling breathlessness, and cough and wheeze are almost invariably present. Because mental state and attitudes can influence breathlessness and exercise capacity, it is perhaps not surprising that in severe lung disease there is a poor correlation between lung function, breathlessness and exercise capacity.[7] COPD is often associated with social isolation, economic disadvantage and fear. The associated uncertainty concerning prognosis can contribute to psychological distress. There is a much greater than expected psychiatric morbidity in COPD, with depression being common.[7-9] Unlike patients with lung cancer, those with COPD may have one crisis after another over some years before dying. In one study, people with end-stage COPD were actually more likely than terminal lung cancer patients to suffer from depression and/or anxiety.[10]

As breathlessness is a frightening symptom, many people with chronic respiratory impairment become progressively less active and less 'fit'. This can contribute to further isolation and development of a 'vicious circle'. As with other chronic diseases, there may be significant co-morbidity. Patients who have been admitted to hospital with an exacerbation of their respiratory condition often have a poor quality of life and low physical functioning.[2,10] Extreme breathlessness is experienced by almost all, but pain, fatigue, difficulty sleeping and thirst are also common.[2]

TREATMENT OF ADVANCED COPD

The medical management of COPD is outlined in Table 15.2. The FEV_1 declines with age, and falls more rapidly in people who continue to smoke. Patients should

Table 15.2 Medical management of chronic obstructive pulmonary disease

---

Smoking cessation
Antibiotics for infective exacerbations
Inhaled bronchodilators
    Beta-stimulants
    Anticholinergics
Vaccination against influenza
Corticosteroid reversibility trial
Assessment for long-term oxygen
Pulmonary rehabilitation
Treatment of exacerbations (including non-invasive ventilation)

---

be persuaded to try to stop smoking, as this will slow the rate of decline of FEV_1. This is important, as in severe COPD a further small reduction in FEV_1 can lead to a disproportionate decrease in the ability to perform daily activities. Participation in an active smoking cessation programme leads to a higher sustained quit rate, especially when nicotine replacement therapy is included.[11]

Bronchodilators are the most important aspect of treatment for the reversible component of airways obstruction. Inhaled agents are preferable to oral preparations. Short-acting beta-2-receptor agonists or inhaled anticholinergics are used as required depending upon symptomatic response. Inhaler technique should be optimized and an appropriate device selected to ensure adequate lung penetration. Combination therapy with a regular beta-agonist and anticholinergic can be helpful. There is increasing evidence of benefit from inhaled long-acting beta-2-agonists. A new long-acting anti-cholinergic inhaler, Tiotropium, is also useful.[12] Oral theophyllines may produce minor improvements in COPD symptoms, but can cause side effects such as nausea, even at recommended therapeutic blood levels. Mucolytic drug therapy should be considered in patients with a chronic cough productive of sputum.

The results of recent studies suggest that treatment with inhaled corticosteroids does not modify the rate of decline of lung function.[13] However, there is a suggestion that in patients with more severe disease there may be a reduction in the number of exacerbations.[13]

There is uncertainty concerning the use of home nebulizer treatment in patients with COPD. Most patients can be treated with bronchodilators delivered by metered-dose inhalers and spacers or by dry powder devices. Ideally, a nebulizer should only be prescribed after a home trial with peak expiratory flow measurements.

There is no evidence to support the use of prophylactic antibiotics given either continuously or intermittently. There is no role for other anti-inflammatory drugs or anti-histamines in COPD.[4] Yearly influenza vaccination is recommended, but the role of pneumococcal vaccine is uncertain. Exercise is to be encouraged in patients with all degrees of severity. Although breathlessness on exertion may be distressing, it is not dangerous, and helps improve general health.

OXYGEN

Long-term oxygen therapy (LTOT) improves survival in advanced hypoxic COPD.[1] Non-smoking patients with stable, severe COPD ($FEV_1 < 1.5$ L) and arterial hypoxia (<7.3 kPa, i.e. 55 mmHg), with or without hypercapnia, may benefit from low-flow domiciliary oxygen used in excess of 15 hours per day. LTOT can also be prescribed in COPD if the clinically stable PaO_2 is between 7.3 and 8 kPa in association with secondary polycythaemia, nocturnal hypoxia, peripheral oedema or evidence of pulmonary hypertension.[14] LTOT is not recommended with a PaO_2 above 8 kPa. It is usually prescribed via an oxygen concentrator, which is cheaper and more convenient than cylinders and acts as a 'molecular sieve' to produce oxygen-enriched gas from air. Patients should be assessed by a respiratory specialist prior to prescription of LTOT.

Short-burst oxygen therapy is frequently used for pre-oxygenation for exercise, breathlessness during recovery from exercise, and control of breathlessness at rest. Despite extensive prescription of short-burst therapy, there is no adequate evidence available for firm recommendations, but ideally it should only be used for patients not on LTOT if any improvement in breathlessness and/or exercise tolerance can be documented.[14]

Ambulatory oxygen therapy employs lightweight oxygen cylinders worn by the patient, carried by another person or pushed on a trolley. It can be prescribed for patients on LTOT who are mobile and need to leave the home on a regular basis. Patients without chronic hypoxia can be considered for ambulatory oxygen therapy if they show evidence of exercise oxygen desaturation, improvement in exercise capacity and/or dyspnoea with ambulatory oxygen therapy, and the motivation to use the ambulatory oxygen outside the house.[14] Patients who are continuing to smoke cigarettes should not be prescribed ambulatory oxygen, as the benefits are debatable in this situation and risks from burns are considerable. Ambulatory oxygen therapy can also be prescribed for patients with cystic fibrosis, interstitial lung disease, chest wall and neuromuscular disorders where there is demonstrable exercise desaturation.

SURGERY

In selected patients, lung transplantation (often single lung) can dramatically improve symptoms. However, there is a severe shortage of donor organs, and problems with late bronchiolitis obliterans after transplantation remain. Rarely, surgical removal or ablation of a large bulla (air sac) may be helpful. Recent reports, predominantly from the USA, have described lung volume reduction surgery in which various forms of surgical ablation of severely affected areas of emphysematous lung have been used. Surprising improvements in lung function can be seen, particularly in patients with severe disease and very marked air trapping.[15] Improvement persists for at least 1–2 years, but it seems that by 3 years lung function is often back to baseline.[16] This 'palliative' major surgery should still be regarded as experimental pending further research.[15]

ACUTE EXACERBATIONS OF COPD

The home treatment of acute exacerbations is to add or increase bronchodilators and to prescribe an antibiotic if infection is likely. Oral corticosteroids can also be prescribed. In hospital, the treatment of an acute exacerbation is similar, with the addition of nebulized beta-agonist or ipratropium bromide. Where there is no response, one would consider intravenous aminophylline. Controlled oxygen, 24–28 per cent via mask or 2 L/min by nasal prongs, is given, with regular checks on arterial blood gases. With exhaustion and respiratory failure, intubation and artificial ventilation may be needed. Artificial ventilation may not be appropriate in some patients with terminal lung disease. The decision whether or not to ventilate is a sensitive one and ideally should be made by a senior doctor, preferably after consultation with the patient and family.

Increasingly, non-invasive positive pressure ventilation (NIPPV) is being used. NIPPV is ventilatory support delivered via nasal mask or facemask, triggered by the patients' own inspiration, and with patients monitoring their own airways. A meta-analysis of eight trials of NIPPV used in exacerbations of COPD has shown that the number of patients requiring endotracheal intubation is significantly reduced (58 per cent risk reduction, with a number needed to treat (NNT) of 5) and that the length of stay in hospital is reduced by 3 days.[17] NIPPV also reduced short-term mortality (59 per cent risk reduction, NNT 8).[17]

The use of NIPPV is rapidly becoming more common in British district general hospitals,[18] and, apart from obviating the need for intubation and ventilation, in some patients it is useful for palliating severe breathlessness and distress even when a decision has been made not to intubate and ventilate. In COPD and other terminal respiratory conditions for which NIPPV is used primarily to relieve distress rather than to prolong survival, it may be thought of as a palliative procedure.

When patients with lung disease suffer from the sleep apnoea syndrome, the use of nocturnal continuous positive airway pressure may markedly improve daytime somnolence. The use of nocturnal NIPPV in people with chest wall and neuromuscular disorders is well established,[5,6] but it is currently uncertain just which patients with COPD may benefit from nocturnal respiratory assistance with NIPPV.[5] The improvement in individual patients can certainly be dramatic.

TREATMENT OF BREATHLESSNESS

Breathlessness is a complicated sensation and is perceived following input from receptors in the lungs, chest wall, upper airways and trigeminal nerve. There are also inputs to the cortex from peripheral chemoreceptors, the brainstem and motor cortex. It is perhaps not surprising that treatment of the symptom of breathlessness is difficult. Distraction, reassurance, breathing exercises, cold air on the face, and nebulizers seem useful, but hard evidence to support these treatments is lacking. If bronchodilators fail to relieve breathlessness, are there any drugs that can reduce the sensation? Reports in the 1980s suggested that oral diazepam was useful in treating breathlessness in 'pink and puffing' patients with COPD. However, a later study found that diazepam had no effect on breathlessness and that it reduced exercise tolerance.[19] Many drugs have been tried for breathlessness but, in general, the therapeutic benefit has been marginal and side effects considerable.[20] Initial reports suggested nebulized morphine might improve exercise endurance and breathlessness in patients with chronic lung disease, but further studies have not borne this out.[21]

Oral morphine might have some effect on COPD breathlessness,[22] but further evidence is needed. All chest physicians have seen patients with respiratory failure (alveolar hypoventilation) resulting from the injudicious use of benzodiazepines and opioids. The use of these drugs in severe COPD therefore needs close monitoring. Generally, 'pink puffers' tend to be more breathless than 'blue bloaters', and the risk of respiratory depression is less in the former. Diazepam 2 mg 4-hourly as necessary can be tried or, alternatively, morphine 2.5–5 mg 4-hourly, carefully increasing the dose if necessary. Anecdotally, patients seem to prefer frequent low doses of morphine rather than twice-daily slow-release preparations, as one might use for pain control, possibly because of the sense of 'control' this gives them over their breathlessness. Because of the long half-life of diazepam, long-term use is best avoided. Lorazepam (0.5–1 mg sublingually) can also help respiratory panic attacks.

The principles of the treatment of dyspnoea in the dying are similar whether one is dealing with end-stage lung disease or cancer. There is little scientific evidence about which drug is best for terminal breathlessness, but subcutaneous midazolam or diamorphine is frequently used.

PULMONARY REHABILITATION

A major advance in the management of patients with severe lung disease has been the introduction of 'pulmonary rehabilitation'. Pulmonary rehabilitation uses a multi-disciplinary programme of education, exercise training, physiotherapy and psychotherapy to help the patient return to the highest possible functional capacity. Most programmes involve a team including a doctor, physiotherapist, occupational therapist, dietician, social worker or psychologist. All successful programmes involve both exercise and education. Topics generally covered include:

- exercise (including walking and strength exercises),

- management of symptoms,

- coping techniques,

- breathing control and relaxation,

- smoking cessation,

- nutritional advice,

- energy conservation,

- drugs and oxygen,

- advice on social support and financial benefits.

Pulmonary rehabilitation has been shown to be effective in prospective randomized clinical studies and in a meta-analysis of the literature.[23] Survival is probably not improved, and there is usually no change in spirometry values or arterial blood gases. However, there is evidence that rehabilitation reduces symptoms and number of hospital admissions and improves performance, exercise endurance and quality of life. Better exercise endurance in the absence of objective cardiopulmonary improvement suggests that a reduction in breathlessness perception is important.[24] It is interesting that a multi-faceted intervention programme for breathlessness in *cancer* has also been shown to be useful.[25]

Most studies of pulmonary rehabilitation have looked at moderately severe disease, but in one study that involved a severely disabled group, who were largely housebound owing to breathlessness, there was no improvement following individualized exercise training.[26] Similarly, there was little improvement in 'health status' in the severely breathless treated group.[26]

PROGRESSION OF COPD

The best guide to the progression of COPD is the change in FEV_1 over time. Individual susceptibility to cigarette smoking is very wide, such that approximately 15 per cent of smokers will develop clinically significant COPD, whereas approximately half will never develop any symptomatic physiological deficit. Prognosis is related to both age and FEV_1. Thus, 3-year survival figures have been estimated as:[4]

- aged <60 and FEV_1 >50 per cent predicted = 90 per cent,

- aged >60 and FEV_1 40–49 per cent predicted = 75 per cent.

In patients with severe disease and hypoxia, prognosis can be worse than with metastatic prostate or breast cancer. In the Medical Research Council LTOT study, the 5-year survival in patients not given oxygen was only 25 per cent (41 per cent with 15 hours of oxygen therapy per day).[1] Unlike patients with lung cancer, patients with COPD may go from one crisis to another over some years before a fairly rapid final event.

PALLIATIVE CARE NEEDS IN COPD

The palliative care needs of patients aged over 55 years with chronic lung disease who had been admitted to hospital for 7 days or more with an exacerbation of their respiratory condition were studied.[2] Following discharge from hospital, 63 individuals were interviewed. The findings revealed a poor quality of life, relating to a high degree of social isolation and emotional distress, associated with low physical functioning and disability, and physical symptoms. As would be expected, the most distressing and debilitating symptom was extreme breathlessness. However, the extent of other symptoms reported was considerable, such as pain in 68 per cent, fatigue in 68 per cent, difficulty sleeping in 55 per cent, and thirst in 54 per cent.[2] Most patients expressed satisfaction with their acute treatment in hospital. Deficits in service provision in the community were identified. The authors concluded that there was a need to shift the emphasis from reactive ad hoc provision towards managing the health and social care interface more effectively.[2]

Another study compared 50 patients with severe COPD (and at least one previous hospital admission for respiratory failure) and 50 patients with unresectable non-small-cell lung cancer.[10] The patients with COPD had significantly worse activities of daily living and physical, social and emotional functioning than those with cancer. No patient with COPD had received help from specialist palliative care services.[10] A recent review has pointed out that, in addition to depression, there is a high prevalence of feelings of low self-esteem in patients with COPD.[9] They are also often deficient in various coping skills.

Symptom control in hospital is not always adequate. Studies in the USA have revealed shortcomings in communication with, and pain control for, patients with advanced COPD.[27] Invasive treatment including mechanical ventilation is frequent, even shortly before death.[27] Hospital support teams can have a significant role to play in symptom control of end-stage lung disease. Some of the palliative care needs in severe COPD are summarized in Table 15.3.

MODELS FOR PALLIATIVE CARE INVOLVEMENT

The palliative approach in severe end-stage lung disease does not necessarily need to involve *specialist* palliative care. The advantages of 'pulmonary rehabilitation' have been mentioned. Patients who have attended these courses usually feel better, with improved quality of life and exercise tolerance and less breathlessness. A review of the psychosocial support in pulmonary rehabilitation programmes for patients with COPD concluded that virtually all identified studies showed

Table 15.3 Palliative care needs in chronic obstructive pulmonary disease

Symptom control
Help with daily activities
Coping skills/relaxation/breathing control
Social and financial support
Emotional support
Information
Support for carers

significant improvements in the psychosocial domain, i.e. self-efficacy, perceived shortness of breath, and quality of life.[9]

Increasingly, respiratory specialist nurses are being appointed in the UK. Nurses are often based in hospitals, but will make community visits. As yet, there is insufficient knowledge about what kind of nursing care makes a difference to patient outcomes and how much quality of life is improved.[28] Some centres in the UK have set up 'hospital at home' respiratory support for patients with exacerbations of COPD. Various models are being evaluated, which should clarify the success of these schemes in avoiding hospital admission and/or improving quality of life. In recognition of the physical and social problems associated with living with long-term lung conditions, the British Lung Foundation has set up a club, 'Breathe Easy', to help to relieve anxiety and isolation.

Some domiciliary palliative care teams will see people with terminal lung disease, but in many of these teams, priority is given to those with cancer. Similarly, although hospices are increasingly accepting patients with non-cancer diagnoses, cancer still remains the most common reason for admission to a hospice. Patients dying of COPD may spend a large proportion of their last 6 months in hospitals, but it is still the exception for hospital palliative care teams/support teams to be involved in advising on symptom control. In Britain, lung cancer nurse specialists are increasingly being appointed, and perhaps it could be part of their remit to review distressed in-patients with end-stage lung disease.

Current service provision in COPD is focused on acute exacerbations and there is a need to manage the health and social care interface more effectively.[2,10] Perhaps this is where the palliative approach to care is best suited to meet the needs identified. Overall care of the patients would remain with general practitioners, chest physicians and respiratory nurse specialists. Palliative care specialists could assist by providing a coherent approach to assessment, facilitating access to community services and assisting in the management of symptoms such as pain, constipation and cachexia.

LIMITATIONS OF PALLIATIVE CARE

The ideal model of palliative care in terminal respiratory disease has yet to be devised. There are limitations to the existing models of service delivery and large gaps in our knowledge.

- Patients in the community and in hospital who might benefit from specialist palliative care often do not receive it.

- There is no systematic record or register of these patients and there may be a large 'unmet need'.

- Custom (and sometimes charitable status) of some hospices/support teams precludes involvement in non-malignant conditions.

- General support for people with end-stage lung disease (charity shops, support organizations, volunteer groups etc.) is markedly less than for cancer sufferers.

- The role of respiratory and lung cancer nurse specialists in the management of these patients needs clarifying.

- The uncertain prognosis during acute exacerbations in a chronic illness can make it difficult to switch from an 'active treatment' to a 'palliative' mode.

- Pulmonary rehabilitation works well in ambulant patients but does not appear to work in severely ill, housebound patients.

- Compared with the treatment of pain, the treatment of breathlessness remains extremely unsatisfactory.

- Further development is required in designing lightweight, portable oxygen cylinders and in deciding which patients will benefit from these.

The palliative approach to the care of patients with severe respiratory disease will inevitably differ from that in cancer. The debate has started, but much more research is needed to improve symptom management and evaluate different approaches to care.

KEY POINTS

- Chronic respiratory disease is often associated with significant co-morbidity and non-respiratory symptoms, but facilities for support are less well developed than for cancer patients.
- Emphasis needs to switch from the treatment of acute exacerbations to a more systematic approach to managing chronic symptoms and psychosocial problems.
- Multi-disciplinary 'pulmonary rehabilitation' has been shown to be of benefit.
- It is never too late to stop smoking.
- Inhaled bronchodilators are the mainstay of treatment for COPD.
- Patients with hypoxia should be assessed for suitability for long-term domiciliary oxygen treatment.
- Non-invasive ventilation is increasingly being used for exacerbations of COPD. It is important to document resuscitation status.
- People with respiratory impairment due to musculoskeletal or neurological causes should be reviewed at a specialist centre.

REFERENCES

1. Report of the Medical Research Council Oxygen Working Party. Long-term domiciliary oxygen therapy in chronic hypoxic cor pulmonale complicating chronic bronchitis and emphysema. *Lancet* 1981; **1**, 681–5.
2. Skilbeck J, Mott L, Page H, Smith D, Hjelmeland-Ahmedzai S, Clark D. Palliative care in chronic obstructive airways disease: a needs assessment. *Palliat Med* 1998; **12**, 245–54.
3. Rijcken B, Britton J. Epidemiology of chronic obstructive pulmonary disease. Management of chronic obstructive pulmonary disease. *Eur Respir Monogr* 1988; **7**, 41–73.

4. British Thoracic Society. Guidelines for the management of chronic obstructive pulmonary disease. *Thorax* 1997; **52**, Suppl. 5.

5. Turkington PM, Elliott MW. Rationale for the use of non-invasive ventilation in chronic ventilatory failure. *Thorax* 2000; 55, 417–23.

6. Schneerson J. Quality of life in neuromuscular and skeletal disorders. *Eur Respir Rev* 1997; 7(42), 71–3.

7. Morgan AD, Peck DF, Buchanan DR, McHardy GJR. Effect of attitudes and beliefs on exercise tolerance in chronic bronchitis. *BMJ* 1983; **286**, 171–3.

8. Heaton RK, Grant I, McSweeney AJ, Adams KM, Petty TL. Psychologic effects of continuous and nocturnal oxygen therapy in hypoxemic chronic obstructive pulmonary disease. *Arch Intern Med* 1983; **143**, 1941–7.

9. Kaptein AA, Dekker FW. Psychosocial support. *Eur Respir Monogr* 2000; **13**, 58–69.

10. Gore JM, Brophy CJ, Greenstone MA. How well do we care for patients with end-stage chronic obstructive pulmonary disease (COPD)? A comparison of palliative care and quality of life in COPD and lung cancer. *Thorax* 2000; **55**, 1000–6.

11. West R, McNeill A, Raw M. Smoking cessation guidelines for health professionals: an update. *Thorax* 2000; **55**, 987–99.

12. Joos GF, Bruselle G, Derom E, Pauwels R. Tiotropium bromide: a long-acting anticholinergic bronchodilator for the treatment of patients with chronic obstructive pulmonary disease. *Int J Clin Prac*, 2003; **57**, 906–9.

13. Van Schayck CP. Is lung function really a good parameter in evaluating the long-term effects of inhaled cortico-steroids in COPD? *Eur Respir J* 2000; **15**, 238–9.

14. *Domiciliary oxygen therapy services.* London: Royal College of Physicians, 1999.

15. Young J, Fry-Smith A, Hyde C. Lung volume reduction surgery (LVRS) for chronic obstructive pulmonary disease (COPD) with underlying severe emphysema. *Thorax* 1999; **54**, 779–89.

16. Roue C, Mal H, Sleiman C *et al*. Lung volume reduction in patients with severe diffuse emphysema. *Chest* 1996; **110**, 28–34.

17. Lightowler JV, Wedzicha JA, Elliott MW, Ram FSF. Non-invasive positive pressure ventilation to treat respiratory failure resulting from exacerbations of chronic obstructive pulmonary disease: Cochrane Systematic Review and meta-analysis. *BMJ* 2003; **326**, 185–7.

18. Shee CD, Green M. Non-invasive ventilation and palliation: experience in a district general hospital and a review. *Palliat Med* 2003; **17**, 21–6.

19. Woodcock AA, Gross ER, Geddes DM. Drug treatment of breathlessness: contrasting effects of diazepam and promethazine in pink puffers. *BMJ* 1981; **283**, 343–6.

20. Stark RD. Breathlessness: assessment and pharmacological manipulation. *Eur Respir J* 1998; 1, 280–7.

21. Jankelson D, Hosseini K, Mather LE, Seale JP, Young IH. Lack of effect of high doses of inhaled morphine on exercise endurance in chronic obstructive pulmonary disease. *Eur Respir J* 1997; **10**, 2270–4.

22. Light RW, Stansbury DW, Webster JS. Effect of 30 mg of morphine alone or with promethazine or prochlorperazine on the exercise capacity of patients with COPD. *Chest* 1996; **109**, 975–81.

23. Lacasse Y, Wong E, Guyatt GH, King D, Cook DJ, Goldstein RS. Meta-analysis of respiratory rehabilitation in chronic obstructive pulmonary disease. *Lancet* 1996; **348**, 1115–19.

24. Belman MJ. (1993). Pulmonary rehabilitation in chronic respiratory insufficiency: 2 – Exercise in patients with chronic obstructive pulmonary disease. *Thorax* 1993; **48**, 936–46.
25. Bredin M, Corner J, Krishnasamy M, Plant H, Bailey C, A'Hern R. Multi-centre randomised controlled trial of nursing intervention for breathlessness in patients with lung cancer. *BMJ* 1999; **318**, 901–4.
26. Wedzicka JA, Bestall JC, Garrod R, Graham R, Paul EA, Jones PW. Randomised controlled trial of pulmonary rehabilitation in severe chronic obstructive pulmonary disease patients, stratified with the MRC breathlessness scale. *Eur Respir J* 1998; **12**, 363–9.
27. Hansen-Flaschen J. Advanced lung disease. Palliation and terminal care. *Clin Chest Med* 1997; **18**(No. 3), 645–55.
28. Littlejohns P, Baveystock CM, Parnell H, Jones PW. Randomised controlled trial of the effectiveness of a respiratory health worker in reducing impairment, disability and handicap due to chronic airflow limitation. *Thorax* 1991; **46**, 559–64.

PSYCHOSOCIAL, SPIRITUAL AND ETHICAL ISSUES

chapter 16

PSYCHOSOCIAL DIMENSIONS OF CARE

Barbara Monroe and Frances Sheldon

Cancer can affect a family in much the same way as it invades the body, causing deterioration if left untreated.

Colin Murray Parkes

[Psychosocial care is] concerned with the psychological and emotional wellbeing of the patient and their families/carers including issues of self esteem, insight into and adaptation to the illness and its consequences, communication, social functioning and relationships.

National Council for Hospice and Specialist Palliative Care Services[1]

The burden of terminal illness is not just physical. Dying individuals are facing loss at every level: physical health, independence, career and status, usual family and friendship relationships, predictability in future plans, motivation and meaning. They will experience a draining diminution in their self-confidence and in their belief in their ability to control their own lives. These losses are often experienced in parallel by families, friends and carers. Everyone will express their grief through a powerful, unfamiliar and often frightening mixture of confused emotions, which may include shock, denial, anxiety, anger, guilt, sadness and fear. All need information so that they are aware of the options, and support to reassert their own sense of dignity and self-worth by making decisions and regaining control wherever possible.

Psychological distress is key in the individual's experience of illness and interacts with physical distress.[2–4] Psychological distress is influenced by perceptions of family and social support, attributions of meaning and hope, and the perceived degree of personal control. In Barkwell's study, for example, patients with cancer were divided into three groups according to the meaning they attributed to their disease: challenge, punishment, enemy.[5] More pain and depression were experienced by those who saw their illness as a punishment. Herth's important studies on the concept of hope demonstrate links between high levels of hope and high levels of coping and identify areas that promote or threaten the maintenance of hope in the dying individual.[6,7]

THE IMPORTANCE OF CONTEXT

Each individual exists in a context in which body, mind and spirit interact with both family and friendship networks and with broader relationships with community and society.[8] Families provide a sort of micro-culture. The family can be regarded as a complex system that changes over time. It has a history that contributes to shaping expectations and behaviour in the present, but is also dynamic, developing and changing as each member passes through their life cycle. As one member of the family approaches death, changes may already be occurring in the distribution of the roles and relationships of others. The dying individual will also connect to other networks containing significant relationships, some of which may be more important to them than those with biological links.

The entire network is placed within a social and cultural context that will have an impact on the possibilities available to both the individual and the family and will include formal and informal care resources, e.g. neighbours, church, social care agencies. Those helping families also become part of the system and it is important to reflect on the effect of this.[9] For example, access to care, truth telling and treatment may be influenced by the cultural perspective of healthcare professionals.[10]

Cultural expectations within the family and its immediate circle about the rights and responsibilities of individual family members may affect decisions about care giving.[11] Field has argued that the use of the portmanteau word 'psychosocial' rather than 'psychological and social' has diminished the understanding and importance of the 'social' in people's lives: 'for palliative care to be fully effective its practitioners must recognise that for its clients the meaning, experience and expression of their terminal illness are shaped and influenced by the communities within which they live.'[12] Hence the failure of palliative care services to reach disadvantaged sectors of society may be the result of inadequate attention to the needs and values of certain communities. Spruyt's study of community-based palliative care for Bangladeshi patients in London found poorly controlled symptoms and severe pain in the majority of patients, with little access to bereavement support for their relatives.[10] Inequality of access to specialist palliative care has also been demonstrated among black people of Caribbean origin.[13]

The extent and availability of resources such as financial, social and medical support will influence the adaptation of the dying individual. The availability and choice of coping mechanisms and styles will also be affected by variables such as social class, socio-economic status, culture, ethnicity, age, gender, education and the phase and nature of the illness itself. Social support appears to be a key factor in maintaining coping and promoting adaptation. For example, higher mortality rates have been recorded for cancer patients in the first year after the loss of a spouse,[14] and it has been noted that those who are married survive longer than single patients.[15]

WHAT IS THE UNIT OF CARE?

Whatever the place of care immediately prior to death, most palliative care will take place at home, where family life may well be deteriorating along with that of the dying person. There is substantial evidence for links between the dying individual and family functioning.

- A majority of cancer patients express most concern about their own loss of independence and their family's future.[16] The number of concerns is related to the degree of their psychological distress.

- Unsatisfactory pain relief in dying people has been correlated with relatives who had limited information about the illness and found it hard to discuss issues with clinical staff.[17]

- There is concordance between levels of anxiety in family and patient.[18]

Over time, families develop patterns of relating to one another, often adopting certain fairly fixed roles and following accepted codes of behaviour in order to fulfil the tasks they face and cope with the problems that confront them. The balance of the family will come under enormous pressure at a time of terminal illness. The medical journey that ends with terminal care may have created a breakdown in communication between patient and family, who may have seen a series of different professionals, who may have told them different things at different times. The transition to palliative care may itself have created uncertainty and ambiguity. Many carers will be struggling with rapid and frightening changes in the physical needs and capacities of the ill person. Old relationship difficulties will be placed under even greater strain. Comforting routines of interaction at work and leisure will be shattered as the illness progresses. Familiar roles will have to be renegotiated and the panic of assuming new roles dealt with.

Forty-two-year-old Sally was dying of advanced breast cancer. She had two sons aged 4 and 6. She struggled with the pain of relinquishing some of her parenting role to her visiting mother-in-law, with whom she had never had a close relationship. Her mother-in-law sensed her resentment but felt powerless to address it. Sally's husband was considering a frightening future of life as a single parent. He had agreed to have children to please Sally; now he would be looking after them alone. Sally was worrying about his motivation and whether she could trust him with her children.

Both family and patient want to protect themselves and one another from further hurt and it may begin to seem safer to avoid talking about difficult emotions and decisions. In the face of such powerful separating forces, healthcare professionals should attempt to provide support and opportunities for the patient and family to talk together, recognizing that the heightened emotion accompanying potential loss can be a powerful driver for change, even when there is a very limited time frame. Most families want to say important things to one another, to be involved in patient care, and to plan for the future, both short and long term. It is just that they do not know where to begin or what to say. Most families will manage well with just a little help. They will need information about what usually happens and what their options are, e.g. what services might be available to support the patient's return home or possible responses to expect from an adolescent facing bereavement. Some may want support as they struggle with the meaning of life itself.

THE IMPORTANCE OF THE TEAM

It is important for professionals in palliative care to work within a team culture. Patients and families choose to whom they want to talk and from whom they find help most acceptable. This does not depend on what professionals themselves define as appropriate. Co-ordination of the professional team involved with the family is vital if the family is not to be swamped and confused. Too little help reduces their options; too much help delivered by a whole range of concerned and worried professionals can leave them exhausted and de-skilled, convinced that the problems are beyond their power to resolve.

Betty's 5-year-old daughter was dying of leukaemia. She spoke of the time absorbed by the visits and sometimes conflicting advice of the family doctor, the district nurse, the health visitor, the hospital psychologist and the Macmillan nurse, and said despairingly 'I need to do it my way'.

THE FAMILY AS CARER

Numerous studies emphasize the importance of social and practical support provided by families to dying individuals.[19] It is vital that families receive support if they are to continue with their tasks. The burden of caring is attested to in many studies, along with reports of increased risk of physical and psychological morbidity.[20] Recent changes in the structure of families, geographical distance, divorce, split and reconstituted families may add to the difficulties. Care givers often have to put their own lives on hold while facing conflicting advice and demands.[21] Eighty-four per cent of informal carers during the palliative care phase have been found to report above-normal levels of psychological distress.[22] Many studies describe unmet practical service needs along with the failure of healthcare professionals to meet carers' learning needs adequately.[23] The literature is clear about the needs of informal carers:[24-26]

- co-ordinated care from confident, committed family doctors with 24-hour community nursing support;

- knowledge of available support, including practical help with household tasks, personal care, equipment loan and financial support;

- advocacy to obtain support when it is needed,

- the availability of respite care, either as an in-patient or a home sitting service;

- knowledge about the illness and training in skills to enhance patient comfort;

- access to specialist palliative care where appropriate;

- emotional support directed specifically at the carer.

Table 16.1 Factors predisposing families to emotional risk[28]

Anger about delays in diagnosis or treatment
Rapid deterioration in the patient
Carer isolated with little perceived support
Practical problems such as housing and finance
Other dependants in the family, e.g. children, elderly parents
Previous or current mental health problems or previous losses
History of abuse or trauma
Evidence of dependency on drugs or alcohol
Close dependent relationship with the ill person
Estranged family members or significant conflict within the family
Particularly strong family myths or rules, e.g. 'somebody must be to blame', 'life must go on exactly as usual'

THE FAMILY AS CLIENT

Care for the family has an important preventive health component, as family members and friends will live on into a future shaped in part by their experience of the dying person's illness and death. There is relatively little published information on the pre-death psychological state of families, although Kristjanson has published a useful review.[27] Most studies have been about morbidity after bereavement and there are no clear formal models to predict family psychological status during the illness trajectory. Oliviere *et al.* have produced a helpful summary of factors that may predispose a family to emotional risk (Table 16.1). The rights of families and carers to support and an assessment of need separate to that of patients are now enshrined in the *Guidance on cancer services: improving supportive and palliative care for adults with cancer* published by the National Institute for Clinical Excellence in the UK.[29]

ASSESSMENT OF FAMILY FUNCTIONING

Good clinical care of families affected by cancer must include an assessment of family functioning, because such functioning influences subsequent grief outcomes.[30] A spouse's perception of overall family coping as poor correlates with greater grief intensity, depression and poor social adjustment. Conversely, family coping perceived as adaptive is linked with a good outcome. Open communication has been clearly demonstrated to be a strong, positive determinant of good coping.[31]

Kissane and colleagues are beginning to assess the impact of limited, focused family sessions provided to at-risk families.[32] They have identified five classes of families: supportive, conflict-resolving, intermediate, sullen and hostile. This classification (first derived from a cohort of 102 families in which an ill member was receiving palliative care) proved stable over time when the cluster analytic approach was repeated with a further cohort of 115 bereaved families. Over half the families fell into the first two categories, where overall psychosocial outcomes were good. About a third fell into the last two categories, reporting high rates of depression and chaotic adaptation to grief. Kissane's group use their typology, in which cohesiveness is the major determinant, to identify families at risk of a poor outcome in the palliative care setting. They stress the importance of creating a collaborative partnership between professionals and the family, describing the use of a short, self-administered family relationships index based on the Family Environment Scale devised by Moos and Moos.[33]

The objective of an assessment is to maximize effective intervention that will be aimed at:

- reducing the impact of existing losses,
- preventing further losses,
- promoting coping,
- providing a sense of engagement in the decision-making process.

If an assessment does not take place, it will be difficult to identify individuals and families at particular risk who could benefit from an increased level of support. It may also diminish the options available to the individual and family.

OBTAINING INFORMATION

An assessment should create a partnership between the ill person and those close to him or her, and the healthcare team. This demands that professionals explain the reason for their enquiries, obtain consent and check on it at regular intervals: 'Please let me know if there is something I ask about that you would rather not discuss'. The dying individual should always be asked if he or she would like to be seen alone or with someone else and, if so, with whom. Discussions about with whom information may be shared, both within the patient's family and friendship network and within the professional team, are vital.

Since the quality of life of dying individuals and the network of those close to them is intertwined, it is evident that the individual and the network should be treated as the unit of care. However, assumptions that dying people and their carers can act as proxies for one another should be avoided. For example, patients underestimate the distress that pain causes to their spouse,[34] and carers are likely to score patients' dependency and disability more highly than do the patients themselves.[35] The dying individual and network members will have different needs at different times. They may require different types of support and sometimes have conflicting agendas. Assessment is not a one-off process: people change their minds, and circumstances alter. Assessment is part of an indistinguishable cycle with intervention, and the assessment process itself will often be therapeutic.[36]

RECORDING

Good professional recording and communication are important if effective care is to be achieved and duplication of enquiry avoided. Genograms and ecomaps have widely been found useful aids to recording information in a clear, easily updated manner that leaves the dying individual in control of the material disclosed.[36,37] Such pictorial mapping can generate additional information about patterns of communication, losses and gaps in care.[38,39] Assessments will vary in their formality and format. However, most will contain four main perspectives:[40]

- the individual,
- the family and those close to the individual,
- physical resources,
- social resources, including cultural and spiritual issues.

More information will be found in the chapters on cross-cultural and spiritual care (see Chapters 17 and 20).

WORKING WITH FAMILIES

Helping families to communicate can achieve very rapid results. The cliché of the deathbed reconciliation is a real image, and late is always better than never. However, meeting family members on a one-to-one basis is often an important prelude to work within the whole family. Individual difficulties and perspectives may need to be understood before their communication and potential resolution is sought within a wider group.

For example, the elderly wife of a dying husband may need to express her fears of waking to find him dead beside her before she can listen to his urgent desire to return home from hospital. It is important that individual time for an assessment and response to carers' needs should be negotiated at the start of the relationship between the professional and the dying individual and family so that it is accepted as a normal part of the contract. If separate meetings are suggested only when difficulties arise, guilt and suspicion may be aroused.

PREPARATION FOR COMMUNICATION WITH GROUPS

The training of most healthcare professionals in communication is limited to one-to-one skills. Preparation can help professionals to feel more confident when meeting with family groups. It is often helpful to have two colleagues of different disciplines present to share the tasks of observing, offering information and time-keeping. Issues to consider include the following.

- What do you know about individual objectives within the family?
- What do you want to achieve?
- Who should attend the meeting?

- How and when will the patient be involved?

- How will you involve those whose views are significant but who cannot be physically present?

- Who should start the session and how?

- How do the family see you? Do you need to make a clear statement of your role?

- Adapt your linguistic style and vocabulary to that of the family.

- Structure the session: people feel safe with clear boundaries about time and confidentiality – 'We've got about half an hour together today'.

- Emphasize that everyone will have an opportunity to speak.

- Be neutral: each individual will need to feel that the professional understands his or her point of view.

SUPPORTING FAMILY PROBLEM SOLVING

The professional working with families has three main tasks:

- to ensure a clear and adequate flow of information,

- to acknowledge emotional pain and facilitate its expression and sharing,

- to support people in discovering and acting upon what is important to them.

It is important to remember that externally imposed solutions seldom stick. The aim of the professional is to help families resolve the issues they identify as significant in a way that feels reasonably comfortable to them, not to assume responsibility for sorting everything out for them.

ADOPT AN OPEN STYLE

Check frequently on pace, comprehension and permission: 'Am I going too fast?', Do we need to recap on that?', 'Does this feel comfortable?'. If you do not know what to say, say so. Everyone will be struggling with uncertainty and it will help to acknowledge this. If you say something that upsets someone, acknowledge it. Use simple 'feeling' words such as sad, angry and frightened; they help people to say difficult things.

FIND OUT HOW EACH INDIVIDUAL DEFINES THE ISSUES

- What concerns you most about the illness?

- What's the worst thing at the moment?

- What else do you need to know about the illness?

- What do you worry about not coping with?

- Who's close to whom in your family?

- What is the most difficult thing to agree on at the moment?

- Is there anyone you are especially worried about?

- What's helping most at the moment?

NORMALIZE AND ANTICIPATE FEARS AND PROBLEMS

- Describe how difficulties might be managed, for example symptoms as death approaches.

- Acknowledge conflicts of need: 'You want to help your mother but you're worried about giving up your job'; 'You'd like to go home to your daughter but you're anxious about the burden it might be for her'.

- Recognize and permit differences: 'John wants to go off on his own, Peter wants you all to stay together and talk. It's normal for illness to affect everyone differently'.

- Point out similarities: 'The important thing is that you all love your mother and want to do your best for her'.

- Use inclusive statements: 'A lot of people worry about ... What's it like for you?'.

ENCOURAGE CHANGE

- Define problems in a positive form, particularly if you want to challenge them: 'You love your children and you want to protect them'.

- Help people compromise and negotiate, which often means helping them to find a dignified way to retreat from fixed positions: 'It's always good to hope for the best, but planning for the worst creates a safety net you can then forget about, like taking out an insurance policy'.

- Outline clearly the resources available to the family and find out what they would like to use. Many will have experienced a dramatic change in what is achievable and may need help to adjust expectations, to segment problems and to focus on one or two at a time. Successful action depends on concrete and achievable goals.

STAND BACK

- Do not get too obsessed with the detail of history taking. Unravelling the minutiae of past relationships can act as a distraction to the family.

- Try to bring unspoken feelings into play: 'You say you're all right, but you look very tense'.

- Gently challenge non-involvement and try to recognize over-protection or conflict.

- Try to recognize and name anger – it is often the energy people need to take action: 'Something has happened to make you very angry'. Remember anger often masks more painful feelings and naming these can provide the necessary pivot for family members to recognize their shared anguish: 'It sounds very lonely, too'.

- Anger is frightening for the family as well as for the professional, who may need to set limits, either by using a firm, slow tone of voice or by suggesting stopping the meeting for a period, 'While everyone cools down'.

- Allow silence: do not make premature attempts to put everything right. An uncomfortable silence can represent important thinking and feeling time and also generate the emotional depth necessary to achieve change.

END THE MEETING IN A SAFE WAY

- Offer the opportunity to rehearse difficult situations: 'Who are you most worried about telling?', 'How do you think you might do that?'.

- Summarize any decisions and agreements clearly and affirm the next opportunity for meeting.

- Write down any important pieces of information such as names and telephone numbers.

- Time warnings are often helpful: 'We have about 5 minutes left. Is there anything else that's important for you to mention?'.

- It may help to acknowledge the emotional intensity of a conversation: 'We've talked about a lot of painful things today. You may find yourself going over them in your mind, but we'll be meeting again on …'.

- Always validate the family's contribution to patient care, their strength and achievements.

- Try to close meetings by moving on to more everyday topics, remembering that an appropriate touch on the shoulder or shaking hands can convey a great deal.

INTIMACY AND SEXUALITY

Issues of intimacy and sexuality are about much more than acts of intercourse. They confirm people's fundamental need to feel some sense of ease with their bodies, to experience physical closeness, to communicate and receive love. Sexuality remains an important quality-of-life issue for very ill people and their partners,[41] but sexual behaviour, self-concepts and relationships are deeply affected in many adults with life-threatening disease.[42] Partners may find that physical changes in the patient, or their own change of role to carer, alters their feelings and sexual desires. In some relationships the physical dependency needs created by the illness can distressingly disturb a well-established pattern of separation. Professionals should also be alert to the possibility of violent or abusive relationships: for example a woman profoundly physically disabled by motor neurone disease reported sexual activity by her husband that she experienced as 'nightly rape'.

Although healthcare professionals appear to agree that discussion of sexuality should be an integral part of their responsibility towards seriously ill people and those close to them,[43,44] studies show that they seldom address the issues.[45,46] Although it would be inappropriate to expect every healthcare professional to have specialist skills in psychosexual counselling, all have a responsibility to offer and respond to cues about sexuality, to provide first-line help and to know how to refer on for specialist support.

Most people will not ask for help spontaneously, so learning to ask is the professional's responsibility. Eighty per cent of women being treated for cancer of the cervix wanted more information about the impact of the disease on their sexuality, but 75 per cent said they would not raise the question first.[45] People often give cues when they are trying to test out whether the professional is safe enough to try discussing such personal topics by making such comments as: 'He won't even let me kiss him', or 'He just doesn't seem to love me any more'. All too often, faced with these shyly uttered statements, professionals retreat into bland reassurances or change the subject quickly: 'Don't worry, illness brings lots of changes, I'm sure he does love you'. Such responses can confirm people's worst fears that this subject is indeed too dangerous and too painful to discuss.

If professionals remove sex from the standard agenda, they can isolate people even further from the help they may need to gain the love and acceptance that will support them in facing losses in so many areas of their lives. In practice, the communication skills required are the same as those needed for approaching any other sensitive topic.

OPENING A DIALOGUE

- See partners separately and together.

- Give information in advance wherever possible, e.g. prior to surgery or treatment.

- Remember the value of mentioning sexuality in appropriate written materials to give permission for verbal discussion.

- Avoid assumptions, for example that sex is less important to older people, or that an individual not in an obvious partnership does not want to discuss issues of sexuality and intimacy.

- Try to find the right vocabulary for the individual and remember that the appropriate use of humour can diffuse potentially embarrassing situations: 'I often blush when I discuss sex, so just ignore this'.

- Think about professional boundaries and limits: rights and respect need to exist on both sides of the client/professional contract.

Nurses gave much-appreciated cucumber massages to a middle-aged man with motor neurone disease suffering from itch. They should perhaps have not been so surprised when his wife became jealous of his pleasure in their attention. It might have been better for them to have trained her to deliver the massage.

Concerns may be expressed about body image, sexual function or both. Physical and psychological issues are closely intertwined. Directly illness-related issues may include pain, fatigue, disfigurement, hair loss, incontinence, smell, nausea, vomiting, sterility, fertility, impotence, weight change, the use of appliances. Psychological issues may include change of role, feeling unfeminine or masculine, fear of being repulsive, fear of abandonment, loss of self-confidence.

Many dying people feel anxious about changes in the way their body behaves and looks. Anxiety about rejection can lead to retreat and a wall of silence, which may be eased by a facilitated discussion. Some couples will appreciate advice about alternative positions, or alternative methods of love making such as mutual caressing. Others will want to talk to the professional alone about their changes in feelings for their partner.

June had had a double mastectomy and now had bony metastases. She was thin, in a lot of pain, nauseated, with very little hair. In the middle of discussing child care with the professional and her husband, she suddenly asked: 'Have you got any suggestions for improving our sex life?'. The professional needed to remember that she was talking to a couple, and to check out whether the other partner also wanted to discuss the issue and whether the comment was really one about sex: 'I can see this is an important issue for you. Are things the same for you, too, Patrick? Are you okay to talk about this together, now?'. The couple confirmed that they would both like to talk about it, and now. The professional asked: 'What's actually more difficult now? When do you get the time and space to make love at the moment?'. For this couple, suggestions about alternative positions and the use of pillows, as well as making love in the day when the children weren't around and June was less exhausted, were helpful. Most importantly, however, this couple wanted to talk about what a central part of their lives together the act of making love had been and continued to be.

SENSITIVE SCREENING

- Create a sense of partnership: 'Are you comfortable to talk about this? Please stop me if I talk about something you would rather not discuss'.

- Find questions that people can respond to on a wide variety of levels: 'In what ways has your illness changed the way you can get close to your friends, to your partner, to your family?'.

- Generalize in order to give permission: 'People often have questions they'd like to ask about the sexual side of life'.

- Always remember that most people want to talk about their feelings rather than physical details, which means that elaborate sexual histories are usually inappropriate: 'How long have you been together? Has the physical side of your relationship been important to you, to your partner? What do you want most from your partner at the moment? What do you think your partner's reaction would be?'.

- It may help to remind people that good sex is built on good communication, not wonderful bodies.

ISSUES FOR CHILDREN

CHILDREN FACING BEREAVEMENT

The care offered to the family by professionals is incomplete without consideration of the needs of children facing bereavement. Terminal illness causes enormous changes within the family, and children quickly sense that something very serious is happening. However, many adults, parents and professionals alike, in their desire to protect children actually succeed in isolating them, excluding them from the family concerns and leaving them alone with their fantasies. Children cannot ultimately be protected from the truth. They will be sad. If they are involved in the impending death, the adults around them can offer them support in their sadness. Ideally, children will receive preparation before the death, an opportunity to ask questions, to receive reassurance and to express feelings.

Children facing bereavement have similar needs and emotions to adults but may express them differently. The quiet child who becomes aggressive at school, the child who refuses to go to school or wets the bed may be expressing grief through their behaviour rather than in the words with which adults are more familiar. Children can sometimes upset adults by seeming casual or callous, like the little boy who greeted his brother's death with the announcement: 'I always wanted my own bedroom anyway'. Such behaviour does not mean that they are not also very sad.

IT IS IMPOSSIBLE NOT TO COMMUNICATE

Many parents have good reasons for their reluctance to share information about illness and death with their children. They are anxious about what their children understand about death and about what words to use. They worry that saying the wrong thing will make an already difficult situation worse. They themselves will be grieving and may be worrying about their ability to maintain control. Children also want to protect their parents. They may try to obey an unspoken rule of 'not talking about it' by pretending that nothing is happening.

External helpers need to reassure parents that they understand and share their concerns for their children. However, they must also gently remind parents that there is no choice about whether or not to tell children. Children are aware of changes in routine. They will read the emotions around them, respond to body language and overhear conversations. What is at issue is whether they will receive consistent and regularly updated information from their carers, whom they trust, or misleading and sometimes contradictory snippets of information from a variety of possibly unreliable sources.

Professionals need to acknowledge with parents that it is not easy to talk to children when what you say is going to hurt them: 'This is probably the most difficult thing you are ever going to have to do'. Parents may appreciate advice about explanations of death and what vocabulary would be appropriate to their children's age, and about the kind of reactions they may anticipate.

They may want lists of appropriate books to read with their children, or leaflets on childhood grief to read for themselves in order to gain some intellectual mastery over an emotionally unfamiliar subject. For many parents this will be sufficient and they will want to speak to their children alone. Others will welcome sharing the task with a professional. Parents want to do what is best for their children and they learn fast. Being part of just one direct conversation between a child and a professional can help to give parents the confidence to continue for themselves.

WORK WITH PARENTS

Many research studies have made clear the cost of inadequate support and involvement for children facing serious illness in someone close to them.[47–50] Children may respond with emotional and behavioural disturbance at the time, throughout childhood and on into adulthood. The outcome of bereavement is strongly influenced by pre-death experiences.[51] For example, children who are given information about parental illness display less anxiety than those who are not.[52] Significant factors include the relationship of the child with the ill person before the death, the openness of communication within the family, the availability of community support and the extent to which the child's parenting needs have continued and will continue to be met.

In the seminal Harvard Child Bereavement Study, the functioning of the surviving parent was the most significant influence on the outcome of the child's bereavement.[51] Christ has shown that positive factors in children's outcomes are parents who can accept help and show active coping styles, and families with parental warmth and cohesiveness where continuing stability and routine are offered. Particular risk factors are pre-existing poor parenting skills and parents so overwhelmed by their own grief that they are unable to relate to their child's grief.[53] Parents must understand their children's developmental needs at different ages so that they can help to prepare, inform and guide them through their experiences. Christ gives clear pointers for helping based on developmental observations.

It is vital that professionals treat parents as colleagues: they are not helped by staff who take over from them. They know their own children best and the aim must be to help them to help their children. Children need the understanding of their families, who will be around long after the professionals have disappeared. It is often necessary to work with parents on their own before children's needs can be addressed. A couple who cannot openly acknowledge impending death between themselves are not well placed to help their children. Parents may also need encouragement to widen their children's support network by involving other adults close to them, rather than feeling they have to do everything themselves. Teachers, clergy, a close relative or friend may all help to offer the child another listening ear.

CHILDREN'S UNDERSTANDING OF DEATH

It is important to know something about the development of the concept of death in children in order to communicate with them at an appropriate and effective level. Children's death concepts evolve from the concrete to the abstract, culminating in 9–11 year olds beginning to develop a full death concept with the elements of inevitability and universality.[54] However, Lansdown and Benjamin found that one-third of 5 year olds had a virtually complete concept of death,[55] and Reilly et al. found that half the 5 year olds and all the 8–10 year olds they interviewed believed that they, too, would die some day.[56] Many much younger children understand more about death than adults are prepared to accept. Of course, this is not a comfortable idea. It places less responsibility on adults if they believe that young children are incapable of understanding death. One of the issues is that they do not have complete death concepts and therefore need help to fill out their thinking.

Seven-year-old Martin's father was admitted to a hospice with a terminal brain tumour. Martin's mother told medical staff that he did not know what was actually wrong with his father, just that he was ill. She agreed that Martin could ask the doctor questions about his father's illness. He did. 'Can you stop the bad thing in Daddy's brain? Will it grow inside the rest of his body? Can Daddy come home?'. If Martin had not received simple and honest answers to his questions, he would have made up his own.

HELPING PARENTS TO TALK TO CHILDREN

- Reassure them that it does not have to be a one-off conversation. Information should be simple, clear and repeated, about what is happening and why and what will happen next. It is all right to say 'I don't know'.

- Acknowledge that it will feel uncomfortable and distressing, but that waiting for the right time for a conversation may mean that it never happens.

- Warn parents that children may respond by changing the subject or focusing on the practical, such as asking immediately 'What's for tea?', and that this does not mean that they are not concerned and involved.

- Help parents to think about what their children know already. It may help to start with their own observations, for example 'Why do you think Mummy is ill?'.

- Parents need to think about what they want their children to know, e.g. what the doctors have said, what the treatment might be.

- Parents may need advice about what the children themselves might want to know, remembering that they may not ask. For example: 'Is cancer catching?', 'Will Daddy die?', 'Is it my fault?'.

- Parents may need help in thinking about where they will find their own support.

- It is important to work within the family's values and with what seems manageable and comfortable to the parents or carers themselves. There is no right way, only the way that is right for this particular family and children.

- Professionals working in in-patient units can assist parents by creating an environment that positively welcomes the presence of children:
  a designated area with small chairs and a toy box;
  toy medical kits, puppets, dolls in beds and telephones can help younger children to act out their concerns and questions;
  children will respond positively to being shown where they can display their pictures and cards by the bed;
  children who find conversation difficult may respond to suggestions that they bring their homework in or write a letter to the ill parent;
  simple explanations about equipment such as syringe drivers are always appreciated.

TAKING RISKS

Parents want to help their children. Although professionals are understandably anxious about suggesting words and phrases, this is particularly helpful when talking to parents about speaking to their children. It is important to be aware of the family's own belief system and not offer explanations that conflict with it, but to make suggestions about simple factual information: 'When somebody dies their body stops working. It is not the same as being asleep. A dead person can never wake up. Their body is no more use to them'; 'A funeral is where everyone who cared about Mummy will get together to say goodbye. Mummy's body will be put in a special box called a coffin'.

Workbooks for children to complete with their parents' help are often a less threatening way of beginning difficult conversations:[57] 'Draw a picture of Mummy. Which bit of her is ill?'. Children facing the death of someone important in their lives also need reassurance about their own continuing care. They will have all sorts of practical anxieties: 'Who will take me to school?', 'Will I still be able to go to football on Saturdays?'. It can be an enormous relief to them and their parents when these painful issues are openly addressed. Bereaved children need to know what will not change in their world as well as what will. They also need explicit reassurance about the fact that their own behaviour or thoughts could not have caused the death. Young children in particular sometimes believe that they can make things happen by thinking about them or saying them out loud: 'I hate you and I wish you were dead'.

Children learn to grieve by observing others. They are often uncertain about what is allowed and need to see others crying. They may also need reassurance about the behaviour of adults around them: 'I'm sorry I was cross. I'm not angry with you. I'm just terribly upset because Granny has died'. Children need a chance to talk about their feelings with adults who are prepared to share theirs. The work of Klass *et al.* on continuing bonds emphasizes the importance of memories and remembering.[58] Children need to find out who the dead person was and will be in their lives. This is an active process that requires support. The choice to attend rituals such as the funeral can help, as can looking at photographs together, or having something that belonged to the person who has died – a watch, a photograph, some tools, a piece of jewellery or a book. This can provide the child with reassurance that life goes on and with a tangible reminder of the existence of the dead person and their continued importance in the child's life.

THINKING ABOUT DEATH IN THE MIDST OF LIFE

At all stages, but especially as death approaches, the ill person and those close to him or her may wish to discuss both the process of dying and the death itself. It is important to indicate a willingness to talk about difficult topics, but not to press the point with those who are reluctant: 'You've really been through a lot. Has it made you wonder what it's all about? Some people who've got an illness like yours feel it's very unfair. Have you ever had that sort of feeling?', 'What do you hope for? What do you find yourself thinking about when you're alone or you can't get to sleep?'. Individuals will answer at the level they want to, but the professional will have demonstrated a willingness to discuss issues of meaning and purpose.

Bereavement begins before the death of an individual and much can be achieved for those close to him or her by providing help in advance. As death approaches, family members need incorporating into the caring team to whatever extent they feel comfortable. Their concerns about what to expect need addressing: 'When will death happen?', 'What will it be like?', 'How will the symptoms be controlled?', 'Who will I call if I'm at home and need help?', 'Do I have to get the funeral director straight away?'. Some families will appreciate help with legal, financial or funeral planning. Clear explanations in advance are important if issues about injections or a failure to eat or drink contributing to the patient's deterioration are not to become troublesome stumbling blocks.

However much it is anticipated, death is always a profound emotional and often physical shock. If professionals maintain a sense of dignity and identity for the dying person, even when he or she is unconscious, relatives will feel encouraged to say what they want to. Suggestions about the value of holding hands, stroking hair and a reminder that although the dying person is unable to show any response he or she may well be able to hear, are all helpful. Some individuals can be profoundly frightened of sitting with a dying person and may welcome company and support. No one should be pressed to do so.

Everyone needs to hold the past, present and future in some sort of continuity. Sometimes this means helping people to do what they can for the person who is dying, sometimes helping the dying to leave something behind. Professionals can suggest or acknowledge ways of creating a legacy. One mother chose to write lists of possible Christmas presents for her sons at different ages. Some dying individuals are struggling with issues of guilt, forgiveness and a desire for reconciliation. We must respect people's capacity to choose. People are not helped by professionals who avoid or deny reality.

Fifty-year-old Tom was helped to write to his teenage son. Tom and his son's mother had been divorced and Tom hadn't been in contact with his son for years. It was important to remind him that his son might not want to reply, and in fact he did not. Sometimes the professional's task is to help individuals to see that their good intentions must be enough.

BEREAVEMENT: PROCESS AND INTERVENTION

INTRODUCTION

Bereavement – here used in the sense of facing the loss of someone close through death – is one of the most dreaded of human experiences. It brings major changes to the bereaved person. Death may rob you of the main person who makes you feel worthwhile, who puts you first. It may change your status in your community or friendship group. It may challenge long-held religious convictions. It may bring sole responsibility for a child or vulnerable adult that was previously shared. It can alter your financial position for the better or for the worse. Of course it can also be a relief from a heavy burden of care, or from a lifelong painful and difficult relationship – or from both. This section of the chapter considers factors that influence how an individual experiences bereavement, theoretical models of the process, and the thorny issue of assessing who is at risk in bereavement. It then discusses ways professionals may support people facing bereavement and draws on examples of current good practice in this field.

The experience of bereavement is profoundly influenced by the wider society in which the bereaved person lives, by their cultural heritage, by the beliefs and behaviours current within their kinship and friendship groups. Inextricably interwoven with this are an individual bereaved person's psychological responses to major loss, which are rooted in the particular significance of the relationship with the person who has died and previous life experience, including experience of earlier losses. Drawing on these influences, the bereaved person develops the personal meaning of this death for him or her. A wife's death may represent yet another rejection and loss of control to one man. To another, the death of his wife may be affirming of him as a loveable person in that their partnership has lasted despite challenges at different times. In any work with people facing bereavement, the particular influences of these three factors – the social context, the psychological response and the individual meaning of the loss for this bereaved person – need to be considered in assessing what intervention might be appropriate.

BEREAVEMENT IN A SOCIAL CONTEXT

In recent years there has been a much greater appreciation of the role of culture in determining the response to bereavement. Research like that of Wikan comparing Egyptian and Balinese approaches shows this clearly.[59] In Egypt, mourners may be encouraged to concentrate on their grief; in Bali friends and family will try to distract them. The purpose is the same: to reduce the risk to health from an event that is recognized as a danger. However, cultures are dynamic. They change in the same geographical location over time, so some members of that society may be adhering to what is seen as the standard approach, whereas other groups may be challenging old ways and trying out new. People from one culture and country who migrate to live in another may particularly be called on to adapt. Firth has described the ways Hindus from the Indian subcontinent living in one town in the UK have sought to preserve the essentials in rituals brought with them, while taking account of the regulations and customs of the host country.[60] Even in a small country like the UK, there are marked variations between different groups within the majority white population in rituals and expressions of grief, which may relate to religion, cultural heritage or social class. The style of an East End of London working-class funeral with imposing hearse and floral tributes might not appeal to a middle-class group of environmental activists looking for a woodland burial. No professional can be aware of all the permutations that might occur within one culture, let alone be an expert on bereavement and mourning practices in several. Indeed, there has been criticism of the attempt to develop 'factfiles' on different cultures, which give a false picture of stability and uniformity.[61] The only respectful approach to those from a different culture is to make no assumptions, but to ask them what they believe and want in relation to this particular death. For the death of an older person, they may want to follow a very traditional path out of respect for that person's wishes; for a teenage son killed in a motorcycle accident who himself did not accept such views, they may wish to alter both behaviour and ritual.

The first section of this chapter discusses the micro-culture of the family, and the impact of a family member having a life-threatening illness. There are similar considerations once that person has died.

Gender is becoming recognized as a factor that shapes the experience of bereavement.[62,63] Generally in Western societies:

- widowers have higher rates of psychological distress than widows, though as there are more bereaved women than men because of women's greater longevity, the actual number of distressed widows is greater;

- while both bereaved men and women suffer more physical illness and disability than their married counterparts, on the whole men are more vulnerable;

- there are higher mortality rates for bereaved men than for bereaved women, suicide being an important factor, particularly for older men.

An explanation of some of these differences may lie in the common experience in Western society that, on the whole, men will seek practical tasks and restrain their emotions in distress, whereas women will express them, and in the greater likelihood of women having a confidante other than their dead husband, and thus being more socially integrated. However, Martin and Doka warn about categorizing men and women too rigidly, and prefer to characterize grief as 'intuitive' or 'instrumental' to maintain an individualized approach.[64] These insights have implications for bereavement practice, which is considered later in this section.

As in all aspects of palliative care, the professionals or volunteers supporting bereaved people are themselves part of a social context, and their thinking and behaviour, and thus their interaction, is influenced by their cultural and family backgrounds. In addition, their contact with the deep and painful emotions of bereavement can recall memories of their own past losses and create anxiety about the safety of themselves and their loved ones. So having access to a system of supervision and support that promotes self-awareness and reflection and helps to maintain appropriate boundaries is equally important in bereavement work.

MODELS OF PSYCHOLOGICAL RESPONSES TO BEREAVEMENT

Drawing on our cultural and family experience, we develop expectations about the way people may/should behave in bereavement. A number of writers and researchers have described the process of bereavement and derived models of common patterns and responses from this. Particularly influential in recent years have been stage or task models, with Parkes[65] and Worden,[66] respectively, being the best known. Kübler-Ross's work is not included here since she studied dying people, rather than those facing the loss of a loved one through death. Although her work is often elided to include bereaved people, there are many differences between these two experiences, and this is theorizing beyond the data. There is an examination of her contribution in the chapter on communication (see Chapter 2).

Parkes described from his research in the UK and the USA:[65]

- an initial response of shock, numbness and denial, most intense if the death is unexpected, but present to some degree even with expected deaths;

- a release of often overwhelming emotion, the pangs of grief, which may include yearning, sadness, anger, guilt and remorse, fear and insecurity; restlessness and agitation may be a feature, even searching for the lost person; somatic symptoms are common, which may be those associated with severe anxiety or may mimic those of the deceased;

- a period of despair and withdrawal as the permanence of the loss is fully grasped;

- over time, an adjustment to the new world without the dead person.

Freud's psychodynamic approach and Bowlby's work on attachment underpinned Parkes' thinking, and he drew particularly on Freud's concept of *griefwork*.

Through recall of the events around the death, a preoccupation with the person who is lost, and attempts to understand the meaning of what has happened, the bereaved person detaches from the dead person, incorporates them into themselves in a different way and thus makes the adjustment to living life without that person.

Worden built on Parkes' work but preferred to characterize the bereaved person as an active participant in the process, hence his description of tasks for the bereaved to tackle in their journey through bereavement:[66]

- task 1 – accept the reality of the loss,

- task 2 – experience the pain of grief,

- task 3 – adjust to a world in which the deceased is missing,

- task 4 – emotionally relocate the deceased appropriately in the bereaved person's life.

Parkes' and Worden's models have become absorbed into everyday conceptualizations of the bereavement process and are frequently reproduced in magazines and popular texts, often without attribution and in ways that are unfair to the subtlety of their thinking. Both were clear that there are not discrete stages or tasks and that people may move backwards and forwards in the process. There has also been a tendency, not only confined to the popular press, to use the models as a prescription for how people *ought* to behave, rather than a description of common experiences. Much of the description has value and implications for practice that are explored later in this chapter.

However, there has recently been some reappraisal of their work and its interpretations. Some of this has emerged from the greater recognition of the importance of culture and gender in determining psychological responses to bereavement. While there are some fairly universal responses to bereavement such as crying, it has become evident that there are no universally applicable models of the process. Culture helps to determine not only behaviour but also modes of thought and even which physiological responses gain attention, so it is impossible to separate feelings and expressions of grief from culturally required mourning. It has also become clear that these models of the process have been drawn from research in which white Western women's experience of spousal loss predominated. There was only a small proportion of widowers in Parkes' key research studies. Stroebe's work suggests that, because of the Western expectation that men control their emotions, fewer men come forward to participate in bereavement research and those who do are less distressed than those who decline.[62]

In Wortman and Silver's view, there is no evidence that griefwork or overt distress are essentials of the grieving process.[67] Instead, there are three predominant patterns of grief in Western societies rather than one:

- moving from high distress to low distress over time,

- never experiencing high distress,

- continuing high distress for years.

Responding to this challenge, Stroebe proposes a new model – the Dual Process model – which offers a more flexible approach and accommodates cultural and gender differences. She suggests that bereaved people are working both on paying attention to the loss (loss-orientated coping) and on adjusting to the consequences of the loss (restoration-orientated coping), and that they oscillate between these in varying proportions, depending on individual and cultural variations. In loss orientation they focus on what they have lost, ruminating, yearning and crying about the death. In restoration orientation they take on new tasks, develop new relationships, and distract themselves from distress through hobbies or work. So restoration orientation has room for both the man who conforms to the Western cultural male stereotype and the woman who has lost a partner from whom she had long ago detached herself emotionally, even though this was previously concealed from the world, without pathologizing either. The reason for oscillation into loss orientation might be the imminence of an anniversary or a conversation with a friend about times past, and this oscillation may occur several times during the day as well as over longer periods.

The earlier models were often interpreted as requiring a detachment and moving on from the old relationship, but there is now a new interest in the bonds that still bind the bereaved person to the deceased. Evidence is emerging from studies of both adults and children that continued engagement is not necessarily detrimental to emotional health, and is much more common than previously thought.[68] Continuing to refer to the dead person, keeping some clothes or telling them about family events need not be viewed as pathological in the majority of situations. Just as with children, mementoes and rituals that maintain the link are important, and in some cultures ancestors play a significant role in daily life.

Related to this is Walter's biographical model.[69] Taking a cognitive approach grounded in his own experience of the death of his father and a close friend, he suggests that the purpose of grief is to construct a durable biography of the dead person that enables the living to integrate him or her into their life. He argues that in the contemporary Western world, where longevity is combined with geographical mobility, those who mourn the death may each have very different experiences of the person who died. Talking with the range of people who had these different knowledges helps mourners to construct a new biography of the dead person, and retain that person in all his or her reality. There is as yet no empirical evidence to support this biographical model, and perhaps its most useful contribution at present is that it emphasizes the importance of supplementing a psychological analysis of bereavement with a sociological perspective.

RISK ASSESSMENT IN BEREAVEMENT

In considering whether to set up a preventive or therapeutic intervention for a bereaved person, it is important to review whether they need it. Unnecessary or inappropriate intervention can do more harm than good by making that person dependent on professionals or volunteers, or by deskilling friends and family.[70] Parkes' studies have identified factors that may risk the bereaved person's health and well-being.[65] He divides these into antecedent, concurrent and subsequent factors.

Antecedent

- Childhood experiences, particularly of loss – especially the loss of a mother under the age of 11 for girls.

- Previous mental illness, especially depression.

- A life crisis prior to the bereavement, e.g. divorce, loss of employment.

- The nature of the relationship with the deceased, e.g. kinship, strength and security of attachment, degree of reliance, intensity of ambivalence. Stigmatized or hidden relationships, gay partnerships for example, may carry an extra weighting here.[71]

- Mode of death: timeliness, previous warnings, preparation for bereavement. In the Western world, we expect to raise children to adulthood and so the death of a child or young person may be felt to be untimely and wrong, whereas the death of an older person after a full life may be seen as part of the natural order and thus more acceptable.

In advanced disease there have often been earlier crises that warn that death is possible, and it is well established[65] that as a group, those who are prepared for a death are likely to do better in bereavement than those who experience a sudden and unprepared-for death. An element in this finding may be that sudden death may be associated with suicide, violence or accident, and in some cases this may have been preceded by a period of turbulence and crisis as well.

Concurrent

- Gender (see above).

- Age: there is conflicting evidence here. Some studies show older widowers more at risk, others younger. Older widows may seek help for physical ailments, whereas younger widows look for emotional support. These effects may well be cohort effects – linked to individuals who have lived at a particular time and in a particular environment and shared many life experiences as a result – rather than related to age.

- Personality: there has been some discussion of whether there is a 'grief-prone' personality and of the influence of personality factors in general. It may be that grief is a risk factor for developing anxiety or depression rather than vice versa, or that bereavement exposes a pre-existing personality disorder.[72]

- Religion: religion may be a buffer against problems in bereavement, but it is unclear whether it is the faith itself or the experience of being part of a supportive community that is important here.

- Cultural and familial factors (discussed earlier in this section and in previous sections).

Subsequent

- Social support: lack of this is one of the most reliable factors in predicting difficulties in bereavement, but it is *perceived* lack of support by the bereaved person, not the existence or otherwise of a network of family and friends.

- Secondary stresses: bereavement may bring a whole series of losses in its train, e.g. home, a secure income, membership of a social group.

- Life opportunities: these may be greater for a fit young widow than for a widower of 80 with hearing and mobility problems.

The key issue in reviewing these factors to decide whether an individual might be at risk in bereavement is not whether to the external observer the factor is present, but its weight as perceived by that bereaved person.

- Although to outsiders this death seems to have been well signalled and well prepared for, is it perceived like that by the bereaved person?

- Has this person a faith that enables him or her to see these horrific, multiple losses as part of a divine plan, or has this experience challenged such a faith for the first time in that person's life?

This personal element is why there are no defining risk factors that inevitably produce mental or physical ill-health, and why some bereaved individuals deal serenely with apparently the most trying circumstances but others unexpectedly succumb.

WHAT IS 'NORMAL GRIEF'?

Those in contact with the bereaved, whether family and friends or professionals, often want to know how to judge whether their emotional state and behaviour are 'normal' for a bereaved person. There is no simple test for this. Indeed, the very question poses the problem of whether 'normal' and 'abnormal' or 'pathological' are possible concepts in a postmodern world where old certainties and authorities have been challenged and individuals may construct their own death and bereavement.[73]

Nevertheless, this certainly feels like a question that needs an answer when confronted with the deep distress or worrying behaviour of a bereaved person.

It should be clear from earlier discussion that this is a complex judgement. It will depend both on the model of the process of bereavement being used by the person making that judgement, by the bereaved person, and on an assessment of how that person is functioning, taking into account their cultural and family background, the risk factors and their previous functioning.

Bill's son asked a bereavement service whether his father was behaving normally because each year on his birthday Bill wrote himself a card from his wife, who had been dead for 5 years. Bill was functioning well – he ate and slept well and had joined a bowls club, where he had made new friends.

In one sense, it was abnormal because rather few bereaved people do this. Within either the stage model or the Dual Process model, this behaviour could be accommodated. Even if he was regularly deeply distressed around his birthday but recovered his equilibrium within a week, this would be acceptable within the Dual Process framework, but less so within a stage model, where greater detachment might have been expected after 5 years.

Professionals have often associated complicated grief with intense distress of long duration (chronic grief) or, conversely, with no reaction (absent or delayed grief). Length of time or presence or absence of reaction is an insufficient guide on its own. As indicated above, understanding the meaning of the loss for the bereaved person is significant in making this judgement. Stroebe has suggested it is a matter of balance. Within her own model, a bereaved person who at no time oscillated from one orientation to another after the early days would be considered to be in difficulty. Middleton and colleagues observe: 'It is less and less possible to think that pathological grief will become a unitary concept. Instead, future research will likely adopt a multidimensional framework in conceptualising what may appear to be similar consequences, or pathologies, but which derive from very different sources and develop along very different paths'.[72] Very varying estimates have been made of the proportion of bereaved people whose grief is complicated by one or more of the factors identified, since this is so dependent on the basis of the judgement. Different studies have assessed between 16 per cent and 36 per cent of bereaved people as suffering from depression.

SUPPORTING BEREAVED PEOPLE IN PRACTICE

The importance of the time before the death cannot be over-emphasized in any consideration of how to support bereaved people. Whatever the disease, good palliative care should:

- provide information that is timely and appropriate;

- give opportunities to say goodbye and deal with any unfinished business between the dying person and those who will be left;

- support those facing bereavement in considering any questions they may have about the future, with or without the dying person.

These issues are discussed in an earlier section of this chapter and in other chapters in this book.

The implication of earlier discussions about the range of factors to be taken into account in considering whether an individual is at risk or is grieving 'normally' must be that there is no one approach or service that will meet all the needs in this situation. Parkes has made a distinction between services that are proactive and services that are reactive.[70]

Bereavement services that are part of a hospice or specialist palliative care service will generally be proactive in assessing for risk and will offer a service to those identified. Indeed, some may offer telephone contact or an invitation to a social event or memorial celebration to all who have used their service. Though it is important to beware of creating dependence, even those who do not give cause for concern are likely to value human expressions of support and continued interest.

The service in touch with the majority of bereaved people in the UK, the primary health care team, is much more varied in its approach. Some teams take a particular interest and have a death book and a protocol for bereavement follow-up.[74] Where there are counsellors attached to GP practices, they are likely to be regularly engaged in supporting bereaved people.

Voluntary groups such as Cruse Bereavement Care or local-authority-supported bereavement services are likely to be reactive, waiting for clients to seek them out.

Issues to consider

Gender   Acknowledging the potential different coping strategies of Western men and women in bereavement – men being more problem focused, women more emotion focused – Schut and colleagues developed an intervention programme that taught women to focus more on problem solving, men on their emotions.[75] They reported a reduction in distress in both groups. It is important to incorporate these insights in a bereavement service, while maintaining an individualized approach.

The place of cognitive therapies   Many interventions in bereavement care have concentrated on providing emotional support. However, cognitive therapies have a useful place. Examples might be the use of Walter's biographical approach, where there is regret at the loss of an opportunity to know in adulthood a father who separated from the family years ago, or a cognitive therapy programme designed to help a bereaved person deal with overwhelming intrusive thoughts. Those providing a bereavement service may need to consider how they can access staff or volunteers with these skills.

Tackling tasks   While it is important not to use Worden's framework too rigidly, his task approach has some useful pointers. For those who are having difficulty taking in the reality of the death, perhaps because it occurred at a distance, participation in ritual can be helpful. Attendance at the funeral, memorial services or at specially devised rituals affirms reality. However, an essential is that the bereaved person chooses to be present – forced participation will be counterproductive. Permission to experience the pain of grief for those who wish to let their emotions go, but fear they will be overwhelmed, can be offered by providing a safe environment.

Jean's husband had died 3 months ago. Her only daughter was at college and preoccupied with student life. Her friends preferred her to have a cheerful face, yet she was carrying a huge pain inside. It was agreed with her bereavement counsellor that during their sessions she could concentrate on talking about her husband and her loss. By the third session she was already starting to cry as she opened the door to the counsellor but was able to compose herself at the end of the session. In a few months she was beginning to take more interest in restoration activities.

Use of the arts   A regular feature of bereavement work with children is the use of drawing, painting and modelling, and art therapies are increasingly being incorporated in programmes for patients with advanced disease. The arts are seldom a formal part of an adult bereavement service, yet they can offer so much to the expression and working out of deep feelings and existential questions. There is potential for development here both in individual and group work.

Post-traumatic stress disorder   Even in advanced disease where death is well prepared for, some deaths may be particularly traumatic – from a massive bleed, a fit, or even as a result of suicide. Parkes has reminded us that a bereaved person who has witnessed such an event may well be suffering from post-traumatic stress disorder (PTSD), with intrusive memories and avoidance behaviour, and that bereavement counselling will be ineffective unless the PTSD has been tackled first.[70] This should be undertaken only by an appropriately trained professional.

Sexual issues   Among the many losses of bereavement may be that of a heterosexual or homosexual partner. MacElveen-Hoehn, drawing on her experience as a psychologist, has identified the potential for a range of sexual responses following bereavement.[76] For some it is a time of reduced activity, but for others it may be a time of heightened interest. It may act as a solace, it may be heightened activity with or without feeling, and she gives examples of bereaved people feeling attracted to or having sex with strangers, often much to their dismay. A sensitive exploration and non-judgemental approach are required to support bereaved people in this aspect of their experience.

Modes of intervention   Modes of intervention are various, and few have been rigorously evaluated.

- Information leaflets on common feelings in bereavement with details of helpful organizations are produced by many specialist palliative care and voluntary bereavement services. There has been no assessment of their value, though a study of the readability of hospice leaflets, including 168 bereavement leaflets, found that many had small fonts, glossy paper that is difficult for sight-impaired readers, and used unfamiliar or long words.[77]

- Anniversary cards: a rather blunt instrument that is often welcomed but, like any unsolicited intervention, may be perceived as inappropriate by some. A very small-scale evaluation has been carried out by Hutchinson.[78]

- Memorial celebrations: using symbols such as candles, balloons or trees and often associated with a religious festival. These are usually open to any bereaved person who has used the service that stages them.[79]

- Individual befriending/counselling /therapy: careful distinctions need to be made between these activities, as they require different levels of training and skills from providers. Worden, in the USA, distinguishes between grief counselling – facilitating uncomplicated grief – and grief therapy – designed to help those who feel stuck or who are struggling with unusual difficulty.

In the UK, the first would probably be a volunteer befriender who had had a course on listening skills and the bereavement process. The second might either be a counsellor with a counselling qualification or, for more serious situations, a psychologist or a psychiatrist. There has been some evaluation of the efficacy of bereavement counselling. Relf showed that support from a well-trained group of volunteers had reduced the use of health care services, particularly GPs, and had lowered anxiety for her sample.[80] Raphael demonstrated the positive effect of psychiatric interventions on those identified as at risk.[81]

- Groupwork: many specialist palliative care services run groups for bereaved adults, often for those who have lost a partner, usually in mixed-sex groups. These may provide a reasonably safe way of testing out socializing as a single person, as well as an opportunity to explore the bereavement experience with others in the same situation. Time-limited groups avoid the problem of how to detach a bereaved person who has become very dependent on the group, since an ending is planned from the start. They also avoid the difficulty of a clique developing among longstanding members, which may be off-putting to a newly bereaved person seeking to join. There have been groups for adult bereaved children and Williams has done innovative group work with bereaved men at St Christopher's Hospice. McFerran-Skewes and Erdonmez-Grocke report on running a group for bereaved teenagers using music therapy to make contact with this often challenging group.[82] Many bereaved people find it therapeutic to participate in voluntary groups focusing on curing the disease that killed the deceased, or improving conditions for those who suffer from it.

- The Internet: bereaved people are now beginning to seek information and companionship through the Internet, just as many dying people do. Martin has provided a useful guide to sites and an assessment of the benefits and dangers of use of the Internet.[83]

CONCLUSION

In the past, there has often been a concentration on the problems of bereavement and insufficient recognition of the strengths that bereaved people bring to dealing with the pain and the losses. Increasingly we are realizing that an individual assessment and approach is needed from professionals rather than trying to make people fit a pattern. Helping each bereaved person to consider how he or she has met crises in the past and what they have learnt from this can be a valuable intervention in itself. Encouraging an approach that takes small, manageable steps rather than big leaps in dealing with problems is supportive. Above all, it is important for the professional to maintain a sense of confidence that it is possible to live with bereavement.

KEY POINTS

- Psychological distress is key in the individual's experience of illness.
- Remember social context and culture.
- Wherever possible, treat the individual and his or her network as the unit of care.
- Provide information.
- Anticipate fears and uncertainties; encourage sharing of feelings.
- Recognize concurrent stressors but do not just identify problems; also work with strengths and resources.
- Financial and practical assistance is vital.
- Carers need attention to their own emotional support.
- Remember children and their needs.
- Care should extend into bereavement.
- Culture, family experience, age and gender all have an impact on the process of bereavement and bereavement practices.
- The crucial factor for professionals to understand is how the bereaved person perceives what is happening.
- Any assessment of whether an individual's grief is 'abnormal' must take into account a complex range of factors personal to that individual.

REFERENCES

1. National Council for Hospice and Specialist Palliative Care Services. Feeling better: psychosocial care in specialist palliative care. A discussion paper. Occasional Paper 13. London: NCHSPCS, 1997.
2. Fawzy FI, Fawzy NW, Arndt LA, Pasnau RO. Critical review of psychosocial interventions in cancer care. *Arch Gen Psychiatry* 1995; **52**, 100–13.
3. Fawzy FI, Fawzy NW, Canada AL. Psychosocial treatment of cancer: an update. *Curr Opin Psychiatry* 1998; **11**(4), 601–5.
4. Vachon M, Kristjanson L, Higginson I. Psychosocial issues in palliative care: the patient, the family and the process and outcome of care. *J Pain Symptom Manage* 1995; **10**, 142–50.
5. Barkwell DP. Ascribed meaning: a critical factor in coping and pain attenuation in patients with cancer-related pain. *J Palliat Care* 1991; **7**, 5–14.
6. Herth K. The relationship between level of hope and level of coping response. *Oncol Nurs Forum* 1989; **16**(1), 67–72.
7. Herth K. Fostering hope in terminally-ill people. *J Adv Nurs* 1990; **15**, 1250–9.
8. Oliviere D, Hargreaves R, Monroe B. Assessment. In: *Good practices in palliative care: a psychosocial perspective*. Aldershot: Ashgate, 1997, 48.
9. Daniel G. Family problems after a bereavement. *Bereave Care* 1998; **17**(3), 35–8.
10. Spruyt O. Community-based palliative care for Bangladeshi patients in East London. Accounts of bereaved carers. *Palliat Med* 1999; **13**, 119–29.

11. Oliviere D. Culture and ethnicity. *Eur J Palliat Care* 1999; **6**, 53–6.

12. Field D. *What do we mean by psychosocial?* National Council for Hospice and Specialist Palliative Care Services Briefing Paper No. 4. London: NCHSPCS, March 2000.

13. Koffman J, Higginson IJ. Accounts of carers' satisfaction with health care at the end of life: a comparison of first generation black Carribeans and white patients with advanced disease. *Palliat Med* 2001; **15**, 337–45.

14. Redd WH, Silberfarb PM, Andersen BL. Physiologic and psychobehavioural research in oncology. *Cancer* 1991; **67**(Suppl.), 813–22.

15. Goodwin JS, Hunt WC, Key CR, Samet JM. The effect of marital status on stage, treatment and survival of cancer patients. *JAMA* 1987; **258**, 3125–30.

16. Heaven CM, Maguire P. The relationship between patients' concerns and psychological distress in a hospice setting. *Psycho-oncology* 1998; **7**, 502–7.

17. Miettinen T, Tilvis R, Karppi P, Arve S. Why is the pain relief of dying patients often unsuccessful? The relatives' perspectives. *Palliat Med* 1998; **12**, 429–35.

18. Hodgson C, Higginson I, McDonnell M, Butters E. Family anxiety in advanced cancer: a multicentre prospective study in Ireland. *Br J Cancer* 1997; **76**, 1211–14.

19. Panke J, Ferrell B. Emotional problems in the family. In: Doyle D, Hanks G, Cherny N, Calman K (eds), *Oxford textbook of palliative medicine*, 3rd edn. Oxford: Oxford University Press, 2004, 985–92.

20. Kinsella G, Cooper B, Picton C. A review of the measurement of caregiver and family burden in palliative care. *J Palliat Care* 1998; **14**(2), 37–45.

21. Hull M. Sources of stress for hospice care-giving families. *Hospice J* 1990; **6**, 29–54.

22. Payne S, Smith P, Dean S. Identifying the concerns of informal carers in palliative care. *Palliat Med* 1999; **13**, 37–44.

23. Kristjanson L, Leis A, Koop P, Carriere K, Mueller B. Family members' care expectations, care perceptions, and satisfaction with advanced cancer care. *J Palliat Care* 1997; **1**, 5–13.

24. Sykes N, Pearson S, Chell S. Quality of care: the carer's perspective. *Palliat Med* 1992; **6**, 227–36.

25. Thorpe G. Enabling more dying people to remain at home. *BMJ* 1993; **307**, 915–18.

26. Neale B. Informal palliative care: a review of research on needs, standards and service evaluation. Occasional Paper No. 3. Sheffield: Trent Palliative Care Centre, 1991.

27. Kristjanson LJ. The family's cancer journey: a literature review. *Cancer Nurs* 1994; **17**(1), 1–17.

28. Oliviere D, Hargreaves R, Monroe B. Working with families. In: *Good practices in palliative care: a psychosocial perspective*. Aldershot: Ashgate, 1998, 54.

29. National Institute for Clinical Excellence. *Guidance on cancer services: improving supportive and palliative care for adults with cancer*. London: NICE, 2004.

30. Kissane D, Bloch S, McKenzie D. Family coping and bereavement outcome. *Palliat Med* 1997; **11**, 191–201.

31. Kissane D, Bloch S. Family grief. *Br J Psychiatry* 1994; **164**, 728–40.

32. Kissane D, Bloch S, McKenzie M, McDowall A, Nitzan R. Family grief therapy: a preliminary account of a new model to promote healthy family functioning during palliative care and bereavement. *Psycho-oncology* 1998; **7**, 14–25.

33. Moos RH, Moos BS. *Family Environment Scale manual*. California: Consulting Psychologists Press, 1981.

34. Dar R, Beach CM, Barden PL, Cleeland CS. Cancer pain in the marital system: a study of patients and their spouses. *J Pain Symptom Manage* 1992; 7, 87–93.

35. Field D, Douglas C, Jagger C, Jagger D, Jagger P. Terminal illness: views of lay patients and their carers. *Palliat Med* 1995; 9, 45–54.

36. Oliviere D, Hargreaves R, Monroe B. Assessment. In: *Good practices in palliative care: a psychosocial perspective.* Aldershot: Ashgate, 1997, 25–48.

37. Sheldon F. Mapping the support networks. In: *Psychosocial palliative care: good practice in the care of the dying and bereaved.* Cheltenham: Stanley Thornes, 1997, 79–80.

38. Kirschling JM (ed.). *Family-based palliative care.* New York: Howarth Press, 1990.

39. McGoldrick M, Gerson R. *Genograms in family assessment.* New York: Norton, 1985.

40. Monroe B. Social work in palliative care. In: Doyle D, Hanks G, Cherny N, Calman K (eds), *Oxford textbook of palliative medicine*, 3rd edn. Oxford: Oxford University Press, 2004, 1008–9.

41. Fallowfield L. The quality of life: sexual function and body image following cancer therapy. *Cancer Topics* 1992; 9, 20–1.

42. Schover LR. Sexual dysfunction. In: Holland JC (ed.), *Psycho-oncology.* Oxford: Oxford University Press, 1998, 494–9.

43. Jenkins B. Oncology patients' reports of sexual changes after treatment for gynaecological cancer. *Nurs Forum* 1988; 15, 349–54.

44. Gamel C, Davis BD, Hengeveld M. Nurses' provision of teaching and counselling on sexuality: a review of the literature. *J Adv Nurs* 1993; 18, 1219–27.

45. Vincent CE, Vincent B, Greiss FC, Linton EB. Some marital concomitants of carcinoma of the cervix. *South Med J* 1975; 68, 552–8.

46. Wright P. Unpublished MSc dissertation. University of Southampton 1996.

47. Black D. Psychological reactions to life-threatening and terminal illnesses and bereavement. In: Rutter M, Taylor E, Herson L (eds), *Child and adolescent psychiatry modern approaches*, 3rd edn. Oxford: Blackwell, 1994.

48. Black D, Young B. Bereaved children: risk and preventative intervention. In: Raphael B, Burrows G (eds), *Handbook of studies on preventative psychiatry.* Amsterdam: Elsevier, 1995, 225–44.

49. Weller RA, Weller EB, Fristad MA, Bowes BM. Depression in recently bereaved prepubertal children. *Am J Psychiatry* 1991; 148, 1536–40.

50. Silverman PR. *Never too young to know. Death in children's lives.* Oxford: Oxford University Press, 2000.

51. Worden WJ. *Children and grief. When a parent dies.* New York: Guilford Press, 1996.

52. Rosenheim E, Reicher R. Informing children about a patient's terminal illness. *J Child Psychol Psychiatry* 1985; 26(6), 995–8.

53. Christ GH. *Healing children's grief. Surviving a parent's death from cancer.* Oxford: Oxford University Press, 2000.

54. Kane B. Children's concepts of death. *J Genet Psychol* 1979; 134, 141–53.

55. Lansdown R, Benjamin G. Development of concept of death in children 5–9 years. *Childcare Health Educ* 1985; 1, 13–20.

56. Reilly TP, Hasazai JE, Bond LA. Children's conceptions of death and personal mortality. *J Pediatr Psychol* 1983; 8(1), 21–31.

57. *My book about.* London: St Christopher's Hospice, 1989.

58. Klass D, Silverman P, Nickman SL. *Continuing bonds.* New York: Washington, 1996.

59. Wikan U. Bereavement and loss in two Muslim communities. *Soc Sci Med* 1988; **27**, 451–60.
60. Firth S. *Death, dying and bereavement in a British Hindu community.* Leuven: Peeters, 1997.
61. Gunaratnam Y. Culture is not enough: a critique of multiculturalism in palliative care. In: Field D, Hockey J, Small N (eds), *Death, gender and ethnicity.* London: Routledge, 1997, 166–86.
62. Stroebe M. New directions in bereavement research: exploration of gender differences. *Palliat Med* 1998, **12**, 5–12.
63. Thompson N. Masculinity and loss. In: Field D, Hockey J, Small N (eds), *Death, gender and ethnicity.* London: Routledge, 1997, 76–88.
64. Martin T, Doka K. *Men don't cry – women do.* Philadelphia: Brunner, Mazel, 1999.
65. Parkes CM. *Bereavement: studies of grief in adult life*, 3rd edn. London: Routledge, 1996.
66. Worden W. *Grief counselling and grief therapy*, 2nd edn. New York: Springer, 1991.
67. Wortman C, Silver R. The myths of coping with loss. *J Consult Clin Psychol* 1989; **57**, 349–57.
68. Klass D, Silverman P, Nickman S. *Continuing bonds.* Philadelphia: Taylor and Francis, 1996.
69. Walter T. A new model of grief. *Mortality* 1996; **1**, 7 –25.
70. Parkes CM. Counselling bereaved people – help or harm? *Bereave Care* 2000; **19**(2), 19–21.
71. Doka K. *Disenfranchised grief: recognizing hidden sorrow.* San Francisco: Jossey Bass, 1989.
72. Middleton W, Raphael B, Martinek N, Misso V. Pathological grief reactions. In: Stroebe M, Stroebe W, Hansson R (eds), *Handbook of bereavement: theory, research and interventions.* Cambridge: Cambridge University Press, 1993, 44–61.
73. Walter T. *The revival of death.* London: Routledge, 1994.
74. Charlton R, Dolman E. Bereavement: a protocol for primary care. *Br J Gen Pract* 1995; **45**, 427 –30.
75. Schut H, Stroebe M, van der Bout J, Keijser J. Gender differences in the efficacy of grief counselling. *Br J Clin Psychol* 1997; **36**, 63–72.
76. MacElveen-Hoehn P. Sexual responses to the stimulus of death. In: Morgan J (ed.), *Personal care in an impersonal world: a multidimensional look at bereavement.* Amityville: Baywood, 1993, 95–119.
77. Payne S, Large S, Jarrett N, Turner P. Written information given to patients and families by palliative care units: a national survey. *Lancet* 2000; **355**, 1792.
78. Hutchinson S. Evaluation of bereavement anniversary cards. *J Palliat Care* 1995; **11**, 32–4.
79. Foulstone S, Harvey B, Wright J, Jay M, Owen F, Cole R. Bereavement support: evaluation of a palliative care memorial service. *Palliat Med* 1993; **7**, 307–11.
80. Payne S, Horn S, Relf M. *Loss and bereavement.* Buckingham: Open University Press, 1999.
81. Raphael B. Preventive intervention with the recently bereaved. *Arch Gen Psychiatry* 1977; **34**, 1450–4.
82. McFerran-Skewes K, Erdonmez-Grocke D. Group music therapy with young bereaved teenagers. *Eur J Palliat Care* 2000; **7**(6), 227–9.
83. Martin D. Internet support for bereaved people. *Bereave Care* 2000; **19**(3), 38–40.

FURTHER READING

Field D, Hockey J, Small N (eds). *Death, gender and ethnicity.* London: Routledge, 1997.

Oliviere D, Hargreaves R, Monroe B. *Good practices in palliative care: a psychosocial perspective.* Aldershot: Ashgate, 1997.

Parkes CM. *Bereavement: studies of grief in adult life*, 3rd edn. London: Routledge, 1996.

Parkes CM, Laungani P, Young B. *Death and bereavement across cultures.* London: Routledge, 1997.

Payne S, Horn S, Relf M. *Loss and bereavement.* Buckingham: Open University Press, 1999.

Sheldon F. *Psychosocial palliative care: good practice in the care of the dying and bereaved.* Cheltenham: Stanley Thornes, 1997.

Worden W. *Children and grief. When a parent dies.* New York: Guilford Press, 1996.

chapter 17

CULTURAL ISSUES IN PALLIATIVE CARE

David Oliviere

The 'art and science' of palliative care lies in considering every aspect of people's lives which may be important in providing 'total care'. An integral part of this consideration is the person's culture. Each patient or family displays a different set of mores, expectations, patterns of relationship and verbal and non-verbal reactions to situations. These responses are partly defined by cultural patterns learnt from babyhood and evolved by exposure to other cultural influences. Good cultural care and appreciation of 'cultural pain' must be part of the holistic approach delivered in the management of advanced disease.

> No one can ever be categorised solely in terms of their cultural and religious background, but there has been a heightened interest in how these factors may, sensitively understood, much enhance the quality of care.[1]

CULTURE

Inherited values, ways of behaving, beliefs, styles of living, tastes and rituals all make up culture and are shaped by it. According to Helman:[2]

> Culture is a set of guidelines (both explicit and implicit) which individuals inherit as members of a particular society, and which tell them how to view the world, how to experience it emotionally, and how to behave in it in relation to other people, to supernatural forces of gods, and to the natural environment. It also provides them with a way of transmitting these guidelines to the next generation – by the use of symbols, language, art and ritual. To some extent, culture can be seen as an inherited 'lens', through which individuals perceive and understand the world that they inhabit, and learn how to live within it.

Culture can be experienced as a basic set of rules – some very explicit; others quite subtle – about different aspects of living and, of course, dying. Some of these 'rules' are rejected, reinforced or amalgamated with other sets of rules during one's lifetime.

Many Western societies are now 'multi-cultural', 'multi-ethnic' and 'multi-faith'. Religion and culture are often inextricably linked and give 'meaning' to body and mind. Their understanding in making the person who they are is imperative. Even though many people from minority ethnic groups do not practise specific religious rituals or engage in active worship, their traditions and culture are shaped by a Christian, Hindu, Jewish, Muslim or other religious background. For some patients and relatives, the approach of death initiates new and richer meaning in their religious rituals and traditions. For others, these will be less meaningful.

Respect for the person whatever their complex make-up has always been important in palliative care. In order to understand patients and their families as well as their wishes, we must understand their culture as well as ours.

Basic to palliative care philosophy are principles of acceptance of the individual (e.g. the patient who displays customs and habits quite unlike our own), non-judgemental attitudes (e.g. towards the family who will not talk about cancer and death because their religion suggests that this may take away hope), and confidentiality (e.g. over the lifestyle of the Chinese Buddhist patient who could easily become a curiosity).

The modern hospice movement has always cherished the idea of being a community. (St Christopher's Hospice, for example, has, since its inception, included provision for local young children to have a presence in the hospice through its nursery. It then pioneered the first home care service, establishing a pattern for community-based services to develop.) It is important that the palliative care service is seen as part of the range of provision in the community and that the service is available to all the different groups/cultures in society irrespective of class or creed. This can only happen if the service is set up to give the appropriate message that all groups are welcome and if we as individuals are as comfortable as possible in working with people of differing cultural experiences and backgrounds.

This chapter considers racism and society's attitudes that affect culture as well as key areas to be considered in providing a culturally sensitive palliative care service.

RACISM AND SOCIETY

Individual care of patients and families cannot be divorced from the inequalities and discrimination existing in the structures of society. Currently, there is concern that palliative care should be a reality and available to *all* groups and communities, and discussion of 'excluded groups' is increasingly common. Issues of access to palliative care and services catering for a culturally and ethnically diverse population are frequently voiced.

Palliative care has to address how much its provision might be 'institutionally racist' by (inadvertently) discriminating against certain groups. The 1999 Macpherson Report into the circumstances surrounding the death of Stephen Lawrence, a young black man from London who was murdered, defined institutional racism as:[3]

> ... the collective failure of an organisation to provide an appropriate and professional service to people because of their colour, culture or ethnic origin. It can be seen or detected

in processes, attitudes or behaviour which amount to discrimination through unwitting prejudice, ignorance, thoughtlessness and racist stereotyping which disadvantage minority ethnic people.

Just some of the ways palliative care can be providing a less than adequate service are the failure to recognize cultural patterns that are important to patients and families, to provide appropriate meals, to value diversity, to train staff adequately or to have clear policies to enhance equality.

Living in a society where there can be a tendency to value commonality rather than difference, palliative care workers can be faced with fears about people from minority groups getting preferential treatment or they may be exposed to basic discomfort and prejudice. There can be real dilemmas: how much does one allow a large family to take up a constant vigil around the patient's bed with other patients in close proximity? Surprisingly, the experience for some staff has not included relating to people who display different looks, dress, accent, preferences or humour. We have to adapt services to meet the various needs of different cultures rather than just help minority groups make use of the service as provided.

Underlying all this is a need to value diversity as giving pleasure, excitement, interest and enquiry. We are all an amalgamation of different cultural influences. We are not just referring to people who look or seem to be 'different'.

One of the challenges in working with people from various cultural backgrounds is assessing where people are in their culture, i.e. which aspects of, and to what extent, their cultural background are important to them. Migration to a new country may have strengthened or diluted cultural practices and beliefs.

In the family context, there may be conflicts between members of different generations who have varying perceptions of and attachments to their own culture, even though these are people who share the same ethnic customs. Hence Jews born and bred in north-west London may live in quite a different style from those in Iraq and Egypt. Furthermore, 'knowledge of a country may not represent the subculture and religious denomination from which a patient comes';[4] 'Among Asians, attitudes to death and bereavement vary with different religions, caste, and socio-eonomic backgrounds'.[5]

In palliative care it is vital to acknowledge the special needs of asylum seekers and refugees or patients and families who have been subjected to persecution as a result of political, religious or racial differences. Whether the experience is recent or in the distant past, they may have experienced numerous losses and emotional trauma, which are likely to be resurrected in their present situation.[6] This sense of trauma, guilt or loss will not be confined to the generation who live through it, but is experienced by the next generation, as illustrated by the children of holocaust survivors.[7]

AREAS TO BE CONSIDERED IN ENSURING MULTI-CULTURALLY SENSITIVE PALLIATIVE CARE

If you were terminally ill, which aspects of your culture would be important for you? For teaching purposes, we sometimes ask students to imagine they are entering a palliative care unit in China and to identify the ten main aspects about which they would be concerned, apart from specific medical care. In palliative care, different cultural attitudes will be held towards:

- the disease – cancer, acquired immunodeficiency syndrome (AIDS),

- hospice environment – food, climate, pictures/symbols/objects, types of staff (ethnicity, gender),

- physical care – pain, analgesia, modesty,

- talking/counselling – honesty, privacy,

- family – who's included; roles of men, women, parents and children,

- point of death – rituals, prayers, those present,

- death – washing, dressing, display of body,

- funeral – type of disposal, open/closed coffin,

- bereavement – open expression of grief.

ACCESS TO SERVICES

Research has repeatedly shown that there is unequal access to health services by black and minority ethnic and migrant workers.[8–11] Services are often linguistically and culturally inaccessible to people from minority ethnic groups; there is a lack of knowledge of the services available. There is no evidence to suggest hospice services are any different.

Indeed, the indications are that people from minority cultures are not adequately accessing palliative care services,[12] and are under-represented. Considerable research is needed on the best strategies to improve take-up of palliative care services from members of minority cultures. It is still unknown whether the numbers of patients served are consistent with the incidence of certain illnesses and other demographic variables with the majority population. This is, in turn, dependent on services recording accurately the ethnic origins of those referred. Ethnicity data are poor.

Part of making a service more accessible involves actively reaching out to potential users and making the image of the service more acceptable to them. In order to make known the palliative care services, various measures for marketing and communicating the service to minority groups will need to be considered. These include the following.

- Translating some literature into the main local languages and ensuring comprehensive dissemination.[13]

- Making personal contact with local leaders or providing 'open days' to discuss what is on offer. This is particularly important, as minority cultures can often view palliative care services as being provided mainly by white people from the established culture or being part of a religious movement and not particularly welcoming of the minority. It is easy for people from a minority culture to be uncomfortable about the service and, therefore, engaging interest is crucial.[14]

• Addressing the image of the service. The fact that many hospices are named 'St' and are staffed predominantly by white staff, even in very mixed areas, can, for some, reinforce the image of not being available equally for people from minority cultures. Therefore staff should include members of local ethnic minorities. We know that patients seem to experience the service very positively once sampled, but the above factors can pose barriers and create initial anxieties.[15]

• Targeting local general practitioners from areas of the main minority ethnic groups.[16]

HOSPITALITY

Hospitality is the basis of good palliative care. It puts patients, relatives and friends at ease so that professionals and volunteers can use their skills and the person they are helping can feel safe and comfortable enough to use the help on offer.

We welcome patients, families and visitors from many cultures and religions or none, trying to communicate a deep respect for them and their customs. We want them to feel at home because their needs and wishes regarding diet, care and rituals and the whole approach to the dying person and to people during bereavement are being met – not as an extra bonus but as their right and expectation to experience care that is in keeping with the way they have lived. They should not be made to feel 'over-special'.

Basic good practices with any patient are particularly important when dealing with the person from a different ethnic group: ensuring their names are accurately understood and recorded and also what they prefer to be called, or checking that they have understood what has been said, who is who and what plans have been agreed. Recording the patient's first language or language spoken at home in the notes can communicate care and concern.

The quality of staff is important irrespective of race, but if personnel reflect the local range of ethnic groups, a powerful message is conveyed regarding the respect for difference. This does not mean that a Jewish patient should automatically have a Jewish nurse or an Asian patient an Asian nurse.

LANGUAGE AND COMMUNICATION

'In a way I am disabled. I can see but I cannot read. I can hear but I cannot understand'. 'No agency can provide a fair or effective service to people with whom it cannot communicate'.[17]

A patient who does not speak the same language as the professional or volunteer carer (or has limited understanding) experiences a handicap and poses one for the carer. We would not try to help a patient who is deaf and has no speech without seeking assistance. Similarly, when seeing a patient with whom there are language difficulties, time must be taken to find and work with interpreters where possible. Otherwise we are left with a greater reliance on working assumptions, guesswork and intuition. Even people who can speak some English may forget most of it when they are ill or worried or under stress.[18]

Misinterpretation of people from ethnic groups has resulted in wrong diagnosis, e.g. the Gujerati-speaking patient from India was seen as having 'stomach pain' when he was basically indicating general 'upset'. People from some cultures nod their head to mean 'no' and shake their head to mean 'yes'.

The points to remember when 'communicating across a language barrier' include the following.

- Speak clearly and simply and at the pace you sense is right for your patient/ relative. Take care not to raise your voice as if the person were deaf! Choose words the patient is likely to know. Listen for the words the patient uses and use them yourself. If necessary, use mime and pictures to help to get the meaning across.

- Check that you have been understood and signal clearly that you are moving on to a new subject, e.g. 'Now I want to ask you about...'.

- People who are stressed and unwell are only likely to be able to remember or absorb a very limited amount of the information discussed. The effort of concentrating to understand a foreign language can seriously affect the memory. You may need to write down one or two key points to which the patient and family can refer.

- Coping across the language barrier can also affect the way people behave. People can be extra nervous knowing they cannot explain their thoughts and feelings and deal with someone in authority. The behaviour you see does not necessarily reflect the personality of your patient. Be aware of any judgements you make about the behaviour or personality of someone whose first language is not your own. Intonation is the most difficult aspect to master in a foreign language, and what may sound excitable, angry or abrupt in one language may sound perfectly acceptable in other languages. Again, beware of making judgements based on intonation or tone of voice.

- Non-verbal communication and body language are strongly culture bound. Signals and movements that convey one thing in one culture may convey something completely different in another. For example, in English culture it is important to indicate that you are listening to someone by nodding and making eye contact and encouraging noises. In some other cultures it is not necessary to do anything special. Beware of making automatic judgements about behaviour or personality on the basis of non-verbal signals. Bear in mind, too, that your attempts at non-verbal communication may sometimes be misunderstood.

- Write down important instructions about how to take medications, and involve relatives and friends here. Important points about drugs and treatment should be translated, if possible.

- Using an interpreter is not an easy option, as it involves:
  building up a list of appropriate interpreters,
  negotiating funding or input from your local interpreting service,
  providing some preparation on the topics you are likely to cover,
  allocating extra time for the interview,
  debriefing time afterwards for the interpreter.

Counselling and communication must, if possible, be done in the language in which the patient thinks. The use of an experienced interpreter, where possible and appropriate, has advantages, although this has to be negotiated with sensitivity. We need to be careful that, as professionals, we are not usurping the roles of family members and ignoring their concerns by imposing an interpreter and Western expectations of the primacy of the patient's autonomy over their identity as a member of the family group. However, using relatives/friends as interpreters severely limits what can be achieved, as they are emotionally involved and would subjectively filter the communication you wish to have. It is important to remember that in some cultures family members are mediators of information.[19] Up to twice as much time has to be allowed for an interview using an interpreter. Remember that, however professional, interpreters can also become very personally concerned about the painful issues often discussed in palliative care.

FAMILY

What 'family' means to an English person may be quite different from what it may mean to someone from another culture. Our understanding of family referring to parents and children, perhaps grandparents, may to another culture include cousins, uncles, aunts, nieces, nephews and others such as fellow members of a religious group. This will also determine who is present near the time of death and afterwards.

Expectations of how the old and the young behave within the family may be very different from our own in terms of respect, unwillingness to express anger or of younger women rather than men being the carers.

Roles, especially of women, are often different. We must be careful not to automatically bring Western values to cultures in which women's roles are very much defined in terms of motherhood and home making.

Some staff in a home care team were upset and critical of Mrs M's family, from India. With breast cancer, bony secondaries and a very oedematous arm, she struggled with all the housework and shopping despite her husband and two grown-up children being at home. However, Mrs M passively accepted the expectation of her role in the family.

Cultural factors influence beliefs concerning communicating with children about death and how much children are allowed to participate in the care of family members. As professional carers, we have to be careful to work through and with the adults in the family in communicating with the children.

STEREOTYPING AND GENERALIZING

'She can cope with the suppositories, she's French'; 'He's a typical Greek'; 'Muslims do it like this'. Although people tend to categorize or generalize to 'make sense' of their experience of other cultures, it is important to avoid becoming rigid, unrealistic, denying people's individuality and increasing the assumptions about the group concerned. Every culture may have its 'tendencies', but many people are subject to several cultural influences and personal characteristics.

We have to confront prejudice and stereotypical thinking and attitudes in ourselves, our colleagues and others. There is sometimes as much difference within groups as between them. As professionals in palliative care, we have never been reluctant to stand for high standards of practice. This is no less important in this area of work.

For example, we are so often exposed to images of Muslims in the media as aggressive and condemnatory of Western influences that we have to try to become aware of how one-sided images can influence our attitude towards the individual Muslim family in our care.

GETTING TO KNOW THE PERSON

In addition to trying to understand the richness and requirements of different cultures, we need to clarify the particular preferences on certain practices of our patient or relative from a specific culture or group. We must remember that, for example, not every Jewish person keeps kosher or every Catholic wants to say the rosary.

Just because someone is categorized as African, Chinese, Hindu etc., it does not automatically mean that they have taken on all the traditions and practices of that culture or faith: 'If we are not sensitive to this fact we may structure things in such a way that we do not allow the person to express what they are feeling in the way most appropriate to them and can sometimes actually induce guilt by implying that they ought to be refusing pork or lighting candles, etc'.[20] Do not assume, either, that the patient now in front of you will match the same pattern as a previous one from the same culture.

The view that 'Asians are helped by having extended family support' did not apply to Nina. She continued to feel very isolated after the death of her mother. With a family business and three young children, she had no space to express her grief and needed the support of the hospice bereavement service.

We cannot possibly know everything about every cultural or religious group in front of us. Remember:

- Often the faith/religion given (Jew, Hindu, Muslim, Sikh) may identify the culture of the person rather than just their religious practices or beliefs.

- Try to understand how important the culture or faith is to the individual. Not everyone from that culture automatically adheres to the conventional practices. There are many shades and variations within each cultural group, from the more orthodox to the more liberal. Do not impose your understanding of their cultural practices – listen to what is wanted.

- Do not assume one person from a particular culture will resemble the next person of the same culture in preferences.

- Many people will be 'in transition' between the family's culture and a local cultural identity and practices. There may be conflict over adherence to cultural traditions between generations.

- Enquire of patient and family or friends whether there are any specific needs and requirements that you should know in respect of the particular person. They are usually very happy that someone is troubling to find out their needs.

OUR OWN ATTITUDES

Our own culture will colour the way we assess the particular needs of people from other cultures.

It should be evident from earlier discussion that to help people from other cultures, we have to understand our own culture, race and religion or non-religion. We have to be aware of our attitudes towards people who are different from us and take care not to transfer our ideas onto the other person. We must be aware of our own assumptions as to what is helpful or unhelpful behaviour for people in crisis.

There are potential conflicts between some palliative care principles which we hold dear and cultural influences, for example that bereaved people should not express their emotions, or that very ill people be urged by anxious relatives to keep eating, or that openness and truth-telling could take away hope.[21] Only with a secure basis to one's own thinking can one really learn about and understand other people's cultures.

CONCLUSION

For each patient and family, 'the journey' from life to death will be different. In palliative care, it is vital we ensure that the journey is in accordance with the person's

Table 17.1 Framework for achieving accessible and appropriate palliative care services

	Principle	Practice
Mission statement	Commitment to equality in value base and in stated aims	All staff aware
Policy and procedures	Management committed to Equal Opportunities Policy	Staff clear on expectations Staff and service users understand
Staff selection	Staff matching ethos Community participation as volunteers	Careful selection Diversity of staff — paid and unpaid
Training	Skilled workforce	Induction and ongoing training Annual appraisal
Environment	User-friendly/hospitable/trust	Furnishings and décor reducing unfamiliarity
Written material	Good communication	Understandable language/offer of interpreter
Language	Good communication	Prepare list of interpreters Training/debriefing essential Consider health advocates
Community development	Trust building Equal access	Personal contact Identify community leaders Visits to unit Work with local GPs Use community's own media
Ethnic monitoring	Information on those currently accessing	Incorporating into database Staff training vital
Patient notes	Accurate information to plan care	Record first language, spoken/written name, dietary/religious requirements, family
Resources	Patient comfort	Availability of books, cassettes with appropriate images and language
Diet	Good care	Availability of other foods
Pastoral care	Respect for individuals	Develop contacts from main faiths Ensure training
Personal care	Individuality and respect	Staff understanding of gender, modesty, personal hygiene
Family and community	Support for patient's network	Understand culture of wider family, death and bereavement customs and rituals
Bereavement	Prevention	Discerning culturally appropriate patterns from risk Counsellors from local communities
Feedback and evaluation	Service improvement	Seeking views Consulting individuals and groups User and carer participation

Reproduced from Oliviere D, Hargreaves R, Monroe B. (1998) *Good practices in palliative care*. With kind permission from Ashgate Publishing Ltd.

individual cultural values and expectations. In this way, staff can find their own experience enriched and enhanced as patient and family are allowed to be themselves.

Indeed, when it comes to basics, we are not just talking about labels – African-Caribbean, Asian, Chinese, Hindu, Jew, Muslim etc. – but about people: people experiencing the deepest human emotions of love and pain linked to attachment and loss. In producing good palliative care, we have to listen sensitively to where people are in their culture and give them permission to live this time using the aspects that support them most securely.

KEY POINTS

- 'Cultural pain' can be real.
- The structures within society discriminate and disadvantage minority ethnic individuals and communities.
- We have to adapt services to meet the various needs of different cultures and minority groups.
- Professionals and services need to be culturally sensitive and structurally aware.
- Numerous factors vary the experience of a person's culture (generation, class, geography).
- There is commonality and differences between people of a range of cultures. It is important to identify a person's individuality.

REFERENCES

1. Ainsworth-Smith I. Foreword. In: Neuberger J (ed.), *Caring for dying people of different faiths*. London: Austen Cornish and The Lisa Sainsbury Foundation, 1987, viii.
2. Helman C. *Culture, health and illness*, 2nd edn. London: Butterworth-Heinemann, 1990.
3. Macpherson W (Sir William of Cluny). *The Stephen Lawrence Inquiry: report of an inquiry*. London: Home Office, February 1999.
4. Clarke M, Finlay I, Campbell I. Cultural boundaries in care. *Palliat Med* 1991; 5, 63–5.
5. Rees D. Terminal care and bereavement. In: McAvoy BR, Donaldson LJ (eds), *Health care for Asians*. Oxford General Practice Series 18. Oxford: Oxford University Press, 1990, 304.
6. Schriever SH. Comparison of beliefs and practices of ethnic Veit and Lao Hmong concerning illness, healing, death and mourning: implications for hospice care with refugees in Canada. *J Palliat Care* 1990; 6(1), 42–9.
7. Baider L, Sarell M. Coping with cancer among holocaust survivors in Israel: an explanatory study. *J Human Stress* 1984; 10(3), 121–7.
8. Baxter C. *Cancer support and ethnic minority and migrant worker communities*. London: Cancerlink, 1989.
9. Firth S. *Wider horizons*. London: The National Council for Hospice and Specialist Palliative Care Services, 2001.
10. Cabinet Office. *Involving users. Improving the delivery of health care*. London: National Consumer Council, Consumer Congress and Service First Unit, 1999.

11. Mount J (ed.). *Palliative care services for different ethnic groups.* London: National Council for Hospice and Specialist Palliative Care Services, 2000.

12. Firth S. Minority ethnic communities and religious groups. In: Oliviere D, Monroe B (eds), *Death, dying and social differences.* Oxford: Oxford University Press, 2004.

13. Oliviere D. Culture and ethnicity. *Eur J Palliat Care* 1999; 6(2), 53–6.

14. Simmonds R, Sque M, Goddard J, Tullett R, Mount J. *Improving access to palliative care services for ethnic minority groups.* Crawley: St Catherine's Hospice, 2001.

15. Oliviere D, Hargreaves R, Monroe B. *Good practices in palliative care.* Aldershot: Ashgate, 1998.

16. Karim K, Bailey M, Tunna K. Non-white ethnicity and the provision of specialist palliative care services: factors affecting doctors' referral patterns. *Palliat Med* 2000; **14**, 471–8.

17. Shackman J. The right to be understood. In: *London Interpreting Project (LIP) Directory of Community Interpreting Services and Resources in the Greater London Area.* London: LIP, 1989.

18. Henley A. *Caring in a multiracial society.* London: Bloomsbury Health Authority, 1987.

19. Nunez Olarte J. Cultural difference and palliative care. In: Monroe B, Oliviere D (eds), *Patient participation in palliative care.* Oxford: Oxford University Press, 2003, 74–87.

20. Speck P. Cultural and religious aspects of dying. In: Sherr L (ed.). *Death, dying and bereavement.* Oxford: Blackwell, 1989, 36–47.

21. Abeles M. Features of Judaism for carers when looking after Jewish patients. *Palliat Med* 1991; 5, 201–5.

chapter 18

EMOTIONAL IMPACT OF PALLIATIVE CARE ON STAFF

Barbara Monroe

Palliative care makes difficult, personal demands on those who provide it.

In early palliative care literature, much was made of the concept of 'burn out' developed by Maslach.[1] It was suggested that there was probably a 'shelf life' for those working in the field, a point beyond which negative self-concepts and job attitudes and a loss of concern for patients were almost inevitable. Vachon's important review of staff stress in hospice/palliative care concludes that this is not so.[2]

Staff stress experienced in the specialist setting has been demonstrated to be less than that experienced by professionals in many other working environments. Death anxiety was found to be higher in medical and surgical nurses than in hospice nurses,[3] while oncology and intensive care nurses were found to experience more stress and to be more likely to leave than those in specialist palliative care.[4] Nurses in specialist palliative care experience less stress in working with the dying than district nurses and health visitors.[5] A recent study of female hospice nurses concludes that despite the difficult nature of the care provided, the hospice is a positive environment in which to work.[6]

Part of the reason for all this was the early recognition in most specialist settings of the potential stress inherent in the field and the development of appropriate organizational and personal coping strategies, such as staff support programmes, education and team development.[2] Palliative care is not a uniquely stressful profession. Many of its pressures are to be found in other environments and require similar solutions: professional attention to staff support, which includes issues of recruitment, orientation, training, appraisal, communication and team building.

Care givers are widely reported to feel that far more of their stressors derive from their work environment and occupational role than from their direct work with dying patients and families. In Vachon's study, 48 per cent reported stress from organizational issues, 29 per cent from role issues, 17 per cent from difficulties connected with the care of patients and families, and 7 per cent from illness-related variables.[7] Particularly emphasized were lack of time, lack of recognition and having to work with and around the emotional state of colleagues.

Nonetheless it is also clear that professionals need to feel comfortable with themselves and their own losses if they are to listen attentively to the problems of others. Professionals must recognize their own needs for support and their responsibility for self-care. An effective support system will include both personal and organizational mechanisms.

WHAT IS OCCUPATIONAL STRESS?

It has been said that: 'job stress results when the individual's supplies and resources do not mesh with the demands of the work environment'.[2] However, most existing studies of occupational stress have been carried out with female participants who have generally been nurses, usually in either the UK or North America.

Researchers are now emphasizing interactive processes between the individual and the organization, with some writers also beginning to examine the impact of culture and inter-professional differences. Papadatou's studies of professionals working with dying children note that:

- physicians are more likely to grieve over their inability to achieve clinical goals and see their grief as private and lonely;[8,9]

- nurses tend to grieve the loss of their special relationships with patients and to identify with the pain of relatives and rely more on one another to find meaning in their loss;

- Greek nurses displayed their emotions more openly in comparison with Hong Kong nurses, who suppressed grief more often by retreating into practical duties.[10] The Greek nurses reported a strong sense of anger towards a God they saw as all-powerful and loving. Chinese nurses, on the contrary, tended to accept death as a form of salvation.

If professionals are to transcend death experiences and invest in living and new professional goals, both individuals and teams must be able to create meaning. Meaning making is a social as well as a personal process: individual values and assumptions may be supported or undermined by the implicit and explicit values and rules of the workplace. Particular stress may be caused when organizational rules about how professionals should behave in the face of death and dying are experienced as contradictory. An example would be when an organization expects a formalized group sharing of difficulties but frowns upon any individual expression of grief.

The emphasis on organizational factors in creating stress might also be due to professionals in palliative care displacing their existential anxieties about working with death and dying. Nimmo contrasts the idealistic objectives of hospices with their vulnerability in terms of bed capacity, funding and the power to alleviate all pain:[11] 'Embodied in the idealism of hospice and staff was a sense that there was nothing they could not do, that they had magical solutions to intractable problems ... The unbearable pain of reality was unconsciously denied and converted into an attack on the discharging doctor, the social worker and the District Nursing Service'.

Speck has also reflected on what lies behind the apparent 'niceness' of hospices and their staff.[12] He suggests that when any experience is especially painful, staff may seek to avoid it by projecting their bad feelings onto others who are deemed not to understand or care, often a 'persecutory management'. Effective consultation between staff and management is therefore especially important so that unconscious processes can be addressed openly.

Lawton argues that a significant proportion of patients are admitted to hospices because of the way in which their disease affects the 'boundedness' of their bodies and undermines their identities as people.[13] She proposes that setting the 'dirty dying' of such patients apart from mainstream society enables the rest of society to maintain certain ideas about living, personhood and hygienic, sanitized bodies. Patients, carers and staff members alike were often observed to employ animal metaphors to describe and account for the physical experiences of patients: 'You wouldn't put a dog through this'; 'He smelt like dog shit'. If this analysis is even partially correct, there are serious challenges to respond to in the support of staff working in these circumstances. Research is needed into the impact upon nurses working in specialist in-patient units of an increasingly dependent and short-stay patient population with complex clinical problems.

Changes in health care policy and planning are potentially stressful.[2,14] The transition of specialist palliative care services from the pioneer phase to greater integration into general health and social care systems may cause tensions between the unboundaried giving of pioneering staff members and the dispassionate attention paid to work–life balance by later recruits.[15] Issues of funding, service specification and an increasing regulatory burden may well become important factors in the hospice load.

SOURCES OF STRESS

PERSONAL VARIABLES AND VALUE SYSTEMS

Risk factors for stress include the following.

- Low self-esteem.

- A tendency to derive identity through the job alone.[16]

- Patients and families with whom professionals most readily identify, perhaps because of age or life situation, can trigger powerful reactions, raising unexpected and unresolved personal issues relating to loss. On the other hand, personal losses may help nurses to be more understanding of carers.[17]

- Over-reliance on social support – partners and friends may become resentful.[18]

- Concurrent emotional demands such as relationship difficulties.[2]

- Possession of an unrealistic set of attitudes and objectives, e.g. expecting to be thoroughly competent in every situation, to feel warmth towards every patient and family member and to be appreciated by all their colleagues. Such 'supermen' not only diminish the patient and family, but also disable the rest of the team, as apparent infallibility is very daunting.

  Stress can be minimized by factors such as the following.

- Loss of confidence in newer members of staff can be avoided if others share 'helper secrets'.[19] For example, most staff feel speechless in front of the anguished patient who declares: 'Talking can't help'.

- A personal philosophy regarding illness and death is important. It may or may not be related to spiritual or religious beliefs.[7]

- Congruence between personal professional ideals and the goals and environment of the workplace.

- Length of experience in the specialist work role.[2]

WORKPLACE STRESSORS

The chapter on teamwork in this book (Chapter 22) highlights the value of a team approach to palliative care. It also emphasizes that poorly managed teams themselves become a source of stress as a result of:

- communication problems,

- role ambiguity,

- inter-disciplinary conflict – the role blurring and overlap that frequently occur in palliative care can be threatening as well as stimulating and challenging,[2]

- uncertain or unrealistic objectives,

- lack of clear leadership.

Difficulties may be exacerbated by poor managerial and administrative practices in the institution as a whole. Problems in teams may result from exhaustion, a failure to match workload to resources. Environmental factors such as poor office space or inadequate equipment also impose a toll. Perhaps most damaging of all is an organizational failure to set clear goals and to give all staff regular recognition for their achievements and regular opportunities to develop new skills against known gaps and deficiencies. Regular team meetings and attention to developing a team philosophy emerge as important coping supports.[2]

There may also be inter-professional differences: a recent survey found that very few doctors felt that their skills and talents were not being adequately used, compared to 80 per cent of nurses.[20] More nurses than doctors had thought of leaving; more doctors had worked in other specialist settings. Such contrasting experiences can make building multi-professional teams difficult.

CONTACT WITH PATIENT AND CARERS

Professionals find it hard to assess the results of their work when patients die. They receive much of the anger and fear carried by patients and those close to them and often feel that they are being asked to solve the insoluble. In this atmosphere, unexpected behaviour by patients and family members can upset the team: relatives who refuse to visit, patients who will not communicate. Patients and families who respond to their illness in a way that differs from 'the norm' present particular problems, and staff find it more difficult dealing with psychiatric symptoms than with physical symptoms.[18] Changes in the attitudes of consumers of health care may also mean that staff increasingly find themselves the recipients of critical comment.

SIGNS OF STRESS

Organizations with a high level of employee stress will be characterized by:

- conflict,
- power struggles,
- rivalry,
- hostility towards team leaders and management,
- unrecognized conflict displaced onto convenient scapegoats,
- rapid staff turnover,
- high sickness rates,
- a general lack of enthusiasm, particularly for new initiatives.

The individual may exhibit stress through:

- irritability,
- depression,
- loss of self-esteem,
- over-involvement in work,
- sleep disturbance,
- weight loss or gain,
- headache and minor illnesses,
- rigidity, cynicism, apathy and a general sense of feeling overwhelmed,
- difficulties in job–home interactions.[2]

WHAT HELPS?

BALANCING POLICIES AND PEOPLE

Organizations wishing to avoid such negative consequences will attempt to find a balance between uniformly applied policies and a personalized, sensitive and flexible response to particular individuals for whom work and personal pressures have coincided. This balance can be difficult to achieve. For example, bereavement in a staff member may well benefit from a personally adjusted amount of time off related to the needs of the individual. However, this can give rise to claims of managerial partiality. Creativity can help, e.g. the timing of bereavement leave can be flexible. Some staff may find that they need time off 2 or 3 months after the death rather than immediately, when work colleagues and routines may represent an important source of support. For others, the opposite will be true. Professionals experiencing a personal bereavement often report a sense of exhaustion in responding to colleagues' thoughtful enquiries. A brief recognition of their circumstances may be more valued – a touch on the arm, a note.

A nurse whose daughter had died after a lengthy illness wrote a document with details about her daughter's last days and some information about her funeral. She asked her manager to circulate it before she returned to work, saying that she wanted people to know what had happened and how she felt, but not to be overwhelmed by a lot of questions and comments. Both she and her colleagues found this approach helpful.

SETTING LIMITS

Many studies point to the central importance of individuals experiencing a sense of competence, control and pleasure in their work.[2] Sheldon's study of the role of the specialist social worker in palliative care emphasizes the importance of recognizing limits and working creatively within them:[21] 'Caregivers can be taught how to do what they can while letting go of the need to control the outcome ... Caregivers may need instruction in letting go and in maintaining clear limits and boundaries'.[22] Davies and Oberle's study of home care nurses in the USA demonstrates that the core dimension in their supportive role was that of preserving their own integrity.[23] They did this by maintaining self-awareness and a critical approach to their own practice. They used particular strategies such as humour and sharing frustrations with colleagues to maintain or regain self-control.

CLINICAL SUPERVISION

The Department of Health describes clinical supervision as 'a formal process of professional support and learning which enables individual practitioners to develop knowledge and competence, assume responsibility for their own practice and enhance consumer protection and safety of care in complex clinical situations'.[24] This claim is unproven, but there are many anecdotal accounts of the value of clinical supervision as a support.[25] Evidence on outcomes is mainly based on indirect evidence of benefit such as the perceptions of supervisees and narrative accounts of the content of supervision sessions.[26] Where outcomes have been identified, they centre around feeling valued and appreciated, a supportive environment, and the opportunity to explore and change practice,[27] although a beneficial effect on sickness rates has been reported.[28]

AN OPPORTUNITY TO SHARE

Talking things over with a colleague, either formally or informally, is one of the most widely used and effective coping mechanisms.[2] The recent requirements of clinical governance are helpful in their insistence on the review and management of near-misses and critical incidents, but the 'no-blame' culture must be made to work so that mistakes can be seen as positive learning opportunities. Serious critical incidents may also require a specific de-briefing to prevent the formation of post-traumatic stress disorders.[29]

A patient committed suicide in a palliative care unit. The following day the unit's psychiatrist got everyone together to share the facts and to talk about their care of the patient and how they felt. All staff involved were included, from doctors and nurses to stewards and domestics. It was very important in containing what had been a very distressing incident for all involved and later in helping staff to make recommendations about changes in practice.

Opportunities need to be found to develop enough intimacy that in a crisis staff feel safe enough with one another to take short cuts. Examples might be away days or undertaking joint training and education. Teaching and writing can become important counterbalancing activities to work with dying patients, as they are creative and allow both overview and sense of control. In a professional area where so much unfinished business is inevitable, it is vital to find activities that have a beginning, a middle and an end. Effective appraisal and training policies also support more informal methodologies.

SUPPORT GROUPS

Support groups can make a contribution to staff well-being, although evidence for their efficacy is limited.[30] Important considerations are:

- clear aims,
- careful consideration of membership,
- clear rules about the group's boundaries,
- effective leadership,
- attention to the group life cycle.[31]

Vachon suggests that time-limited groups are most helpful, often with a defined purpose, for example supporting staff through a major change in work practice.[31]

A 2-day multi-professional staff support training course aiming to help staff recognize their ability to deal with stress and grief was found to increase participants' sense of self-confidence, understanding of stress and grief, and awareness of the need for support.[32]

MANAGING ENDINGS

Palliative care professionals are in the business of endings. They need to take them seriously, not just for patients and families, but also for themselves. All staff will need an institutional framework within which to express their grief and learn how to let go. Rituals can assist, as long as they do not become organizational strait jackets. This will be approached differently in different settings. For example, some hospices have a regular slot in ward meetings to remember the dead; in others it may occasionally be possible for staff to attend the funeral of someone to whom they have become particularly close. It must be remembered by those working within organizations that all staff are affected: a receptionist may have become particularly attached to a family she has spoken to every evening, for example.

Administrative staff expressed their sense of being excluded from the support of seeing the 'thank you' comments in letters that went to clinical staff. Reporting in the staff newsletter helps to spread these more widely. A specially designed training course on working with loss also recognized their involvement with patients and families and increased their level of confidence.

Professionals need to be clear at the end of the working day about which of the feelings stirred up in them belong to the patients and those close to them, and which are properly their own. Time must be taken to separate the two. Good written recording helps in leaving things behind. Professionals must also develop the ability to trust colleagues to carry on in their absence.

RECOGNIZING STAFF GRIEF

It is important to recognize that palliative care workers experience grief as well as stress.[8] Potential losses include:

- a close relationship with a particular patient,

- unmet professional goals,

- losses related to personal belief systems,

- reactivated unresolved past losses or anticipated future losses,

- the realization of personal mortality.

Papadatou builds on Stroebe's dual process model, describing the grieving reactions of health professionals as following a similar fluctuation between experiencing grief feelings by focusing on the loss experience, and avoiding them by distracting themselves from the loss experience. Both activities are necessary and both require support in the workplace.

SPIRITUAL CARE

Moments of special intimacy between patient and professional in palliative care often represent the height of professional aspiration and may move the patient or carer significantly forward.[33] However, they also arouse fears of being over-whelmed by suffering and chaos. Individuals need to find personal balancing strategies, which may include the practice of a particular faith or a recognition of the importance of fostering hope and creativity for both patients and themselves.[34,35]

Staff members valued the offer of the aromatherapy sessions that had benefited patients and carers. They also enjoyed attending art and pottery classes after work in the day centre.

Individual professionals need to be open to ways of strengthening personal resources and finding renewal. These might include the following.

- Developing a particular area of work as a personal specialism in which particular satisfaction can be taken, even when compromises have to be made elsewhere.

- Physical activity, such as yoga or hill walking.

- Cultivating a sense of humour and the occasional act of delinquency. After a difficult home visit, an ice cream in the park with a colleague before the return to work can make a lot of difference.

The attention paid by professionals to spiritual care for the dying and those important to them must also extend to themselves and their colleagues. No one can function effectively at the spiritual level if it is one-way traffic. There is currently less focus on training in spiritual care, at the same time as fewer professionals are joining palliative care motivated by a strong personal faith and a commitment to active witness. Without training that permits self-exploration alongside skills acquisition, staff may continue to feel unprepared and uncertain. If professionals let their own inner lives become underused and unvisited, they may actively avoid cues that indicate that patients and carers want to discuss issues of meaning and belief: 'Why me?'

CONCLUSION

Organizations delivering palliative care must be realistic. The major goal of the team is to support patients and their families, not to be endlessly sensitive to the personal needs of team members. Professionals must avoid letting their vision of total pain, their desire to treat the whole person, trip them into thinking that they can or should treat every problem. Most people are seeking support, not protection: someone willing to listen to their difficulties rather than someone who can achieve a miracle. Probably the most important element in maintaining personal and institutional morale is a sense of job satisfaction and competence in the work role. This requires organizational affirmation and a personal acceptance that 'good enough' care linked to a knowledge that things are better than they would have been without the team's intervention often represents enormous achievements.

KEY POINTS

- Palliative care is not a uniquely stressful profession.
- Good staff support requires professional attention to recruitment, induction, appraisal and training.
- Healthcare professionals experience grief as well as stress.
- All staff members need opportunities to reflect on the meaning, purpose and value of what they do.
- Attention to effective teamwork delivers dividends.
- Clinical supervision is a valuable framework for the development of self-awareness, knowledge and competence.
- More training in spiritual care is required.

REFERENCES

1. Maslach C. *Burnout: the cost of caring.* New Jersey: Prentice Hall, 1982.
2. Vachon M. Staff stress in hospice/palliative care: a review. *Palliat Med* 1995; **9**, 91–122.
3. Bene B, Foxall MJ. Death anxiety and job stress in hospice and medical–surgical nurses. *Hospice J* 1991; 7, 25–41.
4. Bram PJ, Katz LF. Study of burnout in nurses working in hospice and hospital oncology settings. *Oncol Nurs Forum* 1989; **16**, 555–60.
5. Dunne J, Jenkins L. *Stress and coping strategies in Macmillan nurses.* London: Cancer Relief Macmillan Fund, 1991.
6. Payne N. Occupational stressors and coping as determinants of burnout in female hospice nurses. *J Adv Nurs* 2001; **33**(3), 396–405.
7. Vachon M. *Occupational stress in the care of the critically ill, the dying and the bereaved.* Washington: Hemisphere, 1987.
8. Papadatou D. The grieving healthcare provider. Variables affecting the professional response to a child's death. *Bereavement Care* 2001; **20**(2), 26–9.
9. Papadatou D. A proposed model of health professionals' grieving process. *Omega* 2000; **41**(1), 59–77.
10. Papadatou D, Martinson I, Chung B. Caring for dying children: a comparative study of nurses' experience in Greece and Hong Kong. *Cancer Nurs* 2001; **24**(5), 402–12.
11. Nimmo S. On being a counsellor in a hospice. *Psychodynamic Counselling* 1997; **3**(2), 133–41.
12. Speck P. Unconscious communications. *Palliat Med* 1996; **10**, 273–4.

13. Lawton J. Contemporary hospice care: the sequestration of the unbounded body and 'dirty dying'. *Sociol Health Illness* 1998; **20**(2), 121–43.

14. Sheldon F. *Psychosocial palliative care. Good practice in the care of the dying and bereaved.* Cheltenham: Stanley Thornes, 1997, 108.

15. James N, Field D. The routinisation of hospice: charisma and bureaucratisation. *Soc Sci Med* 1992; **14**, 488–509.

16. Schneider J. Self-care: challenges and rewards for hospice professionals. *Hospice J* 1987; **3**, 255–76.

17. Pitcher P. The personal bereavement experience of nurses working in palliative care. Unpublished MSc dissertation, 1996, University of Southampton. Cited in Sheldon F. *Psychosocial palliative care. Good practice in the care of the dying and bereaved.* Cheltenham: Stanley Thornes, 1997, 110.

18. Vachon M. The stress of professional caregivers. In: Doyle D, Hanks G, MacDonald N (eds), *Oxford textbook of palliative medicine*, 2nd edn. Oxford: Oxford University Press, 1998, 919–29.

19. Larson D. Helper secrets: invisible stressors in hospice work. *Am J Hospice Care* 1985; Nov./Dec., 35–40.

20. Addington-Hall J, Karlsen S. *Summary of the national survey of health professionals and volunteers working in voluntary hospices.* London: Help the Hospices, 2001.

21. Sheldon F. Dimensions of the role of the social worker in palliative care. *Palliat Med* 2000; **14**, 491–8.

22. Carmack B. Balancing engagement and detachment in caregiving. *J Nurs Scholarship* 1997; **29**(2), 139–43.

23. Davies B, Oberle K. Dimensions of the supportive role of the nurse in palliative care. *Oncol Nurs Forum* 1990; **17**, 87–94.

24. Department of Health. *A vision for the future. The nursing, midwifery and health visiting contribution to health and health care.* London: HMSO, 1993.

25. Jones A. A 'bonding between strangers': a palliative model of clinical supervision. *J Adv Nurs* 1997; **26**, 1028–35.

26. Gilmore A. *Review of U.K. evaluative literature on clinical supervision in nursing and health visiting.* London: UKCC, 1999.

27. Scanlon C, Weir WS. Learning from practice? Mental health nurses' perceptions and experiences of clinical supervision. *J Adv Nurs* 1997; **26**, 295–303.

28. Dunn C, Bishop V. Clinical supervision: its implementation in one acute sector trust. In: Bishop V (ed.), *Clinical supervision in practice.* London: Macmillan, 1998, 85–107.

29. Walker G. Crisis-care in critical incident debriefing. *Death Studies* 1990; **14**(2), 121–33.

30. Lewis A. Reducing burnout: development of an oncology staff bereavement program. *Oncol Nurs Forum* 1999; **26**(6), 1065–9.

31. Alexander DA. Staff support groups: do they support and are they even groups? *Palliat Med* 1993; **7**, 127–32.

32. Blanche M. Running a hospice staff support course. *Eur J Palliat Care* 1997; **4**(6), 200–2.

33. Barnard D. The promise of intimacy and the fear of our own undoing. *J Palliat Care* 1995; **11**, 22–6.

34. Herth K. Fostering hope in terminally ill people. *J Adv Nurs* 1990; **15**, 1250–9.

35. Kennett CE. Participation in a creative arts project can foster hope in a hospice day centre. *Palliat Med* **14**(5), 419–25.

chapter 19

EQUAL ACCESS IN PALLIATIVE CARE

Jonathan Koffman and Irene J. Higginson

THE DEVELOPMENT OF PALLIATIVE CARE SERVICES IN THE UK: EXTENDING CARE TO ALL?

Palliative care now encompasses a wide range of specialist services, but commenced in the 1960s with the development of the modern hospice movement by Dame Cicely Saunders when she founded St Christopher's Hospice in Sydenham, London. The number of hospices and specialist palliative care services has increased rapidly since that time. In 1980, there were fewer than 80 in-patient hospices and 100 home support teams. By the end of the millennium this had increased to 212 in-patient hospices comprising 3205 beds, 433 home care and extended home care support teams, and 243 day care centres.[1] In addition, there are more than 260 hospitals with palliative care nurses or teams and many offer a shared model of care.

Whilst the actual supply of specialist palliative care plays a vital role in defining which patients and their families with advanced disease receive care, concerns have been raised about other factors that influence the accessibility of care at the end of life for those who might benefit from it. This chapter examines the available evidence to determine in what ways age, sex, ethnicity, economic disadvantage, clinical diagnosis and clinical symptoms influence palliative care at the end of life (Fig. 19.1).

SOCIO-DEMOGRAPHIC CHARACTERISTICS AND ACCESS

AGE

It has long been suggested that the palliative care movement has not afforded elderly patients adequate care, preferring to devote more its resources to relatively younger people, although some research has, in part, rebutted this accusation.[2] The 1990 Regional Study of the Care of the Dying (RSCD)[1] demonstrated that age does represent an important influence in determining which patients receive hospice

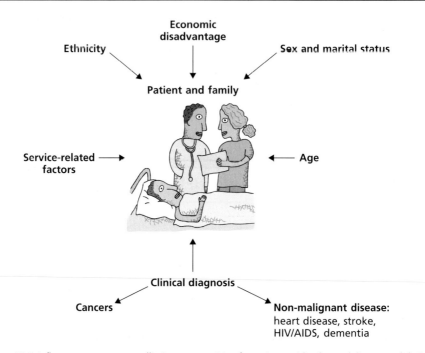

Figure 19.1 Influences on access to palliative care provision for patients with advanced disease and their families.

in-patient care.[3] Analysis of this large data set demonstrated that patients admitted to hospices with a cancer diagnosis were shown to be, on average, younger than those who were not. Although further examination of the data controlled for the possibility that this may have been due to more elderly patients being in residential or nursing homes, the difference still remained significant. A number of reasons have been advanced to account for fewer elderly patients making use of this provision, including:

- elderly cancer patients are less troubled by their diagnosis than younger people;
- many elderly cancer patients' physical symptoms are due to other co-morbidities related to ageing in general;
- many of the physical restrictions elderly cancer patients experience are due to the ageing process;
- elderly cancer patients are more accepting of death.

However, many elderly patients do experience significant distress from their illness and associated symptoms.[3] Patients with cancer in particular and advanced disease in general should not be excluded from specialist palliative care input on the basis of their age alone.

The Regional Study of the Care of the Dying

The RSCD made use of retrospective survey methods originally developed by Anne Cartwright in 1967. The RSCD was undertaken to provide a contemporary account of dying and bereavement in 20 health authorities (inner city, semi-urban, and rural) in England. Approximately 10 months after the patient's death, and following a letter of introduction, interviewers contacted the address of the deceased in order to identify the person best able to recount the deceased's last 12 months of life. They then conducted structured interviews that covered the deceased's health problems and restrictions, sources of formal and informal care, and the respondent's experience of caring for the deceased, the deceased's use of and satisfaction with health care services, information and communication with healthcare professionals, and the respondents' experience of bereavement and bereavement care.

SEX AND MARITAL STATUS

Sex and marital status can be considered important influences on the type and location of care patients with advanced disease receive. Although studies have indicated that being married is positively associated with death at home for both sexes, this is far more pronounced for males, for whom caregivers are more likely to be wives or daughters.[4] This rarely applies to women, who are more likely to be widowed by the time they die and consequently have a far greater chance of dying in a nursing home or a residential home.[4]

ETHNICITY

The impact of ageing on black and minority ethnic groups now means larger numbers of older members within these communities will require health services for advanced disease. The palliative care movement has aspired to extend care services widely and inclusively and *The new NHS: modern, dependable* has stated that: 'black and minority ethnic groups should not be disadvantaged in their access to healthcare provision'.[5] However, anecdotal reports have levelled criticism at care at the end of life for its lack of attention to the provision of culturally sensitive services and access to appropriate care. Although many studies have explored the needs of patients with advanced disease during their last year of life and of their caregivers, few have focused on the needs of black and minority communities. This is consequently a neglected area, where little research has been undertaken. Most recently, a study in an inner London health authority demonstrated that black Caribbean patients with advanced disease experienced restricted access to specialist palliative care services compared to white patients in the decedent's last 12 months of life,[6] yet an analysis of local provision revealed no lack of palliative care services.[1] Various explanations have been postulated to account for the apparently lower utilization of services.

- Knowledge among the black and minority ethnic groups on how best to make use of local health care services may be restricted.

- There is evidence that some general practitioners are more likely to act as 'gatekeepers' to services among black and minority ethnic groups, contributing to lower referral rates.

- The demand for services may have been influenced by the 'ethnocentric' outlook of palliative care services, discouraging black and minority ethnic groups from making use of relevant provision.

More research is required to determine the accessibility, cultural acceptability and appropriateness of palliative care services among other minority ethnic groups. This is particularly important in light of the development of *Guidance on supportive care* for the National Cancer Programme, which highlighted their social exclusion from services at the end of life.[7]

ECONOMIC DISADVANTAGE

In areas of higher social deprivation, people die at younger ages, often having had an inferior quality of life. Furthermore, services require considerably more resources to achieve the same level of care as provided in less disadvantaged areas. Several studies have shown that cancer patients who have a higher education, are more skilled or live in higher socio-economic areas of residence are far more likely to die at home than their poorer counterparts.[4] Figure 19.2 illustrates the wide variation in deaths at home by deprivation band.[8]

Social disadvantage also impacts significantly on the ability of healthcare professionals to deliver effective care to patients who live in deprived areas. One study in London compared the activity of home palliative care nurses in deprived and more affluent areas. It found that in order to achieve similar levels of home

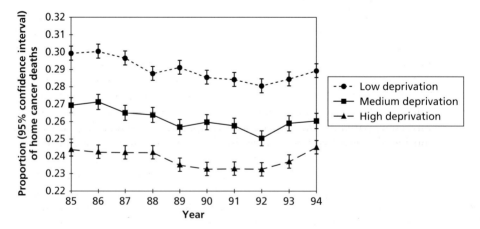

Figure 19.2 Trends in deaths at home from cancer by deprivation band (1/3 population sorted by score of deprivation). (Reproduced from Higginson IJ. Jarman B. Astin P. Dolan S. Do social factors affect where patients die: an analysis of 10 years of cancer deaths in England. *Journal of Public Health Medicine* 1999; 21: 22–28, with permission from Oxford University Press.)[8]

death rates, at least twice the number of visits was needed in the deprived areas.[9] The authors also stated that the area they surveyed was characterized by problems raising voluntary funding for hospice and home care. In addition, although little evidence is actually available as to their actual preferences for place of care and death, choices remain limited for patients from lower occupational groups.

CLINICAL DIAGNOSIS AND ACCESS TO PALLIATIVE CARE SERVICES

CANCER

Of all patients with advanced disease, cancer patients are more likely to receive specialist palliative care services: approximately 96 per cent of individuals cared for in all hospice settings in 1995 in the UK had cancer.[4] The reasons for this situation are historic (the development of hospice services and the palliative care movement) and also patient based. It has been suggested that cancer patients are very different from other patient groups with advanced disease. First, age-related symptoms such as mental confusion and long-term disability are considered less common. This is important because patients with non-malignant disease are therefore more likely to have other incidental co-morbidities associated with old age, for example mental confusion, breathlessness and incontinence. All these symptoms may considerably exacerbate their care agenda. In addition, younger patients with human immunodeficiency virus/acquired immunodeficiency syndrome (HIV/AIDS), multiple sclerosis and motor neurone disease may exhibit neurological deficits resulting in similar symptoms, which in turn present challenges. Second, the incidence, duration and severity of these symptoms follow a different course – the terminal phase of advanced cancer can frequently be predicted with far greater certainty.

However, despite the growth in hospices and specialist palliative care services, a number of population-based studies have revealed that care for patients with advanced cancer has not been universal. Evidence suggests that many patients are denied access to appropriate palliative care, or have significant unmet needs for symptom control and psychosocial support. According to the findings from the RSCD, patients who received hospice in-patient care provision were more likely than other patients to have been diagnosed with breast cancer or colorectal cancer. Conversely, patients who experienced lymphatic or haematological cancers were considerably less likely to receive this form of provision at the end of life.[3] Possible explanations to account for this might be that patients with breast cancer are a relatively more politicized group, and that they also may be more accepting of the hospice concept. It is more common for patients with haematological cancers to die in acute hospital settings,[4] where they may have developed longer-term relationships with the healthcare professionals associated with their care. Furthermore, patients with head and neck cancers and with primary cerebral tumours, which are frequently associated with mental confusion, also tend to be more likely to die in hospital settings.[4] In addition, evidence has shown that they are also less likely to receive palliative home care, despite the considerable stress this may place on their caregivers. If adequately supported, it may be possible to care for these patients at home.

NON-MALIGNANT DISEASE

Although an increasing number of patients with a limited range of neurological conditions and patients with advanced HIV/AIDS are now in receipt of hospice care, until recently little attention has been paid to the palliative care needs of people who die from other non-malignant disease. This may be due to the previously accepted wisdom that cancer patients experienced a wider range of symptoms, and that many of these symptoms were considered to be very distressing, particularly pain. However, an increasing body of research is beginning to refute this assertion and has demonstrated considerable unmet need for the provision of care, and in turn the inadequate control of symptoms and poor psychosocial support of patients who die from other causes and their caregivers.[10]

Circulatory disease

Heart disease is as frequent a cause of death as cancer in the UK, and whilst many patients with heart disease die suddenly, a large number experience significant poor health beforehand. Findings from the RSCD demonstrate that less than half of the respondents representing deceased patients with heart disease felt that they were provided with an adequate choice about where the deceased died.[11] This would strongly suggest that healthcare professionals in both acute and primary care settings need to have a shared understanding of the range of hospital and community support available to this patient group.

Stroke

Although many stroke patients are admitted to hospital for care and treatment, a sizeable number remain in the community, cared for by family members. The limited information available suggests that health and social care services are failing to meet the needs of stroke survivors. Despite the fact that many stroke patients die within the first 3 weeks after a stroke, between a third and two-thirds may survive with the consequences of their disease for up to a year. Further, the RSCD revealed that the majority of deceased patients had spent some time in residential or nursing home care during their last year of life. The authors suggest this may have reflected the paucity of alternative services to support this patient group at home with family members.[12] The caregivers that managed stroke patients at home reported needing help with domestic chores and personal care. In many instances they were assuming responsibility for procedures and treatments that, until recently, were confined to specialist in-patient care settings. These responsibilities are frequently performed with little or no education and little emotional support. Many caregivers consequently reported being anxious or depressed during this period. This evidence strongly suggests that there is some way to go before the palliative care needs of stroke patients can be considered to be being met effectively and appropriately.

Dementia

Dementia is a major concern for the UK and impacts greatly on the use of health and social care services.[13] The population prevalence of dementia increases with age, rising to one in four people aged 85+ years. Supportive management and help for caregivers are the main objectives of health services. Patients die with dementia, if not directly because of it. Recent research has indicated that many patients with dementia have symptoms and health needs comparable to those of cancer patients. Mental confusion, urinary incontinence, pain, low mood, constipation and loss of appetite were frequently reported symptoms, and many of these were experienced for longer periods of time than by patients with a cancer diagnosis.[14] Respondents describing the experiences of deceased patients with dementia reported that the levels of assistance required at home were far higher than for patients with cancer. Furthermore, the lives of the dementia patients had been restricted for a longer period of time than those of the cancer patients, 50 per cent having needed help for more than a year with five or more activities of daily living, compared with 9 per cent of cancer patients. These results indicate that many patients with dementia have unmet disease-related concerns that could be dealt with by generalist health and social services support but that would also be ameliorated by palliative care.

HIV/AIDS

In recent years, fewer patients with HIV infection have required palliative care for advanced AIDS-related illness. This has been largely due to developments in combination drug therapies that significantly reduce the viral load in potentially compromised individuals. However, a London-based review of the care of patients with HIV/AIDS revealed that many health care providers were concerned that the substantial cost of combination therapies may lead to cuts in funding for HIV palliative care services.[15] It was felt that a significant proportion of these patients would continue to need palliative care, and that this should continue to be funded. Furthermore, service users and providers indicated that some needs were not being met for members of the gay community. Gay service users continue to experience stigma, judgemental attitudes/behaviour and a lack of cultural awareness from non-HIV specialist services.

Many health care providers in London have expressed concerns that the many members of the various African communities with advanced AIDS-related disease are less likely to make use of palliative care services, and a number of potential barriers have been identified. Two principal problems identified were:

- a limited understanding of palliative care and the difficulty of maintaining confidentiality about diagnosis among the family when using specialist HIV hospices;

- language difficulties and a perceived lack of cultural awareness from service providers (see also 'Ethnicity' above).

Bereavement services were considered inaccessible and unco-ordinated for homosexual men, Africans and children. The general consensus was that if services were to be developed, they should be culturally aware and have a non-judgemental ethos.

FACTORS INFLUENCING DYING AT HOME

It has been argued that acute hospitals are frequently geared towards the healing and restoration of health in the acutely sick. Many doctors regard chronic illness and death as a failure and, even with good training, the psychological strains of dying and death are not easily handled by nursing staff. It therefore comes as no surprise that a recent systematic review of 15 studies in different developed countries, primarily the UK, revealed that between 50 and 70 per cent of patients would prefer to be cared for at home for as long as possible, and to die at home.[16] However, many patients with advanced disease still die in acute settings, although there is strong evidence to demonstrate that palliative home care is often more cost-effective than acute hospital care. Therefore, although patients are often cared for in hospital at the end of life, this is not what they would wish, and is probably not cost-effective for the NHS. Inappropriate interventions at this time will lead to increased suffering. However, access to specialist palliative care services and the ability to die at home are unequally distributed.

Referral to palliative care services is also likely to be a key factor in home death. Indeed, users of home care services are more likely than other patients to die at home.[4] Importantly, however, the type of home care can be considered a contributory factor and the best predictor of place of death. Patients receiving home care attached to in-patient services are less likely to die at home than patients receiving care from services not attached to in-patient services.[4] Once the type of hospice had been taken into consideration, patients' characteristics and the support they can potentially draw on contribute little to the ability to predict place of death.[4] Geography and inequalities in referral may therefore impact greatly on preferred place of death.

CONCLUSIONS

Thirty years since the inception of the modern hospice movement, with laudable aspirations to extend care as widely as possible, access to care has been demonstrated as inequitable on a number of fronts. The influences include age, sex, ethnicity, economic disadvantage and clinical diagnosis, specifically non-malignant disease. Elderly cancer patients appear to present with a host of co-morbidities that are often unrelated to their presenting diagnosis and that represent additional challenges to healthcare professionals. Research has shown that social deprivation impacts on which patients with advanced disease, and particularly cancer, are likely to be admitted to hospices and have a choice about their place of death. Although the evidence is currently sparse, black and minority ethnic groups have been shown to be less likely to receive palliative care services than would be expected. However, the growing number of older members within these communities, many of whom will experience advanced disease, dictates that greater resources are focused on them in future. Also, although not all cancer patients have received palliative care, patients with non-malignant disease appear to have fared considerably worse. In many instances, the problems of this latter group of patients may be even more severe or debilitating because the duration of their illness is frequently longer and more unpredictable, interspersed with periods of great uncertainty. The challenge for palliative care in the future will be to develop adequate and appropriate support to address the many issues highlighted in this chapter. Not investing more has the potential of costing service providers more dearly as delicate care networks have the potential to become compromised.

KEY POINTS

- Since the introduction of the National Health Service, health care has been more widely extended to sections of the population, many of whom were previously excluded from arrangements under the National Insurance Act.
- However, universal access to care and treatment for the dying and their families still remains elusive.
- This must remain a concern, given that there is no second chance to improve the care of individuals who are dying, and it is practically and emotionally extremely difficult for them to raise concerns or to complain about the lack of services they receive.
- Solutions to these problems come in many forms, none of which will be successful in isolation. This involves raising public awareness of palliative care services and providing public education about care to reduce misconceptions about services; improving health and social care professionals' knowledge and attitudes about engaging socially excluded populations; and a greater emphasis on exploring strategy at an epidemiological and corporate level.

REFERENCES

1. Hospice Information Service. *2000 directory of hospice and palliative care services.* London: St Christopher's Hospice, 2000.
2. Smith J. *Going well.* London: Council and Care, 1995.
3. Addington-Hall J, Altmann D, McCarthy M. Which terminally ill cancer patients receive hospice in-patient care? *Soc Sci Med* 1998; **46**, 1011–16.
4. Grande GE, Addington-Hall JM, Todd C. Place of death and access to home care services: are certain patient groups at a disadvantage? *Soc Sci Med* 1998; **47**, 565–79.
5. Secretary of State for Health. *The new NHS: modern, dependable* (Cm 3807). London: HMSO, 1997.
6. Koffman J, Higginson IJ. Accounts of satisfaction with health care at the end of life: a comparison of first generation black Caribbeans and white patients with advanced disease. *Palliat Med* 2001; **15**, 337–45.
7. Department of Health. *National cancer programme – supportive care guidance: draft proposals for external comment.* London: Department of Health, October 2000.
8. Higginson IJ, Jarman B, Astin P, Dolan S. Do social factors affect where patients die: an analysis of 10 years of cancer deaths in England. *J Public Health Med* 1999; **21**, 22–8.
9. Clark C. Social deprivation increases workload in palliative care of terminally ill patients (Letter). *BMJ* 1997; **314**, 1202.

10. Lynn J, Teno JM, Phillips RS *et al*. Perceptions by family members of the dying experience of older and seriously ill patients. SUPPORT Investigators. Study to Understand Prognoses and Preferences for Outcomes and Risks of Treatments. *Ann Intern Med* 1997; **126**, 97–106.
11. McCarthy M, Addington-Hall J, Altmann D. Dying from heart disease. *J R Coll Phys* 1996; **30**, 325–8.
12. Addington-Hall J, Lay M, Altmann D, McCarthy M. Symptom control, communication with health professionals, and hospice care of stroke patients in the last year of life as reported by surviving family, friends, and officials. *Stroke* 1995; **26**, 2242–8.
13. Koffman J, Fulop NJ, Pashley D, Coleman K. No way out: the use of elderly mentally ill acute and assessment psychiatric beds in north and south Thames regions. *Age Ageing* 1996; **25**, 268–72.
14. McCarthy M, Addington-Hall J, Altmann D. The experience of dying from dementia: a retrospective study. *Int J Geriatr Psychiatry* 1997; **12**, 404–9.
15. Higginson IJ. *The palliative care for Londoners: needs, experience, outcomes and future strategy.* London: The London Regional Strategy Group for Palliative Care, 2000.
16. Sen-Gupta GJA, Higginson IJ. Home care in advanced cancer: a systematic literature review of preferences for and associated factors. *Psycho-Oncology* 1998; **7**, 57–67.

chapter 20

SPIRITUAL CONCERNS

Peter W. Speck

INTRODUCTION

If you undertake a literature search using the term 'spiritual' or 'spirituality', you will soon find yourself submerged in a wide variety of literature, ranging from orthodox religion to the very broad and at times bizarre. If you add the words 'health' or 'palliative care' to your search, the number of responses diminishes but is still extensive, and you become aware of the number of new books and articles entitled 'Spirituality and ...' or 'Spirituality in ...'. All of this indicates the enormous growth in interest in spirituality and spiritual care, which still remains for many an awkward topic to explore for themselves, and a very intrusive area to explore with others. As Cobb comments:

> Spiritual ... may suffer from being used in such a generic form that it has become too malleable and therefore lost its distinguishing features. This points to a further aspect of the conundrum: the ambiguity of spirituality and the elusiveness of clarification. Spirituality therefore becomes a self-fulfilling prophecy, respectfully ring-fenced and considered out of bounds to examination, research and exposition.[1]

There has also been a shift in our understanding of the term 'spiritual' because of the differentiation and widening of its identification with religion.[2] However, this has sometimes led to the accusation that the concept of spirituality is now nebulous and only of relevance to those philosophically minded or in need of a crutch to help them cope with life. The differentiation of spiritual from religious has, for some, led to a complete split of one from the other rather than a varying degree of interrelatedness.

The UK 1947 Act of Parliament that introduced the National Health Service ensured that the religious/faith needs of people entering health care featured as a key part of that care. This was re-enforced in the Patient's Charter, and in the Department of Health guidance letter 'The provision of spiritual care to staff, patients and relatives' (HSG(92)2), which has been re-cast in a multi-faith mode.[3] Spiritual care also features in a whole raft of standards documents issued in respect of cancer care, palliative care and elderly care. Respect for religious and spiritual belief has become an important part of the Nursing and Midwifery Council (NMC) code for nursing and in other professional codes of practice.

However, the diffidence felt by many in engaging with this aspect of care has led to much 'lip service' or a narrow focusing on religion and culture, with a consequent lack of perception of people's wider needs in the presence of illness or death.

In the mid-1960s, Cicely Saunders introduced the concept of 'total pain' and in doing so highlighted the need to review a variety of influences in the patient's life which might affect the perception and experience of pain.[4] Dame Cicely also indicated that failure to recognize and give due attention to these aspects of someone's life could result in ineffective care being given. In her 'total pain' model she suggests that we should assess psychological, social, spiritual and sexual aspects. In more recent times, we might also add cultural and bureaucratic aspects. How one makes this assessment is also felt to be difficult for caregivers. Randall and Downie suggest that non-medical/nursing aspects of care have no place in palliative care (being an extrinsic component), but should only be assessed with the express permission of the patient.[5] However, in the context of the understanding that specialist palliative care is essentially a multi-professional approach, there should be an holistic approach to the patient which includes these other components of care. This would not force people to address issues they are clearly unready or unwilling to discuss, but would present opportunities and make known the availability of other services to the patient and family.

One of the problems in addressing spiritual care with patients is that many of those attempting to make an assessment are themselves unclear about their own personal beliefs. This can lead staff to feel ill-equipped to deal with any of the existential issues that the patient may wish to explore. It can be difficult to go confidently to places you have not been to yourself. In an unpublished Bachelor of Nursing thesis, Dukes found that nurses who had a strong belief system that was religious were very effective at discerning religious needs for patients and ensured that they accessed chaplaincy or were able to attend chapel worship.[6] However, in the absence of religious requests, she found that the staff were less able to discern any wider spiritual need. Nurses with a strong spiritual, but non-religious, belief were best at recognizing and responding to the wider spiritual agenda but often missed the religious unless the patient specifically requested help. Those who had a low strength of belief (whatever its nature) rarely assessed the religious or spiritual needs of patients. There were parallels between these findings and those of Ross[7] who described some of the barriers to the assessment of spiritual need, of which the nurses' own belief system was a powerful filter.

Recent research by Koenig and colleagues within the USA shows that there is a positive correlation between religion and health in terms of outcome, protectiveness and sense of well-being.[8,9] In the UK, studies are beginning to show that, in the absence of religion, belief (especially if it is spiritual) is important to a large proportion of people entering health care.[10,11] Thus, if approximately 70 per cent of newly admitted patients have a belief system that is important to them, it should be taken into account when writing a care plan or preparing a care pathway. Since many of the 70 per cent may not practise a religion any more, the challenge is that much greater. There is a growing evidence base for the importance of belief and it is therefore increasingly important to recognize and respond if we are to provide a truly holistic approach within palliative care.

WHAT IS SPIRITUAL CARE?

In a study day held at a large teaching hospital, a wide cross-section of staff was invited to identify the key components of spiritual care. The group ($n = 84$) included a range of health care occupations, age, gender and belief. Central in much of their thinking was an understanding that spirituality is about:

- affirming the humanity of the other person, especially when that person is not capable of doing so for her/himself,

- relatedness,

- hope,

- the ability to transcend or rise above the current situation,

- finding some sense of meaning and purpose in life, especially as it relates to who and what we are (i.e. an existential dimension).

None of this necessarily requires a religious belief, although most of the major world faiths would address these points within their teachings and religious writings. However, someone who followed a humanistic philosophy would also be able to affirm these core aspects, albeit outside of a religious framework.

Spirituality is often described in terms of a search for meaning. Frankl, in his book of this title,[12] describes against the background of the Holocaust how people survived such experiences by finding some form of meaning that could help them understand the experience, and enable them to continue to function and retain a sense of personal identity. This was especially important given the de-personalizing experiences many were undergoing. There are perhaps parallels with the effect of some illnesses in later life and their potential for undermining personhood. Many authors have linked spirituality to meaning and this is helpful. However, I believe that what we are talking about is actually *existential* meaning. Does the fact that you and I exist have any meaning and purpose at all in the context of my life and eventual death? If so, what is that meaning, how do I discover it and does it change over time? These are ultimate questions that can challenge us in a variety of different ways and may only be addressed at key moments in people's lives, when perhaps their very existence is being threatened, or they are undergoing some significant life change that touches on their identity.

In much of Western society, technological advances may seem to have displaced the role of religion in people's lives. People may, therefore, be invited to place their trust in the rituals of modern science rather than in those of the religious life. However, it is interesting to see that, for a sizeable proportion of people, a belief system, however expressed, is important in their lives.[11] Many people seek this existential understanding with reference to the existence of a power other than themselves, which may not be defined too precisely. If we are concerned with finding existential meaning within any particular life experience, and if this is usually linked to an understanding of a relationship to some power other than oneself, can that power be influential when coping with normal life events and transitions as well as illness? In particular, can that power enable us to transcend the difficulties of the 'here and now' experience and foster hope for a future?

In a survey of the way 33 women aged 65 years coped with breast cancer, one respondent said:

> It's almost as if, throughout this entire breast cancer thing, I felt that I was going to come out of it okay. It was only because of my faith in a higher power that I felt I'm going to come out okay because my God is going to take care of me, one way or the other my family can verbalize comfort but my higher power gives me more than that, more reassurance.[13]

Not everyone wishes to describe this power as a deity or God, and many people are usually much more general in their understanding (e.g. a 'higher power', 'a power in the universe' or a 'force for good or evil' etc.). However, out of a large number of patients interviewed in a UK acute health care setting, and in the external healthy population interviewed, approximately 79 per cent claimed to have a spiritual belief system that was very important to them, even though many of them were not religious.[11]

The Oxford English dictionary has defined spiritual as: 'A vital life principle that integrates other aspects of the person and is an essential ingredient in interpersonal relationships and bonding'.

There are several key words in this definition. *Vital* and *integrating* imply that we are multi-faceted as people and it is this vital life principle that holds it all together and enables us to become whole people. The words *relationship* and *bonding* refer to the way in which we can discern that this vital life force is present by the extent and quality of the relationships we have. We all develop affectional bonds with people, animals, places or objects in the course of our life. Events that threaten to separate or damage those bonds have the potential to threaten our spiritual health and well-being. Illness and admission to hospital can have this potential effect, as hospitalization may lead to an experience of loss of freedom, independence, bodily function or body part, with the consequent impact that such loss has on body image and self-worth.[14] At times when that bonding is threatened, or actually severed, we may feel the event at a very deep level. Psychologically we may experience a period of mourning and grief.[15] In addition, we may also feel as if our very existence as a person is under threat.

This approach is helpful when thinking of the way in which we view people who may be struggling to come to terms with a life-threatening disease. It is also relevant for those who have lost, or are in process of losing, their identity as a result of dementia, Alzheimer's disease or stroke or experiencing social isolation. In this context it is important that others affirm our personhood, especially when we are unable to do so, as one aspect of offering spiritual care and of responding to us as a whole person when we may feel fragmented. By 'personhood' I am thinking of that status bestowed upon one human being by others within the context of relationship and social being. In this definition,[16] there is an implied recognition, respect and trust between carer and cared-for, which can be affected by degenerative changes consequent to mental or physical illness. A process of alienation can commence, which can be experienced internally as well as externally and socially. It is a sense of dis-connectedness from oneself, which can have a marked effect on our sense of a continuing identity, the ultimate dis-connectedness being that experienced in the process of dying. Prior to death, it is often the treatment process and the side effects of that treatment that can trigger this feeling of being dis-connected. Patients sometimes describe this in terms of 'my whole life seems to be falling apart. I don't know if I'll ever get it together again', and 'I feel as if my body is outside of my control'.

The experience of major changes within one's physical body, as well as socially and psychologically, may trigger many existential questions for people. The *existential* dimension is often expressed in terms of questions such as 'Who am I?', 'Does my life have any purpose?', and 'Has this illness the power to destroy me?'. We may not, however, wish to use the term 'God' to describe the power, but may talk about natural or cosmic forces, a sense of the other, a power in the universe etc. Whatever description is used concerning that power, it is often explored and understood in and through relationship.

SPIRITUAL AND RELIGIOUS ARE NOT NECESSARILY THE SAME

Distinguishing spiritual care from religious ministry is important and there are many people who would claim to have a deep spirituality but choose not to give expression to it in a religious way.[17,18] The absence of a religious expression or activity in a person's life should not be taken as indicative of a lack of spirituality, as the needs associated with this aspect of the person may continue to exist but in a less recognizable or accessible form.

Spiritual may be described as the vital essence of human life, often enabling us to transcend life circumstances and foster hope. We may not be conscious of its presence or perceive it as an area of need at all times. The outward expression of this vital force or principle will be shaped and influenced by life experience, culture and other personal factors. Spirituality is a dynamic, and will, therefore, be unique for each individual.

> **Spiritual** relates to: a search for *existential* meaning within a life experience, usually with reference to a power other than the self, which may not necessarily be called 'God'. It is the sense of a relationship or connection with this power or force in the universe that can enable us to transcend the present context of reality. It is more than a search for meaning or a sense of unity with others.

Religion may be understood as a system of faith and worship that expresses an underlying spirituality. This faith is frequently interpreted in terms of particular rules, regulations, customs and practices as well as the belief content of the named religion. There is a clear acknowledgement of a power other than self, usually described as 'God', though some faith groups may not have a specific deity but a higher state of being that they will seek to achieve, as in Buddhism. In some religious understandings, this power is seen as an external controlling influence. In others, the control is more from within the believer, guiding and shaping behaviour. The importance of either an external or internal 'locus of control' within a faith context has been the subject of much research, especially in the USA, where a Religious Orientation Scale has been developed, although the scale is really only of relevance in religious populations.[19,20]

When talking about religion, one would not usually separate religion from spirituality. Neither should one use these terms interchangeably or assume that people who deny any religious affiliation have no spiritual needs, since you can be spiritual without being religious.

> **Religious** relates to: a particular system of faith and worship expressive of an underlying spirituality and interpretive of what the named religion understands of 'God' and the individual's response to the deity.

Therefore, some people would choose to express their *spiritual* belief within a *religious* framework, which might bring with it a measure of social integration. On this basis, all religious believers would be spiritual but not all spiritual believers would be religious. This distinction is important when thinking about needs assessment and provision of services.

Sometimes people adopt a set of religious practices without any underlying spiritual belief system. This can lead to forms of superstitious practice whereby the ritual must be performed or bad luck will follow. At its extreme, it is displayed as part of the 'religious' behaviour and obsessive rituals in psychotic illness. There can, therefore, almost be a sliding scale from healthy religion (with a developed underpinning spirituality) to a potentially unhealthy 'religion' (without a deeper spirituality). This latter can lead to restrictive, if not crippling, practices and rituals that can be associated with poor mental health for the individual.

Philosophical: the existence of a power other than self which can be influential is not acceptable to some people who would still wish to assert that they had a belief system of importance. Usually such people would claim to have developed a *philosophical* belief – such as existentialism, humanism, agnosticism or 'free thinking'.

Atheism, which is the denial of the existence of God, should be distinguished from agnosticism, which allows for a degree of uncertainty as to whether or not a deity exists. Some philosophical people would claim to be spiritual and to have an appreciation of aesthetic experiences and, in particular, to be able to transcend their present situation, especially through achieving connectedness with themselves, others and the world around them. They would, however, usually exclude any reference to a power other than themselves that might be influential.

> **Philosophical** refers to: the search for existential meaning that excludes any reference to a power other than themselves, life events and the destiny of the individual being seen as manifestations of the individual's own personality as expressed individually and corporately.

A wider understanding of the word spiritual, as relating to the search for existential meaning within any given life experience, allows us to consider spiritual needs and issues in the absence of any clear practice of a religion or faith, but this does not mean that they are to be seen as totally separated from each other.[2]

If we consider a Venn diagram to illustrate a possible interrelationship between these three main belief systems, the outer circle would represent the *spiritual set*, with an inner circle representing the *religious sub-set*. A third circle representing *philosophical* might be partly within the spiritual and partly outside. The religious circle may also extend outside of the spiritual circle and represent those who follow rituals independent of any spiritual belief. Thus, most of those belonging to the sub-set 'religious' would belong also to the set 'spiritual'. But those who are 'spiritual' will not necessarily express that in a religious way and so may not belong to the 'religious' sub-set.

Similarly, some of those within the philosophical set will also be 'spiritual' and others will not. This becomes important when trying to assess 'spiritual' need, since people may, incorrectly, deduce that those who decline anything religious have no spiritual needs. Frequently, however, the questions that have been asked only relate to religious practice and need, and therefore little attempt has been made to explore the spiritual dimension. In planning for the provision of services in hospitals or residential care, this distinction becomes important, as it recognizes the need for 'spiritual care providers' to be broad, interactive and flexible in their approach.

The assessment of spiritual need often relates to trying to assess the extent to which the sick person feels dis-connected from those people or powers that enable the person to retain some sense of existential meaning and purpose in their life under more normal circumstances (as reflected in the existential domain of the McGill quality of life questionnaire).[21] The extent to which we are, or wish to be, connected will depend on previous life experience as well as on the present situation or our prognosis for the future. People who do not profess any form of religious faith may still wish to have opportunity to be quiet, to reflect, to commune with whatever forces or powers they feel are beneficial to them. In the various ways in which palliative care is made available to people there needs to be opportunity to explore the impact of the illness and its consequences for both the quality of life and the ultimate quality of the death event. Spiritual well-being may be a valuable resource to support people as they come to terms with terminal illness and try to retain this sense of identity in the face of illness and treatments that may threaten to fragment it. Failure to identify and sustain this resource may contribute to the experience of spiritual pain or distress.

SPIRITUAL PAIN AND DISTRESS

Spiritual pain is linked to many of the factors that might lead to a brokenness in our relationship with others, with God or an external power, or with ourselves:

- a sense of hopelessness,

- focus on suffering rather than pain,

- feelings of guilt and/or shame,

- unresolved anger,

- inability to trust,

- lack of inner peace,

- sense of dis-connectedness or fragmentation.

Spiritual pain, or distress, is often identified in people whose physical/emotional pain fails to respond adequately to recognized approaches to symptom relief. It is frequently linked to issues relating to a sense of hopelessness or meaninglessness. Spiritual pain may be expressed as 'suffering' rather than 'pain', indicating that there seems to be no meaning or purpose to the pain and the experience is all-encompassing rather than localized or specific. Feelings of guilt or shame may be expressed as well as an inability to trust – other people, oneself or 'God'. This can lead to breaking away from a previous religious or belief position, or from other people, which can result in greater disease or lack of inner peace. While some of these things can be tackled from a psychosocial perspective, when they assume an ultimate or existential significance, the intervention needs to be of a spiritual nature.

It is significant that many of the complementary forms of therapy have a clear focus on the individual person and on trying to assist that individual in his or her search for what many describe as 'inner peace' and well-being within oneself, which is therefore related to spiritual need and development. It is often the experience of dis-connectedness that causes most anxiety to people.

A friend broke his arm when he was knocked off his bike. The arm was in a plaster cast for a long time. The fingers were exposed and he had to move them as an exercise at regular intervals. He described that he felt the fingers were no longer owned by him – they felt dis-connected. When the day came for the plaster cast to be removed, the consultant orthopaedic surgeon took hold of my friend's arm and gently stroked it from shoulder to fingertips several times. My friend said he had the very strange feeling that the action reunited his fingers, not only with his arm, but also with his whole body.

In a similar way, aromatherapy, head or foot massage, visualization or art therapy may all enable people to explore and express aspects of themselves and their experience of illness and treatment in the hope of transcending some of the more difficult aspects. Touch in a safe context is a not insignificant factor in these approaches that often serve to re-connect the dis-connected and restore a greater sense of wholeness. Reminiscence (written and spoken) and guided imagery are also important aspects of care that may help to ease spiritual pain in terms of allowing some healing or reconciliation of people with their past. Most patients wish to engage in activities which they believe address them more clearly as a person, or which nourish the non-material aspects of their life.

It must not be forgotten that there are also many patients who may not wish to be active but who still value having an aesthetically good setting. For such patients especially, touch, smell, views through a window and beauty can become very important. In this situation it is especially important to focus on the art of *being with* rather than always wanting to be active and *do to*.

SPIRITUALITY IS EVERYONE'S CONCERN – OR IS IT?

While in many cases spiritual care will be the specific remit of properly appointed faith leaders, anyone willing to listen to the patient's story and stay alongside can provide spiritual care in its general sense. There is also a responsibility to liaise with the multi-disciplinary team concerning any perceived spiritual needs.[22] However, the questions that arise may become quite challenging to the listener, who may then find the faith leader/chaplain a useful resource in knowing how best to respond. Assessment can be a source of difficulty to some, but three simple questions can open the door to an understanding of where the person is spiritually.

- Do you have a way of making sense of the things that happen to you in life?

- What helps you cope when life is difficult?

- Would you like to talk to someone about the way the disease is affecting you and your family?

The answers to these three questions may not be in terms of belief or faith, but in terms of family support, strength of character etc. However, the questions can also help to identify spiritual strength and health and lead to discussion of whether the patient wishes to maintain contact with these resources while in hospital or hospice.

Where the need is for a non-Christian spiritual resource, those appointed specifically to provide spiritual care should establish links with the various faith communities and try to obtain the services of people who can confidently offer supportive care and spiritual support to terminally ill people.[22]

For some faith communities, pastoral care may not be understood in the same way as it is interpreted in Christianity. For example, in Judaism and Islam, the faith leader (Rabbi or Imam) would primarily be a teacher who would instruct what to read, what to eat or not eat, what rituals to follow around the time of death. It would be the family or other designated community members who would visit to offer support. In the case of Judaism, however, many of these visitors would studiously avoid talking about the imminent death and direct the individual to thoughts of the goodness of God and the blessings of this life.

Interpreting the approaches of another culture and faith is fraught with difficulty and we need always to remember that we speak from an ethnocentric context, however well informed we may be. In all cases the patient should be our guide in terms of needs and of who should meet them.

In many cases spiritual care will be provided by the very staff who have assessed it, as the patient will have developed a relationship of trust with that individual or group. The role of the official pastoral care givers may then be to support the staff as they follow through with the patient rather than taking over. Where very specific rituals are required, the faith leader and staff could also work together and complement each other's role at such times.[23]

CONCLUSION

Amidst the complexity of the spirituality which pervades the modern hospital, a pastoral ministry rooted in the narratives of communities of faith, nurtured by the rituals and symbols of these communities, and open to the spiritual needs of people and places, is well worth aiming for.[24]

To know who you are and what you believe in is an essential prerequisite to the development of that spirit of openness that allows you genuinely to 'be there' for the other person, whatever their beliefs. It also guards against personal agendas getting in the way of responding to the patient's expressed need and can become truly reflective of a holism that is central to palliative care.

KEY POINTS

- Spirituality suffers from ambiguity and an elusiveness of clarification.
- It is now more widely accepted that spirituality is related to, but not always identical to, religion.
- Evidence for the relevance of spirituality in health care is growing.
- A key component of spiritual distress is loss of any sense of meaning in life, together with a growing feeling of inner fragmentation. This can lead to alienation from self and others, loss of hope and (if religious) loss of God.
- Personal agendas should not get in the way of assessing the needs of the patient.
- While all staff should be alert to spiritual need, and may be able to offer supportive care, palliative care should have easy access to trained spiritual care providers/faith leaders.

REFERENCES

1. Cobb M. *The dying soul: spiritual care at the end of life.* Buckingham: Open University Press, 2001.
2. Speck PW. *Being there: pastoral care in time of illness.* London: SPCK, 1988.
3. Department of Health. *NHS chaplaincy: meeting the religious and spiritual needs of patients and staff.* London: HMSO, 33830, 2003.
4. Saunders C. *The management of terminal illness.* London: Arnold, 1967.
5. Randall F, Downie RS. *Palliative care ethics: a good companion.* Oxford: Oxford University Press, 1996.
6. Dukes C. Nurses' assessment of spiritual need. Unpublished Bachelor of Nursing thesis submitted to University of Southampton, UK, 1999.
7. Ross L. Spiritual aspects of nursing. *J Adv Nurs* 1994; **19**, 439–47.

8. Koenig HG, George LK, Peterson BL. Religiosity and remission from depression in medically ill older patients. *Am J Psychiatry* 1998; **155**(4), 536–42.

9. Koenig HG, Pargament K, Nielsen J. Religious coping and health status in medically ill hospitalized older adults. *J Nerv Ment Dis* 1998; **186**(9), 513–21.

10. King M, Speck P, Thomas A. Spiritual and religious beliefs in acute illness – is this a feasible area for study? *Soc Sci Med* 1994; **38**(4), 631–6.

11. King M, Speck P, Thomas A. Spiritual belief and outcome from illness. *Soc Sci Med* 1999; **48**, 1291–9.

12. Frankl V. *Man's search for meaning*. London: Hodder & Stoughton. 1987.

13. Feher S, Maly RC. Coping with breast cancer in later life: the role of religious faith. *Psycho-Oncology* 1999; **8**(5), 408–16.

14. Speck PW. *Loss and grief in medicine*. London: Baillière-Tindall, 1978.

15. Parkes CM. Psycho-social transitions: comparison between reactions to loss of a limb and loss of a spouse. *Br J Psychiatry* 1975; **127**, 204–10.

16. Kitwood T. *Dementia reconsidered: the person comes first*. Buckingham: OUP, 1997.

17. Speck PW. Spiritual issues in palliative care. In: Doyle D, Hanks G, MacDonald M (eds), *Oxford textbook of palliative medicine* 2nd edn. Oxford: Oxford University Press, 1998, 805–17.

18. Coleman PG, McKiernan F, Mills M, Speck P. Spiritual beliefs and existential meaning in later life: the experience of older bereaved spouses. *Quality in Ageing – Policy, Practice and Research* 2002; **3**(1), 20–6.

19. Allport GW, Ross JM. Personal religious orientation and prejudice. *J Personal Soc Psychol* 1967; **5**, 432–43.

20. Kirkpatrick LA, Hood RW Jr. Intrinsic–extrinsic religious orientation: the boon or bane of contemporary psychology of religion. *Journal for the Scientific Study of Religion* 1990; **29**, 442–62.

21. Cohen SR, Mount BM, Bruera E *et al*. Validity of McGill Quality of Life Questionnaire in the palliative care setting: a multicentre Canadian study demonstrating the importance of the existential domain. *Palliat Med* 1997; **11**, 3–20.

22. National Institute for Clinical Excellence (NICE). Spritual support services. In: *Supportive and palliative care guidance*. London: NICE, 2004, Chapter 7.

23. Walter T. The ideology and organization of spiritual care: three approaches. *Palliat Med* 1997; **11**, 21–30.

24. Lyall D. Spiritual institutions. In: Orchard H (ed.), *Spirituality in health care contexts*. London: Jessica Kingsley, 2001, 55.

chapter 21

ETHICAL ISSUES

Andrew Thorns, John Ellershaw and Nigel Sykes

INTRODUCTION

Ethical issues in palliative care often present a more difficult challenge to teams than clinical ones. In this chapter we explore some of these challenging areas, providing some of the moral argument, research evidence and practical approaches to their management.

LIVING WILLS

The advance directive or statement, often known as a 'living will', was originated in 1965 by Luis Kutner. It was a response to a perception that advances in medical technology were keeping increasing numbers of people alive in situations in which their quality of life was poor. Had these people been able to express an opinion, they would not, Kutner felt, have consented to the treatment that was now sustaining them in this state. The logical basis of the advance directive was the extension of the right possessed by competent adults to determine what medical treatment they were given forward through time to encompass the moment when they would not be able to express themselves.

However, it has become recognized that advance directives can be more subtle than simply a method to forbid certain treatments. Instead, they can be statements of individuals' life values or a description of how they would wish their life to end. In this way, relatives and medical staff can be helped to judge what the patient would probably have wanted in the circumstances that have now arisen. They may help to identify the appropriate management of some of the complex problems described later in this chapter.

FORMS OF ADVANCE DIRECTIVE

Advance directives do not have to be written down, although the term is usually applied to formal written statements. An oral statement to next of kin or to care staff (in which case it should be recorded in the patient's notes), or an audiotape or video recording is also a possible format. A clear recollection by close relatives or friends of a patient's consistently expressed view regarding particular treatments in the clinical situation that has now occurred should be accepted by medical staff. This is not the same as the appointment of a health care proxy, a person who is appointed by patients to give instructions about medical treatments on their behalf if they should become incompetent. Such proxies exist in the USA and elsewhere but are not currently legal in English law, although the Law Commission has proposed a Continuing Power of Attorney.[1] This provision would encompass the role of a health care proxy in addition to that of a proxy for property matters which is included in the present Enduring Power of Attorney.

People are free to write a living will themselves in any style they choose, which may be appropriate if the advance statement is very specific, for example the absolute refusal of any blood transfusions. Most living wills are not so specific and can leave much doubt as to what treatment would be wanted in which situation. To an extent, such vagueness is hard to avoid, given the variety of events that might occur to an individual in the future, and might actually be desirable in that it allows carers some discretion. The best way of avoiding unwanted doubt about what is desired is to use a well-prepared model advance directive such as that prepared by the Terence Higgins Trust and the King's College Centre for Medical Law and Ethics.

The basic requirements of an advance directive

- Full name.
- Address.
- Name and address of general practitioner.
- Whether advice was sought from health professionals.
- Signature.
- Date of original signature (and dates of reviews, if any).
- Witness signature.
- Clear statement of wishes, either specific or general.
- Details of nominated contact person.

(Patients' Association, 1996.)

CAPACITY

The key decision regarding living wills is that of capacity – did the person have mental capacity when they made the will and do they have capacity now when treatment decisions have to be made? An advance directive only applies if the patient has become incompetent. Whatever they might have written previously, the carers of a person with mental capacity must always be bound by what that individual is saying *now*. It is therefore vital to be able to decide capacity, and case law has given guidance on how this might be done (see the box below). Chapter 4.4 (Confusion and psychosis) looks at the issue of capacity in more detail.

Deciding capacity

Capacity has nothing to do with whether another person would regard a decision as sensible. Decisions may be made for reasons that are rational, irrational or non-existent.
   Capacity is assumed unless there is evidence to the contrary.
   To have capacity, a person must be able to:

- understand the nature and purpose of a medical treatment when it is explained in clear, simple terms;
- understand the main benefits and risks of the treatment and what alternatives there are;
- understand what would be likely to happen if the treatment were not given;
- retain the above information long enough to be able to reach a decision based on it;
- be in a position to make a free choice, without coercion or undue influence.

LEGAL STATUS OF ADVANCE DIRECTIVES

The first statute relating to advance directives was the California Natural Death Act of 1976. Since then, numerous American states have enshrined living wills in law, and since 1990 there has also been federal legislation in the form of the Patient Self-Determination Act. This act requires hospitals, nursing homes and hospices to advise patients on admission of their right to accept or refuse medical care and to execute an advance directive. There is also a requirement to document whether patients have advance directives. Compliance with the act is a condition of Medicare and Medicaid reimbursement. It appears that this provision has had little practical effect on patients' knowledge or behaviour, possibly because the tasks it imposes are usually delegated to clerks rather than being carried out by healthcare personnel.[2]

In Britain, advance directives do not yet have the enforcement of statute law. Despite the reservations of the 1993 House of Lords Select Committee on Medical Ethics, the Law Commission has proposed such legislation, with penalties for disobeying, concealing or destroying a living will. However, where an advance directive exists and it is clear that its provisions apply to the situation that has now arisen, it will be recognized under common law. Such recognition can only apply to a directive that refuses particular types of treatment. It is never legal to force a doctor to prescribe or carry out treatment that he or she considers to be inappropriate, and so directives cannot demand specific treatments. Neither can a directive seek to impose a duty upon another person to do something illegal, and hence a living will cannot request euthanasia.

Certain safeguards are envisaged in the proposed legislation. No one would be able to refuse basic care, which includes maintenance of hygiene, the provision of oral food and fluids, and relief of pain and other distressing symptoms. Neither would an advance directive apply if it might lead to the patient's death, or if the patient were pregnant, unless the directive had specifically envisaged these circumstances.[3] However, in some quarters there is concern that the ability of advance directives to refuse *artificial* hydration and nutrition might result not in the patient's death, as might have been supposed when the directive was made, but in a level of disability that could have been avoided had doctors had unfettered access to all therapeutic options.

In the absence of a living will, clinicians are expected to continue to treat patients on the basis of their best interests. This means that the risks and benefits of various treatments and their alternatives will be assessed in the light of the pain and other suffering the patient is exposed to by his or her condition, and the likelihood of restoration or further loss of functioning. The legal responsibility for deciding about best interests and what line of treatment would best serve them rests with the doctor who is caring for the patient and not, as is often supposed, that patient's relatives.

USE OF ADVANCE DIRECTIVES

The House of Lords Select Committee on Medical Ethics recommended against giving living wills greater legal force than they already possess, because to do so might deprive 'patients of the benefit of the doctor's professional expertise and of new treatments and procedures which may have become available since the directive was signed'. The committee's area of concern is one of a number of potential difficulties that arise from the implementation of advance directives.

The possibility of the advent of new treatments is a reason why it is recommended that advance directives be reviewed regularly, perhaps every 3 years, in order to ensure that their provisions are still appropriate.[4] For the same reason, it has also been suggested that the text of directives be lodged with the patient's general practitioner or solicitor, who could trigger and facilitate the periodic reviews. Beyond this, however, anyone who wishes to restrict the options of their doctor has to recognize that in doing so they run the risk of outcomes that are different from those that might have been achieved or perhaps different from what had been intended.

A circumstance frequently envisaged in living wills is the onset of dementia. It is a complex and unresolved philosophical question as to whether an apparently content demented person should be denied life-saving treatment on the instructions of their previously competent self. Legally the two are the same person, but to anyone who has known them well, everything may seem to have changed. The fear of such radical change may, indeed, have been the motivation for writing the directive in the first place.

The first advance directive emerged under the auspices of the Euthanasia Society of America and ever since it has had an association with movements for the legalization of euthanasia. This is in part because the provisions of directives do not have to have any rational basis and may be heavily restrictive. Conversely, a request in a living will cannot legitimize an act of euthanasia where it remains illegal.

A major question relates to the effectiveness of advance directives in obtaining the outcomes their holders intended. Potentially life-saving treatment is often given as an emergency and, if it is to be applied, the advance directive must be immediately available to the medical staff. In practice this is frequently not the case. Even if they are known to exist, living wills may not be invoked because the patient is not considered to be ill enough for them to apply.[5] Where proxies are valid in end-of-life decision-making, it appears that earlier communication has too often not been good enough for the proxy to have a clear understanding of the patient's wishes.[6] In addition, some proxies feel the weight of their responsibilities too keenly and opt for life-sustaining treatments that the patient would not have desired.

To counter these problems of accessibility and misunderstanding it would seem better for advance directives to be viewed as an aid to ongoing communication between patient, clinicians and carers rather than as the prime vehicle for such communication. Directives are poorly effective if those closest to the patient do not know of their existence or are uncomfortable with their contents. On the other hand, directives hold the possibility of enabling a form of health care towards the end of life that is more in accord with a patient's wishes than might have occurred in the past. Directives might also absolve next of kin from decisions that they would find onerous. The acceptance of advance directives might be taken as helpful evidence of the medical profession's readiness to hear and respond to the patient's voice in the formation of management plans.

KEY POINTS

- In Britain, advance directives are recognized under common law.
- An advance directive can refuse treatment but cannot demand it.
- Hygiene measures, oral food and fluids, and symptom control cannot be refused by advance directive.
- A competent person's contemporaneous decision always overrides any advance directive he or she may previously have made.
- In the absence of an advance directive, decisions about a patient's best interests rest legally with the doctor, not the relatives.

ARTIFICIAL HYDRATION

In the normal adult, oral intake of fluids maintains the physiological fluid balance. In palliative care it is important that patients take adequate oral fluids to ensure hydration and to prevent symptoms, including constipation.

INDICATIONS FOR ARTIFICIAL HYDRATION IN PALLIATIVE CARE

There are a number of situations that arise in palliative care which can prevent adequate oral intake of fluids and therefore artificial hydration needs to be considered. These include recurrent aspiration, vomiting, total dysphagia and intestinal obstruction. In these situations, encouraging oral fluids may produce overall harm, including the symptoms of increased vomiting and aspiration, leading to potential respiratory tract infection. In such situations open discussion with the patient should take place regarding the benefits and burdens of artificial hydration. In some cases, with small volumes of oral fluid and adequate mouth care, the patient can maintain hydration with minimal side effects.

However, in some situations patients become centrally dehydrated and symptomatic, with thirst and dry mouth, and in these cases artificial hydration should be considered for the relief of symptoms. Another situation in which consideration of artificial hydration may arise is that of a patient who becomes confused and is unable to take fluids. This may be due to metabolic disturbances, including hypercalcaemia or infection, and treatment of the underlying problem and antibiotics for respiratory tract infection can lead to resolution of the confusion and an improvement in the patient's condition. If the patient is taking inadequate oral fluids, artificial hydration may be indicated. The patient may not be competent to give consent and the physician must act in the best interest of the patient. Discussion with the relatives plays an important part in the decision-making process, but the final decision rests with the clinician in charge. In making such a decision, a full history, examination and relevant investigations should be undertaken.

METHODS OF PROVIDING ARTIFICIAL HYDRATION

If artificial hydration is indicated, it can be administered subcutaneously or intravenously or, if *in situ*, via nasogastric tube or percutaneous endoscopic gastrostomy (PEG) tube. If the subcutaneous route is chosen (hypodermoclysis), 750 units of hyaluronidase in 1 L of fluid will aid absorption. If the underlying cause is treated successfully leading to recovery of the patient, artificial hydration can be discontinued and the patient can resume oral fluids.

ARTIFICIAL HYDRATION IN THE DYING PHASE

The considerations relating to artificial hydration of the patient in the dying phase are somewhat different. Patients with cancer often have a history of weight loss, fatigue and weakness, which have developed over a number of weeks or months. There is a decrease in the food and fluid intake of the individual, but generally no associated symptoms of dehydration or hunger. This natural physiological process associated with the last months and weeks of life is part of the process of progressive disease. The body appears to compensate for this diminution of food and fluid. As patients enter the dying phase, they are able to take only sips of fluid, become bed bound and often semi-comatose before death.

This gradual process is different from the more acute picture of a patient whose deterioration is due to a mechanical, metabolic or infective cause that may be reversible with artificial hydration. The diagnosis of the dying phase is not always clear, and in such situations the benefits of active treatment as opposed to the burdens that this may bring need to be balanced. Full consideration of the issue of artificial hydration also needs to be given when the patient is clearly in the dying phase.

ARGUMENTS IN FAVOUR OF ARTIFICIAL HYDRATION

It is argued by some that artificial hydration in the dying patient decreases the distress for relatives and healthcare professionals.[7,8] It acts as a source of hope for the relatives and may decrease symptoms, including dry mouth, thirst, headache, confusion and exhaustion.

ARGUMENTS AGAINST ARTIFICIAL HYDRATION

However, it is a common experience in other care settings, including the hospice setting, that patients can die with dignity and peacefully without artificial hydration. A number of studies have demonstrated no relationship between oral and artificial hydration and the symptoms of thirst and dry mouth in a palliative care population.[9-11] These symptoms may well be related to iatrogenic causes, including opioids and anti-emetics and the mouth breathing that often predominates in the dying phase. In this situation it may well be futile to treat the patient for their symptoms of thirst and dry mouth with artificial hydration. Further evidence has demonstrated relatively normal biochemical profiles of patients in the last days of life,[9] again suggesting artificial hydration may well be inappropriate when it appears that the physiological mechanisms of the body are compensating with decreased fluid intake.

COMMUNICATION WITH CARERS AND RELATIVES

Healthcare professionals may find it easier to continue active treatment such as artificial hydration and avoid discussing openly with the patient and relatives that the patient is entering the dying phase. The relatives are given false expectations of the likelihood of recovery and do not understand that the patient is dying. It is the duty of all healthcare professionals to acquire the knowledge, skills and attitude necessary to communicate such sensitive information to patients and their relatives and in difficult situations to seek assistance from specialists in this area.

COMPLICATIONS OF ARTIFICIAL HYDRATION

A study of hypodermoclysis in a palliative care population showed that 16 per cent of the patients had their treatment stopped for various reasons, including fluid overload, and on average each patient had two complications associated with the hypodermoclysis.[12]

SUMMARY

When decisions are being made regarding the appropriateness of artificial hydration, the patient's cultural and religious background should be taken into consideration, as should the views of the relatives. If artificial hydration is thought to be appropriate in the dying phase, this should be limited to 1 L over 24 hours. A decision to give fluid in the dying phase should not override the need to discuss with the patient and family the fact that the patient is now entering the dying phase and appropriate consideration and care should be given to symptom control, psychological and spiritual support.[13,14]

ARTIFICIAL NUTRITION

In patients with a progressive terminal disease, e.g. cancer, the requirement for oral nutrition declines in the last months, weeks and days of life. Good symptom control, including treatment of nausea, vomiting and dysphagia, enables patients to maintain adequate nutritional levels. It is important that the patients' wishes are respected regarding the quantity and frequency of food they are given, as it can be counterproductive continually to face them with more food than they can cope with. It is often the anxiety of relatives that leads to this behaviour pattern. The belief that we must eat to survive is part of the basic human instinct. Therefore the less patients eat, the more their relatives are concerned that this is contributing to their decline. It is important to communicate clearly to patients and their relatives that a decline in food intake is part of the natural course of the disease.[15,16]

INDICATIONS FOR ARTIFICIAL NUTRITION

In some situations, symptoms can prevent patients from taking an adequate oral nutritional intake, for example postoperatively, when delayed recovery may lead to total parenteral nutrition being initiated to maintain adequate nutritional status of the patient. This is normally seen as a temporary measure and, as the patient recovers, oral intake of nutrition is restored. A more difficult situation arises when the patient develops irreversible dysphagia, for example due to motility problems in motor neurone disease or due to obstructive problems in carcinoma of the oesophagus. In such situations, the patient may well develop the symptom of hunger and not be able to relieve it due to the dysphagia.

Careful discussion should be undertaken with the patient regarding the possibility of artificial feeding. This can be done via a nasogastric tube or, increasingly commonly, by a PEG tube. The benefits and burdens to the patient must be carefully discussed. The benefits include the relief of the symptom of hunger and the fact that with adequate nutrition the patient may feel less weak. However, some patients may be concerned about the insertion of the tube and the potential disfigurement and inconvenience of artificial nutrition. They may also be concerned that artificial nutrition may prolong life unnecessarily, which they may feel is inappropriate. In these cases when artificial nutrition is being considered, it is vital that the patient's autonomy is respected. This cannot be achieved unless the patient is fully involved in the discussion and decision-making.

ARTIFICIAL NUTRITION IN THE DYING PHASE

As the patient approaches the dying phase, i.e. the last days and hours of life, if artificial nutrition is being delivered via a nasogastric or PEG tube, consideration should be given to reducing and withdrawing feeding. To continue with high volumes of feeding at this time may lead to fluid overload, which may compound underlying medical problems of peripheral oedema and cardiac failure. If this is the case, it may well be appropriate to reduce the volume of the feed to a maximum of

1 L a day or discontinue feeding altogether. Again, careful discussion needs to be undertaken, not only with the patient but also with the relatives, who may perceive this as 'giving up on' or 'abandoning' the patient.

It is important in the dying phase that the focus of care is on good symptom control and psychosocial and spiritual support. The issue of feeding must be dealt with in a sensitive manner, in the context of this care.

NUTRITION WITHDRAWAL FOR PATIENTS IN LOW CONSCIOUSNESS STATES

Different issues need to be considered when artificial nutrition has been initiated in a patient whose death is not imminent and whose wishes are not known, for example if the patient does not have a terminal disease but is incapable of maintaining adequate nutrition, such as a patient who has had a stroke or is in a persistent vegetative state. In these situations, the British Medical Association (BMA) believes that the following additional safeguards should be applied.

- All proposals to withhold or withdraw artificial nutrition and hydration, whether in hospital or in the community, should be subject to formal clinical review by a senior clinician who has experience of the condition from which the patient is suffering and who is not part of the treating team.

- In England, Wales and Northern Ireland, where it is proposed to withdraw artificial nutrition and hydration from a patient in (or in a state closely resembling) a persistent vegetative state, legal advice should be sought and a court declaration is likely to be required until such time as the courts have stated that this is no longer necessary.

- All cases in which artificial nutrition and hydration have been withdrawn should be available for clinical review to ensure that appropriate procedures and guidelines were followed. Anonymised information should also be available to the Secretary of State on request and, where applicable, to the Commission for Health Care Audit and Inspection.[17]

KEY POINTS

- There are a number of strong indications for the use of artificial hydration and nutrition in palliative care.
- The balance of benefit against burden must always be carefully assessed and communicated to relatives and carers.
- In the dying phase, evidence suggests that artificial hydration and nutrition are unlikely to provide benefit.
- The BMA has provided guidance on the withdrawal of such measures.

VENTILATION

Assisted ventilation is currently a rare technique in British palliative medicine but is much more common in some other countries, particularly in relation to the management of advanced amyotrophic lateral sclerosis or motor neurone disease (ALS/MND), which is characterized by respiratory failure.

In the USA, 5–10 per cent of ALS patients undergo tracheostomy ventilation, and significant numbers of such patients receive this treatment in Japan and Germany. This form of mechanical ventilation is expensive and also imposes particular burdens on carers, up to a third of whom may feel that their own quality of life is actually less than that of the severely disabled patient.[18] Approximately 25 per cent of patients on tracheostomy ventilation have it initiated in an emergency, without an opportunity for prior discussion. Some patients will request withdrawal of ventilation, but others may continue for many years until they are in a 'locked in' state. In some centres, the onset of such a condition is a previously agreed trigger for the withdrawal of ventilation.

Much more widespread (and set to become yet more so) is non-invasive positive pressure ventilation (NIPPV). This technique has shown effectiveness in relieving the symptoms of nocturnal hypoventilation and daytime breathlessness. Eventually users require it almost constantly, but generally it does not prevent a final increase in breathlessness, which has to be dealt with pharmacologically. Occasionally, however, NIPPV can maintain an end-stage ALS/MND patient in a moribund condition for some days, to the distress of relatives and carers.

Ventilation is one of the treatments doctors are least likely to withdraw,[19] particularly if they are relatively unfamiliar with its use.[20] The decision to do so can be greatly facilitated by a clear advance statement from the patient defining the circumstances in which he or she would want this to be done. Ideally, this discussion should take place before commencement of tracheostomy ventilation, and it can be a potential benefit of the prior involvement of a palliative care service with ALS/MND patients that they can stimulate this discussion and anticipate the onset of respiratory failure so that ventilation is the result of a properly informed decision rather than a crisis intervention. Where acceptable to the patient, it would also be good practice to discuss the eventual outcome of NIPPV before it was commenced, so that expectations are clear on the part of both the patient and the family.[21]

Withdrawal of ventilation of whatever form involves the provision of sedation to avoid distress. A staged withdrawal allows prompt control of any distress that might appear after each adjustment of the ventilator, using further doses of the same drugs. However, there is no place in this context for the very slow weaning from ventilation sometimes practised,[22] as there is no prospect that patients will be able to resume breathing on their own.

CARDIOPULMONARY RESUSCITATION IN PALLIATIVE CARE

Cardiopulmonary resuscitation (CPR) is an important topic for palliative care to consider because of the concerns raised by the press and public, the change in hospice population in terms of diagnosis and stage of illness, the misperceptions of patients, families and healthcare professionals regarding the role of CPR, and the influence hospital palliative care teams can have in decision-making.

OUTCOMES FROM CPR AND THE VIEWS OF PATIENTS, CARERS AND HEALTHCARE PROFESSIONALS

Most patients believe CPR to be always successful. Discussion has been shown to decrease requests for CPR and it was found in one study that 25 per cent of patients would not want CPR even if it had a 100 per cent success rate.[23] All healthcare professionals overestimate the chances of success, including hospice staff.[24]

Success rates are approximately 15 per cent in hospital and between 1 and 5 per cent in the community. Currently it is debatable whether these results have been significantly altered by the advent of automatic external defibrillators (AEDs).[25]

CURRENT GUIDELINES ON CPR

In the UK, the National Council for Hospice and Palliative Care Services and the Association of Palliative Medicine guidelines advise:[26]

- decisions should be based on the likely outcome, quality of life and competent wish of the patient;

- there is no obligation to discuss CPR if it is believed to be futile;

- if the outcome is uncertain, sensitive discussion is appropriate;

- decisions relating to quality of life should be made by the patient.

The original guidance of the BMA and the Royal College of Nursing (RCN) was similar to that of the National Council, but a more recent revision moved towards more open discussion of CPR, even when considered futile:[27]

> When the basis for a DNR ['do not resuscitate'] decision is the absence of any likely medical benefit, discussion with the patient, or others close to the patient, should aim at securing an understanding and acceptance of the clinical decision that has been reached.

DISCUSSION OF CPR

To discuss the withholding of futile CPR makes it unusual, if not unique, in medicine because discussion of a treatment that will offer no benefit is encouraged whilst a non-futile CPR treatment you plan to initiate requires no discussion.

It should be normal practice to discuss issues around the end of life with all patients, including quality of life, treatment options and future wishes. It is probably inappropriate to raise futile CPR specifically with patients or their families, as this preserves the misperception of CPR being life prolonging.

In discussion of CPR with patients or relatives, the points to be covered include the likely outcome, the description of the procedure and practical aspects such as the need for transfer to an acute unit.

POLICIES IN PALLIATIVE CARE

A number of policies relating to CPR in palliative care units could be considered.

Blanket ban

A policy of no CPR would protect the hospice philosophy of a peaceful death avoiding excess medical intervention. This would effectively deny access to the small number of patients for whom CPR is appropriate, and it may be difficult to justify morally or legally why an effective treatment is being denied to a patient because of his or her hospice location.

Patient choice

Respect for autonomy requires all patients to make a competent choice. A doctor is under no obligation to provide a treatment offering no benefit. If futile CPR is offered to a patient, unnecessary harm and excess use of resources would result. A patient considered to be suitable for CPR should be allowed to consider such an intervention in advance.

Medical decisions

The route that would seem most appropriate is somewhere between these two approaches, with a decision being made by the healthcare professionals as to which patients would have a reasonable chance of surviving CPR. Quality-of-life decisions could be offered to the patient.

FACTORS TO BE CONSIDERED IN DESIGNING POLICIES

Consideration should be given to the possible effect on the hospice environment and other patients of performing CPR and to who should make decisions regarding futility and at what stage.

The central theme should be that active treatment is inappropriate for the majority of patients because of the futile outcome, the poor resulting or ongoing quality of life or that the intervention is not in keeping with the patient's wishes.

When implementing such a policy, consideration should be given to the overestimation of success by patients, relatives and professionals, the need for education of staff, the provision and maintenance of basic equipment and the need for regular training of staff expected to perform CPR.

KEY POINTS

- Patients and healthcare professionals overestimate the survival from CPR, which is usually negligible in palliative care patients.
- Discussion of end-of-life issues is important with all patients, but it is unlikely that CPR specifically needs discussion.

SEDATION

The issue of sedation in palliative care can be viewed from two different perspectives. The first and least contentious is when the patient is in the dying phase. The second concerns the agitated or confused patient who is not yet in the dying phase.

THE USE OF SEDATION IN THE DYING PHASE

The issue of diagnosing dying has been discussed already in the section on artificial hydration. When a patient is in the dying phase and is expected to live for hours, possibly days, and develops agitation, obvious interventions such as relieving urinary retention and repositioning of the patient should be undertaken. If reversible causes have been excluded and the patient remains agitated, the use of sedative drugs is appropriate. This should be undertaken using the lowest doses appropriate on an as-required basis. If three or more doses are required over a 24-hour period, the drugs can be given as a constant infusion over 24 hours subcutaneously via a syringe driver.

Clear guidelines should be agreed regarding the dose of sedation prescribed, which should be within the bounds of what is considered good medical practice. There needs to be a clear explanation to the family that the patient is in the dying phase and that the symptom of agitation will be relieved by the use of sedative drugs. Relatives are often in attendance in the dying phase and it is important to empower them to alert the healthcare professionals if the patient does become agitated and requires reassessment and, if appropriate, sedative medication.

Literature review indicates that the proper use of sedatives at the end of life does not further shorten prognosis.[28] However, if excessive doses of sedative drugs are given in a situation that falls outside what is considered acceptable medical practice and the patient dies a premature death, the doctor may be responsible for foreshortening life.[29,30]

THE USE OF SEDATION OUTSIDE THE DYING PHASE

The second perspective is that of patients who are not in the dying phase, but have become agitated or confused and require sedation to protect them from causing harm – either to themselves or to other people. Again, in this situation the minimal amount of sedative necessary to sedate the patient should be used.

As in the previous scenario, the sedative may be given on an as-required basis and, if necessary, converted into a 24-hour dose delivered subcutaneously via a syringe driver after the first 24 hours. The cause of agitation/confusion should be ascertained and psychiatric advice sought in such situations. It is not uncommon that following 24–48 hours of sedation, the sedative medication can be reduced and the patient will become lucid and no longer agitated. However, if the patient requires sedation extending beyond 24–48 hours, consideration should be given to artificial hydration in order to maintain fluid balance.

Once more, in this situation prolonged sedation of a patient who is not in the dying phase and who is not given artificial hydration may lead to premature death, for which the doctor could be considered to be responsible.

KEY POINTS

- Sedation has an important role in controlling symptoms of agitation, anxiety and confusion.
- Moral and legal considerations require careful monitoring of indications and dosages used.
- Good communication with carers and other professionals is vital.

EUTHANASIA AND PHYSICIAN-ASSISTED SUICIDE

Euthanasia and physician-assisted suicide (PAS) remain one of the most contentious issues around the end of life. Here, the term physician-assisted death (PAD) is used when referring to the combination of both issues.

DEFINITIONS

Euthanasia is the intentional bringing about of the death of a patient for his or her own sake, either by killing (active) or by allowing to die (passive).

Euthanasia can be classified as:

- *voluntary*: the patient is both sufficiently informed and competent to consent to euthanasia and does in fact request it;

- *non-voluntary*: the patient is not sufficiently competent to consent to euthanasia;

- *involuntary*: the patient, although sufficiently informed and competent to request or consent to euthanasia, does not in fact do so.

Intention to kill is the key distinction from other end-of-life decisions such as the doctrine of double effect or the provision of non-beneficial treatments to dying patients. Here, although shortening of life may be a possible or even probable result, it is not the intention of the person undertaking the act.

MORAL ARGUMENTS

The arguments in favour of PAD are simple and powerful:

- it would prevent needless suffering,

- it would affirm patients' autonomy in choosing how to direct their lives,

- allowing patients to die ('passive' euthanasia) is philosophically no different from directly causing their death, so 'active' euthanasia should also be permitted.

The arguments against are more complicated and are partially based on morals that not all members of society may share:

- killing the innocent is always wrong,

- human life has intrinsic value and should not be taken away,

- appropriate palliative care can relieve suffering,

- PAD would weaken our commitment to improving the lives of the terminally ill,

- PAD would damage the professional–patient relationship,

- PAD is irreversible and allows no possibility of error,

- PAD may place undue pressure on patients,

- the risk that allowing intentional killing in very specific circumstances will be abused and lead to a more generalized acceptance (the slippery slope argument).

IS THERE A DISTINCTION BETWEEN PAS AND EUTHANASIA?

Physician-assisted suicide would appear to offer less risk of abuse as patients take the lethal dose themselves, although they may experience difficulty in completing the act successfully and require the doctor's active assistance.[31] However, the intention in both PAS and euthanasia is the same – the death of the patient. Therefore PAS and euthanasia are morally indistinguishable.

WHAT DO PATIENTS THINK AND WANT?

Surveys of both public and professionals show a large degree of support for PAD. Ward and Tate found that 46 per cent of UK doctors said they would consider taking active steps to bring about a patient's death if it were legal to do so.[32] However, surveys can be misleading, depending on the exact question asked and whether hypothetical answers match actual behaviour.

THE CURRENT SITUATION WORLDWIDE

UNITED KINGDOM

In the UK, both euthanasia and PAS remain illegal. A House of Lords Select Committee looked at this area extensively in 1993 and recommended no change in the law because of the difficulties in setting limits, the pressure that would be placed on vulnerable individuals and the fact that palliative care offers a real alternative. Leading organizations such as the BMA, the National Council for Hospice and Palliative Care Services and the Association of Palliative Medicine support this view. At the time of writing, the formation of a new Select Committee has been agreed, prompted by proposed euthanasia legislation.

HOLLAND

Euthanasia and PAS remain illegal, although they have been depenalized in certain circumstances. The main consideration relates to quality of life and degree of suffering rather than length of life.

OREGON, USA

The state of Oregon legalized PAS (not euthanasia) in 1997, provided certain conditions are met:[33]

- the patient should request PAS on three separate occasions over 15 days,
- the final request should be written,
- two doctors should determine that the patient has a terminal illness with a life expectancy of less than 6 months.

NORTHERN TERRITORY, AUSTRALIA

Euthanasia and PAS were temporarily legalized in 1996. Four patients died under the act before it was repealed because of concerns over the risk from the 'slippery slope'.

SWITZERLAND

Aiding suicide is legal as long as the motives of the assistant (doctor or otherwise) are altruistic.

STUDIES LOOKING AT CURRENT EXPERIENCE

Rates of physician-assisted death

In Holland, the reported deaths from PAD increased from 1.7 per cent of all deaths in 1990 to 2.4 per cent of all deaths in 1995 and 2.6 per cent of all deaths in 2001.[34] Most episodes of euthanasia are performed on cancer patients, but relative to their numbers, people with AIDS or ALS/MND are the most likely to receive euthanasia. It has been estimated that about 50 per cent of PADs are unreported and these are less likely to have met all the legal requirements.[35]

In Oregon, 129 people died legally by assisted suicide between 1998 and 2002, making up 0.1 per cent of deaths in the state.[36] Although this is not a high percentage of all deaths, 5 per cent of deaths amongst ALS/MND patients have been reported to occur by assisted suicide.[37]

Competency of requests

No explicit request for PAD was received in 0.6 per cent of Dutch deaths; 13 per cent of Dutch doctors had ended life without the explicit request of the patient.[34]

Reasons for requesting physician-assisted death

The risk factors for suicide are depression, pain and poor social support;[6] these may also be factors associated with requests for PAD. Concern has been raised that the poorly educated and financially less well off may be more vulnerable, although studies have not suggested such a link.[36]

In Oregon, the most common reasons for PAS were:

- wish for autonomy

- loss of control

- loss of enjoyment of life

- suffering

- burden on families.

Doctors were more likely to agree to requests if the patient was already in a hospice programme, had a wish to be in control or had a cancer diagnosis. Twenty-one out of the 27 patients who died were in hospice programmes, but despite this, 26 per cent reported uncontrolled pain as a reason for requesting PAS.[36]

These results are open to different interpretations and no clear trends have emerged. It will be interesting to follow the developments in Holland and Oregon.

Practical problems

Evidence from Holland shows that side effects of spasm, myoclonus, cyanosis, nausea and vomiting, excessive mucus production, hiccups, perspiration and extreme gasping were experienced in 4 per cent of cases of PAD.[31] Problems with completion occurred in 7 per cent of cases, with death occurring sometimes days after the administration of the lethal drugs.

Problems were more likely to occur with PAS than with euthanasia, if a non-specialist was involved and if oral or rectal routes were used rather than parenteral.

HOW TO RESPOND TO REQUESTS TO END LIFE

Forty-five per cent of UK doctors have received requests from patients to end their lives.[32] An estimated 8.5 per cent of terminally ill patients will have an unequivocal desire for death at some time in their illness.[38] It is therefore important to be able to respond appropriately to these situations.

Requests should be treated with respect, explored carefully and discussed reasonably. The following areas may need to be covered.

- Recognition of the patient's wishes: often requests are a plea to be listened to.

- Exploration of reasoning: the commonest factors behind such requests revolve around physical distress from unrelieved symptoms, the fear of being a burden or experiencing a 'high-tech' lingering death, social isolation and depression.

- Addressing precipitating factors: provide appropriate symptom control, encourage communication regarding fears and emphasize the role of autonomy in deciding future treatment. Increase social contact, e.g. day centre, and treat any underlying depression.

- Patients with a competent, enduring wish not to go on living: there is a small number of patients who have no desire to continue living despite addressing all the above factors. For these, the answer to their request is more difficult, but reassurance may be provided by reminder of their right to refuse treatment or discussion of the prognosis, as some patients may not realize their time is already limited and may be more fearful of long-term incapacity. Sedation may be considered as a treatment of distress. You should explain that you respect the patient's wish but that your own autonomy and legal restraints prevent you from complying. The final justification for not legalizing PAD is the potential damage that could result to the rest of society. Allowing intentional ending of life in one circumstance could result in a more general acceptance by means of the 'slippery slope' putting vulnerable individuals at risk.

- Consideration of the team: such requests are stressful and can be damaging to team functioning, so encouraging open discussion amongst members and offering debriefing sessions may be helpful.

REFERENCES

1. Lord Chancellor's Department. *Making decisions.* London: Lord Chancellor's Department, 1999.
2. Lamont EB, Siegler M. Paradoxes in cancer patients' advance care planning. *J Palliat Med* 2000; 3, 27–35.
3. Lord Chancellor's Department. *Who decides?* London: Lord Chancellor's Department, 1997.
4. British Medical Association. *Advance statements about medical treatment.* London: BMJ Publishing, 1995.
5. Teno JM, Stevens M, Spernak S, Lynn J. Role of advance directives in decision making. *J Gen Intern Med* 1998; 13, 439–46.
6. Pearlman RA, Cain KC, Starks H, Cole WG, Uhlmann RF, Patrick DL. Preferences for life-sustaining treatments in advance care planning and surrogate decision making. *J Palliat Med* 2000; 3, 37–48.

7. Collaud T, Rapin CH. Dehydration in dying patients: study with physicians in French-speaking Switzerland. *J Pain Sympt Manage* 1991; **6**, 230–9.
8. Micctich KC, Steinecker PH, Thomasma DC. Are intravenous fluids morally required for a dying patient? *Arch Intern Med* 1983; **143**, 975–8.
9. Ellershaw JE, Sutcliffe JM, Saunders CM. Dehydration and the dying patient. *J Pain Sympt Manage* 1995; **10**(3), 192–7.
10. Burge FI. Dehydration symptoms of palliative care cancer patients. *J Pain Sympt Manage* 1993; **8**(7), 454–64.
11. Musgrave CF, Bartal N, Opstad J. The sensation of thirst in dying patients receiving iv hydration. *J Palliat Care* 1995; **11**(4), 17–21.
12. Fainsinger RL, MacEachern T, Miller MJ et al. The use of hypodermoclysis for rehydration in terminally ill cancer patients. *J Pain Sympt Manage* 1994; **9**(5), 298–302.
13. Ellershaw JE, Murphy D, Shea T, Foster A, Overill S. Development of a multiprofessional care pathway for the dying patient. *Eur J Palliat Care* 1997; **4**(6), 203–8.
14. National Council for Hospice and Specialist Palliative Care Services. *Changing gear: guidelines for managing the last days of life in adults.* London: National Council for Hospice and Specialist Palliative Care Services, December 1997.
15. Dunlop RJ, Ellershaw JE, Baines MJ, Sykes N, Saunders CM. On withholding nutrition and hydration in the terminally ill: has palliative medicine gone too far? A reply. *J Med Ethics* 1995; **21**(3), 141–4.
16. Craig GM. On withholding nutrition and hydration in the terminally ill: has palliative medicine gone too far? *J Med Ethics* 1994; **20**, 139–43.
17. British Medical Association. *Withholding and withdrawing life-prolonging medical treatment: guidance for decision making.* London: BMJ Books, 1999.
18. Kaub-Wittemer D, von Steinbuchel N, Wasner M, Laier-Groeneveld G, Borasio GD. Quality of life and psychosocial issues in ventilated patients with amyotrophic lateral sclerosis and their caregivers. *J Pain Symptom Manage* 2003; **26**, 890–6.
19. Christakis NA, Asch DA. Biases in how physicians withdraw life support. *Lancet* 1993; **342**, 642–6.
20. Christakis NA, Asch DA. Medical specialists prefer to withdraw familiar technologies when discontinuing life support. *J Gen Intern Med* 1995; **10**, 491–4.
21. Borasio GD, Voltz R. Discontinuation of mechanical ventilation in patients with amyotrophic lateral sclerosis. *J Neurol* 1998; **245**, 717–22.
22. Gilligan T, Raffin TA. Withdrawing life support: extubation and prolonged terminal weans are inappropriate. *Crit Care Med* 1996; **24**, 352–3.
23. Murphy DJ, Burrows D, Santill S et al. The influence of the probability of survival on patients' preferences regarding CPR. *N Engl J Med* 1994; **330**, 545–9.
24. Thorns AR, Ellershaw JE. A survey of nursing and medical staff views on the use of cardiopulmonary resuscitation in the hospice. *Palliat Med* 1999; **13**, 225–32.
25. National Council for Hospice and Specialist Palliative Care Services, and the Association of Palliative Medicine. *CPR: policies in action.* Proceedings of a seminar to inform best practice with cardiopulmonary resuscitation (CPR) policies within palliative care. London: National Council for Hospice and Specialist Palliative Care Services, April 2003.
26. National Council for Hospice and Specialist Palliative Care Services and The Association for Palliative Medicine. *Ethical decision making in palliative care: Cardiopulmonary Resuscitation for people who are terminally ill.* London: National Council for Hospice and Specialist Palliative Care Services, January 2002.

27. Decisions relating to cardiopulmonary resuscitation. A statement from the BMA and RCN in association with the Resuscitation Council (UK), June 1999.
28. Sykes NP, Thorns A. The use of opioids and sedatives at the end of life in palliative care. *Lancet Oncol* 2003; **4**, 312–18.
29. Gillon R. Palliative care ethics: non-provision of artificial nutrition and hydration to terminally ill sedated patients. *J Med Ethics* 1994; **20**, 131–2.
30. Fainsinger RL, Waller A, Bercovici M *et al.* A multicentre international study of sedation for uncontrolled symptoms in terminally ill patients. *Palliat Med* 2000; **14**, 257–65.
31. Groenewoud JH, van der Heide A, Onwuteaka-Philipsen BD, Willems DL, van der Maas PJ, van der Wal G. Clinical problems with the performance of euthanasia and physician-assisted suicide in the Netherlands. *N Engl J Med* 2000; **342**, 551–6.
32. Ward BJ, Tate PA. Attitudes among NHS doctors to requests for euthanasia. *BMJ* 1994; **308**, 1332–4.
33. Ganzini L, Nelson HD, Schmidt TA, Kraemer DF, Delorit MA, Lee MA. Physicians' experience with the Oregon Death with Dignity Act. *N Engl J Med* 2000; **342**, 557–63.
34. Onwuteaka-Philipsen BD, van der Heide A, Koper D *et al.* Euthanasia and other end-of-life decisions in the Netherlands in 1990, 1995 and 2001. *Lancet* 2003; **362**, 395–9.
35. van der Maas PJ, van der Wal G, Haverkate I *et al.* Euthanasia, physician-assisted suicide, and other medical practices involving the end of life in the Netherlands. *N Engl J Med* 1996; **335**, 1699–705.
36. Ganzini L, Dobscha SK, Heintz RT, Press N. Oregon physicians' perceptions of patients who request assisted suicide and their families. *J Palliat Med* 2003; **6**, 381–90.
37. Sullivan AD, Hedberg K, Fleming DW. Legalized physician-assisted suicide in Oregon – the second year. *N Engl J Med* 2000; **342**, 598–604.
38. Chochinov HM, Wilson KG. The euthanasia debate: attitudes, practices and psychiatric considerations. *Can J Psychiatry* 1995; **40**, 593–602.

ORGANIZATIONAL ISSUES FOR PALLIATIVE CARE PROFESSIONALS

chapter 22

MULTI-PROFESSIONAL
TEAM WORK

Penny Hansford and Barbara Monroe

INTRODUCTION

The needs and wishes of the dying and those close to them can be complex. They will need support with practical, emotional and spiritual issues as well as attention to symptom control. No one health professional has the monopoly of skills needed to deliver such care. The concept of the multi-professional team has been an accepted essential in the delivery of palliative care since its inception in the late 1960s. The term needs clarification. It is a dynamic concept that is growing and changing with the specialism and the term inter-professional is now gaining wider use. Carrier and Kendal have defined it in the following way:[1]

> ... multi-professional work is a co-operative and enterprising approach to work in an environment in which traditional forms and divisions of professional knowledge and authority are retained. More radically, inter-professional work implies a willingness to share and give up exclusive claims to specialised knowledge and authority over those clients' needs that can be met more effectively by other professional groups.

This chapter examines the following issues.

- What are the benefits of multi-professional working?

- What are the difficulties?

- What characterizes an effective multi-professional team?

- What makes multi-professional teams work?

WHAT ARE THE BENEFITS?

In recent years the concept of multi-professional team working has been taken up by policy makers and it is becoming increasingly common practice in mainstream health care. For example, in the British National Health Service Plan, the concept of clinical governance is introduced: 'Clinical governance is about changing the way people work, demonstrating that leadership, teamwork and communication is as important to high quality care as risk management and clinical effectiveness'.[2] In the UK, the implementation of clinical governance via the Care Standards Act[3] in April 2002 specifically demanded that services demonstrate effective multi-professional working, a position reinforced by the publication of the National Institute for Clinical Excellence's *Guidance on cancer services: improving support-ive and palliative care for adults with cancer.*[4]

Users of health care are increasingly recognized as team members. Walters suggests that British society is in a postmodern era:[5]

> ... post modernism celebrates the private ... the feelings of the dying, deceased or bereaved person become paramount ... the patient opts for the treatment that best accords with his or her values or that he or she feels most comfortable with, not the treatment that doctors believe is most effective.

Patient autonomy implies that the patient should be central to the decision-making process and that those who are important to the patient are also part of the team. As Sheldon notes, however, these principles are difficult to maintain in practice.[6] Ethical issues are also becoming more complex, with the introduction of living wills and debates about euthanasia and resuscitation.[7] The views of users can be of enormous benefit in service evaluation and development.[8]

There is very little research concerning the impact of the multi-professional team on the quality of patient care. A study by Jones in 1993 indicated that better symptom control and satisfaction were achieved for palliative care patients at home when the general practitioner (GP), district nurse and specialist palliative nurse were all involved.[9] Those visited by the full team including the social worker were better informed about local support and finance and had improved domestic support. Fountain outlines four important considerations in developing the multi-professional team:[10]

- define the purpose of the team,
- develop standards for best practice,
- let the needs of consumers guide the programme,
- each member should be 100 per cent responsible and accountable for the team's success.

There is some evidence suggesting that the sharing of skills and information in multi-professional teams leads to:[11]

- improved decision-making, accountability and co-ordinated use of resources,
- a more integrated and holistic experience of care for patients and those close to them and an expanded range of options,
- greater support and learning opportunities for team members.

WHAT ARE THE DIFFICULTIES?

Vachon's study of occupational stress in palliative care reported that key stressors were related to team dynamics and to issues concerning role ambiguity rather than to direct patient and family contact.[12] Finlay found that British hospice medical directors rated their relationships with hospice nursing directors as being the most problematic.[13] In the same study Finlay found that doctors encountered difficulties in their working relationships with nurses generally. This was the only aspect of work about which the palliative care specialists reported more stress than did their medical colleagues in other specialties. It is important therefore that the potential problems with multi-professional teamwork are understood and addressed.

McGrath carried out a large study of multi-professional teamwork amongst community mental handicap teams.[14] The research examined areas such as size, composition, activities and caseload, inter-professional differences, management and organizational context, accountability and achievements.

The results mirrored the earlier experiences of palliative care teams. Team members' concerns included role blurring, joint accountability, too little delegated authority and poor team relationships. Management issues highlighted were bureaucracy and the inflexibility of local authority structures.

STEREOTYPES

All health professionals have stereotypical images that are reinforced by media portrayals. Stereotypes develop because they contain recognizable elements of reality. However, as Robertson states, stereotypes can be misused in order 'to safeguard professional identity and maintain interdisciplinary difference'.[15] All team members need to remember that just as they are bound by the stereotypes given to them, they in turn can limit the efficacy of other professionals by the stereotypes they themselves use.

Most palliative care teams have an immediate numerical imbalance of professionals. Most will have more nurses than any other discipline. Team members need to feel confident enough in their roles to be able to coach others in their skills. A social worker can teach a doctor how to respond to the questions of a child facing bereavement. A doctor can teach a nurse how to examine a swollen abdomen for ascitic fluid. This inter-professional trust is the basis for good team working. As Bliss observes, gate-keeping can occur if the role and expertise of the profession are not well understood and may result in the individual not accessing the most appropriate care.[16]

PROFESSIONAL VALUES AND CODES OF ETHICS

Each discipline has a different professional culture, including codes of ethics, which will pervade all aspects of inter-professional working. For example, nursing is a rule-based profession concentrating on the needs of individuals, whereas social work tends to place the individual client within a family and societal context. Unexplored, such differences can become a source of tension rather than a mechanism for maximizing the options available to patients and their families.

LANGUAGE

Implicit in the different professional cultures are language differences. Pietroni suggests that communication difficulties encountered between different professionals arise more from misunderstandings of others' languages than from personality clashes, power struggles or role confusion.[17] He proposes that these problems may be overcome through team exploration and increased opportunities for inter-professional education. Palliative care teams need to develop a common culture and vocabulary. For example, social workers in a specialist palliative care team must have an understanding of common symptoms and associated drugs. Doctors need to pay attention to the needs of children. Both will need to respect the use of terms such as 'patient' and 'client'. Opie[11] reflects helpfully on the need to attend to and work with different 'professional knowledges' and to add to these those of the client and family, which may also differ from one another.

WHAT CHARACTERIZES AN EFFECTIVE MULTI-PROFESSIONAL TEAM?

Within palliative care there exists a variety of models of the multi-professional team and virtually no research to demonstrate which model is most appropriate and effective in each setting. Øvretveit offers a descriptive framework for the multi-professional team:[18]

- degree of integration,

- extent of collective responsibility,

- membership,

- client pathway and decision-making,

- management structures.

He suggests that at one end of the spectrum is:

> a loose knit association, which some people would not call a team at all because membership changes and is voluntary. At the other end is a closely integrated team where team members' workload and clinical decisions are governed by a collective multidisciplinary policy and by decisions made at team meetings.

Teams are dynamic and inevitably move through stages of development. Tuckman identifies five distinct stages: forming, storming, norming, performing and mourning.[19] McGrath[14] and Onyett[20] draw on various authors' perspectives to describe the components of effective and mature teams:

- competent and committed staff,

- agreed goals and priorities,

- agreed definitions of members' roles,

- open communication system and shared information,

- task-centred, problem-solving approach,

- participative management,

- creative, stimulating environment,

- supportive environment,

- staff self-critical, self-managing and able to cope with conflict.

West and Field's study of primary healthcare teams offers some suggestions for increasing team effectiveness:[21]

- there should be clear goals and in-built performance feedback,

- individuals need to be actively managed, with supervision and appraisal systems in place,

- teams should have interesting tasks to perform.

West and Field found that a recurring theme of poor teamwork was 'a lack of regular meetings to define objectives, clarify roles, apportion tasks, encourage participation and handle change'. Multi-agency teamwork can be vitiated by managerial conflict and poor resource allocation.

CONFLICT MANAGEMENT AND COMMUNICATION

The capacity to manage conflict is vital for effective team working; it is the responsibility of every team member. Developing the capacity and maturity to lose the battle in order to win the war is paramount. Some issues are best left alone; others need to be addressed. Conflict can be creative and, if properly managed, may bring a team to a new level of working practice. Ajeman offers useful guidelines for resolving conflict between two colleagues.[22] These include:

- deal with the issue as soon as possible after it arises, but not until the emotions have cooled,

- find a private place to talk,

- describe what has happened and the subsequent consequences in personal terms,

- protect the self-respect of the other individual.

Ajeman emphasizes that what is at issue is behaviour, and not the credibility or integrity of others. She suggests that each party should:

- specify what they would like to see happen and how they can help the process,

- work with the other team member(s) to generate all possible solutions,

- agree to settle on one solution and review it after an agreed time.

Conflict within a team may require facilitation from a professional who is not part of the team. It is important that the facilitator ensures that one individual or discipline is not backed into a corner, but is given a respectful exit in this public setting. This approach is affirmed by Randall and Downie, who assert that: 'Respect for the autonomy of others demands that we recognise that they may have moral values which differ from our own and therefore we must respect their right to reach different conclusions in clinical decisions'.[23] However, once a joint decision has been reached, all team members must abide by it.

Teams also need good formal communication systems, both written and verbal. These should include agreements about confidentiality, frequency and timing of meetings and required outcomes.[11]

As well as clarity around clinical decisions and communication, wider team and organizational issues will be important. Briefings, newsletters, open meetings and staff forums are all possible ways of consulting and communicating with multi-professional staff groups. Team rituals such as celebrating events, recognizing and marking personal or national loss will all help teams to form and relate positively.

WHAT MAKES MULTI-PROFESSIONAL TEAMS WORK?

LEADERSHIP AND MANAGEMENT

'Teams don't just happen, they are a by-product of good leadership'.[24] Teams need an appointed manager who has vested authority as well as responsibility. The tasks of the manager are to develop the individual, achieve the task and build and maintain the team. Many multi-professional teams lack a defined and agreed leadership and management structure. Assumed leadership is often given to the doctor, which can create further conflict and difficulties.

DECISION-MAKING AND COMMUNICATION

Apart from the core clinical disciplines, teams need to be alert to who else should be involved in either making the decision or communicating a decision. Many teams have important key professionals who are not full-time members of that particular team or organization, for example a psychiatrist or physiotherapist. Multi-professional teams need to have agreed policies and procedures for their formal lines of communication, which will need regular review. An important tool to aid this process can be the development of multi-professional[25] and patient-held notes,[26] demonstrating the working together of professionals, acknowledging role overlap and aiding communication between professionals of different disciplines.

CASE STUDY

A community palliative care team with a core membership of several clinical nurse specialists, a consultant and a social worker, struggled with the conflicting approaches of the consultant and the lead clinical nurse. Both were experienced and senior in their roles. The consultant expected a detailed and objective report of the patient's symptoms. She was visibly irritated by the nurse's addition of her intuitive thoughts about the patient and her insistence on a comprehensive report on the patient's family and physical environment.

The issue was resolved following a series of team-building exercises related to individually preferred styles. Once these two professionals realized that they viewed the world from different ends of the personality spectrum and that neither of them was wrong, as both perspectives were needed in the team, a new level of respect and understanding emerged.

TEAM BUILDING

All team members need to develop respect for the individual professional's discrete area of responsibility and expertise in decision-making. A significant way to break down the barriers between professionals is by joint education and training. This should ideally begin at undergraduate level.[27] In 1995, the Council of Europe identified the following rationale for multi-professional education:[28] 'By sharing skills, experiences and attitudes the undergraduate student or professional in their continuing education gets an insight into the similarities and dissimilarities between the different health professionals. An increased respect and mutual understanding of each other is thus facilitated'.

It has also been suggested that there may be important parallels to be drawn between the experience of learners in taking the risk of exposing themselves to learning with an unfamiliar group and the experience of the dying person making contact with the palliative care service.[29] Koffman emphasizes the importance of the experiential elements in such training programmes.[30]

CLINICAL REVIEW

Clinicians can learn from reviewing cases that went well or badly. It can be helpful to review cases on a regular basis in a formal setting. Gaps in knowledge and training or policy can be recognized and addressed. Staff will particularly recognize the value of such a review if training is organized following the identification of learning needs.

Taking the time for an away day can be important in reviewing objectives and forming new ones. Away days must include all members of the core team. Facilitation by someone external to the team may be helpful in allowing the team leader to participate. However, a review of research into team building suggests that although it has a positive effect on members' attitudes and perceptions of each other, it does not increase team performance.[31]

SUPERVISION

Effective development of the individual will mean regular supervision and appraisal. Being managed by a person with a different professional background remains a pertinent and sometimes contentious issue in the healthcare setting.

HAVING A CLEAR TASK

Central to the effective performance of the team is the challenge of the task. Participating in the achievements of agreed objectives can energize a team. Finding ways of objectifying personal disagreement into a team task can bring about positive change.

Katzenbach and Smith summarize the key issues concerning teams and team performance as follows.[32]

- Significant performance challenges energize teams regardless of where they are in an organization.
- Concentration on a strong performance ethic is more likely to deliver effective results than attention paid to team-building activities.
- Work to develop individuals need not get in the way of team performance.
- Organizations with clear structures and boundaries provide the conditions for effective team performance.

EFFECTIVE MANAGEMENT AND INTEGRATION OF VOLUNTEERS

Many palliative care services that have grown out of the voluntary sector use volunteers to maximize resource and service delivery. Multi-professional organizations need clear protocols for working with volunteers. There can be anxiety about the substitution of volunteers in tasks previously undertaken by professionals.[33] Clear understandings about information and confidentiality are also important. Volunteers should be aware of team and organizational strategies and efforts should be made to involve them appropriately in planning service improvements.

CONCLUSION

Teams have intangibles. To work well they demand trust, honesty and respect between individuals and a level of generosity and flexibility towards different professional groups. It is important to share vulnerabilities. All team members have a responsibility to respond appropriately rather than react automatically. Everyone needs to learn how to say sorry. Difficult conversations benefit from prior practice and wherever possible should be conducted face to face. 'Thank you' really matters – and actions speak louder than words.

KEY POINTS

- The dying individual (and, where appropriate, those close to him/her) should be central to the decision-making process.
- Good co-ordination is vital.
- Avoid professional stereotyping.
- Be aware of different professional cultures, languages and codes of ethics.
- Make clear agreements about goals, priorities and roles.
- Adopt a task-centred, problem-solving approach.
- Individual supervision and appraisal remain important.
- Develop good formal communication systems. Remember those 'outside' the team.

REFERENCES

1. Carrier J, Kendal I. Professionalism and interprofessionalism in health and community care: some theoretical issues. In: Owens P, Carrier J, Horder J (eds), *Issues in community and primary health care*. London: Macmillan, 1995, 9–36.
2. Department of Health. *The NHS: modern and dependable*. London: Her Majesty's Stationery Office, 1997.
3. Department of Health. Hospices. In: *Independent health care (Care Standards Act 2000)*. London: Department of Health, 2000, 145.
4. National Institute for Clinical Excellence. *Guidance on cancer services: improving supportive and palliative care for adults with cancer*. London: NICE, 2004.
5. Walters T. Traditional, modern and neomodern death. In: Walters T. (ed.), *The revival of death*. London: Routledge, 1994, 47–65.
6. Sheldon F. *Psychosocial palliative care: good practice in the care of the dying and bereaved*. Cheltenham: Stanley Thornes, 1997, 114.
7. NCHSPCS. *Vital judgements – Ethical decision making at the end of life*. London: National Council for Hospice and Specialist Palliative Care Services, 2002.
8. Monroe B, Oliviere D. *Patient participation in palliative care. A voice for the voiceless*. Oxford: Oxford University Press, 2003.
9. Jones RVH. Teams and terminal cancer at home: do patients and carers benefit? *J Interprofessional Care* 1993; 7, 239–44.
10. Fountain MJ. Key roles and issues of the multidisciplinary team. *Semin Oncol Nurs* 1993; 9(1), 25–31.
11. Opie A. *Thinking teams/thinking clients: knowledge-based teamwork*. New York. Columbia University Press, 2000.
12. Vachon M. Staff stress in hospice/palliative care: a review. *Palliat Med* 1995; 9, 91–122.
13. Finlay I. Sources of stress in hospice medical directors and matrons. *Palliat Med* 1989; 4, 5–9.
14. McGrath M. *Multi-disciplinary teams*. Aldershot: Gower, 1991.
15. Robertson NA. Opportunities and constraints of teamwork. *J Interprofessional Care* 1999; 13(3), 311–18.

16. Bliss J, Cowley S, While A. Interprofessional working in palliative care in the community: a review of the literature. *J Interprofessional Care* 2000; **14**(3), 281–90.

17. Pietroni PC. Towards reflective practice, the languages of health and social care. *J Interprofessional Care* 1992; **6**(1), 7–16.

18. Øvretveit J. Five ways to describe a multidisciplinary team. *J Interprofessional Care* 1996; **10**(2), 163–71.

19. Tuckman B. Development sequence in small groups. *Psychol Bull* 1965; **63**, 384–99.

20. Onyett S. *Teamworking in mental health*. Basingstoke: Palgrave, 2003.

21. West M, Field F. Teamwork in primary health care. Perspectives from organisational psychology. *J Interprofessional Care* 1995; **9**(2), 117–22.

22. Ajeman I. The interdisciplinary team. In: Doyle D, Hanks G, MacDonald N (eds), *Oxford textbook of palliative medicine*. Oxford: Oxford University Press, 1993, 17–28.

23. Randall F, Downie RS. *Palliative care ethics. A companion for all specialities*, 2nd edn. Oxford: Oxford University Press, 1999.

24. Adair J. *Effective teambuilding*, 2nd edn. London: Pan, 1998, 117.

25. Jones K, McIntyre M. A multidisciplinary approach to terminal care. *Eur J Palliat Care* 2002; **9**(1), 21–4.

26. Finlay I. Use of unstructured patient-held records in palliative care. *Palliat Med* 1998; **12**(5), 397–8.

27. Wee B, Hillier R, Coles C, Mountford B, Sheldon F, Turner P. Palliative care: a suitable setting for undergraduate interprofessional education. *Palliat Med* 2001; **15**, 487–92.

28. Council of Europe. *Multiprofessional education health personnel*. Strasbourg: Council of Europe Press, 1995.

29. Sheldon F, Smith P. The life so short, the craft so hard to learn: a model for post basic education. *Palliat Med* 1996; **10**(2), 93–8.

30. Koffman J. Multiprofessional palliative care education: past challenges, future issues. *J Palliat Care* 2001; **17**(2), 86–92.

31. Guzzo RA, Shea GP, Dunnette MD, Hough LM (eds). *Handbook of industrial and organizational psychology*. Palo Alto, CA: Consulting Psychologists Press, 1992, 269.

32. Katzenbach JR, Smith KS. The wisdom of teams. In: *Why teams?* Boston: Harvard Business School, 1993, 11–14.

33. Relf M, Couldrick A. Bereavement support: the relationship between professionals and volunteers. In: Gilmore A, Gilmore S (eds), *A safer death: multidisciplinary aspects of terminal care*. New York: Plenum Press, 1988, 133–7.

THE PRIMARY HEALTHCARE TEAM

Brian Fisher*

The primary healthcare team is involved throughout the patient's illness and has a key role to play at a number of stages in the patient's final journey.

DIAGNOSIS OF THE TERMINAL PHASE OF ILLNESS

It can be difficult to be sure when palliative care should begin.[1] Frequently it is the hospital that informs the primary healthcare team and, sometimes, the patient, that active treatment will no longer be pursued. This can be a difficult transition for both the patient and the primary care professionals, sometimes necessitating a re-evaluation of prognosis and always a shift in emotional gear. It is usually helpful to contact the palliative care team early rather than late: it is easier for everyone to build relationships if there is more time to do so. This contact is often initiated by the hospital as it relinquishes responsibility, or by the practice as it recognizes the need to contribute more, and to become the focus of care.

The primary healthcare team can provide a clear approach here, ensuring that the patient, carers and other agencies know what the practice can offer and how it will work with other agencies. One approach is to put this in writing so that the patient and family have a record they can refer to. Our practice leaflet is attached as an appendix to this chapter, as an example of documentation to facilitate this process.

It is also helpful to assure patients that their wishes will be carried out as far as possible and to answer any questions they may have. Common questions concern pain, fear of pain and other predictable symptoms and what support will be available for patients and their families.

Our work with patients, through contact with a community development organization, has also highlighted the need for continuity. This is managed better by regular visits from two doctors, visiting alternately, thus spreading the emotional load and reducing absence due to leave and other commitments. It also means that patients have two clinical opinions regarding their symptoms and disease progression.

It is important for the primary healthcare team to create an atmosphere of caring, but also clarity of purpose and flexibility with regard to patient and family needs. Terminal care should never mean 'nothing can be done'.

Difficulties can arise when hospital information is unclear to either the patient or the practice. It can be difficult to put across to patients the new situation; from their point of view, all hope of cure is now lost. While acknowledging this, those aspects that are most positive can be emphasized: symptom control, closeness with and support for the family. In addition, many patients are relieved that some degree of clarity enters the outlook, even if the news is bad. Patients often cope better with bad news than they do with uncertainty.

MANAGEMENT AT HOME

There are wide variations between practices during this time. Some will take on the majority of the care and others will share with a hospice or palliative care team to variable degrees.[2] This will partly depend on the availability and structure of such services.

To make this time most beneficial for the patient, a number of facilities need to be available.

- Rapid advice from a hospice or palliative care team when needed: this may be prescribing or other management advice.[3]

- Good communication with out of hours (OOH) agencies: there needs to be a system that allows primary healthcare teams to alert an OOH co-operative, for example that a particular patient is terminal, either facilitating more focused and appropriate care or allowing the practice to be alerted so that they can carry out care themselves.

- Rapid admission to a hospice, if necessary: there is nothing more demoralizing than a rapidly deteriorating situation that cannot be relieved by admission when needed.

There are suggestions that GPs could have direct access to beds in a hospice. There are mixed feelings in the hospice movement about this and often the primary care team does not feel that the hospices are responsive enough to patient need and are inflexible about unplanned admissions at times other than Monday to Friday 9 a.m.–5 p.m.[4]

One essential aspect of care at this time is a discussion about both the nature of the symptoms around death and the place of death chosen by the patient. These aspects need sensitive discussion, naturally, but it is usually a great relief to the patient and family to talk about these topics: significant fantasies and fears are generated about symptoms and lack of support and it is important not only to air these, but also to reassure that support will be available and wishes will be respected.

Despite excellent support from a hospice, it seems clear that patients and their families welcome continued input from the GPs in the primary healthcare team. GPs are often still seen as the central figure in a sometimes-confusing whirlwind of clinicians and helpers.[5] General practitioners have often known the patient and family the longest of all the professionals involved. Confusion can sometimes follow multi-disciplinary involvement.

The last few years have seen significant changes in the structure of care delivered in the community. Most of these changes have widened the focus of the primary healthcare team from individual demand-responsive care to a more population-focused approach. The time demands of audit and screening mean individual care and continuity are likely to suffer. This tendency is aggravated by an increase in part-time working of all primary healthcare team staff. Other factors contributing to this process include less face-to-face and more telephone contact, often with NHS Direct or with OOH co-operatives.

Although the shift towards multi-disciplinary working is likely to improve evidence-based care, it also fragments care and puts a premium on communication, which may be difficult in busy primary healthcare teams. It becomes possible for hospice home care staff to offer excellent support almost without interaction with primary healthcare team clinicians, apart from leaving messages about prescription changes. Another consequence of these changes is the de-skilling of generic clinicians.

Thus, although the technical quality of care has almost certainly improved, and there is less demand for visits and for frequent personal attention from the primary healthcare team, in other respects new developments place more strain on the primary healthcare team.

DYING

The diagnosis of dying can be difficult.[3,6] Too optimistic and vigorous an approach can lead to number of problems:

- unnecessary intervention assuming benefit, such as transfer into hospital for extra care or investigation towards the end;

- too little anticipation and intervention, such as putting up a syringe driver too late;

- poor preparation of the patient and family.

However, once the diagnosis of dying has been established, quiet relief often seems to follow. Many of the anticipated difficulties in decision-making are avoided and helped by the first decision being an agreement by all involved in the care that the patient is dying.[7] However, a number of key interventions need to be available, such as flexible home care and carer support. Symptoms and feelings can change rapidly at this time and the whole team needs to be able to change tack when necessary. Different members of the family may be in different emotional states. Frequent communication is always helpful here and the often long pre-existing association between the practice and the family is a real asset in this situation. The contribution this relationship makes to the situation should not be underestimated or supplanted by the specialist team that may now also be involved.

Again, there is a wide variation in approach between practices and between partners within a practice – some doctors would give their private number to a patient, while others would delegate their OOH care to the co-operative or equivalent agency. There are no right ways to do this sort of thing, but clarity and understanding of what has been agreed are essential. However, it is vital that if a promise is made, it should be delivered.

The recent changes in primary care organization, with a new GP contract in England and Wales, mean that many practices are no longer responsible for the OOH care of their patients. This makes communication and liaison with the primary care team and the providers of OOH services most important. An essential factor in good symptom relief is the immediate availability of appropriate drugs. This is key to patient care and has to be organized across the primary care team, the OOH service and the palliative care team, which may all be involved. The Liverpool Pathway for the Care of the Dying[8] and the *Gold standards framework*[9] offer a model of one way to address these difficulties. The National Institute for Clinical Excellence (NICE) guidelines for supportive and palliative care for adults with cancer encourage the use of such tools and models of care.[10] The primary healthcare team can be prime movers in setting up and maintaining such support, but it is often delegated to the hospice or community palliative care team.

Apart from the clear benefit to the patient, regular visiting by a GP makes it easy to complete death certification, it being necessary in the UK to have seen the patient in the previous 14 days.

AFTERCARE

Both the primary healthcare team and the hospice can offer support at this stage. Depending on the situation and the family, a number of people may be in need of support: these often include the spouse, other close members of the family and children. There is a common feeling among the bereaved that there is a correct way to grieve and, also commonly, that the bereaved person is doing it wrong in some way. The popular notions of a set of stages through which a person commonly passes may have reinforced this idea. It is therefore useful to make it clear to those left behind that there is no right and no wrong way to grieve, whatever their friends and relations may say.

The position of children is particularly delicate. Apart from common sense advice, most GPs will be happy to delegate the care of dying children to the expertise of the hospice, if available. However, the vast majority of families will manage their own process of bereavement without the help of a professional. Allowing the family's own healing without intervention is often best. There is a risk that professionals muscle in and interfere with 'good enough' caring to deal with their own emotions and feelings.

Sometimes, with difficult bereavements, the primary healthcare team's knowledge of years of the family's life and relationships can make support considerably easier. On the other hand, it may also be true that that an insider view may hinder honesty and openness in some situations. It is always helpful to be able to offer another opinion on the situation – in the primary healthcare team this can be another doctor or nurse, or a counsellor. There is also often a number of local voluntary agencies that can be of assistance.

Particular problems tend to arise when:

- there were difficulties in the relationship with the dead person;

- caring and dying have taken such a long time and so much effort that, when it is all over, bereaved people have virtually to reconstruct a life for themselves;

- the bereaved person lacks key skills in running a household, for instance when a surviving wife has never handled the finances;

- this death resurrects memories of a previous death and attendant traumas;

- the dying process was more traumatic, or perceived to be so, than expected.

A number of these issues can be predicted and catered for in advance.

However, even if great care is taken over management throughout the process of dying, the primary healthcare team may need to work with the family through their complex of feelings after the death. These feelings can often manifest as anger, guilt and depression, sometimes directed at the agencies involved. In rapidly changing situations such as these, where emotions can run high and substantial demands are placed on the primary healthcare team and others, mistakes can be made; it is important not to dismiss complaints as misplaced family emotions, but to respond to them formally. The leaflet in the appendix at the end of this chapter was the result of such feedback.

The primary care team has an important role in the palliative care of patients and, although the skills and expertise of palliative care specialists are very important, the true collaborative and integrated working of both together often offers the best care to patients and their carers.

KEY POINTS

- Communication:
  All involved need to know what others are doing.
  Who does what should be in writing for the patient and family.
  Patient's wishes should be recorded.
  Never true that nothing can be done.
- Out of hours services need to know:
  Who is terminally ill.
  Who is under a palliative care service.
  When hospital admission is not necessary.

When admission is not the patient's choice.

If a hospice bed is available.

- Diagnosis of dying:

  Recognize the patient is dying.

  Avoid admission or investigation.

  Have drugs available in the house.

  Anticipate common problems.

  Make family aware of what to do when a patient dies.

- Bereavement:

  Identify at-risk carers.

  Anticipatory problems.

  Avoid symptomatic deaths.

  Involve and notify carer's GP.

ACKNOWLEDGEMENTS*

This chapter was written in collaboration with Dr Carol Cheal MB BChir, Dr Tony Adegoke MB BS, Dr Ruth Williams MB ChB, Dr Shona Lidgey MB BS and Dr Adrian Munn MB BS.

REFERENCES

1. Farquhar M, Grande G, Todd C, Barclay S. Defining patients as palliative: hospital doctors' versus general practitioners' perceptions. *Palliat Med* 2002; **16**, 247–50.
2. Shipman C, Addington-Hall J, Barclay S *et al*. How and why do GPs use specialist palliative care services? *Palliat Med* 2002; **16**, 241–6.
3. Lloyd-Williams M. Out-of-hours palliative care advice line. Letter. *BJGP* 2001; Aug, 677.
4. Munday D, Dale J, Barnett M. Out-of-hours palliative care in the UK: perspectives from general practice and specialist services. *J R Soc Med* 2002; **95**, 28–30.
5. Thomas K. *Out-of-hours palliative care in the community*. London: Macmillan Cancer Relief, 2001.
6. Ellershaw J, Ward C. Care of the dying patient: the last hours or days of life. *BMJ* 2003; **326**, 30–4.
7. Higgs R. The diagnosis of dying [comment]. [Editorial.] *J R Coll Physicians Lond* 1999; **33**(2), 110–12.
8. Ellershaw JE, Wilkinson S. *Care of the dying: a pathway to excellence*. Oxford: Oxford University Press, 2003. (Also available online at: www.lcp-mariecurie.org.uk.)
9. Thomas K. *The gold standards framework – a programme for community palliative care*. London: Macmillan Cancer Relief, 2003.
10. NICE. *Improving supportive and palliative care for adults with cancer*. London: National Institute for Clinical Excellence, 2003. (Also available online at: www.nice.org.uk.)

APPENDIX: CARE YOU CAN EXPECT FROM WELLS PARK PRACTICE

Dear ....

The surgery would like you to feel that, during your illness, you have as much control as you would like over your care.

We have therefore produced this leaflet which will tell you what you can expect from members of our team and other organisations who may be involved, where you can obtain advice, support and help should you need it.

1. Whilst you are at home, there will be two GPs assigned to you. These are .... One of them will visit you a minimum of once every two weeks at his or her discretion.
2. The District Nurses will be involved in your care early on. They will visit regularly as needed and will communicate any concerns they or you may have to your GP or other caring agencies as appropriate. If after discussion with you or your family, you feel that you will benefit from the support of St Christopher's or the Macmillan Team, a referral will be made to them and they will be able to offer you a further level of care.

Out of hours you will be under the care of SELDOC. This is a GP cooperative – all visits will be done by a GP who works in the area. SELDOC will be informed in advance of your medical condition, which will help them make informed decisions about your treatment. Your GP will be informed about all the visits or advice you needed.

The contact numbers of these services are as follows:

GP	0208 699 2840
District Nurses	0208 778 1333
St Christopher's	0208 778 9252
Macmillan Team	0208 333 3017
SELDOC	0208 693 9066

We aim to make managing your illness as easy and worry-free as possible. If there are any problems, questions or worries, do not hesitate to let us know.

The Wells Park Practice

THE HOME CARE TEAM

Penny Hansford

Whilst having devoted my life to hospital work, I have come to the conclusion that hospitals are not the best places for sick people except perhaps for a few surgical cases.

Florence Nightingale, Chicago 1893

INTRODUCTION

Since the 1950s there has been a developing trend towards the hospitalization of death. Studies based on random samples of deaths that had a recognized terminal period showed that the proportions of patients in England who died in institutions increased between 1969 and 1987 from 46 per cent to 50 per cent (hospitals) and from 5 per cent to 18 per cent (hospices and other institutions). Meanwhile the proportion of those who died at home reduced from 42 per cent to 24 per cent. However, despite these trends, patients spend 80–90 per cent of their last year of life at home.[1]

Evidence from both population and patient surveys shows that the majority of cancer patients would prefer to die in their own homes.[2,3] Remaining at home enables patients to live out their lives in privacy and in familiar, comfortable surroundings. They are also able to continue their familial relationships.[4] Caring may give family members an opportunity to begin working through the grieving process, in addition to the satisfaction they often gain from the caring itself.[5] However, staying at home will not be appropriate for everyone, and specialist palliative care at home will need access to in-patient beds if it is to offer a comprehensive, quality service. Indeed, recent preliminary evidence suggests that greater emotional distress is experienced by carers of patients who have died at home,[6] and further work is urgently needed on this key issue.

This chapter gives a résumé of the historical context of the development of specialist palliative care at home and describes the current models available. It looks at factors that influence the place of care and death and describes the factors that ensure best practice in the delivery of care. The chapter concludes with a discussion of the key challenges facing palliative care at home in the twenty-first century.

HISTORICAL BACKGROUND

The first specialist palliative care service at home was set up at St Christopher's Hospice in London in 1969, with support from the Department of Health. The service aimed to extend hospice services into the community, enabling more patients to be cared for at home and to remain there if that was their choice. Other community palliative care services developed over the next few years aimed at complementing existing primary care services by providing additional information, support and expertise. There was no intention to take over from the patient's own general practitioner (GP) or community nurse. This partnership with the primary healthcare team has remained the basis for sharing the care of people dying at home.

During the late 1970s, the charity formerly known as Cancer Relief Macmillan Fund and now known as Macmillan Cancer Relief initiated its Macmillan Nurse scheme, in which home care nurse posts in the National Health Service (NHS) were funded for 3 years, with the health authority, hospital trust or hospice agreeing to continue the funding. In 1980, the Wilkes Report recommended that palliative care be disseminated throughout the health service.[7] At that time, there were 32 community palliative care teams in the UK.

This combination of funding and political strength led to a rapid expansion of specialist nursing posts and home care teams. Nevertheless, the modern hospice movement developed out of the voluntary sector, and there was little strategic planning from the statutory sector or involvement of other stakeholders. This led to overlap of services in some areas, whereas others have little or no service, thus causing inequalities in health care. In the last large data collection in 1995, it was estimated that 347 home care teams cared for about 90 000 new patients per annum.[8] The survey by Addington-Hall and McCarthy gave an estimate that 29 per cent of cancer patients dying at home in 1990 were seen by a community palliative care nurse. This was an estimated 46 000 patients in the UK.[9]

MODELS OF SPECIALIST PALLIATIVE CARE PROVISION AT HOME

Boyd surveyed the structure and working arrangements of 12 urban hospice-based home care teams in the UK.[10] From this study, the operational workings of specialist palliative care teams at home fall into two main models.

The first and more traditional model is a *participatory* one, in which direct involvement with patients and families is a major component of the home care nurse's work. The nurse would hope to educate the primary healthcare teams by example, and more formally if time allowed. For this model to work well, effective communication has to be established and maintained between generalist and specialist services. Palliative care offered through the participatory model is more likely to be provided by a multi-professional specialist team.

The second model is an *advisory* service, in which the home care team offers advice, support and education to the primary healthcare team without necessarily having ongoing involvement with patients and families. The advisory model is more likely to be nurse based, with limited input from other disciplines. Many of the nurses appointed to such posts had undertaken only a short course in the care of the dying (Enrolled National Board 931) and were considered specialists. Today, these short courses are being replaced by a more substantial training at diploma, degree or masters level.

More recent developments of care in the home include the growth of *hospice at home* or *respite care* teams. These are usually teams of nurses offering practical nursing care that augments existing community nursing services. These services often work in conjunction with the Marie Curie Cancer Foundation nurses. Marie Curie nurses formed the first community nursing service for people dying of cancer. They began in 1952 and deploy registered and auxiliary nurses to offer practical nursing care in the home during the whole 24-hour period. The service is now widely available and continues to be jointly funded by Marie Curie Cancer Care and local health authorities or independent palliative care services.

With the reorganization of cancer care services following the Calman Hine Report in 1991, specialist palliative care services were expected to be more integrated into the oncology setting, a policy confirmed by the National Cancer Plan in 2000:[11]

> New funding, in partnership with the voluntary sector, will expand specialist palliative care services in the community, hospitals and in hospices, and tackle past inequalities, enabling cancer patients to live and die in the place of their choice wherever possible.

A needs assessment by Lidstone of the provision of specialist palliative care in oncology out-patient clinics showed that doctors found the presence of community palliative care nurses in the clinics particularly beneficial because it provided a link with the community and an opportunity for information exchange.[12]

EFFECTIVENESS OF SPECIALIST PALLIATIVE CARE AT HOME

In an era of clinical governance and evaluation of services, the impact of specialist palliative care in the community needs to be explored. It is difficult to conduct prospective studies that identify and collect information from people so close to death,[13] and research in the form of randomized controlled trials is rare. Observational studies or retrospective studies of carers are carried out more often.

A systematic literature review found that the use of specialist multi-professional teams in palliative care improves the satisfaction of both patients with advanced cancer and their carers.[14] Such teams appear more able to identify and deal with patient and carer needs and to provide access to other services. There is also evidence of improved pain control and symptom management as a result of the involvement of a specialist team. Specialist palliative care teams can also affect cost by reducing the number of in-patient days required.

Principal factors that influence the place of death[15]
• Older people are less likely to die at home.
• People with haematological and lymphatic cancers are less likely to die at home.
• People from lower socio-economic groups are less likely to die at home.
• People from black and ethnic minority groups are less likely to die at home.
• People who have good access to hospice beds are less likely to die at home.
• Men are more likely to die at home.
• People who express a strong desire to die at home are more likely to do so.
• Relatives who want the patient to die at home are more likely to achieve this.
• People with lung and colorectal cancers are more likely to die at home.

CARE PROVISION

The National Health Service Community Care Act of 1990 recognized the changing pattern of care away from institutions and towards the community setting. Without appropriate practical nursing and social care, many patients would not be able to stay at home, and in palliative care the boundaries between health and social needs tend to become blurred. Unfortunately, the resource implications of decisions continue to cause conflict between service providers. In order to give guidance on this issue, the National Council for Hospice and Specialist Palliative Care Services (NCHSPCS) published a report.[16] It states that there should be 'clear agreement between social services and health authorities as to their respective responsibilities to ensure a total integrated package of care'. Sadly, this remains an unresolved issue in many areas.

ACCESS TO EQUIPMENT

In nursing a patient with a deteriorating condition in the home setting, the provision of equipment can be vital to both the comfort of the patient and the support of the carer. A commode, an electrically operated bed and a pressure-relieving mattress can all be essential items. It is often inappropriate to order the equipment before the patient has deteriorated and it is needed. Therefore people at home need rapid access to obtaining these items at the point of need. Addington-Hall[17] and Sykes et al.[18] have shown that problems are caused by the late arrival of equipment and the failure of professionals to advise on the financial support available.

CARE FOR THE CARERS

Increasingly, studies are revealing the needs of carers and the importance of informal care in the patient's illness. A prospective cohort study of patients on a hospice home care programme found that, by the interview that preceded the death, 17 per cent of their carers were clinically depressed and 14 per cent were very anxious and suffering more emotional distress than the dying person.[19] Neale identified six areas of activity that define the support carers say they need:[20]

- practical help with household tasks or personal care for the dying person, equipment or home modifications;

- enabling help that provides advice and information on what services are available and assistance in securing them;

- respite care, which may be offered by admission to a home, hospital or hospice or by providing a sitting or nursing service in the home to relieve the carer;

- financial support to maintain an income for the carer as well as meet the extra everyday costs for heating, telephone and food when someone is ill at home;

- palliative care for the dying person that offers indirect help to the carer by, for example, securing good symptom control or regular monitoring of changes in the situation;

- psychological and emotional help directed specifically at the carer, which for a minority comes through carers' groups or formal counselling, but much more often from friends, neighbours and family members.

In a smaller survey of the needs of 50 patients and their carers, carers outlined four key areas of need:[21]

- to see the same clinical nurse specialist and have continuity of personnel;

- to have their own time with the professional, separate from the patient;

- to have access to training in practical tasks of nursing care;

- to know whom to call for help and have indicators as to when help should be summoned.

If palliative care teams are to offer effective and high-quality services, they must heed the needs of carers, on whom most of the burden of caring falls when the patient is at home.

CALL OUT

Whether or not a specialist service offering 24-hour assistance is necessary or desirable remains a contentious issue. Macmillan Cancer Relief's early guidelines for those planning new home care services suggest that, in general, out of hours calls should first be dealt with by community services.[22] However, a more recent report by the NCHSPCS recommends that a 24-hour specialist service is a measure of good quality.[23]

In a survey of the views of GPs in South London, 71 per cent thought that a home visiting service out of hours is desirable.[24] In the light of the use of deputizing services or co-operatives to provide GP out of hours cover and the decreasing provision of community out of hours nursing services, there seems little doubt that a 24-hour specialist service is an essential part of palliative care for people at home. In a study of an out of hours specialist team in South London,[25] the findings supported the view that an out of hours service is a vital component of effective palliative care and can at times prevent unnecessary hospital admissions.

There is increasing evidence that primary healthcare teams feel that specialist palliative care should be available in the community over the 24-hour period.[26] What is not clear from studies is whether this should take the form of telephone advice only, or phone advice and the prospect of specialist assessment by a visit. Barclay showed that GPs were keen to access more Marie Curie services and hospice in-patient beds at night, but that communication between GPs and co-operatives is poor for terminally ill patients.[27,28] Thirty-five per cent of calls received by a specialist team come from healthcare professionals.[29]

The National Institute for Clinical Excellence (NICE) has now incorporated 24-hour access to palliative care (which may be by telephone out of hours) into its guidance for palliative care.[30]

Offering a 24-hour community palliative care service has resource implications for many teams that are small in size. On the other hand, it gives an opportunity for palliative care providers to work in partnership and offer a service across the health authority divides.

ORGANIZATION AND MANAGEMENT OF COMMUNITY TEAMS

Nurses provide the majority of the workforce offering specialist palliative care at home. However, there is no defined training path to follow to become a 'specialist'. Today, many specialist palliative care nurses working in the community are educated to diploma or degree level. There are approximately 400 community-based teams, of which about a third are attached to in-patient hospice services.[31] One of the issues faced by a number of teams is of not having a line manager in close proximity and no direct team leader. This means that active managerial supervision can be lacking. With the advent of clinical governance, it is important the services are able to demonstrate their effectiveness and value. The training and development of individual nurses are essential for developing and maintaining standards of clinical practice in the community.

CONCLUSION

Access to responsive, flexible and effective primary and specialist care alongside good support for carers will help narrow the gap between where patients want to die and what actually happens. Specialist palliative care faces many challenges. Services must begin to develop working partnerships both within and across health authority boundaries. As has already been described, small independent teams have inevitable limitations. The challenge is to develop innovative ways of providing service equality both geographically and to all users. Specialist palliative care teams must work in partnership with health authorities, primary care groups and primary care trusts to strategically plan and deliver care. They must deliver evidence-based care where the cost of the service can be justified through its effectiveness.

Research is needed into which models of specialist palliative care deliver best practice. Differences between urban and rural areas may become apparent. People dying of diseases other than cancer do not yet have adequate access to specialist palliative care. The task could seem daunting but, in the words of Dr Samuel Johnson, 'Nothing will be attempted if all possible objections must be overcome'.

Above all, practitioners must respond to the challenge of developing services in partnership with the patient's and carer's agenda rather than by the paternalistic imposition of that of the professional. Palliative care was built on listening to patients and carers.[32] This is relevant as much today as it was at the start of the modern hospice movement.

KEY POINTS

- Multi-professional specialist palliative care teams:
  improve satisfaction of both patient and carers,
  improve pain and symptom control,
  reduce the number of in-patient days required,
  provide access to other services.
- Patients with palliative care needs require rapid access to equipment.
- Good-quality specialist palliative care at home offers an advice and visiting service to patients out of hours.

REFERENCES

1. Cartwright A. Changes in life and care in the year before death 1969–1987. *Public Health Med* 1991; **13**, 81–7.
2. Townsend J, Frank AO, Fermont D *et al*. Terminal cancer care and patients' preference for place of death. A prospective study. *BMJ* 1990; **301**, 415–17.
3. Hinton S. Can home care maintain an acceptable quality of life for patients with terminal cancer and their relatives? *Palliat Med* 1994; **8**, 183–6.
4. Addington-Hall J. *Regional study in care of the dying*. London: Department of Epidemiology and Public Health, King's College Hospital, 1993.
5. Thorpe G. Enabling more dying people to remain at home. *BMJ* 1993; **307**, 915–18.
6. Addington-Hall J, Karson S. Do home deaths increase distress in bereavement? *Palliat Med* 2000; **14**, 161–2.
7. Wilkes E. *Department of Health and Social Security. Report of the working group in terminal care*. London: HMSO, 1980.
8. Eve A, Smith A, Tebbit P. Hospice and palliative care in the UK 1994–5 including a summary of trends 1990–5. *Palliat Med* 1997; **11**, 31–43.
9. Addington-Hall J, McCarthy M. How do cancer patients who die at home differ from those who die elsewhere? *Palliat Med* 1999; **13**, 169–70.

10. Boyd K. The working patterns of hospice-based home care teams. *Palliat Med* 1992; **6**, 131–9.
11. NHS. *NHS National Cancer Plan 2000*, Section 40. London: Department of Health, 2000.
12. Lidstone V, Richards M, Sinnot C, Beynon T. Provision of specialist palliative care in cancer out-patient clinics; a needs assessment. Research abstract. *Palliat Med* 1999; **13**, 513.
13. McWhinney IR, Basi MJ, Donner A. Evaluation of a palliative care service, problems and pitfalls. *BMJ* 1994; **309**, 1340–2.
14. Hearn J, Higginson I. Do specialist palliative care teams improve outcomes for cancer patients? A systematic literature review. *Palliat Med* 1998; **12**, 317–32.
15. Grande G, Addington-Hall J, Todd CJ. Place of death and access to home care services: are certain patients at a disadvantage? *Soc Sci Med* 1998; **47**, 565–79.
16. NCHSPCS. *Care in the community for people who are terminally ill: guidelines for health authorities and social service departments* London: NCHSPCS.
17. Addington-Hall J, Macdonald L, Anderson HR, Freeling P. Dying from cancer: the views of bereaved family and friends about the experiences of terminally ill patients. *Palliat Med* 1991; **5**, 207–14.
18. Sykes N, Pearson S, Chell S. Quality of care, the carer's perspective. *Palliat Med* 1992; **6**, 227–36.
19. Hinton J. Can home care maintain an acceptable quality of life for patients with terminal cancer and their relatives? *Palliat Med* 1994; **8**, 183–96.
20. Neale B. *Informal palliative care. A review of research on needs standard and service evaluation.* Occasional Paper No. 3. Sheffield: Trent Palliative Care Centre, 1991.
21. Hansford P. *Gaining user feedback to develop a palliative care service at home.* Abstract. Geneva: European Association of Palliative Care, 22–24 September, 1999.
22. Cancer Relief Macmillan Fund. *The operation and management of Macmillan nursing services.* London: NSCR, 1988.
23. NCHSPCS. *Palliative care 2000. Commissioning through partnership.* London: NCHSPCS, 1999, **9**.
24. Shipman C. *Working together in palliative care: the challenges for specialist and primary care services.* Abstract. Geneva: European Association of Palliative Care, 1999, 22–4.
25. Boyd K. The role of specialist home care teams' views of GPs in south London. *Palliat Med* 1995; **9**, 138–44.
26. Addington-Hall J. *Care in the last year of life in Lambeth, Southwark and Lewisham.* Report for the Health Authority, 1 Lower Marsh, SE1. 1999.
27. Barclay S, Todd C, McCabe J, Hunt T. General practitioners' and district nurses' views of the adequacy and importance of local palliative care services, a comparative study. *Palliat Med* 1997; **11**, 68.
28. Barclay S. Letter. *BMJ* 1997; **3**, 15.
29. Hatcliffe S. Open all hours. *Health Service J* 1997; **107**, 40–1.
30. National Institute for Clinical Excellence. Specialist palliative care services. In: *Improving supportive and palliative care for adults with cancer.* London: National Institute for Clinical Excellence, 2004, 122–3.
31. *Hospice information service directory 2001.* London: St Christopher's Hospice and Cancer Relief Macmillan Fund, 2001.
32. Saunders C. Introduction – history and challenges. In: Saunders C, Sykes N (eds), *The management of terminal malignant disease*, 3rd edn. London: Arnold, 1993, 1–14.

THE HOSPITAL PALLIATIVE CARE TEAM

Claire Butler

INTRODUCTION

The modern hospice movement has established a new model of care for the dying. Initially this model was developed outside the hospital setting, which was perceived to be failing to meet the needs of dying patients. There has been an enormous and rapid expansion in the number of hospice beds available in the UK (and to a lesser extent worldwide) over the past 30 years, yet hospices do not have the physical capacity to care for all the dying. When questioned, most patients would prefer to die at home, but the majority continue to die in acute hospitals. It has therefore been a logical step to try to import the increasingly well-developed practices of palliative care as modelled in the hospice setting into the care of patients in hospital. The first teams designed with this purpose in mind appeared in the mid-1970s in New York, Montreal and London. There are now 208 hospital-based palliative care (PC) teams in the UK alone.

THE PROBLEMS WITH GENERAL HOSPITAL CARE FOR DYING PATIENTS

- The priorities of palliative care are different from those of general hospital care.

- There is evidence of high levels of inadequately managed symptom problems and psychosocial issues in hospital patients and their families.

  It is of utmost importance to recognise the misalignment between the needs of the terminally ill and the four goals of the general hospital: to investigate, to diagnose, to cure and to prolong life.[1]

It is also of relevance, in the palliative care of cancer patients, to note that the proliferation of palliative chemotherapies for the common solid tumours has taken place over a historical time period similar to that of the development of modern palliative care. For all the good and genuine intentions of shared, collaborative care, these two specialties have perspectives that may be in conflict when they interface in the hospital setting. Crucially, this can result in a lack of clarity for patients about expectations and priorities. It may also result in there being little time to explore holistic palliative care between the ending of an active 'cancer treatment' approach and death.

Research has confirmed the impression that patients with advanced, life-threatening illnesses experience high levels of physical symptoms and psychosocial problems, many of which are poorly controlled in the hospital setting.[2–6] Other research has suggested problems in the provision of even the most basic care for these patients.[7,8] It has also been shown that inappropriate care (e.g. routine patient observations, cardiopulmonary resuscitation attempts, mechanical ventilation)[5,9,10] is being delivered to this group of patients in hospital.

Large numbers of bereaved family members and carers have been interviewed in the quest to evaluate the care of the dying. In the context of many positive comments, some dissatisfaction with the care in hospitals has been expressed by between a third and a half of those interviewed. Common themes have been:

- the lack of staff and how busy and over-worked the staff seem,

- poor information,

- poor communication and co-ordination.[8,11–13]

THE 'NEED' FOR SPECIALIST PALLIATIVE CARE (SPC) TEAMS IN HOSPITAL

- Five to 13 per cent of all hospital in-patients may have 'palliative care needs'.

- Education of healthcare professionals and role modelling are important goals of the work of hospital PC teams.

- Teams individualize the appropriate level of specialist input for each clinical situation.

Recent studies in large teaching hospitals in the UK and France have assessed the need for palliative care by identifying all hospital in-patients with 'palliative care needs', 'advanced' and 'terminal' conditions (not limited to those with cancer).[6,14–16]

Table 23.3.1 suggests that there is under-referral of hospital in-patients to SPC.

No SPC service anticipates being involved in the care of all of those with advanced disease, or in all deaths. From the outset, hospital PC teams have viewed the education of non-specialists in palliative care as an important part of

Table 23.3.1 Assessments of need for palliative care of hospital in-patients

Patients identified	'Palliative care needs'[14]	'Advanced' conditions[15]	'Terminal' conditions[6]	'Palliative care needs' and/or 'terminally ill'[16]
Percentage of hospital in-patients fulfilling these descriptions	5	12	13	23
Percentage of those identified patients who had been referred to hospital PCT or SPC services	54	30	27	–

PCT, palliative care team; SPC, specialist palliative care.

their role. Modelling the skills and attitudes and sharing the knowledge of palliative care should impact on the care of patients beyond the team's immediate caseload.

Most teams have a flexible response to referrals and will offer a range of levels of involvement on an individualized basis. Simple telephone advice only may be appropriate in some situations.

The assessment of a patient and family/carer situation by a PC team often reveals important issues that other teams have not identified or prioritized. Nevertheless, the point of entry (referral) to palliative care services is controlled by those outside the specialty. Hospital teams will invest time in making relationships with appropriate wards, out-patient clinics and departments to facilitate the referral process. Some services have developed guidelines for referral,[17] but these are only of value if they are actively in use. Experience suggests that many factors, beyond the needs of patients and their carers, determine who is referred and who is not.

STRUCTURE AND FUNCTIONING

- Hospital PC teams work primarily on an advisory basis.

- Hospital PC teams aim to be as multi-professional as possible.

- Clinical nurse specialists form the clinical core of most teams.

The structure and operational behaviour of a particular hospital PC team depend upon:

- the nature of the hospital in which it exists,

- the population served,

- the interests and background of those who established the team,

- financial arrangements.[18]

Most PC teams are advisory in the hospital setting and do not aim to take over patient care, but to support, facilitate and educate the primary team responsible for the patient. There is considerable care taken not to 'de-skill' other health carers and to allow them to develop confidence in caring for the very ill and dying. It can be frustrating to work constantly through negotiation and liaison and inevitably compromise. Some teams are complemented by access to palliative-care-run in-patient beds or even a dedicated unit within the hospital;[1] many more have direct links with hospice units locally.

The multi-professional approach is central to the ethos of palliative care, and patients in hospital have a wide range of needs and concerns.[19] Hospital teams strive to be multi-professional and to deliver holistic care rather than just 'symptom control'; nevertheless, there are constraints in this setting. Teams often co-opt professionals from other groups within the hospital who may give a part of their time to the PC team and the rest to other services. Whilst this is enriching, it can make the cohesiveness and strategy of a team difficult to manage.

The Department of Health *Manual of cancer service standards*[20] describes a 'core palliative care team that includes the following members: Consultant in Palliative Medicine; Palliative Care Nurse Specialist'. Palliative care nurse specialists are able to practise with autonomy and authority. They have a broad range of skills and knowledge, enabling them to assess and manage a wide range of problems and concerns. They are also aware of all the other resources (other professionals and services) available to the team.

Table 23.3.2

| Professional group | Areas of skill and expertise | | | |
| | Physical | | Psycho-social | Spiritual |
	Physical functioning	Diagnostics and therapeutics	Communication/ counselling	Spiritual care
Palliative care clinical nurse specialists	++	++	++	++
Doctors (palliative medicine)	+	+++	++	+
Psychological/counselling care professionals	–	+	+++	++
Physiotherapists/ occupational therapists	+++	+	+	+
Spiritual leaders/ chaplaincy	–	–	++	+++

Doctors trained in palliative medicine offer more diagnostic skills for physical symptoms, confidence in recommending and prescribing drugs and regimens and may be more acceptable to some other teams for liaison in difficult situations.

Other groups represented in teams, or liaising closely with them, may include: religious/spiritual leaders, social workers, counsellors, psychologists, psychiatrists, anaesthetic pain services, site-specific cancer nurses, physical therapists, complementary therapists, day care workers and volunteers.

There are areas of overlap between many of the roles on the team (Table 23.3.2) and this can sometimes be a cause of confusion or conflict within a team.

KEY OPPORTUNITIES FOR PALLIATIVE CARE IN THE HOSPITAL SETTING

- Interfacing with 'active treatment' teams to influence the direction of care.

- Readily accessible to patients with non-malignant disease.

- Education of all healthcare professionals (not just those who choose to seek further education in palliative care).

- Training for palliative care specialists.

The hospital setting offers some particular opportunities for SPC that are not encountered elsewhere in the healthcare system.

It may be possible to negotiate for changes in the goals and priorities of patient care towards a more palliative approach directly with the primary team responsible. This is a strong test of positive collaborative working and relies upon well-established professional relationships and mutual respect. Sometimes it is easier for the PC team, as a new team coming into the situation, to see turning points in a patient's illness. It may also be easier for the PC team to take on some of the difficulties as patients and families adapt to different objectives in their care.

Despite the increasingly well-recognized needs of patients with non-malignant disease, referrals of these patients to SPC are growing only slowly. In the general hospital setting, such patients are potentially more readily accessible to PC teams.

There are opportunities for delivering education at every level of activity for hospital PC team staff. Every referral can be used as a teaching exercise if handover, discussion and explanation to the primary ward team are an integral part of the process. More formal educational programmes may be developed, but often suffer from the rapid rate of staff turnover in many hospitals. In teaching hospitals there are also opportunities for undergraduate and postgraduate medical and nursing training.

The hospital provides a robust environment for training palliative care specialists. Unlike a hospice, there is not a shared palliative care agenda or set of objectives across the institution. Hospital PC teams have to front the palliative care ethos and be prepared to be challenged. This encourages the maintenance of a sound, confident grounding in evidence and practice.

HOSPITAL PALLIATIVE CARE TEAMS: EVIDENCE OF EFFECTIVENESS

- Studies indicate improvements in pain relief and some symptoms under hospital PC teams.

- Other evidence for the effectiveness of hospital SPC is not strong.

Several studies have shown (statistically) significant improvements in pain and other physical symptom control under hospital SPC.[21–24]

In terms of other outcomes attributable to SPC in hospital, the evidence is limited. Areas of expected or presumed impact include:

- improvements in communication and insight,[22]

- reductions in length of hospital stay,[18,22,24,25]

- reductions in complaints relating to terminal care in hospital,[3]

- effects on prescribing practices, particularly of opioids and non-steroidal anti-inflammatory analgesics.[24]

What is particularly lacking are data comparing the outcomes with and without PC team involvement.

A systematic literature review of patient and carer satisfaction with specialist models of palliative care showed that consumers are more satisfied with palliative care in in-patient units or in the community than with palliative care provided by general hospitals.[26]

CONCLUSIONS

The general hospital is an exciting and needy arena for specialist palliative care. The limited evidence available suggests that much can potentially be achieved in this setting. Continuing research is essential, as is the development of agreed, systematic ways of ensuring that patients and their families/carers are referred appropriately to receive the care and expertise they need.

KEY POINTS

- The majority of dying patients in the UK die in hospital.
- Evidence shows that hospital patients need SPC and that hospital PC teams can improve the patient experience.
- The core members of the hospital PC team are: nurse specialists and consultants in palliative medicine.
- In order to improve palliative care for all dying patients in hospital, PC teams need to provide education as well as direct patient care.

REFERENCES

1. Mount BM. The problem of caring for the dying in a general hospital: the palliative care unit as a possible solution. *Can Med Assoc J* 1976; **115**, 119–21.
2. Chan A, Woodruff R. Palliative care in a general teaching hospital: 1. Assessment of needs. *Med J Aust* 1991; **155**, 597–9.
3. Hockley JM, Dunlop R, Davies RJ. Survey of distressing symptoms in dying patients and their families in hospital and the response to a symptom control team. *BMJ* 1988; **296**, 1715–17.
4. McQuillan R, Finlay I, Roberts D, Branch C, Forbes K, Spencer MG. The provision of a palliative care service in a teaching hospital and subsequent evaluation of that service. *Palliat Med* 1996; **10**, 231–9.
5. SUPPORT Investigators. Perceptions by family members of the dying experience of older and seriously ill patients. *Ann Intern Med* 1997; **126**(2), 97–106.
6. Morize V, Nguyen DT, Lorente C, Desfosses G. Descriptive epidemiological survey on a given day in all palliative care patients hospitalized in a French university hospital. *Palliat Med* 1999; **13**, 105–17.
7. Mills M, Davies HTO, Macrae WA. Care of dying patients in hospital. *BMJ* 1994; **309**, 583–6.
8. Rogers A, Karlsen S, Addington-Hall JM. Dying for care: the experiences of terminally ill cancer patients in hospital in an inner city health district. *Palliat Med* 2000; **14**, 53–4.
9. Pincombe J, Brown M, Thorne D, Ballantyne A, McCutcheon H. Care of dying patients in the acute hospital. *Progr Palliat Care* 2000; **8**, 71–7.
10. SUPPORT Investigators. A controlled trial to improve care for seriously ill hospitalized patients. *J Am Med Assoc* 1995; **274**(20), 1591–8.
11. Addington-Hall JM, MacDonald LD. Dying from cancer: the views of bereaved families and friends about the experiences of terminally ill patients. *Palliat Med* 1991; **5**, 207–14.
12. Field D, McGaughey J. An evaluation of palliative care services for cancer patients in the Southern Health and Social Services Board of Northern Ireland. *Palliat Med* 1998; **12**, 83–97.
13. Higginson IJ, Wade A, McCarthy M. Palliative care: views of patients and their families. *BMJ* 1990; **301**, 277–81.
14. Skilbeck J, Small N, Ahmedzai S. Nurses' perceptions of specialist palliative care in an acute hospital. *Int J Palliat Nurs* 1999; **5**(3), 110–15.
15. Edmonds P, Karlsen S, Addington-Hall J. Palliative care needs of hospital inpatients. *Palliat Med* 2000; **14**, 227–8.
16. Gott CM, Ahmedzai SH, Wood C. How many inpatients at an acute hospital have palliative care needs? Comparing the perspectives of medical and nursing staff. *Palliat Med* 2001; **15**, 451–60.
17. Leeds Group. Guidelines for referral to palliative care services. *Palliat Med* 2000; **14**, 157–8.
18. O'Neill WM, O'Connor RN, Latimer EJ. Hospital palliative care services: three models in three countries. *J Pain Symptom Manage* 1992; **7**(7), 406–13.
19. Meystre C, Gaskill J, Rudd N. Hospital based palliative care teams – are doctors and pain control teams adequate? Abstract.

20. Department of Health. *Manual of cancer services standards*. London: NHS Executive, December 2000.
21. Edmonds PM, Stuttaford JM, Penny J, Lynch AM, Chamberlain J. Do hospital palliative care teams improve symptom control? Use of a modified STAS as an evaluation tool. *Palliat Med* 1998; **12**, 345–51.
22. Ellershaw JE, Peat SJ, Boys LC. Assessing the effectiveness of a hospital palliative care team. *Palliat Med* 1995; **9**, 145–52.
23. Higginson IJ, Hearn J. A multicenter evaluation of cancer pain control by palliative care teams. *J Pain Symptom Manage* 1997; **14**, 29–35.
24. Higginson IJ, Finlay IG, Goodwin DM *et al.* Do hospital-based palliative teams improve care for patients or families at the end of life? *J Pain Symptom Manage* 2002; **23**(2), 96–106.
25. Woodruff RK, Jordan L, Eicke JP, Chan A. Palliative care in a general teaching hospital: 2. Establishment of a service. *Med J Aust* 1991; **155**, 662–5.
26. Wilkinson EK, Salisbury C, Bosanquet N *et al.* Patient and carer preference for, and satisfaction with, specialist models of palliative care: a systematic literature review. *Palliat Med* 1999; **13**, 197–216.

SPECIALIST PALLIATIVE DAY CARE

Cynthia Kennett

INTRODUCTION

Day care has been developed to meet the needs of patients living at home with advanced terminal illness whose lives have been severely limited by their disease. It is a rapidly expanding area of specialist palliative care: in 1980 in the UK there were 11 day care centres and in 2002 this had increased to 243.[1] A study involving the North and South Thames Health Regions was carried out in 1999/2000 and if the findings from this are projected nationally, it is estimated that there are now more than 12 250 day care places per week.[2]

Quality-of-life issues are commonly the focus of the objectives of day care. They address the physical, psychological, social and existential needs of the patients and respite for carers. Many day centres use Maslow's concept of a hierarchy of needs responsible for human motivation, drive and initiative as a basis for their operational policy. The hierarchy he described begins with basic physical needs and freedom from distressing symptoms and progresses up through the need for safety and freedom from fear, the need to give and receive love and feel accepted in relationships, the need to experience self-esteem, and finally the need to seek meaning and fulfilment. According to Maslow, needs at the lower end of the hierarchy must be at least partly met before others can be addressed.[3]

MODELS OF DAY CARE: MEDICAL OR PSYCHOSOCIAL

Centres providing specialist palliative day care vary considerably. In some the service provision is concentrated on meeting the physical needs of the patients. Medical interventions, such as consultations with a doctor, transfusions, radiological investigations and rehabilitation, take up a significant proportion of the time spent in the centre. Teams offering this type of care have found that the patients benefit from the easy access to these services while being able to remain out-patients.[4-6] This has traditionally been described as a medical model of care.

In contrast to this, a social, or psychosocial, model is provided by centres that focus their specialist palliative day care service on meeting the needs higher up Maslow's hierarchy. A day spent in the centre will have a minimum of medical interventions; rather, the focus is on meeting psychosocial needs. For this to be effective, physical needs must be adequately addressed before the patients attend the centre. Some centres, such as St Christopher's in South London, offer clinic appointments with a doctor, regular symptom control from clinical nurse specialists working with general practitioners (GPs), and day care treatments on an alternative day to the regular day centre attendance. Thus day care can offer an environment in which '... we can try to create an atmosphere in which others find freedom to make their uniquely personal journey'.[7]

More recently, the term 'therapeutic model' of care has been used in relation to centres offering appointments with a range of therapists, nurses and doctors. However, it can also be argued that a psychosocial model of care is therapeutic as it provides a safe, supportive environment in which creative opportunities, social interaction, mutual support and spiritual care can flourish. Maybe the difference in models can be illustrated metaphorically by comparing the patient to a plant: the medical model concentrates procedures on the plant itself, the psychosocial model focuses on providing a rich growing medium, allowing the plant to draw from it what it needs. Higginson et al. concluded that there was not much distinction between the centres describing themselves as mainly medical or social,[2] but the debate continues.

The choice of model operated in any one centre may be related to the location of the unit, the needs of the population served, the stage in their illness at which patients are accepted for care, and the availability of other palliative care services in the area.[8,9]

PROVISION OF SERVICES

STAFFING

There is no universal staffing structure in palliative day care centres. However, there are common patterns that are apparent from the Thames study and descriptions of individual day centres. A manager is usually responsible for the overall running of a centre and commonly a nurse holds this post. However, there are currently centres managed by social workers, occupational therapists, physiotherapists and other healthcare professionals. In addition, most centres have some input from doctors, nurses, aromatherapists, chaplains and hairdressers. The provision of occupational therapy, physiotherapy, social work, hypnotherapy, reflexology, chiropody, arts and crafts teachers, and art and music therapy varies from centre to centre.[2]

Nurses' duties may include assessment, symptom control and ongoing monitoring, running clinics, monitoring transfusions, wound care, bathing, provision of emotional support and encouraging social and creative activities. Where a psychiatric nurse is in post, behavioural management of anxiety and depression can be offered.

The skill mix of staff is a management decision and reflects the focus of care in each centre. For instance there are regular visits from doctors to some centres, whilst others choose to have patients seen in clinics on a different day, prioritizing the provision of creative and social opportunities. Some centres consider rehabilitation to be the main focus of the work, with emphasis on physiotherapy and hydrotherapy, whilst others work closely with a physiotherapy department that is not an integral part of the day centre. Complementary therapies, provided by qualified practitioners, are extremely popular; patients find that the treatments improve their sense of well-being and often report relief of symptoms.

Help from volunteers is widely available in day centres; it is probably true to say that many could not run without their support. These may be people with particular qualifications, such as complementary therapists, hairdressers or arts facilitators who are prepared to give their services for no payment, whilst others give their time to provide hospitality and help with domestic tasks. Commonly, volunteer drivers transport the patients to and from the centres.

REFERRAL

The majority of patients attending palliative day care have cancer. Patients with other diseases are accepted in some centres. These include human immunodeficiency virus (HIV) disease, acquired immunedeficiency syndrome (AIDS), progressive neurological conditions such as motor neurone disease (MND), supranuclear palsy, multiple sclerosis (MS), multi-system atrophy and advanced pulmonary disease.[2,10,11]

The reasons for referral include social isolation, carer stress, need for psychological and/or spiritual support, symptom control and monitoring, and rehabilitation. Most centres offer one attendance a week to each patient, although more may be available in particular circumstances.

The number of places available varies from centre to centre but it is unusual for there to be more than 20 per day. Centres that are attached to in-patient units often encourage anyone who is well enough to leave the wards and join in the activities.

THE ARTS IN SPECIALIST PALLIATIVE DAY CARE

The value of the arts in health care has been recognized from ancient times, although increased technology and financial restraints have often led to their use being seen as an optional extra instead of an integral part of the healing and caring process.[12]

The use of the arts is widespread in palliative day care, although the range offered varies from centre to centre. Broadly speaking, there are three areas in which the arts can be incorporated into the care: first, there is consideration of the environment in which the care is delivered; second, art and music therapies provide a process by which emotions can be externalized within a therapeutic relationship; and third, engaging with the arts in a learning environment can foster feelings of purpose and achievement.[13] There are few evaluated studies, but the organization known as Arts For Health, based in Manchester, has gathered a database of information on a large number of arts projects, many of them in palliative care.[14] In a phenomenological study exploring patients' experiences of participation in a creative arts project at St Christopher's Hospice in South London it was possible to identify hope as the essence of the phenomena.[15] A 10-week sculpture residency in St Joseph's Hospice Lancaster,[16] and an evaluated project which directly involved day centre patients in the metaphor of 'building pyramids' have described the benefits to patients and a useful framework in which to explore their reasons for valuing the activity.[17]

THE ENVIRONMENT

Florence Nightingale recorded in her nursing notes: 'Little as we know about the way in which we are affected by form; by colour and light, we do know this, they have an actual physical effect. Variety of form and brilliancy of colour in the objects presented to patients are an actual means of recovery'.[18] More recently, studies have shown that patients in beds in a surgical ward with a view out of a window leave hospital sooner and require fewer drugs than those who have no outside view.[19] Although no comparative studies on hospice environment have been made, staff report that patients entering an airy, colourful department in which original art works are well displayed immediately show appreciation and signs of reduced anxiety. In St Christopher's Hospice day centre there is a large mobile made by patients and staff, and patients frequently remark on the relaxing effect it has on them.

ART AND MUSIC THERAPY

It is not uncommon for any arts activities involving patient participation to be described as 'art therapy'. This is a misnomer; there is a clear distinction between art therapy and therapeutic arts activities. The focus of the work in art and music therapy is on the *process* of making an image or music within the safe environment provided by the relationship with a qualified therapist. Other creative arts activities focus on accessing an individual's creative process with a *product* as a goal and with instruction from a qualified teacher or facilitator.

The role of the therapist working with people who are terminally ill has been described by one practitioner as a questioning companion assisting patients undergoing palliative care towards a better understanding of their situation.[20] There are accounts of many different ways of delivering art and music therapy in palliative care, the one common theme being the need for flexibility and the ability to adapt the work to each patient's situation.[21,22] Many day centres provide art and music therapy either individually or in a group setting.

ARTS AND CRAFTS

When individuals face terminal illness, they experience multiple losses. The opportunity of acquiring new skills and accomplishments has been seen to foster hope in the last months of life, with resulting comments from patients such as

'It gives me a reason to get up', 'When I am painting I don't feel any pain', 'Since I have been painting again I have been able to talk to my family in a way I could not before', and 'I like it when we repot the plants, spreading out their roots to give them a new lease of life like they give you here'. Being engaged in purposeful activity also provides companionship and the opportunity for patients to encourage and support each other. One patient who had been involved in a mural project said, 'In a group I think you have collective energy, when everybody inspires everybody else'.[15] By encouraging individual projects it is possible to enable patients from minority ethnic groups to celebrate and share their different cultures.

The products of arts and crafts groups – which can include creative writing, painting and drawing, ceramics, gardening, painting on silk and glass, enamelling, jewellery making, dried and fresh flower arranging, mosaics, soft toy making, sugar craft and basketry – provide individuals with a means to redress some of the loss of power they have experienced. When there is a skilled tutor and high-quality materials, patients report how much they appreciate the value afforded to their work. In addition, they relate how important it is for them to be able to give something back to their friends and relatives from whom they have received help and gifts. The recipients frequently refer to the importance of these tangible reminders when they are bereaved.

SOCIAL INTERACTION

The Thames Regions study found that, in answer to the question 'What is the most important thing about day care?', 81 per cent said it was getting out, meeting others and the support they received. Activities that promote social interaction are widely available in palliative day care and, as well as the creative arts groups described above, they may include drama, reminiscence groups, games, outings, discussion groups and visiting musicians and speakers. When activities are skilfully facilitated in a non-patronizing and non-judgemental environment, there is evidence of an increased sense of self-worth being fostered.[23] However, this is probably the most elusive area of day care to evaluate. There is ample anecdotal evidence from patients saying they feel better and have a good day, but to date there are no satisfactory measures available.

Observers in day care often express surprise at the energy and humour apparent among the patients. The value of using humour in palliative care has been recognized.[24] Among staff involved in day care it has been found that by promoting a safe and purposeful environment, there is much spontaneous humour, which is more appropriate than providing 'humorous entertainment' that may appeal to some but make others uncomfortable.

DISCHARGE POLICY

As treatments for cancer improve, it is not uncommon for a patient's disease to stabilize. If an individual no longer requires specialist palliative care he or she will need to be discharged from day care. This needs to be carried out sensitively, with careful planning and preparation. An alternative day centre should be offered if possible, and the patient given the opportunity to make a good ending to the social life he or she has enjoyed in the day care centre.

KEY POINTS

- A common aim of palliative day care centres is to provide patient-centred facilities that improve the quality of life for people with advanced disease and help them achieve realistic goals.
- Day care centres vary: some focus on medical interventions, others on psychosocial care. The geographical area and other available facilities may influence the model chosen in any one unit.
- Complementary therapies are requested by patients and improve their sense of well-being.
- Value is placed on therapeutic activities that improve self-esteem and restore hope and a sense of purpose when much of what constitutes normal life has been lost.
- If a patient's disease stabilizes, she or he should be discharged after careful preparation.

REFERENCES

1. Hospice Information Service at St. Christopher's. *Directory 2002, hospice and palliative care services in the United Kingdom and Republic of Ireland.* London: Hospice Information Service, St Christopher's Hospice, 2002.
2. Higginson IJ, Hearn J, Myers K, Naysmith A. Palliative care: What do services do? *Palliat Med* 2000; **14**, 277–86.
3. Maslow A. *Towards a psychology of being*, 2nd edn. Toronto: Van Nostrand, 1968.
4. Sharma K, Olivier D, Blatchford G, Higginbottom P, Khan V. Medical care in hospice day care. *J Palliat Care* 1993; **9**, 42–3.
5. Noble S, Hargreaves P. Hospice day care. *Eur J Palliat Care* 2002; **9**, 4.
6. Tookman AJ, Scharpen-von Heussen K. The role of the doctor in day care. In: Hearn J, Myers K (eds), *Palliative day care in practice.* Oxford: Oxford University Press, 2001, 79–93.
7. Saunders C. Into the valley of the shadow of death. *BMJ* 1996; **313**, 1599–1601.
8. Faulkner A, Higginson I, Egerton H, Power M, Sykes N, Wilkes E. *Hospice day care: a qualitative study.* Sheffield: Trent Palliative Care Centre and Help the Hospices, 1993.
9. Grafen M. Literature review. In: *Scottish Partnership Agency for Palliative and Cancer Care.* Edinburgh: Scottish Partnership Agency, 1995, 8–9.
10. Eve A, Smith AM. Palliative care services in Britain and Ireland – update 1991. *Palliat Med* 1994; **8**, 19–27.
11. Fisher R. *Palliative day care.* London: Arnold, 1996.
12. Attenborough R. *Arts and disabled people. The Attenborough Report.* London: Bedford Square Press, 1985.
13. Kaye C, Blee T (eds). *The arts in healthcare, a palette of possibilities.* London: Jessica Kingsley, 1997.
14. *Arts for health information pack.* Manchester: Manchester Polytechnic, 1998.

15. Kennett C. Participation in a creative arts project can foster hope in a hospice day centre. *Palliat Med* 2000; **14**, 419–25.

16. Crimmin M, Shand W. *The art of dying.* London: King Edward's Hospital Fund for London and Forbes Trust, 1989.

17. Shaw R, Wilkinson S. Building pyramids: palliative care patients' perceptions of making art. *Int J Palliat Nurs* 1996; **2**, 4.

18. Nightingale F. *Notes on nursing.* London: Harrison and Sons, 1860.

19. Ulrich RS. Effects of interior design on wellness. Theory and recent scientific research. *J Health Care Interior Design* 1991; **3**, 97–109.

20. Connell C. Art therapy as part of a palliative care programme. *Palliat Med* 1992; **6**, 18–25.

21. Pratt M, Wood M (eds). *Art therapy in palliative care. The creative response.* London: Routledge, 1998.

22. Aldridge D. *Music therapy in palliative care. New voices.* London: Jessica Kingsley, 1999.

23. Stevens E. Promoting self-worth in the terminally ill. *Eur J Palliat Care* 1996; **3**, 60–4.

24. Langly-Evans A, Payne S. Light-hearted death talk in a palliative day care context. *J Adv Nurs* 1997; **27**, 1091–7.

TRAVEL ABROAD

Polly Edmonds and John Wiles

It is not uncommon to be asked to comment on a patient with advanced disease's fitness to travel abroad, either on holiday or to return home, frequently involving air travel.

AIR TRAVEL

The International Air Transport Association (IATA) has introduced procedures for 'medical clearance' to travel by air.[1] Passengers are required to notify the airline at the time of booking; assessment of fitness to travel is the responsibility of the airline's medical officer, who may request information from the patient's general practitioner or specialist.

Potential hazards of flying[2]

- Fall in arterial oxygen saturation by 3–10 per cent: this may cause problems for those with respiratory or cardiac disease or anaemia.
- Gas in body cavities expands by 30 per cent: this may cause perforation of the eardrum if blocked, e.g. by infection.
- Inactivity: this increases risk of thromboembolism.

The risk of venous thromboembolism (or 'economy class syndrome') has received much attention of late. A recent study has confirmed that air travel is a risk factor for pulmonary embolism, with a progressive and significant increase in the incidence of severe pulmonary embolism the greater the distance travelled (specifically those travelling a distance greater than 5000 km or who spend approximately 6 hours or more in flight).[3]

Most patients with advanced disease are at high risk of venous thromboembolism and should be advised to take simple precautions if undertaking a long flight, including:

- an adequate fluid consumption, but avoidance of alcohol,

- refraining from smoking,

- avoidance of constrictive clothing,

- use of elastic support stockings,

- frequent changes of position while seated,

- minor physical activity, such as walking around the cabin.

One randomized controlled study of placebo versus aspirin (400 mg daily for 3 days) versus low-molecular-weight heparin (LMWH) demonstrated superior efficacy for LMWH; the authors recommend one dose of LMWH 2–4 hours prior to the flight.[4]

MEDICAL CLEARANCE TO FLY

Several factors influence whether a patient is deemed fit to fly.

- Fitness to cope with the physiological demands of the flight: patients with an exercise tolerance of 10–12 stairs or walking 50 m on the flat without becoming severely breathless are usually deemed fit to fly.[5]

- Fitness to manage the duration of travel.

- Requirement of special provisions, e.g. supplementary oxygen, wheelchair or stretcher, escort. Airlines do not supply nursing care or specialized equipment.

RELATIVE CONTRAINDICATIONS TO FLYING[2]

- Severe breathlessness at rest.

- Neutropenia.

- Marked anaemia.

- Confusion or psychosis that could disrupt the flight or endanger passengers or crew.

- Flying should be avoided for 10 days after surgery to a hollow viscus, 3–4 weeks after uncomplicated chest surgery.

- Suspected pneumothorax or pneumomediastinum.

INSURANCE

It is crucial that patients take out adequate medical insurance; the insurance will usually only cover events that were unexpected at the time of purchase. The insurance company will usually require certain medical details, disclosure of which requires the patient's consent:

- information on prognosis,

- current clinical state,

- stability of disease,

- recent treatment,

- medication,

- whether the doctor expects the patient to require treatment whilst away,

- intended destination and duration of travel.

Cancer BACUP provides a helpful information leaflet on travel insurance for people with cancer, including details of insurance companies.

The majority of countries have no reciprocal agreement for medical costs with the UK. The form E111 (available in post offices) details the medical cover available to patients travelling to countries within the European Economic Community.

TRAVEL WITH CONTROLLED DRUGS

A small amount of controlled drugs can be carried out of the UK under the Open General Licence.[6] If patients need to carry more than the allowance (Table 23.5.1), a Home Office licence needs to be applied for (see 'Useful addresses' on next page). Patients should be advised to carry their medication in its original packaging, fully labelled, and to carry a covering letter from a doctor. It is also important to explore whether the patient's medication is legal in the destination country; this information can be obtained from the relevant embassy or high commission.

Table 23.5.1 Quantities of controlled drugs allowed under Open General Licence

Drug	Total allowance (mg)
Morphine	1200
Hydromorphone	360
Fentanyl	45
Diamorphine ampoules[a]	1350
Oxycodone	900
Methadone	500
	(If patient is carrying more than 2000 mg, require confirmation of travel from doctor, i.e. s/he has seen the air tickets)
Diazepam	900

[a]Diamorphine is illegal and cannot be imported to the USA, Australia, Greece, Germany, Italy, France, Japan, South Africa, Netherlands and Zimbabwe.

Useful contact details

Cancer BACUP
3 Bath Place
Rivington Street
London EC2 3OR
Telephone: 020 7696 9003

Home Office Drugs Branch
Room 239
Queen Anne's Gate
London SW1 9AH
Telephone: 020 7273 3806

Flying home – or on holiday; helping patients to arrange international travel.
Hospice information factsheet F3.
Tel: 0870 903 3 903.
Email: info@hospiceinformation.info
Web: www.hospiceinformation.info

Tripscope
Travel information and advice for people with impaired mobility
Tel: 08457 58 56 41

KEY POINTS

- Assess the patient's fitness to manage the proposed travel.
- Liaise with the insurance company.
- Liaise with the airline.
- Apply for a licence for controlled drugs if appropriate.

REFERENCES

1. International Air Transport Association. Resolution 700. Acceptance and carriage of incapacitated passengers. In: *Passenger services conference resolutions manual*, 14th edn. IATA, 1994.
2. Advising patients about air travel. *Drugs Ther Bull* 1996; **34**(4), 30–2.
3. Lapostolle F, Surget V, Borron SW et al. Severe pulmonary embolism associated with air travel. *N Engl J Med* 2001; **345**, 779–83.
4. Cesarone MR, Belcaro G, Nicolaides AN *et al*. Venous thrombosis from air travel: the LONFIT3 study – prevention with aspirin vs low molecular weight heparin in high risk subjects: a randomized trial. *Angiology* 2002; **53**, 1–6.
5. Byrne NJ. Comparison of airline passenger oxygen systems. *Aviat Space Environ Med* 1995; **66**, 780–3.
6. HM Customs and Excise. *Taking medicines with you when you go abroad*. Notice 4. London: HM Customs and Excise, July 1998.

chapter 24

REHABILITATION

Ann Elfred

The *Oxford English Dictionary* defines rehabilitation as '… to readapt …'. In the context of palliative care, it has been defined as 'making the patient into a person again'.[1]

This chapter looks at the concept of helping patients with advanced disease to re-adapt to their situation and make the most of their potential. This will inevitably involve a team effort, with different professionals having various inputs and perspectives to offer. The emphasis here is on the role of the physiotherapist and the particular skills he or she may have to offer, but a range of specialist services may be required (e.g. occupational and speech and language therapists, dietician) as well as creative therapies in a more social setting, e.g. art, music etc.

The need for rehabilitation is well accepted in many branches of medicine, yet until its recent inclusion in the National Institute for Clinical Excellence (NICE) guidance it had a relatively low profile in oncology and palliative care. This is surprising, given that 50 per cent of cancer sufferers will survive 5 years or more, whereas half of stroke patients will die within a year and 30 per cent of coronary patients will not survive the convalescent period.[2] It is to be hoped that availability of rehabilitation services will improve following the publication of new guidance from the NICE,[3] which cites rehabilitation as a major route to improving quality of life, no matter how long or short the timescale, and integral to patient care. Palliative care is not just about symptom control, but also about affirming life – rehabilitation is one way of helping to achieve this.[4]

Quality of life may be diminished by a number of disabling conditions arising from both the disease and its treatment. An evaluation of 50 cancer patients seen by a rehabilitation service found that:

- 26 per cent had one identifiable problem adversely affecting function,

- 54 per cent had two identifiable problems adversely affecting function,

- 20 per cent had three or more such problems,

- the most common problem was deconditioning,

- lack of awareness of functional compromise was common.[5]

As disease advances, such functional deficits become more marked and may severely affect quality of life. Specialist services are needed to address these needs, aiming to improve quality of life by achieving maximum level of functioning within the limits of disease.[6]

Dietz describes four phases of rehabilitation:[7]

- preventative: to lessen the severity of potential disability;

- restorative: where return to premorbid status is possible;

- supportive: reducing complications of ongoing disease;

- palliative: maximizing quality of life (aiming to make the most of potential by extenuating the effects of disease and complications).

The emphasis of treatment will move through these phases as disease progresses.

ASSESSMENT AND PLANNING A TREATMENT PROGRAMME

It is essential to take an holistic approach, considering physical, psychosocial and spiritual dimensions.

Assessment must be thorough and systematic and include the following.

- History of the disease and its treatment (this may be gleaned from the medical notes, to prevent repeatedly asking the patient the same questions).

- Current symptoms.

- The patients' perception of their problems (what strikes the professional as important may be of little relevance to the patient, and vice versa!).

- Physical assessment; for the physiotherapist, this will include:
  range and quality of movement,
  muscle strength,
  balance and co-ordination,
  transfers and gait.

Comprehensive assessment involves listening, observation, palpation and testing as appropriate. This may have to be spread over more than one session, according to the patient's tolerance.

From this assessment, a problem list can be drawn up, realistic goals discussed and a treatment plan made. Frequently patients have been faced with a long series of losses over which they have had little or no control. Here is an opportunity to give back some control. It has been shown that the majority of patients prefer to participate in their care, and that those who want active information and participation are significantly more hopeful.[8] Also that active coping strategies are associated with increased activity and lower psychological distress.[9]

Goals may be relatively long or short term and subject to frequent modification, as the patient's situation may change rapidly. It is important to remain realistic about possibilities without dashing the hopes of the patient – this requires both skill and sensitivity. It is also important that family, friends and carers are included in treatment planning and delivery, where that is the wish of the patient.

Treatment may be delivered in a variety of settings, for example:

- the home, where domiciliary services are available,

- specialist department (this may have positive connotations for many patients),

- as part of day care,

- in-patient unit/ward.

Input will generally be 'little and often', rather than in prolonged sessions, as patients may tire quickly. As disease progresses, it is important to avoid highlighting deterioration, by scaling treatment down gradually according to the patient's capabilities rather than abruptly ceasing.

PAIN AND SYMPTOM CONTROL

Rehabilitation occurs as part of a total management programme. For it to be effective, good symptom control is essential, and physiotherapy may assist with this.

Whilst analgesic drugs are the mainstay of pain management, optimal relief may only be achieved by a combination of two or more therapies.[10] Modalities such as relaxation and electrophysical agents and the teaching of coping strategies have the particular advantage of returning some degree of control to the patient. It has been stated that passivity in treatment degrades the individual's sense of personal control and adequacy,[11] and that the perception of having control over pain relates to satisfaction with pain relief.[12]

TREATMENT MODALITIES

THERAPEUTIC EXERCISE

It has been estimated that one third or more of the decline in functional capacity experienced by cancer patients, regardless of stage of disease, can be attributed to hypokinetic conditions that develop as a consequence of prolonged physical inactivity.[7]

Therapeutic exercise may be used to improve such deconditioning to maintain the current level of functioning or to minimize deterioration.

Exercise may be part of a general regime for:

- endurance and stamina,

- cardiovascular fitness,

- relaxation or enjoyment.

Or it may be prescribed more specifically for:

- muscle strengthening,

- range of movement,

- balance and co-ordination,

- teaching elements of specific motor skills in order to improve function.

An exercise programme will usually be designed to address several of these aims. Assisted movements and supervised exercise may also help to alleviate symptoms resulting from prolonged bed rest or inactivity, where a vicious cycle as illustrated in Figure 24.1 may become established.

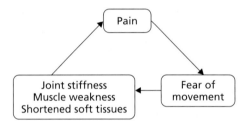

Figure 24.1

Exercises may be:

- passive: i.e. performed by the therapist, not under voluntary control;

- assisted:
  voluntary movement assisted by another force, e.g. the therapist, by the patient themselves (as in auto-assisted movement of hemiplegic arm), or by equipment such as sliding board, sling and pulley systems;

- resisted: by therapist, weights or other equipment, e.g. static bike.

Exercise programmes must be tailored to the individual and monitored, with realistic aims agreed between the patient and therapist. It is helpful if they are backed-up in writing and taught to family and carers, who can provide support and encouragement.

There is evidence of an overall health benefit of exercise in all age groups and more specifically in the management of cardiovascular and pulmonary disease, diabetes, end-stage renal disease and some psychological disorders such as depression.[13]

Studies also show that exercise is an effective strategy for the relief of fatigue[14] and for improving deconditioning[15] and function.[16,17] Professional support has been found to be an important incentive to exercise.[18]

However, many of these studies have been conducted either at an earlier disease stage or without making the disease stage clear, although some include patients with metastatic disease. There is no evidence to direct the design of particular exercise regimes (type, intensity, frequency, duration etc.) in this patient group.

Physiotherapists may also be asked to prescribe exercise programmes for patients suffering from steroid-induced myopathy, a frequently occurring and serious side effect in neuro-oncology patients.[19] Whilst exercise may be helpful and supportive, it is doubtful whether this process can be reversed in advanced disease.

FUNCTIONAL REHABILITATION

Dependency is a major problem for the terminally ill. Research suggests that patients in the last year of life fear dependency more than pain, and that this was the main reason for those who expressed the wish to die early.[20] A symptom audit at St Christopher's Hospice ranked weakness (91 per cent) and immobility (77 per cent) as the most frequent symptoms and with the greatest effect on daily life amongst home care patients. Clearly, symptom burden and dependency are closely linked, and the ability for independent activity is likely to decline with advancing disease.

One study of physiotherapy in a day hospice found that the two main factors contributing to quality of life were:

- positive psychological support,

- the ability to do things for oneself.

Physiotherapy was found to be supportive and to improve function in 80 per cent of those interviewed.[16]

Most patients are keen to remain ambulant for as long as possible. Normal gait is a very complicated process, requiring integrity of both musculoskeletal and nervous systems. Gait re-education aims to:

- prevent pain or injury,

- maximize independence,

- minimize effort.

Walking aids such as sticks, crutches and rollators are frequently helpful, enabling:

- weight to be re-distributed through both upper and lower limbs,

- increased base of support, improving stability,

- a stable rest, e.g. for the dyspnoeic patient,

- increased confidence,

- increased safety, reducing the risk of falls.

A recent national audit has enabled guidelines to be established for the prevention of falls in the elderly – these can be used to guide practice to try and reduce the risk of falls in this vulnerable patient population.[21]

Where ambulation is no longer possible, provision of an appropriate wheel-chair (manual or electric) may enable some degree of independence to be maintained. Arrangements need to be in place for such equipment to be available quickly, as considerable delays may be encountered with statutory services. Where possible, a store of basic equipment should be available for loan. In small units where this is impractical, it may be possible to have arrangements for 'fast-tracking' palliative care patients with local statutory services.

It is important to teach safe transfers, with the minimum of effort, to both patients and carers. Use of the correct positioning and sequence can greatly improve the ability to stand from sitting independently. Advice should also be given for all regular transfers, e.g. to and from bed, toilet, commode etc. The provision of equipment such as a transfer board or glide sheets may be helpful.

Referral to an occupational therapist should also be considered for patients with functional impairments and difficulties with activities of daily living.

There is some evidence for the success of rehabilitation programmes. Studies have shown that brain tumour patients (both primary and metastatic) can make significant functional gains, comparable to those of both stroke patients[22] and traumatic brain injury patients.[23] Both of these studies showed significant functional gains and a discharge rate to the community of more than 85 per cent. Patients suffering from neoplastic spinal cord compression showed significant improvements in dressing, grooming, transfers, wheelchair use, ambulation and stairs, which was maintained or improved at 3-month follow-up.[24] This group was screened to have a prognosis greater than 3 months, and to be able to tolerate 3 hours of daily rehabilitation. These papers originated from specialist physical medicine and rehabilitation centres in the USA. Specific details of the programmes and personnel involved were not given. Another study has developed a scoring system to select neoplastic spinal cord injury patients who may benefit from rehabilitation.[25] A recent audit in an oncology centre has allowed development of a care pathway for suspected malignant spinal cord compression with the possibility of earlier rehabilitation.[26]

A retrospective study of 159 cancer patients undergoing in-patient rehabilitation showed that significant improvements could be achieved in both functional status and motor independence.[15] The presence of metastatic disease did not have a detrimental effect on functional outcome.

ELECTROPHYSICAL AGENTS

The use of electrophysical agents may aid the rehabilitation of the patient by assisting with pain relief in conjunction with other analgesic measures. Electrotherapeutic modalities are not widely used in this field, as there is concern that some treatments (for example ultrasound) may accelerate the growth of metastases.[27] However, transcutaneous electrical nerve stimulation (TENS) is widely available, relatively cheap and easy to use, with few contraindications or side effects. Many units run a loan system for equipment.

Although studies have shown that TENS can give effective pain relief in some chronic pain conditions, they have not been able to demonstrate correlations between particular stimulation parameters or electrode placements and pain relief, or to show which conditions are most likely to respond.

The literature suggests:

- better outcome with well-localized pain,[28]
- greatest relief in those who have had fewer previous interventions,[29]
- psychogenic pain does not respond well,[30]
- visceral pain may respond less well.[30]

There are few studies regarding the use of TENS with cancer patients. Those available suggest:

- initial good pain relief, but with limited long-term effect,[31]
- extremity and trunk pains were relieved more effectively than pelvic and perineal pain,[32]
- good response for myofacial and localized bone pain; variable response for neurogenic pain.[33]

A small series of single case studies carried out by the writer found that TENS could contribute to pain relief in the terminally ill, but that patients' perceptions of its usefulness and acceptability did not always accord with the level of pain relief. It is the writer's experience that some patients respond to the 'paraphernalia' of TENS better than others. For it to be successful, the patient must be prepared to persevere with its use over a trial period, experiment with stimulation parameters, and use long stimulation periods (i.e. several hours).

Both heat and cold have been used for thousands of years for the relief of pain, probably achieving their effect through sensory modulation via a spinal gating mechanism. A number of simple methods of application are available (hot and cold packs, electrically heated pads etc.), their very simplicity making them attractive to patients and suitable for home use. Application of heat is contraindicated where sensation is reduced or absent, or where weakness or paralysis would prevent the patient moving from the heat source should it become uncomfortable.

Simple measures such as TENS, heat and cold may be helpful in reinforcing a rehabilitation approach by returning some control to the patient.

RELAXATION

Relaxation is a state which decreases the activity of the sympathetic and motor nervous systems and has been shown to be effective in the reduction of pain related to cancer treatment.[34] A small study carried out at St Christopher's Hospice identified several potential benefits of relaxation, including:

- perceived reduction in stress and anxiety, which positively influenced other symptoms, e.g. pain and dyspnoea;
- increased comfort from skilled positioning;
- enhanced feelings of control.[35]

A number of methods have been described for teaching relaxation – that chosen will depend largely on the preference and experience of the therapist and the response of the patient. There is no available evidence to suggest that any one method is better than another. It may be useful to back-up relaxation teaching with the loan of an audiotape for practice.

REHABILITATION OF THE BREATHLESS PATIENT

The management of dyspnoea is dealt with elsewhere (see Chapter 4.3), but a chapter on rehabilitation would be incomplete without mention of the breathless patient.

Non-pharmacological approaches have long been used to alleviate breathlessness and other symptoms, resulting in the development of pulmonary rehabilitation programmes for some chronic respiratory diseases. There is evidence that this approach improves function and quality of life.[36] Clinical practice guidelines for the physiotherapy management of breathlessness have been developed by the Association of Chartered Physiotherapists in Respiratory Care (ACPRC), which include details of assessment and strategies such as:

- techniques to clear bronchial secretions,
- breathing control,
- positioning,
- TENS,
- mobilization.

More recently, this kind of rehabilitative approach has been used in the management of lung cancer patients suffering from breathlessness, both by physiotherapists and in the development of nurse-led clinics.[37,38]

CONCLUSION

Rehabilitation should be considered as integral to the management of patients with advanced disease. Rehabilitative interventions may have physical, psychological, social and spiritual benefits.[3] Specialist services may be provided by a range of health professionals, but it is also important that all healthcare professionals encourage efforts to promote well-being and self-management strategies. Evaluation in a hospice setting has shown that rehabilitation is valued by both patients and carers.[39]

KEY POINTS

- Weakness and deconditioning are common functional impairments with a great impact on daily life.
- Exercise may be an effective strategy in:
  alleviating fatigue,
  improving functional capacity,
  improving quality of life.
- Rehabilitation can produce significant functional gains for patients with brain tumours and neoplastic spinal cord compression.
- Physiotherapy in a hospice has been found to:
  improve function,
  give positive psychological support.
- A multi-professional team approach is necessary for effective rehabilitation, to enable individuals to maximize their potential at the end of life.

REFERENCES

1. Doyle D. Rehabilitation in palliative care (Introduction). In: Doyle D, Hanks G, MacDonald N (eds), *Oxford textbook of palliative medicine*, 2nd edn. Oxford: Oxford University Press, 1998, 817–18.
2. Wells R. Rehabilitation: making the most of time. *Nurs Forum* 1990; **17**(4), 503–7.
3. National Institute for Clinical Excellence. Rehabilitation Services. In: *Improving supportive and palliative care for adults with cancer*. London: NICE, 2004; 134–47.
4. National Council for Hospice and Specialist Palliative Care Services. *Fulfilling lives. Rehabilitation in palliative care*. London: NCHSPCS, August 2000.
5. Brennan M, Warfel B. Musculoskeletal complications of cancer. A survey of 50 patients. *J Back & Musculoskeletal Rehabil* 1993; **3**(2), 1–6.
6. Hockley J. Rehabilitation in palliative care – are we asking the impossible? *Palliat Med* 1993; **7**(Suppl. 1), 9–15.
7. Dietz J. *Rehabilitation oncology*. New York: John Wiley, 1981.
8. Cassileth B, Zupkis R, Sutton-Smith K, March V. Information and participation preferences among cancer patients. *Ann Intern Med* 1980; **92**, 832–6.
9. Snow-Turek A, Norris P, Tan G. Active and passive coping strategies in chronic pain patients. *Pain* 1996; **64**, 455–62.
10. Bonica J, Ventafridda V, Twycross R. Cancer pain. In: Bonica J, Ventafridda V, Twycross R (eds), *The management of pain*, Vol. 1, 2nd edn. Philadelphia, London: Lea & Febiger, 1990, 400–58.

11. Chapman C, Hill H. Patient-controlled analgesia in a bone marrow transplant setting. In: Foley K, Bonica J, Ventafridda V (eds), *Advances in pain research and therapy*, Vol. 16. Philadelphia: Raven Press, 1990, 231–47.

12. Pellino T, Ward S. Perceived control mediates the relationship between pain severity and patient satisfaction. *J Pain Symptom Manage* 1998; **15**(2), 110–16.

13. Young-McCaughan S, Sexton D. A retrospective investigation of the relationship between aerobic exercise and quality of life in women with breast cancer. *Oncol Nurs Forum* 1991; **18**(4), 751–7.

14. Graydon J, Bubela N, Irvine D, Vincent L. Fatigue reducing strategies used by patients receiving treatment for cancer. *Cancer Nurs* 1995; **18**(1), 23–8.

15. Marciniak C, Sliva J, Spill G, Neinemann A. Functional outcome following rehabilitation of the cancer patient. *Arch Phys Med Rehabil* 1996; **77**, 54–7.

16. Martlew B. What do you let the patient tell you? *Physiotherapy* 1996; **82**(10), 558–65.

17. MacVicar M, Winningham M, Nickel J. Effects of aerobic interval training on cancer patients' functional capacity. *Nurs Res* 1989; **38**(6), 348–51.

18. Kun Leddy S. Incentives and barriers to exercise in women with a history of breast cancer. *Oncol Nurs Forum* 1997; **24**(5), 885–90.

19. Koehler P. Use of cortico-steroids in neuro-oncology. *Anti-Cancer Drugs* 1995; **6**, 19–33.

20. Seale CF, Addington-Hall J. Euthanasia: why people want to die earlier. *Soc Sci Med* 1994; **39**(5), 647–54.

21. Simpson J, Harrington R, Marsh N. Guidelines for managing falls among elderly people. *Physiotherapy* 1998; **84**(4), 173–7.

22. Huang M, Cifu D, Keyser-Marcus L. Functional outcome after brain tumor and acute stroke: a comparative analysis. *Arch Phys Med Rehabil* 1998; **79**, 1386–90.

23. O'Dell M, Barr K, Spanier D, Warnick R. Functional outcome of inpatient rehabilitation in persons with brain tumours. *Arch Phys Med Rehabil* 1998; **79**, 1530–4.

24. McKinley W, Conti-Wyneken A, Vokac C, Cifu D. Rehabilitative functional outcome of patients with neoplastic spinal cord compression. *Arch Phys Med Rehabil* 1996; **77**, 892–5.

25. Hacking H, Van As H, Lankhorst G. Factors related to the outcome of inpatient rehabilitation in patients with neoplastic epidural spinal cord compression. *Paraplegia* 1993; **31**, 367–74.

26. Pease NJ, Harris RJ, Finlay IG. Development and audit of a care pathway for the management of patients with suspected malignant spinal cord compression. *Physiotherapy* 2004; **90**, 27–34.

27. Low J. Electrotherapeutic modalities. In: Wells P, Frampton V, Bowsher D (eds), *Pain management by physiotherapy*, 2nd edn. London: Butterworth Heinemann, 1994, 140–76.

28. Woolf C. Transcutaneous and implanted nerve stimulation. In: Melzack R, Wall P (eds), *Textbook of pain*, Edinburgh: Churchill Livingstone, 1984, 679–90.

29. Wolf S, Gersh M, Rao V. Examination of electrode placements and stimulating parameters in treating chronic pain with conventional transcutaneous electrical nerve stimulation. *Pain* 1981; **1**, 37–47.

30. Nielzen S, Sjolund B, Eriksson M. Psychiatric factors influencing the treatment of pain with peripheral conditioning stimulation. *Pain* 1982; **13**, 365–71.

31. Ventafridda V, Sganzerla E, Fochi C, Pozzi G, Cordini G. TENS in cancer pain. In: Bonica J, Ventafridda V (eds), *Advances in pain and research therapy*. Philadelphia: Raven Press, 1979, 509–15.

32. Avellanosa A, West C. Experience with TENS for relief of intractable pain in cancer patients. *J Med* 1982; **13**(3), 203–13.
33. Abram S. Electrical stimulation for cancer pain management. In: Abram S (ed.), *The pain clinic manual.* Philadelphia: J.B. Lipincott Co., 1990, 285–8.
34. Syrjala K, Donaldson G, Davis M, Kippes M, Carr J. Relaxation and imagery and cognitive–behavioural training reduce pain during cancer treatment: a controlled clinical trial. *Pain* 1995; **63**, 189–98.
35. Howell W, Kelly M. An exploratory study to consider the benefits of relaxation therapy as carried out by physiotherapists in palliative care. Unpublished 1995. Study carried out at St Christopher's Hospice, London.
36. Shee CD. Palliation in chronic respiratory disease. *Palliat Med* 1995; **9**, 3–12.
37. Corner J. Non-pharmacological intervention for breathlessness in lung cancer. *Palliat Med* 1996; **10**, 299–305.
38. Hately J, Scott A, Laurence V, Baker R, Thomas P. *A palliative-care approach for breathlessness in cancer. A clinical evaluation.* London: Help The Hospices, 2001.
39. Yoshioka H. Rehabilitation for the terminal cancer patient. *Am J Phys Med Rehabil* 1994; **73**(3), 199–206.

RECOMMENDED READING

Flannagan J, Holmes S. Facing the issue of dependence: some implications from the literature for the hospice and hospice nurses. *J Adv Nurs* 1999; **29**(3), 592–9.
Fulton C. Physiotherapists in cancer care: a framework for rehabilitation of patients. *Physiotherapy* 1994; **80**(12), 830–4.
Fulton C, Else R. Physiotherapy. In: Doyle D, Hanks G, MacDonald N (eds), *Oxford textbook of palliative medicine*, 2nd edn. Oxford: Oxford University Press, 1998, 819–28.
Rashleigh L. Physiotherapy in palliative oncology. *Aust Physiother* 1996; **42**(4), 307–12.

SYSTEMATIC REVIEWS

Association of Chartered Physiotherapists in Respiratory Care (ACPRC). *Clinical practice guidelines. Physiotherapy management of the spontaneously breathing, acutely breathless, adult patient – a problem solving approach.* ACPRC, 1996.
Chartered Society of Physiotherapy (CSP). *Physical activity and exercise.* Effectiveness Bulletin, 1999.
Details of CSP Effectiveness Bulletins and ACPRC guidelines are available from: Chartered Society of Physiotherapy, 14 Bedford Row, London WC1R 4ED.
Ellis B. Short report: TENS for pain relief: recent research findings and implications for clinical use. *Phys Therapy Rev* 1998; **3**, 3–8.
Friedenreich C, Courneya K. Exercise as rehabilitation for cancer patients. *Clin J Sports Med* 1996; **6**, 237–44.

chapter 25

ACCESSING INFORMATION: THE ROLE OF THE INTERNET

John Wiles

THE NEED FOR INFORMATION

Patients need information. To consent to treatment or procedures they must be fully informed. The nature of the clinical consultation means that, inevitably, the length of the consultation is constrained by time. Even when the consultation provides an opportunity to discuss issues in depth, the patient and family often do not understand what they are told and wish to review the information later. The tendency not to take information on board is especially true in a consultation associated with an emotionally heightened atmosphere. This is often the case in breaking bad news or in a situation in which the patient is anxious and fearful. The need to understand what has been said may be helped by patient information leaflets focusing on the issues raised. However, patients may seek further information and clarification for themselves and they now have access to more information than ever before via the Internet and the Worldwide Web.[1]

It is essential that professionals are up to date and that their practice should be evidence based. In palliative care, evidence is often not a randomized controlled trial but a professional consensus of best practice. The immediacy of communication via the Internet may facilitate communication of perceived best practice.

Much of the cancer information on the Internet is located in sites in the USA. The culture of that society is reflected in the information available and often in the subsequent behaviour of patients, in that they want a more active role in their treatment, demanding second opinions abroad or requesting treatments not routinely available in the UK. In the cancer field, there has been a rapid growth of the information available.[2] Elderly patients may not use the Internet much themselves, but often receive information from relatives who do. Oncologists are an example of one professional group being challenged by the demands of their patients for more information,[3] which is often from another country.

Patient-specific advice is not available on the Internet. The key role for the physician or healthcare professional may be to make sense of generic and generalized information, interpret it for the specific patient, and apply it to the clinical scenario facing that patient. Only that professional may know the full case history, have examined the patient and have all the test results available. Healthcare professionals may find themselves acting as information counsellors, interpreting the generic information patients have gained from the Internet and making it specific to the unique clinical situation.

The doctor who feared patients arriving at the consultation with a written list of questions may be even more daunted when they arrive with a printout from the Internet!

CAN THIS INFORMATION BE TRUSTED?

A recent survey looked at the information that patients trust.[4] Pew found 72 per cent of health consumers presumed you could believe all or most of the health information online. Half never or hardly ever checked site information details such as source and had little concept of quality assurance. A Health on the Net survey suggested that 83 per cent of users believed in the accuracy of the information they retrieved and 79 per cent believed it was trustworthy;[5] 70 per cent of users felt they were more knowledgeable and 61 per cent in the USA and 45 per cent in Europe felt subsequent consultations were more constructive having retrieved information from the Internet.

WHAT INFORMATION?

If a patient wishes to retrieve information, there are generic health encyclopaedia sites. A patient visiting Yahoo[6] will have an alphabet of subjects to choose from, and the letter A alone offers more than 300 subjects. Using a search engine such as Google.com and enquiring about the Gerson Diet offers more than 8000 sites to visit. The volume of information is overwhelming. The Internet is akin to a very big library where all the books are kept in disarray. However, the greatest danger of the Internet is not the amount of information available but the fact that much of it is not quality controlled and it can be inaccurate. It is time to grasp the nettle.[7]

A key site for patients in the UK is NHS Direct (www.nhsdirect.nhs.uk). This is available as a telephone help line to which patients are often directed when seeking advice when the surgery is closed. Patients may also seek to use self-help groups and these are indexed on www.patient.co.uk/selfhelp/index. A valuable site for cancer patients receiving palliative care in the UK is that of Cancer BACUP (www.cancerbacup.org.uk/questions). This site has the answer to 700 common questions that can be browsed by cancer topic or searched by keywords.

QUALITY OF INFORMATION

The issue of quality is key and it was suggested by Silberg *et al.* in the *Journal of the American Medical Association*[8] that any web page that did not clearly identify the author, with credentials and affiliations, attribute the research evidence, disclose any conflict of interest, advertisers or sponsors and clearly state when the web page was created and last updated should be rejected. We cannot restrict the information that patients have access to, but we should be able to point them to reliable and quality-assured sites to help them – and we should not be afraid to do so.

Quality assurance may be achieved by using only sites that have been approved, e.g. those that have a Health on the Net badge or a Six Senses badge. However helpful these are in aiding selection, the best method may still be personally to critically appraise the sites you use and find most useful. To help you do this there are sites such as QUICK (**Qu**ality **I**nformation **ChecK**list: www.quick.org.uk) developed by the Health Education Authority. This is based around eight questions, including: 'Is the information biased?', 'Can the information be checked?' and 'Is it clear who has written the information?'. Very few Internet users later remember from which websites they retrieved information and who was responsible for the sites.[9]

Researchers at the University of Oxford have developed a more sophisticated online tool. Comprising 15 key questions, the DISCERN instrument www. discern.org.uk enables users to calculate a score to determine whether the information is credible and trustworthy. This surely is what is needed to help us feel confident about the information we are retrieving and then sharing with patients and families. This is the counterbalance to their possible non-discriminatory search for information. Patients often surf the Net until they see what matches what they wish to know, especially if looking for a cure or a better outcome. Quality information is what they may need to make a truly informed choice about their care.

SEARCHING

Patients may use conventional search engines such as Google, Yahoo, Northern Light, Infoseek or AltaVista. It may be helpful to search these sites using the key words and phrases that patients and families use, rather than technical and professional words, to see what they are offered. Search tools often do not help look beyond the front page of a site, and it may be worth browsing chosen sites in more depth if you are seeking particular information. The nature of the site retrieved may instil a higher level of confidence, for example the postscript '.ac' is an academic site, often a university, '.gov' is used by government departments, and '.org' is used by many charities and patient self-help groups.

There are meta search tools that use five or six tools combined. Inference Find (http://www.deafblind.com/search.html) is a meta search tool of six search engines; it removes duplication, and clusters the results into understandable groupings. It may also be worth seeing whether using a search engine yields more useful sites – http://www.allsearchengines.co.uk and http://turbo10.com. However, using multiple search engines is time consuming and may not yield the quality assured by peer review.[10]

DATABASES

Professionals may find the best way forward for medical information is to use a bibliographic database. The core medical databases are:

- Medline: www.ncbi.nlm.nih.gov/PubMed

- Cochrane Reviews: www.update-software.com/ccweb/cochrane/revabstra/ abidx.html

- EMBASE: www.healthgate.com/HealthGate/druginfo

- CINAHL: www.healthgate.com/HealthGate/nursing/

- PsycINFO: www.healthgate.com/HealthGate/behavior/

- CancerLit: http://cnetdb.nci.nih.gov/cancerlit.shtml.

The National Institute for Clinical Excellence (NICE: www.nice.org.uk) is part of the National Health Service and its role is to provide patients, health professionals and the public with authoritative, robust and reliable guidance on current 'best practice'. The website has two areas, one for patients and the other for professionals.

Pub Med was developed by the US National Center for Biotechnology Information in conjunction with the publishers of biomedical literature in 1997. It was upgraded in 2000 to be more user friendly and has subsequently increased the number of full text journals available to over 800. It also provides links to related datasets.

The National Electronic Library for Health (NeLH: www.nelh.nhs.uk) was created as part of the British Government's new information strategy published in September 1998. This was to establish a digital library of evidence-based material to be made available to clinicians during their day-to-day work. The NeLH was also designed to empower patients and meet the need of patients and the public for information.

Another option is to use an evaluated subject gateway. This limits access to only the Internet sites that meet a defined quality threshold. Examples of these are OMNI, Medical Matrix and Healthfinder. Lists of evaluated gateways can be found at http://henry.ugl.lib.umich.edu/megasite/.

OMNI (Organising Medical Networked Information: www.omni.ac.uk) is a health 'gateway' site. It covers medicine, biomedicine and allied health. It is a collaborative project of, among others, the Royal Free Hospital School of Medicine, the National Institute of Medical Research and the Wellcome Trust, funded by the JISC via the Electronic Libraries programme hosted by the University of Nottingham.

Medical Matrix (www.medmatrix.org) is similar to OMNI but aimed primarily at American physicians. Users and an editorial board from the American Medical Informatics Association Internet Working Group rank sites.

Healthfinder (www.healthfinder.org) was developed by the US Government and launched in April 1997. It is a gateway to consumer health resources on the

Internet. Resources are selected in accordance with a clear and explicit policy, which, among other things, states that any selected site that does not get updated within 2 years of being included will be deselected. There are more than 1000 topics, but rather than being a collection of pure data, it attempts to provide a manageable number of links that can answer most questions and point to additional sources of information. The resources used are selected because they are clear, reliable and user friendly.

Health on the Net (www.hon.ch) is an international non-profit organization dedicated to realizing the benefits of the Internet and related technologies in the fields of medicine and health care. MedHunt is a medical search tool available from that site.

If you are interested in retrieving recent data, you can limit the search to those published in the last 30 days (Pub Med) or you can pay for an update of a search each time the database is updated, e.g. OVID (www.ovid.com) or Silver Platter (www.silverplatter.com).

If you are new to the web, search tools or Medline, there are online tutorials, an example of which is available via OMNI.

DISCUSSION GROUPS

Many professional groups or others sharing a particular interest may keep in touch and share information through a discussion or news group. The problem again is that information may express the view of an individual rather than be truly evidence-based or researched. However, the Internet does enable professionals to communicate with each other, and there are subject-specific mailbases to enable this in the UK. A list of subjects including palliative medicine can be found at http://mailbase.ac.uk.

JOURNALS

Many published journals are now available in electronic format. This access may be limited to subscribers of the paper version, but many are free online. For free medical journals consider www.freemedicaljournals.com. However, many journals will offer to e-mail the index page of each issue free of charge. Therefore you can be aware of what is published and is likely to picked up by the press and then presented to you by patients. The *British Medical Journal* (www.bmj.com) is available free to the public, as is the *American Family Physician* (www.aafp.org/afp). The concept of an electronic medical library has been realized by the eMedicine World Medical Library on http://emedicine.com.

WEBSITES

Many organizations have their own websites, either stand-alone sites or within an Intranet that is produced by a hospital or other organization. These may allow desktop access to information, treatment protocols, guidelines and referral forms that can be completed online and e-mailed immediately. Suggestions to help set a standard for a website can be found in the guidelines that the NHS has set itself for websites under its own logo on www.doh.gov.uk/nhsidentity/websites.

TEACHING

Many presentations can be produced in a format such as PowerPoint and are available online. Backgrounds, photographs, X-ray examples and other images and illustrations are readily available to enhance presentation skills. Some can be accessed from Health on the Net or retrieved from search engines using key words.

CONCLUSIONS

The Internet offers unlimited opportunity to help patients, families and professionals by retrieving high-quality information. It will be necessary for us all to learn the skills to navigate the Worldwide Web and retrieve, from the vast mass of data available, the quality information needed to benefit and enhance the care of all our patients.

KEY POINTS

- Increasing numbers of patients and those close to them use the Internet to find medical information and tend to feel empowered by doing so.
- Internet-based medical information is of highly variable quality but is widely trusted by the public.
- Good sites on the web have a designated author with clear credentials, have facts supported with evidence, are regularly updated and declare sponsorship or conflicts of interest.
- Assessment tools such as DISCERN (www.discern.org.uk) are available to help assess the validity of medical information presented on the Internet.
- Palliative care practitioners should know how to harness the Internet for their own updating of knowledge and also how to guide their patients in interpreting web-derived information.
- Clinicians need to be aware of relevant bibliographic databases and of means of accessing them, e.g. Pub Med or, in the UK, the National Electronic Library for Health.

REFERENCES

1. Allum T, Mersey D. Doctors, patients and the search for truth on the Internet. *Clin Med* 2002; 2(4), 346–7.
2. Cotterill SJ. Rapid growth in the provision and usage of cancer related information available on the Internet in the UK. Implications for cancer patients, clinicians, and

researchers. Proceedings of the World Congress of the Internet in Medicine: http://www.staff.ncl.ac.uk/s.j.cotterill/sim97.htm (1997).

3. Chen X, Siu LL. Impact of the media and the Internet on oncology: survey of cancer patients and oncologists in Canada. *J Clin Oncol* 2001; **19**(23), 4291–7.

4. Pew Internet & American Life Project. Vital decisions: how Internet users decide what information to trust when they or their loved ones are sick: www.pewinternet.org/reports/toc.asp?Report=59 (2002).

5. Health on the Net Foundation. Evolution of Internet use for health purposes: www.hon.ch/survey/FebMar2001/survey.html (2001).

6. http://health.yahoo.com/health/encyclopedia/a.html.

7. Sastry S, Carroll P. Doctors, patients and the Internet: time to grasp the nettle. *Clin Med* 2002; **2**(2), 131–3.

8. Silberg J. Assessing, controlling and assuring the quality of information on the Internet: *Caveat Lector et Viewor* – Let the viewer and reader beware. *J Am Med Assoc* 1997; **277**, 1244–5.

9. Eysenbach G, Kohler C. How do consumers search for and appraise health information on the world wide web? Qualitative study using focus groups, usability tests, and in-depth interviews. *BMJ* 2002; **324**, 573–7.

10. Graber MA, Bergus GR, York C. Using the World Wide Web to answer clinical questions: how efficient are different methods of information retrieval? *J Fam Pract* 1999; **48**(7), 520–4.

Appendix 1

DRUG DATA

**Jeanette Parry-Crowther, Jennifer Todd
and Steven Wanklyn**

Drug name	Preparation	Indication for use	Dose	Caution
Adrenaline	1 in 1000 solution	Haemostasis	1 mL applied on gauze pad	
Alfentanil	1 mg/2 mL, 5 mg/10 mL inj.	Opioid-sensitive pain	Variable titration, dependent on previous opioid requirement	None, if titrated carefully against a patient's pain Severe hepatic impairment
Aminophylline	225 mg MR tabs	Reversible airways obstruction	Start at 225 mg b.d. Increase after 1 week based on plasma levels	Elderly, epilepsy, peptic ulcer, cardiac disease, hepatic impairment and hypertension Numerous drug interactions
	350 mg Forte MR tabs (MR preparation preferable)		350 mg (Forte) b.d. for smokers or others with raised theophylline clearance	
Amitriptyline	10 mg, 25 mg, 50 mg tabs 25 mg, 50 mg/5 mL liquid	Antidepressant Neuropathic pain	Start at 10–25 mg nocte and titrate every 3 days against side effects	Elderly, epilepsy, cardiac disease, hepatic impairment narrow angle glaucoma, prostatic symptoms
Baclofen	10 mg tabs 5 mg/5 mL liquid	Skeletal muscle relaxant	Start with 5 mg b.d. or t.d.s., increase by 5 mg b.d. or t.d.s. every 3 days	Peptic ulcer, epilepsy, psychiatric disorders, renal impairment, hesitancy of micturition
		Hiccups	Hiccups: 5–10 mg t.d.s.	
		Spasticity	Spasticity: 20 mg t.d.s.	
Bethanechol	10 mg, 25 mg tabs	Saliva stimulant	10–25 mg t.d.s.	Asthma, intestinal or urinary obstruction, cardiac disorders, peptic ulcer, epilepsy
Bisacodyl	5 mg tabs	Stimulant laxative	5–20 mg o.d. or b.d. orally	Large bowel obstruction
	10 mg suppos		10–20 mg o.d. p.r.	

Common side effects	Interactions	Additional information
		Vasoconstrictive and may result in ischaemic necrosis
Drowsiness, confusion, GI effects (constipation, nausea and vomiting)	Additive sedation with other CNS depressants, reduces absorption of mexiletine Unpredictable CNS stimulation with MAOIs Cimetidine and erythromycin inhibit metabolism of opioids	Synthetic opioid Alternative opioid for patients unable to tolerate diamorphine, e.g. in renal failure Alfentanil 1 mg = diamorphine 10 mg
Nausea, dyspepsia, headache, tachycardia, palpitations, hypokalaemia, anorexia, convulsions	Plasma concentration increased by ciprofloxacin, clarithromycin, erythromycin, fluconazole, calcium-channel blockers and corticosteroids Plasma concentration decreased by carbamazepine, phenytoin	Recommended therapeutic range 10–20 mcg/mL
Antimuscarinic, sedation, delirium, postural hypotension, hyponatraemia and cardiovascular	Co-administration with MAOI causing CNS excitation and hypertension Additive sedation with other CNS depressants Increased muscle relaxation with baclofen	Side effect of sedation may be useful in agitated depression Titrate to a level the individual patient can tolerate
Hypotonia, sedation, altered mood, tremor, insomnia, nystagmus, dry mouth, GI tract and urinary disturbances	Additive sedation with other CNS depressant drugs NSAIDs decrease excretion of baclofen Increased muscle relaxation with TCAs	Discontinue by gradual reduction over 1–2 weeks Some patients use spasticity to maintain posture
Parasympathominetic effects, e.g. nausea, vomiting, blurred vision, colic	Antagonism of anticholinergics	
Intestinal colic, diarrhoea, suppos may cause local inflammation		Acts on both small and large intestine

(continued)

Drug name	Preparation	Indication for use	Dose	Caution
Bupivacaine	0.25% via urethral catheter 10 mL ampoules	Pain due to direct tumour infiltration of bladder	20 mL in bladder, leave for 15 min Repeat 12-hourly	
Bupivacaine (via nebulizer)	0.25% 10 mL ampoules	Cough suppression (acts as a local anaesthetic)	5 mL of 0.25% nebulized t.d.s.–q.d.s.	Bronchospasm
Buprenorphine	200 mcg, 400 mcg SL tabs 35 mcg/h, 52.5 mcg/h, 70 mcg/h transdermal matrix patch	Opioid-sensitive pain	Initially 0.2–0.4 mg t.d.s. SL Initially 35 mcg/h patch changed every 3 days Initial doses may be dependent on previous opioid requirement	Severe hepatic impairment or hypothyroidism
Buspirone	5 mg, 10 mg tabs	Anxiolytic	5 mg b.d. or t.d.s. Increase every 2–3 days Usual dose 15–30 mg daily in divided doses	Epilepsy, hepatic or renal impairment
Calcitonin (Salmon/ salcatonin)	50 units/mL, 100 units/mL, 200 units/mL inj.	Hypercalcaemia Bone pain in neoplastic disease	5–10 units/ kg s.c or. i.m. o.d. to 400 units 6–8-hourly according to response 200 units 6-hourly or 400 units 12-hourly for 2 days, repeated if necessary	History of allergy, renal impairment, heart failure
Capsaicin	0.025%, 0.075% cream	Neuropathic pain Pruritus	Apply 3–5 times daily	Avoid contact with eyes, mucous membranes and inflamed or broken skin
Carbamazepine	100 mg, 200 mg, 400 mg tabs 200 mg, 400 mg SR tabs 100 mg/5 mL liquid	Neuropathic pain Epilepsy	100–200 mg o.d. or b.d. Increase by 100–200 mg every 2 weeks Usual dose 800–1200 mg per day in divided doses	Hepatic or renal impairment

Common side effects	Interactions	Additional information
		Consider radiotherapy where sub-optimal control
Unpleasant taste Bronchospasm: pre-treatment with broncho-dilator is recommended		Reduced sensitivity of gag reflex – avoid eating/drinking for 30–60 min after nebulizer (risk of aspiration) Limited evidence
Drowsiness, nausea, confusion, hypotension, constipation and sweating Allergy to the patch adhesive	Additive sedation with other CNS depressants Reduces absorption of mexiletine Unpredictable CNS stimulation with MAOIs Cimetidine inhibits metabolism of opioids	0.4 mg t.d.s. equivalent to 10–15 mg morphine 4-hourly 52.5 mcg/h patch equivalent to fentanyl 25 mcg/h patch Max. 2 patches applied at any one time Max. dose of combined patches 140 mcg/24 h
Nausea, dizziness, head-ache, light-headedness		Response may take up to 2 weeks Does not alleviate benzodiazepine withdrawal
Nausea, vomiting, diar-rhoea, dizziness, flushing, abdominal pain, tingling hands		Can be used in conjunction with bispho-sphonates in the emergency situation
Transient burning sensa-tion may occur during initial treatment but should lessen over 2–3 days		Avoid taking hot showers or baths just before or after applying capsaicin – burning sensation enhanced
Nausea, vomiting, drowsi-ness, ataxia, confusion, leucopenia, visual disturbance, erythematous rash, constipation or diarrhoea	Effects enhanced by dextroprop-oxyphene and fluoxetine Reduces effect of warfarin, digoxin, tricyclics, haloperidol, steroids, tramadol	SR preps are best taken b.d. SR formulations smooth out plasma levels, so reducing side effects and aiding compliance

(continued)

Drug name	Preparation	Indication for use	Dose	Caution
Carbocisteine	375 mg caps 125 mg, 250 mg/ 5 mL liquid	Mucolytic agent – reduction of sputum viscosity	750 mg t.d.s. Reduce to b.d. when satisfactory response	Active peptic ulcer
Chlorpromazine	10 mg, 25 mg, 50 mg, 100 mg tabs 25 mg, 100 mg/ 5 mL liquid 25 mg/mL, 50 mg/2 mL inj.	Hiccups	25–50 mg t.d.s. or q.d.s. orally (or 25–50 mg deep i.m. inj.	Elderly, hepatic and renal impairement, epilepsy, Parkinson's disease, postural hypotension, cardiac disease, closed angle glaucoma
Chlorpropamide	100 mg, 250 mg tabs	Oral hypoglycaemic (long acting)	100–250 mg o.d. Adjust according to response	Elderly, hepatic and renal impairment
Cimetidine	200 mg, 400 mg, 800 mg tabs 200 mg/5 mL liquid	Sweating (anecdotal)	400–800 mg o.d.	Hepatic and renal impairment
Citalopram	10 mg, 20 mg, 40 mg tabs 40 mg/mL oral drops	Depressive illness or panic disorder	20 mg o.d. Increase to max. 60 mg Panic: 10 mg o.d. Increase to 20–30 mg after 7 days	Epilepsy, cardiac disease, diabetes mellitus, GI or other bleeding disorders, hepatic and renal impairment, closed angle glaucoma
Clobazam	10 mg tabs	Adjunctive treatment of epilepsy	10 mg nocte, increasing at 10 mg increments up to 60 mg in 2 divided doses	Caution in respiratory depression, elderly, renal and hepatic impairment
Clonazepam	0.5 mg, 2 mg tabs 1 mg/mL inj.	Myoclonus Neuropathic pain Anticonvulsant	0.5–2 mg o.d. orally or s.c. Initially 1 mg o.d., increased over 2–4 weeks to 4–8 mg in divided doses 2–8 mg/ 24 h s.c.	Elderly, hepatic and renal impairment Caution in reduced respiration

Common side effects	Interactions	Additional information
Occasional GI irritation, rashes		Beware of copious liquid sputum that weak patient is unable to cough up. Useful with end-stage fibrotic lung disease and COPD
Antimuscarinic, extra-pyramidal, hypotension and interference with body temperature	Additive sedation with other CNS depressants	50 mg orally = 25 mg i.m.
Hypoglycaemia, GI disturbance, headache, hyponatraemia	Steroids, loop and thiazide diuretics antagonize hypoglycaemic effect. Fluconazole enhances hypogly-caemic effect	Longer acting should not be used in anorexic patients. Generally avoid use in favour of shorter acting analogues
Diarrhoea, headache, dizziness, rash	Binds to cytochrome P450. Avoid in patients stabilized on war-farin, phenytoin and theophylline. Inhibits metabolism of opioid analgesics	Altered LFTs. Rarely, liver damage
GI side effects, anorexia, weight loss, hypersensi-tivity reactions, dry mouth, anxiety, headache, insomnia, arthralgia, myalgia	Increased CNS toxicity with tramadol. Increased risk of bleeding with NSAID	SSRI should not be started for 2 weeks after stopping MAOI
Drowsiness, light-headedness, confusion, ataxia	Additive sedative effects with other CNS depressants	Effectiveness may wane on prolonged use. Avoid abrupt withdrawal
Drowsiness, fatigue, dizziness, poor co-ordination	Additive sedative effects with other CNS depressants	Avoid sudden withdrawal. Tolerance develops within 3 months when used as an anticonvulsant, so rarely used long term

(continued)

Drug name	Preparation	Indication for use	Dose	Caution
Codeine phosphate	15 mg, 30 mg, 60 mg tabs 25 mg/ 5 mL liquid	Diarrhoea Mild to moderate pain	30–60 mg every 4–6 h	Caution in renal impairment or hypothyroidism
Codeine phosphate linctus	15 mg/5 mL liquid (also diabetic prep.)	Cough	5–10 mL p.r.n. 4–6-hourly	See codeine phosphate
Colestyramine (cholestyramine)	4 g sachets	Pruritus associated with biliary obstruction	4–8 g daily in plenty of water or flavoured liquid	Intestinal and complete biliary obstruction
Co-proxamol	Combined preparation tabs	Mild to moderate pain	1–2 tabs every 4–6 h	Caution in renal impairment or hypothyroidism
Cyclizine	50 mg tabs 50 mg/mL inj.	Nausea and vomiting	50 mg t.d.s. oral 150 mg/24 h s.c.	Severe heart failure, hepatic disease, renal impairment
Dantrolene	25 mg, 100 mg caps	Skeletal muscle relaxant	25 mg o.d. starting dose Increase by 25 mg weekly Usual effective dose 75 mg t.d.s. Max. dose 100 mg q.d.s.	Hepatic impairment, impaired cardiac or pulmonary function
Demeclocycline	150 mg caps	SIADH	300 mg b.d.–q.d.s. Maintenance 300 mg b.d. or t.d.s.	Hepatic and renal impairment
Desmopressin	100 mcg, 200 mcg tabs 10 mcg metered nasal spray	Refractory nocturia (exclude infection)	200–400 mcg orally o.d. 20–40 mcg intranasally o.d.	Cardiovascular disease, renal impairment and hypertension

Common side effects	Interactions	Additional information
Drowsiness, nausea, vomiting, confusion constipation	Sedation effects with other CNS depressants Reduces absorption of mexiletine Unpredictable CNS stimulation with MAOIs Cimetidine inhibits metabolism of opioids	30 mg codeine p.o = 3 mg morphine p.o.
See codeine phosphate		
GI side effects mainly, especially constipation	Other drugs should be taken 1 h before or 4–6 h after to reduce interference with their absorption	
Drowsiness, nausea, vomiting, confusion, constipation	May increase carbamazepine levels and the risk of bleeding with warfarin Additive sedative effects with other CNS depressants	Paracetamol 325 mg + dextro-propoxyphene 32.5 mg
Antimuscarinic, drowsiness	Additive sedative effects with other CNS depressants Adverse effects increased by tricyclics, haloperidol Blocks prokinetic effects of metoclopramide	Particularly useful for symptoms due to secondary bowel obstruction and raised intracranial pressure
Transient drowsiness, dizziness, muscle weakness, diarrhoea	Calcium-channel blockers (risk of arrhythmias – only with i.v. dantrolene)	Some patients use spasticity to maintain posture Dose should be built up slowly, although some centres increase more rapidly because of patient's limited prognosis
Nausea, vomiting, diarrhoea, dysphagia, oesophageal irritation	Avoid milk, antacids and iron preparations for 1 h after a dose	Photosensitivity risk is very rare
Water retention, hyponatraemia, vomiting, headache and stomach pain		Advise to restrict fluids in evening Use with care if risk of water retention

(continued)

Drug name	Preparation	Indication for use	Dose	Caution
Dexamethasone	0.5 mg, 2 mg tabs 2 mg/5 mL liquid 4 mg/mL inj.	High dose – peritumour oedema	8–24 mg o.d.	Systemic infection, diabetes mellitus
Dexamfetamine (dexamphet-amine)	5 mg tabs	Depression in advanced disease	2.5–10 mg daily	Cardiac disease, history of epilepsy
Diamorphine	5 mg, 10 mg, 30 mg, 100 mg, 500 mg inj.	Opioid-sensitive pain	Variable titration, dependent on previous opioid requirement	Caution in renal impairment or hypothyroidism
Diazepam	2 mg, 5 mg, 10 mg tabs 2 mg/5 mL solution 10 mg supp 5 mg, 10 mg rectal tubes	Anxiolytic Muscle relaxant (lower doses) Anticonvulsant	2–20 mg o.d. in divided doses 10 mg p.r./i.v. stat p.r.n. Common range 10–30 mg daily	Caution in respiratory depression and elderly (half doses)
Diclofenac	25 mg, 50 mg tabs 50 mg disp. tabs 75 mg, 100 mg MR tabs 50 mg, 100 mg suppos 75 mg/3 mL inj.	Pain, especially associated with tissue inflammation	50 mg t.d.s. 75 mg SR b.d. or 100 mg SR o.d. 50–100 mg p.r. 150 mg/24 h CSCI	Active peptic ulceration Hypersensitivity to aspirin or other NSAIDs Renal impairment
Dihydrocodeine	30 mg tablets 60 mg, 90 mg, 120 mg SR tablets 10 mg/5 mL oral liquid 50 mg/mL inj.	Moderate to severe pain	30–60 mg 4–6-hourly For SR, 60–120 mg b.d.	Caution in renal impairment or hypothyroidism

Common side effects	Interactions	Additional information
GI, musculoskeletal, endocrine, neuropsychiatric effects Impaired wound healing	Co-administration with NSAIDs (increased risk of GI bleeding) Phenytoin and carbamazepine may reduce the bioavailability Higher doses may be needed May affect response to warfarin	If given for more than 2 weeks, should not be stopped abruptly
Insomnia, nervousness, raised blood pressure, motor tics, dyskinesias, headache, GI symptoms and psychotic symptoms	Avoid co-administration of MAOIs	Rapid action against severe psychomotor slowing and fatigue (usually 36–48 h) Should be given in the morning to avoid sleep disturbance at night
Drowsiness, confusion, GI effects (constipation, nausea and vomiting)	Sedative effects with other CNS depressants Reduces absorption of mexiletine Unpredictable CNS stimulation with MAOIs Cimetidine inhibits metabolism of opioids	As effective as morphine Ratio 3:1, p.o.:s.c.
Drowsiness, light headedness, confusion, ataxia	Sedative effect enhanced with other CNS depressants, baclofen Cimetidine and omeprazole inhibit metabolism Anti-epileptic levels may vary	In elderly may have prolonged half-life Accumulation of active metabolites may require dose reduction after 7 days
GI side effects (especially dyspepsia), headache, dizziness	Nephrotoxicity increased by diuretics Increases adverse effects of warfarin, phenytoin, steroids, baclofen	Avoid in renal failure Must be given in separate syringe driver – immiscible with other drugs
Drowsiness, confusion, GI effects (constipation, nausea and vomiting)	Sedative effects enhanced with other CNS depressants Reduces absorption of mexiletine Unpredictable CNS stimulation with MAOIs Cimetidine inhibits metabolism of opioids	One-tenth as potent as morphine Increased risk of toxicity in severe renal failure, reduce to 8-hourly

(continued)

Drug name	Preparation	Indication for use	Dose	Caution
Disodium pamidronate	15 mg, 30 mg, 90 mg inj.	Hypercalcaemia Bone pain	15–90 mg by infusion at rate of 1 mg/min depending on serum calcium level (according to SPC)	Renal impairment
Docusate sodium	100 mg caps 50 mg/5 mL solution	Surfactant laxative Partial bowel obstruction	Start at 100 mg b.d., up to 500 mg in divided doses orally	
Domperidone	10 mg tabs 30 mg suppos 5 mg/5 mL suspension	Nausea and vomiting	10–20 mg t.d.s. oral 30–60 mg b.d.– t.d.s. rectal	Intestinal obstruction
Doxepin	10 mg, 25 mg, 50 mg, 75 mg caps	Antidepressant	75 mg o.d. in divided doses or single dose o.d.	Recent MI or arrhythmias, narrow angle glaucoma, prostatic symptoms (see amitriptyline)
	5% cream	Antipruritic: apply t.d.s.–q.d.s., max. 12 g/day		Drowsiness, local irritation
Etamsylate (ethamsylate)	500 mg tabs	Surface bleeding from ulcerating tumours	500 mg q.d.s.	
Fentanyl transdermal	25 mcg/h, 50 mcg/h, 75 mcg/h, 100 mcg/h patches	Opioid-sensitive pain	Variable titration, dependent on previous opioid requirement Change patch every 3 days	Unstable pain

Common side effects	Interactions	Additional information
Approximately 10% of patients develop a transient pyrexia Influenza-like symptoms start within 24–48 h and resolve within 72 h Musculoskeletal, headache and nausea	May cause hypocalcaemia if given concurrently with aminoglycosides	Rate should not exceed 1 mg/min Reduce dose and speed of infusion in renal impairment
Diarrhoea, unpleasant aftertaste or burning sensation, minimized by drinking plenty of water	Enhances absorption of liquid paraffin	Evidence for laxative efficacy is limited
Acute dystonia (rare), rash	Prokinetic effect blocked by antimuscarinics	Poor oral bioavailability 30 mg p.r. = 10 mg p.o. Does not cross blood–brain barrier
Anticholinergic, epilepsy and severe liver disease (see amitriptyline)	Additive sedative effects with other CNS depressants	Titrate to a level the individual patient can tolerate Sedative effect may be useful in agitated depression
Headache, rash, nausea (when taken on empty stomach)		
Drowsiness, confusion, GI effects (constipation, nausea and vomiting) Rare reactions to patch adhesive	Sedative effects enhanced with other CNS depressants Reduces absorption of mexiletine Unpredictable CNS stimulation with MAOIs Cimetidine inhibits metabolism of opioids	Systemic analgesic concentration reached within 12 h Increased absorption in febrile patients or those with other factors changing skin integrity

(continued)

Drug name	Preparation	Indication for use	Dose	Caution
Fentanyl citrate transmucosal	200 mcg, 400 mcg, 600 mcg, 800 mcg, 1.2 mg, 1.6 mg lozenge	Breakthrough pain in patients on regular strong opioids	200 mcg initially over 15 min Repeated if necessary after 15 min of first dose (no more than 2 doses for each pain episode) Adjust dose according to response as per SPC Max. 4 dose units daily once satis-factory dose achieved	Intact oral mucosa
Fluoxetine	20 mg, 60 mg caps 20 mg/5 mL liquid	Depression	20 mg daily to max. 60 mg	Epilepsy, cardiac disease, diabetes mellitus, GI bleeding disorders, hepatic and renal impairment
Gabapentin	100 mg, 300 mg, 400 mg, 600 mg, 800 mg tabs	Neuropathic pain	300 mg o.d. day 1, 300 mg b.d. day 2, 300 mg t.d.s. day 3 Increase by 300 mg as required to max. 1.8 g	Elderly, renal impairment, diabetes mellitus
Glibenclamide	2.5 mg, 5 mg tabs	Oral hypoglycaemic (long acting)	2.5–5 mg o.d. Adjust according to response	Elderly, hepatic and renal impairment
Gliclazide	80 mg tabs 30 mg MR tabs	Oral hypoglycaemic (short acting)	40–80 mg o.d. up to max. 320 mg daily 30 mg MR o.d., adjusted 4-weekly to max. 120 mg	Hepatic and renal impairment
Glycopyrronium bromide (glycopyrrolate)	200 mcg/mL inj.	Bronchial secretions Abdominal colic Sialorrhoea	200–400 mcg s.c. stat or 600–1200 mcg CSCI/24 h	

Common side effects	Interactions	Additional information
See fentanyl transdermal Rarely, mouth ulceration	See fentanyl transdermal	Lozenge should be rubbed up and down the side of the cheek at intervals until dissolved Moistening the mouth may help; do not chew
GI side effects, anorexia, weight loss, hypersensitivity reactions, dry mouth, anxiety, headache, insomnia	Increased CNS toxicity with tramadol Plasma concentration of carbamazepine increased Increased risk of bleeding with NSAIDs	SSRI should not be started for 2 weeks after stopping MAOI
Ataxia, fatigue, drowsiness and dizziness	Reduced absorption with antacids Additive sedation with other CNS depressants	Slower titration with the elderly, or those on other CNS depressants
Hypoglycaemia, GI disturbance, headache	Steroids, loop and thiazide diuretics antagonize hypoglycaemic effect	Longer acting should not be used in anorexic patients
Hypoglycaemia, GI disturbance, headache	Steroids, loop and thiazide diuretics antagonize hypoglycaemic effect	Should be used in preference to a long-acting sulphonylurea
Tachycardia, drowsiness, dry mouth, blurred vision, urinary retention	Increased adverse effects of antidepressants Blocks prokinesis of metoclopramide and domperidone	Less sedating than hyoscine hydrobromide as does not cross blood–brain barrier

(continued)

Drug name	Preparation	Indication for use	Dose	Caution
Granisetron	1 mg, 2 mg tabs 1 mg/5 mL syrup 1 mg/mL inj.	Nausea and vomiting, especially with highly emetogenic chemotherapy	1–2 mg p.o. or s.c. o.d.	Subacute intestinal obstruction
Haloperidol	0.5 mg caps 1.5 mg, 5 mg, 10 mg, 20 mg tabs 10 mg/5 mL liquid 5 mg/mL inj.	Nausea and vomiting Anxiety Confusion	1.5–5 mg/24 h oral or s.c. Higher doses 0.5–1 mg p.o. q.d.s. 3–5 mg stat s.c./i.m., then 1.5–3 mg t.d.s. 5–10 mg CSCI for antipsychotic effect	Parkinson's disease, cardiovascular disease, additive sedation with other CNS depressants
Hydromorphone	1.3 mg, 2.6 mg IR caps 2 mg, 4 mg, 6 mg, 12 mg, 24 mg, 48 mg SR caps	Opioid-sensitive pain	Variable titration, dependent on previous opioid requirement	Prolonged use in renal impairment as metabolites may accumulate
Hyoscine butylbromide	10 mg tabs 20 mg/mL inj.	Bronchial secretions Smooth muscle spasm Renal colic	20 mg s.c. stat dose 20–120 mg/24 h oral or CSCI 20 mg s.c. p.r.n.	
Hyoscine hydrobromide	0.3 mg tabs SL 1 mg/72 h patch 400 mcg, 600 mcg/mL inj.	Bronchial secretions	400–600 mcg s.c. stat 1.2–2.4 mg/24 h CSCI 400 mcg p.r.n.	
Ibuprofen	200 mg, 400 mg, 600 mg tabs 100 mg/5 mL liquid	Bone pain	200–600 mg t.d.s.	Active peptic ulceration Hypersensitivity to aspirin or other NSAIDs Renal impairment
Imipramine	10 mg, 25 mg tabs 25 mg/5 mL liquid	Nocturnal urinary frequency/urge incontinence	10–50 mg nocte	As for amitriptyline

Common side effects	Interactions	Additional information
Constipation, headache, facial flushing, rash, occasional alterations in LFTs	Do not give i.v. concurrently with i.v. metoclopramide	
Extrapyramidal effects, sedation, antimuscarinic effects, hypotension neuroleptic malignant syndrome	Increased adverse effects with fluoxetine, metoclopramide and other CNS drugs Plasma concentration halved by concurrent use of carbamazepine	Reduce dose in elderly
Drowsiness, confusion, GI effects (constipation, nausea and vomiting)	Sedative effects enhanced with other CNS depressants Reduces absorption of mexiletine Unpredictable CNS stimulation with MAOIs Cimetidine inhibits metabolism of opioids	Alternative opioid Hydromorphone 1.3 mg p.o. = morphine 10 mg p.o.
Antimuscarinic	Blocks effects of prokinetics	Poor oral absorption Does not cross blood–brain barrier so does not cause drowsiness/paradoxical hyperexcitation Relieves death rattle in 50–60% of patients
Antimuscarinic	Blocks effects of prokinetics	Can accumulate and result in paradoxical agitated delirium Relieves death rattle in 50–60% of patients
GI side effects (especially dyspepsia), headache, dizziness	Nephrotoxicity increased by diuretics Increases anticoagulation effects of warfarin and levels of phenytoin, steroids, baclofen	First-line NSAID Lower risks of side effects than other NSAIDs but less potent
As for amitriptyline but less sedating	As for amitriptyline	Elderly may not tolerate starting dose above 10 mg

(continued)

Drug name	Preparation	Indication for use	Dose	Caution
Ipratropium bromide	20 mcg/ 40 mcg (Forte) inhaler 250 mcg/mL, 500 mcg/2 mL nebulizing solution	Reversible airways obstruction	1–2 puffs (20–40 mcg) t.d.s. – 250–500 mcg q.d.s.	Glaucoma, prostatic hypertrophy
Ketamine	200 mg, 500 mg, 1000 mg vial for inj.	Neuropathic pain unresponsive to other neuropathic agents	Starting dose 10 mg s.c. or 30 mg p.o. Otherwise s.c. infusion 50–300 mg/24 h or 100–200 mg 6-hourly p.o.	Hypertension, schizophrenia, acute psychosis Raised intracranial pressure, cardiac failure
Ketorolac	10 mg tabs 10, 30 mg/mL inj.	Severe pain associated with soft-tissue and bone metastases	60 mg/24 h CSCI Increase by 15 mg/24 h up to 90 mg/24 h	History of ulcer or GI bleeding, asthma, abnormal renal or liver function, hypersensitivity to aspirin or other NSAIDs
Lactulose	3.1–3.7 g/5 mL liquid	Softening/osmotic laxative	15 mL t.d.s. Adjust according to need	Lactose intolerance, intestinal obstruction
Levomepromazine (methotrimeprazine)	6.25 mg, 25 mg tabs 25 mg/mL inj.	Nausea and vomiting Agitation/terminal restlessness	6.25–25 mg p.o. at night 6.25–12.5/24 h CSCI for nausea/ vomiting Higher doses for agitation (up to 300 mg)	Epilepsy, postural hypotension, Parkinsonism, hypothyroidism
Lidocaine (lignocaine)	2% gel	Pain	Topically as required	
Liquid paraffin	Liquid oral emulsion	Lubricant laxative		Avoid prolonged use

Common side effects	Interactions	Additional information
Dry mouth, narrow angle glaucoma, nausea, constipation and headache		
Dysphoria, hallucinations, sedation, confusion, increased muscle tone In higher doses, tachycardia and hypertension may occur. Erythema and pain at injection site	Increased risk of convulsions with theophylline (higher doses) Raised levels with diazepam	Neuropsychiatric effects may be reduced by the concurrent use of benzodiazepines/haloperidol Opioid-sparing effect
GI side effects (especially dyspepsia), headache, dizziness Increases anticoagulant effect of warfarin Pain and bleeding at injection site	Decreases diuretic response with frusemide Increases risk of renal impairment with ACE inhibitors Nephrotoxicity increased by diuretics Increases anticoagulation effects of warfarin and levels of phenytoin, steroids, baclofen	Co-prescribe misoprostol or lansoprazole Compatible with diamorphine in a syringe driver if used with normal saline as diluent
Flatulence in 20% of users Abdominal bloating, colic		Expensive Large volumes needed if used alone in marked constipation
Sedation, especially over 25 mg/24 h, anti-cholinergic, postural hypotension (dose dependent)		Higher doses may be used with caution May lower fit threshold
		Topical analgesia
Chronic paraffin use can cause fat-soluble vitamin deficiencies Anal seepage can cause local irritation Lipid pneumonia		Liquid paraffin combined with magnesium hydroxide is currently most common form (Milpar) Cheap

(continued)

Drug name	Preparation	Indication for use	Dose	Caution
Lorazepam	1 mg, 2.5 mg tabs	Breathlessness Anxiety Anticipatory vomiting	0.5–1 mg p.r.n. oral or SL	
Magnesium hydroxide	Susp.	Softening/osmotic laxative (also stimulant at higher doses)	25–50 mL	Acute GI conditions, renal and hepatic impairment
Magnesium sulphate (Epsom salts)	Powder 4–5 g/ 10 mL solution (prepared extempora- neously)	Softening/osmotic laxative (also stimu- lant at higher doses)	4–10 g of powder dissolved in warm water and taken with extra fluid	Acute GI conditions, renal and hepatic impairment
Medroxyproges- terone	100 mg, 200 mg, 250 mg, 400 mg, 500 mg tabs	Appetite stimulant	400 mg daily Consider doubling dose if initial poor response (doses of up to 500 mg b.d. have been used)	Epilepsy, hyperten- sion, migraine, asthma, cardiac/ arterial disease, hepatic or renal dys- function, history of liver/genital tumours, diabetes mellitus
Megestrol acetate	40 mg, 160 mg tabs	Appetite stimulant	80–160 mg daily Consider doubling dose if initial poor response (doses of up to 1600 mg have been used; elderly may respond to 80 mg/day max.)	As for medroxy- progesterone
Metformin	500 mg, 850 mg tabs	Oral hypoglycaemic	500 mg t.d.s. or 850 mg b.d.	Hepatic impairment Must not be used if even mild renal impairment
Methadone	2 mg/5 mL linctus	Antitussive	1–2 mg 4–6-hourly	

Common side effects	Interactions	Additional information
Drowsiness, confusion light-headedness, ataxia	Additive sedation with other CNS depressants, baclofen, cimetidine Raises digoxin and lowers carbamazepine levels	Intermediate acting Half-life 10–20 h
Colic		Cheap
Colic, risk of hypermagne-saemia with chronic use		Cheap More potent than hydroxide Can give sensation of distension and cause sudden passage of liquid faeces Difficult to adjust dose
Nausea, fluid retention, weight gain, urticaria, acne, hypertension, consti-pation, fatigue, depression, insomnia		Greatest benefit if used earlier in course of disease Adding a NSAID may enhance efficacy
As for medroxyproges-terone		Weight gain correlates with dose used and length of treatment Max. weight gain can take up to 14 weeks As effective as steroids for weight gain fewer side effects Adding a NSAID may enhance efficacy
Abdominal pain, anorexia, nausea, vomiting, flatu-lence, diarrhoea	Hypoglycaemic effect antagonized by loop and thiazide diuretics Cimetidine raises metformin levels	May exacerbate anorexia, especially if taken on empty stomach
Drowsiness, confusion, GI effects (constipation, nausea and vomiting)	Sedative effects enhanced with other CNS depressants Reduces absorption of mexiletine Unpredictable CNS stimulation with MAOIs Cimetidine inhibits metabolism of opioids	Beware of accumulation with prolonged use

(continued)

Drug name	Preparation	Indication for use	Dose	Caution
Methylphenidate	5 mg, 10 mg, 20 mg tabs	Depression in advanced disease	5 mg b.d., increasing every few days up to 15 mg b.d.	Cardiac disease, history of epilepsy
Metoclopramide	10 mg tabs 15 mg SR tabs 5 mg/5 mL liquid 10 mg/2 mL inj.	Nausea and vomiting Hiccups	10–20 mg q.d.s. 30–120 mg CSCI	Hepatic and renal impairment
Mexiletine	50 mg, 200 mg caps	Neuropathic pain	50 mg t.d.s. up to 10 mg/kg	Hepatic impairment
Midazolam	10 mg/2 mL inj. 10 mg/5 mL inj.	Terminal agitation Anticonvulsant	2.5–20 mg s.c. stat 30–60 mg CSCI (up to 240 mg reported) 10–20 mg s.c. stat p.r.n. 30–60 mg/24 h CSCI	
Morphine	10 mg, 20 mg, 50 mg IR tabs 10 mg/5 mL, 20 mg/mL liquid 5 mg, 10 mg, 15 mg, 30 mg, 60 mg, 100 mg, 200 mg SR tabs; 20 mg, 30 mg, 60 mg, 100 mg, 200 mg oral susp. granules 30 mg, 60 mg, 90 mg, 120 mg, 150 mg, 200 mg XL once-daily caps 10 mg, 15 mg, 20 mg, 30 mg supp	Opioid-sensitive pain	4-hourly 4-hourly 12-hourly 24-hourly Variable titration, dependent on previous opioid requirement	Renal impairment or hypothyroidism

Common side effects	Interactions	Additional information
As for dexamfetamine, also rash and arthralgia	May inhibit metabolism of tricyclics and warfarin Increased plasma concentration of phenytoin	Rapid action against severe psychomotor slowing and fatigue Should be given in the morning to avoid sleep disturbance at night
Extrapyramidal effects, drowsiness, restlessness and diarrhoea	Contraindicated with concurrent administration of antimuscarinic drugs or i.v. administration with 5HT3 receptor antagonists	Antagonizes 5HT3 at higher doses
Nausea, vomiting, constipation, bradycardia, hypotension, atrial fibrillation, palpitations, drowsiness, tremor and nystagmus	Opioid analgesics and antimuscarinics delay absorption Action of mexiletine antagonized by hypokalaemia due to loop and thiazide diuretics Pro-arrhythmogenic drugs (TCAs) should be stopped 48 h prior	Rarely used in palliative care
Drowsiness	If patient does not settle on 30 mg/24 h, an antipsychotic should be added before increasing dose further	Reduce dose in elderly
Drowsiness, confusion, GI effects (constipation, nausea and vomiting)	Sedative effects enhanced with other CNS depressants Reduces absorption of mexiletine Unpredictable CNS stimulation with MAOIs Cimetidine and erythromycin inhibit metabolism of opioids	Morphine p.o. one-third as potent as s.c. diamorphine

(continued)

Drug name	Preparation	Indication for use	Dose	Caution
Nabilone	1 mg caps	Persistent dyspnoea	0.1 mg b.d. to start Increase by 0.1 mg increments every 3–5 days (up to about 1 mg daily in 4 divided doses)	Elderly, psychiatric history, hyper-tension, hepatic impairment, cardiac disease
Naproxen	250 mg, 375 mg, 500 mg tabs 500 mg MR tabs 125 mg/5 mL susp.	Pain associated with tissue inflammation Neoplastic fever	250–500 mg b.d. (up to 500 mg t.d.s.)	Active peptic ulceration, hyper-sensitivity to aspirin or other NSAIDs, renal impairment
Olanzapine	2.5 mg, 5 mg, 7.5 mg, 10 mg tabs 5 mg, 10 mg disp. tabs	Agitation and delirium	2.5–5 mg o.d.	Parkinson's disease, hepatic and renal impairment, epilepsy, narrow angle glaucoma, diabetes mellitus
Ondansetron	4 mg, 8 mg tabs and oral disp. tabs 4 mg/5 mL syrup 16 mg suppos 4 mg/2 mL, 8 mg/4 mL inj.	Nausea and vomiting, especially with highly emeto-genic chemotherapy	4–8 mg b.d. oral 8–16 mg/24 h CSCI	Hepatic impairment
Oxybutynin	2.5 mg, 3 mg, 5 mg tabs 5 mg, 10 mg MR tabs 2.5 mg/5 mL susp.	Bladder spasms and urgency	2.5–5 mg b.d.–q.d.s.	Hepatic and renal impairment, intestinal obstruc-tion or atony, bladder outflow obstruction May worsen CCF and arrhythmias Reflux oesophagitis

Common side effects	Interactions	Additional information
Drowsiness, confusion, dizziness, headache, altered mood, dry mouth, nausea	Alcohol, anxiolytics and hypnotics potentiate sedative effect	1 mg is the lowest strength available The solution for 0.1 mg strength needs to be made up specially by a pharmacy
GI side effects (especially dyspepsia), headache, dizziness	Nephrotoxicity increased by diuretics Increases adverse effects of warfarin, phenytoin, steroids, baclofen	
Drowsiness, weight gain, dry mouth, constipation	Omeprazole, carbamazepine and rifampicin decrease olanzapine plasma concentrations Olanzapine potentiates the sedative effects of alcohol and other CNS depressants	Oral dispersible tablets are placed on the tongue or dispersed in water, orange juice, apple juice, milk or coffee before administration
Constipation, headache, facial flushing, hiccups, occasional alterations in LFTs		8 mg daily in moderate/severe hepatic impairment Oral dispersible tablets should be allowed to dissolve on the tongue
Dry mouth, nausea, abdominal discomfort, other antimuscarinic effects Cognitive function and delirium in the elderly		

(continued)

Drug name	Preparation	Indication for use	Dose	Caution
Oxycodone	5 mg, 10 mg, 20 mg NR caps	Opioid-sensitive pain	4–6-hourly	Renal impairment or hypothyroidism
	5 mg/5 mL, 10 mg/1 mL liquid		4–6-hourly	
	5 mg, 10 mg, 20 mg, 40 mg, 80 mg SR tabs		12-hourly	
	10 mg/mL inj.		4-hourly CSCI/ 24 h Variable titration, dependent on previous opioid requirement	
Paracetamol	500 mg tabs 500 mg disp. tabs 250 mg/5 mL liquid 500 mg suppos	Mild to moderate pain	0.5–1 g 4–6-hourly	Hepatic impairment Hypersensitivity to aspirin or NSAIDs
Paroxetine	20 mg, 30 mg tabs 10 mg/5 mL liquid	Depression and panic disorder	20 mg o.d. up to max. 50 mg Panic: 10 mg o.d., increased to 50 mg daily	As for fluoxetine
Phenobarbital (phenobarbitone)	200 mg/mL	Terminal agitation Anticonvulsant	100–300 mg s.c. 600–1200 mg/24 h CSCI 200–400 mg/24 h CSCI	Elderly, impaired hepatic or renal function
Phenytoin	50 mg, 100 mg tabs 25 mg, 50 mg, 100 mg, 300 mg caps 50 mg chewable 'Infatabs', 30 mg/5 mL susp., 90 mg/5 mL susp.	Anticonvulsant	150–300 mg daily as a single dose, or divided if nausea Increase gradually to 500 mg daily	Hepatic impairment

Common side effects	Interactions	Additional information
Drowsiness, confusion, GI effects (constipation, nausea and vomiting)	Sedative effects enhanced with other CNS depressants Reduces absorption of mexiletine Unpredictable CNS stimulation with MAOIs Cimetidine and erythromycin inhibit metabolism of opioids	20 mg of oral oxycodone is equivalent to 10 mg of injectable oxycodone
Occasional rash	Action increased by metoclopramide and domperidone Action reduced by antimuscarinic agents	
As for fluoxetine	As for fluoxetine	During initial treatment for panic disorder, symptoms may worsen SSRI should not be started for 2 weeks after stopping MAOI Extrapyramidal reactions and withdrawal syndrome are more common with paroxetine Avoid abrupt withdrawal
Drowsiness, mental depression, ataxia, allergic skin reactions	Lowers plasma concentration of carbamazepine, warfarin, clonazepam, phenytoin, valproate and steroids	Do not combine with other drugs in syringe driver
Nausea, vomiting, delirium, dizziness, acne, hirsutism, gingival hypertrophy, ataxia, slurred speech, nystagmus and blurred vision are signs of over-dosage Rash: discontinue	Reduces therapeutic effect of steroids – patients may therefore require higher doses Reduces plasma levels of mirtazapine, paroxetine, TCAs, carbamazepine, clonazepam, lamotrigine, theophylline and valproate Variable effect with warfarin Some enteral feeds and sucralfate may interfere with absorption of phenytoin NSAIDs, aspirin and fluoxetine raise plasma levels of phenytoin	Advantage of once-daily dosing Difficult pharmacokinetics – needs to be monitored closely Avoid sudden withdrawal Care is needed when changing between preparations that contain either phenytoin or its sodium salt due to unequivalent bioavailability

(continued)

Drug name	Preparation	Indication for use	Dose	Caution
Polyethylene glycol (macrogols)	Oral powder	Osmotic laxative Oral treatment for faecal impaction and chronic constipation	2–3 sachets daily in divided doses for up to 2 weeks 8 sachets daily, drunk within 6 h, repeated for 3 days for faecal impaction	Intestinal obstruction
Risperidone	500 mcg, 1 mg, 2 mg, 3 mg, 4 mg, 6 mg tabs 1 mg, 2 mg orodispersible tabs 1 mg/mL oral solution	Acute and chronic psychoses Delirium Behavioural and psychological symptoms in dementia	1 mg b.d., increasing to 2 mg b.d. and 3 mg b.d. on successive days 500 mcg b.d. Increase if necessary 1 mg o.d	Parkinson's disease, epilepsy, hepatic and renal impairment
Salbutamol	100 mcg aerosol inhaler 2.5 mg/ 2.5 mL 5 mg/ 2.5 mL nebulizing solution	Reversible airways obstruction	1–2 puffs t.d.s.–q.d.s. 2.5–5 mg q.d.s. nebulized	Myocardial insuffi-ciency, arrhythmias, hypertension
Senna	7.5 mg tabs 15 mg/5 mL granules 7.5 mg/5 mL syrup	Stimulant laxative	15 mg daily starting dose (b.d. dose often required) Increase if necessary to 15–22.5 mg t.d.s.	Large bowel obstruction
Sertraline	50 mg, 100 mg tabs	Depression	50 mg daily up to max. 200 mg daily	Epilepsy, cardiac disease, diabetes mellitus, GI bleeding disorders hepatic and renal impairment
Sodium clodronate	60 mg/mL 5 ml inj. 400 mg caps 800 mg tabs 520 mg tabs	Hypercalcaemia of malignancy Bone pain due to metastases	1500 mg i.v. 1.6–3.2 g orally o.d. or in divided doses 2 tabs o.d., increased to max. 4 tabs o.d. in single or divided doses	Moderate to severe renal impairment

Common side effects	Interactions	Additional information
Abdominal distension, pain nausea		For impaction, 8 sachets should be dissolved in 1 L of water and taken within 6 h – large volume can prove unacceptable for frailer patients More effective and better tolerated than lactulose
Insomnia, agitation, anxiety, headache, movement disorders, drowsiness, fatigue, dizziness, impaired concentration, blurred vision, dyspepsia, nausea and vomiting, constipation, urinary incontinence	Carbamazepine decreases plasma concentration of risperidone Phenothiazines, tricyclic antidepressants, fluoxetine and some beta-blockers may increase the plasma concentration of risperidone Orodispersible tablets should be dissolved on the tongue, then swallowed	Avoid use in elderly patients
Tremor, palpitations, muscle cramps, headache, tachycardia	Increased risk of hypokalaemia with steroids, diuretics, theophylline	A range of breath-actuated inhalers and spacer devices exist to assist technique and aid patient compliance – see *BNF*
Intestinal colic, diarrhoea		Relies on colonic bacteria for activation, therefore action confined to the large bowel only, and may be unpredictable
GI side effects, anorexia, weight loss, hypersensitivity reactions, dry mouth, anxiety, headache, insomnia	Increased CNS toxicity with tramadol Increased risk of bleeding with NSAIDs	SSRI should not be started for 2 weeks after stopping MAOI Avoid abrupt withdrawal
Skin rashes, dyspepsia, nausea, diarrhoea, transient pyrexia, influenza-like symptoms with i.v. infusion	May cause hypocalcaemia if given concurrently with aminoglycosides Renal dysfunction reported with concurrent NSAIDs	Given i.v. initially due to poor oral absorption and tolerance Food significantly affects absorption – preparation should always be taken on an empty stomach Relatively ineffective orally in prevention of recurrence

(continued)

Drug name	Preparation	Indication for use	Dose	Caution
Sodium picosul-fate (sodium picosulphate)	5 mg/5 mL oral syrup	Stimulant laxative	5–20 mL o.d.	Large bowel obstruction
Sodium valproate	100 mg tabs 200 mg, 500 mg tabs enteric coated 200 mg, 300 mg, 500 mg MR tabs 200 mg/5 mL solution	Anticonvulsant	600 mg daily in divided doses Increase by 200 mg daily to max. 2.5 g daily in divided doses	Liver and renal impairment, bleeding disorders
Spironolactone	25 mg, 50 mg, 100 mg tabs	Sodium and fluid retention (ascites)	25–300 mg o.d. in divided doses if nausea	Hyperkalaemia, hyponatraemia, hepatic and renal impairment
Sucralfate	1 g tabs 1 g/5 mL susp.	Oral inflammation and ulceration	1 g q.d.s.	Renal impairment
Theophylline	200 mg, 300 mg, 400 mg MR tabs Numerous other brands and presentations – see *BNF*	Reversible airways obstruction	200 mg b.d. Increase after 1 week	Elderly, epilepsy, peptic ulcer, cardiac disease, hepatic impairment and hypertension Numerous drug interactions
Tolbutamide	500 mg tabs	Oral hypoglycaemic	500 mg b.d. Increase every 3 days to max. 1 g b.d.	Caution in hepatic and renal impairment
Tramadol	50 mg caps 50 mg, 100 mg effervescent granules 50 mg disp. tabs 50 mg, 75 mg, 100 mg, 150 mg, 200 mg MR caps/tabs	Moderate to severe pain	50–100 mg q.d.s. 100–200 mg b.d. Note: some preparations formulated for o.d. dosing, check SPC	Caution with epilepsy, hepatic and renal impairment, raised intracranial pressure

Common side effects	Interactions	Additional information
Intestinal colic, diarrhoea		Relies on colonic bacteria for activation, therefore action confined to the large bowel only, and may be unpredictable
Gastric irritation, nausea, tremor, ataxia, drowsiness, hepatic toxicity/impairment, oedema and inhibition of platelet aggregation	Raises plasma concentration of carbamazepine, phenobarbitone and phenytoin (but may also lower) Cimetidine raises plasma levels of sodium valproate	Better for primary generalized epilepsy Avoid sudden withdrawal
Nausea, vomiting, headache, lethargy	Potassium-sparing diuretics, ACE inhibitors, NSAIDs all raise risk of hyperkalaemia NSAIDs reduce efficacy	Body weight and renal function should be used to monitor effect Consider adding loop diuretic if underachieving
Constipation, diarrhoea, nausea, indigestion, gastric discomfort, dry mouth, rash, hypersensitivity reactions, dizziness, bezoar formation	Reduced absorption of ciprofloxacin, norfloxacin, ofloxacin, tetracycline, warfarin, phenytoin, cardiac glycosides, levothyroxine and lansoprazole Bezoar formation in those receiving enteral feeds and predisposed to delayed gastric emptying	
Nausea, dyspepsia, headache, tachycardia, palpitations, hypokalaemia, convulsions	Plasma concentration increased by ciprofloxacin, clarithromycin, erythromycin, fluconazole, calcium-channel blockers and corticosteroids Plasma concentration decreased by carbamazepine, phenytoin	Therapeutic range 10–20 mcg/mL Therapeutic index is narrow Numerous preparations available Patients should be maintained on the same brand due to non-bioequivalence
Hypoglycaemia, GI disturbance, headache	Steroids, loop and thiazide diuretics antagonize hypoglycaemic effect	Should be used in preference to a long-acting sulphonylurea, particularly in the elderly
Orthostatic hypotension, hallucinations, confusion, nausea and constipation	Use with caution with tricyclic and SSRI antidepressants as seizure threshold may be lowered Effects reduced by carbamazepine Increases the effect of digoxin and warfarin	Regarded as 'double-strength' codeine It inhibits reuptake of 5HT and noradrenaline and this may have a role in non-opioid-sensitive pain

(continued)

Drug name	Preparation	Indication for use	Dose	Caution
Tranexamic acid	500 mg tabs 100 mg/mL inj.	Surface bleeding from ulcerating tumours	1.5 g stat then 1 g t.d.s. Discontinue or reduce to 500 mg t.d.s. 1 week after bleeding stops	Renal failure, thrombo-embolic disease, DIC Risk of ureteric obstruction and retention with haematuria
Warfarin	0.5 mg, 1 mg, 3 mg, 5 mg tabs	Oral anticoagulant	Depends on INR result	Hepatic and renal disease, recent surgery

ACE, angiotensin-converting enzyme; b.d., twice a day; *BNF, British National Formulary*; caps, capsules; CCF, continuous subcutaneous infusion; DIC, disseminated intravascular coagulopathy; disp., dispersible; e/c, international normalized ratio; IR, immediate release; i.v., intravenously; LFT, liver function test; MAOI, NSAID, non-steroidal anti-inflammatory drug; o.d., once daily; p.o., orally; p.r., rectally; prep., preparation; inappropriate antidiuretic hormone; SL, sublingual; SPC, specialist palliative care; SR, slow release; SSRI, selective antidepressants; t.d.s., three times a day; XL, extra long.

Common side effects	Interactions	Additional information
Nausea, vomiting, diarrhoea, disturbance of colour vision	Increased risk of thrombosis with other thrombogenic drugs	
Haemorrhage, bruising, hypersensitivity and rash	A wide variety of drugs, e.g. cimetidine, diuretics, thyroid hormones, hormone antagonists, certain analgesics and antibiotics, interact with warfarin by either increasing or decreasing the anticoagulant effect NSAIDs and aspirin may prolong or intensify the anticoagulant effect of warfarin SSRI antidepressants increase the risk of bleeding if taken with warfarin	Regular blood tests are necessary to determine INR result Antidote: vitamin K (phytomenadione) List of interactions extensive – see *BNF*

congestive cardiac failure; CNS, central nervous system; COPD, chronic obstructive pulmonary disease; CSCI, enteric coated; GI, gastrointestinal; 5HT3, 5-hydroxytryptamine; i.m., intramuscularly; inj., injection; INR, monoamine oxidase inhibitor; MI, myocardial infarction; MR, modified release; NR, normal release; p.r.n., when required; q.d.s., four times a day; s.c., subcutaneously; SD, syringe driver; SIADH, syndrome serotonin reuptake inhibitor; suppos, suppositories; susp., suspension; tabs, tablets; TCAs, tricyclic

APPENDIX 2

SYRINGE DRIVER DRUG COMPATABILITY GUIDE

Each prescription should be checked to make sure the drug combinations are compatible. Many different combinations have been successfully used in clinical practice without the supporting laboratory data. Experience has shown that few, if any problems arise if attention if paid to the following points:

- Drug combinations should be used within 24 hours of making a mixture.

- The mixture must be inspected visually to detect signs of flocculation or precipitation.

As a general rule, drugs with similar pH are more likely to be compatible than those with widely differing pH.

Saline is recommended as the diluent for granisetron, ketamine, ketorolac, octreotide and ondansetron. For other drugs the recommended diluent for injection is water because there is less chance of precipitation.

DRUGS NOT TO BE USED IN SYRINGE DRIVERS

- Prochlorperazine

- Chlorpromazine

- Diazepam

COMPATIBILITY CHART

Drug	Diamorphine	Levomepromazine	Haloperidol	Hyoscine hydro	Dexamethasone	Buscopan	Cyclizine	Metoclopramide	Midazolam	Diclofenac	Octreotide	Clonazepam
Diamorphine												
Levomepromazine												
Haloperidol												
Hyoscine hydrobromide												
Dexamethasone												
Buscopan (hyoscine butylbromide)												
Cyclizine												
Metoclopramide												
Midazolam												
Diclofenac												
Octreotide												
Clonazepam												

■, Compatible; ■, Not compatible; ■, Caution.

USEFUL REFERENCES

www.pallcare.info – syringe driver drug compatibility database.
www.palliativedrugs.com – you will need to register in order to access full site.

INDEX

Page numbers in **bold** type refer to figures; those in *italic* refer to tables and boxed material. Page numbers preceded by an asterisk (*) indicate entries in the drugs data table (preparation; indication; dose; caution; side effects; interactions etc.) in Appendix 1.